Steroids in Brain Function

Steroids in Brain Function

Editor: Cristin Roth

AMERICAN
MEDICAL PUBLISHERS
www.americanmedicalpublishers.com

AMERICAN
MEDICAL PUBLISHERS
www.americanmedicalpublishers.com

Cataloging-in-Publication Data

Steroids in brain function / edited by Cristin Roth.
p. cm.
Includes bibliographical references and index.
ISBN 979-8-88740-475-2
1. Steroid drugs. 2. Brain. 3. Brain--Effect of drugs on. 4. Neurohormones--Physiological effect.
5. Steroid hormones--Physiological effect. 6. Neuroendocrinology. I. Roth, Cristin.
RM297.S74 S743 2023
615.36--dc23

American Medical Publishers,
41 Flatbush Avenue,
1st Floor, New York,
NY 11217, USA

ISBN 979-8-88740-475-2 (Hardback)

Contents

Preface

Steroids refer to biologically active organic compounds which generally have seventeen carbon atoms that are bonded in four fused rings. They are found in animals, plants and fungi. Steroids are components of cell membranes and also function as signaling molecules. On the basis of function, they can be classified into various types, such as neurosteroids, corticosteroids and sex steroids. Neurosteroids are steroids which interact with cell surface receptors and ligand-gated ion channels to alter neuronal excitability. Corticosteroids are a group of steroids which are produced by the adrenal cortex and are involved in a range of physiological processes such as carbohydrate metabolism, regulation of inflammation, protein catabolism, immune response and stress response. This book includes some of the vital pieces of work being conducted across the world, on various topics related to steroids and their relevance in brain functions. From theories to research to practical applications, case studies related to all contemporary topics of relevance to this area of study have been included herein. This book is a resource guide for experts as well as students.

The information contained in this book is the result of intensive hard work done by researchers in this field. All due efforts have been made to make this book serve as a complete guiding source for students and researchers. The topics in this book have been comprehensively explained to help readers understand the growing trends in the field.

I would like to thank the entire group of writers who made sincere efforts in this book and my family who supported me in my efforts of working on this book. I take this opportunity to thank all those who have been a guiding force throughout my life.

Editor

1

Characteristics of Seizure and Antiepileptic Drug Utilization in Outpatients with Autoimmune Encephalitis

*Qi Huang, Meigang Ma, Xing Wei, Yuhan Liao, Hengchang Qi, Yuejuan Wu and Yuan Wu**

Department of Neurology, First Affiliated Hospital, Guangxi Medical University, Nanning, China

***Correspondence:**
Yuan Wu
nwuyuan90@163.com

Autoimmune encephalitis (AE) is one kind of encephalitis that associates with specific neuronal antigens. Most patients with AE likely suffer from seizures, but data on the characteristics of seizure and antiepileptic drugs (AEDs) utilization in this patient group remains limited. This study aimed to report the clinical status of seizure and AEDs treatment of patients with AE, and to evaluate the relationship between AEDs discontinuation and seizure outcomes. Patients with acute neurological disorders and anti-N-methyl-D-aspartate receptor (NMDAR), γ-aminobutyric acid B receptor ($GABA_BR$), leucine-rich glioma inactivated 1, or contactin-associated protein-like 2 (CASPR2) antibodies were included. As patients withdrew from AEDs, they were divided into the early withdrawal (EW, AEDs used $\leq$3 months) and late withdrawal (LW, AEDs used $>$3 months) groups. Seizure remission was defined as having no seizures for at least 1 year after the last time when AEDs were administered. Seizure outcomes were assessed on the basis of remission rate. The factors affecting the outcomes were assessed through Spearman analysis. In total, we enrolled 75 patients (39 patients aged $<$16 years, male/female = 39/36) for follow-up, which included 67 patients with anti-NMDAR encephalitis, 4 patients with anti-$GABA_BR$ encephalitis, 2 patients with anti-voltage-gated potassium channel encephalitis, and 2 patients with coexisting antibodies. Among the 34 enrolled patients with anti-NMDAR encephalitis who were withdrawn from AEDs, only 5.8% relapse was reported during the 1-year follow-up, with no significant difference in the percentage of relapse between the EW and LW groups ($P = 0.313$). Fifteen patients (an average age of 6.8, 14 patients with anti-NMDAR encephalitis and 1 patient with anti-CASPR2 encephalitis) presented seizure remission without any AEDs. Seventy five percent of patients with anti-$GABA_BR$ antibodies developed refractory seizure. Other risk factors which contributed to refractory seizure and seizure relapse included status epilepticus ($P = 0.004$) and cortical abnormalities ($P = 0.028$). Given this retrospective data, patients with AE have a high rate of seizure remission, and the long-term use of AEDs may not be necessary to control the seizure. Moreover, seizures in young patients with anti-NMDAR encephalitis presents self-limited. Patients with anti-$GABA_BR$ antibody, status epilepticus, and cortical abnormalities are more likely to develop refractory seizure or seizure relapse.

Keywords: autoimmune encephalitis, outpatients, seizure remission, antiepileptic drug withdrawal, refractory seizure

INTRODUCTION

Autoimmune encephalitis (AE) is kind of encephalitis which associates with humoral or cellular responses against specific neuronal antigens (1, 2). The clinical characteristics of these patients include seizure, abnormal behavior, speech dysfunction, movement disorders, and autonomic dysfunction (3). With the development of biochemical assays, several antibodies, such as the anti-*N*-methyl-D-aspartate receptor (NMDAR), anti-γ-aminobutyric acid B receptor ($GABA_BR$), anti-leucine-rich glioma inactivated 1 (LGI1), and anti-contactin-associated protein-like 2 (CASPR2) antibodies, have emerged as the leading causes of AE. Therapeutic regimens included first-line immunotherapy (steroids, intravenous immunoglobulin, plasmapheresis), and second-line immunotherapy (rituximab, cyclophosphamide). Despite the severity of the disease in acute phase, most patients recover after proper immunotherapy and intensive support (4).

In acute phase, seizure is a highly prevalent symptom, and parts of patients develop status epilepticus (SE) (5–7). Hence, multiple anti-epileptic drugs (AEDs) are often necessary to control the attacks. However, based on the previous studies and data from our center, most patients likely recover completely after adequate immunotherapy, and seizure is rarely reported in the chronic phase (5, 8, 9). Considering the adverse events of AEDs, some patients stop taking AEDs at the early stage. However, an instructional database describing the long-term use of AEDs with AE is lacking.

This retrospective study aimed to report the seizure characteristics and long-term use of AEDs in outpatients with AE. Our secondary goals included assessing the outcomes between patients with early and late AEDs withdrawal, and determining the probable risk factors for seizure relapse and refractory seizures.

MATERIALS AND METHODS

Study Population

This study was conducted in compliance with the ethical standards of Guangxi Medical University. Written consents were obtained from the patients.

The antibodies, including NMDAR, $GABA_BR$, LGI1, and CASPR2, were detected in patients' cerebrospinal fluid and serum samples. The anti-NMDAR antibody was detected by specific staining against NMDAR isolated from rat' hippocampus and cerebellum, and positive cell-based assay with HEK293 cells transfected with NR1. Other antibodies were detected using transfected HEK293 cells with the respective target proteins.

Patients with acute neurological disorders of either sex or any age were considered eligible for this study if they presented any positive antibodies from January 2012 to May 2017. The exclusion criteria included (1) patients diagnosed with epilepsy, cerebral infarction, cerebral trauma, cerebral tumor, and other nervous system disease prior to the onset of encephalitis, (2) patients with evidence of infectious encephalitis, for example, viral, bacteria, mycobacterium tuberculosis, or fungal, (3) patients in the acute phase of autoimmune encephalitis and still required hospitalization. Immunotherapies were used in the acute phase (**Figure 3A**). The decisions about the type and duration of immunotherapy were based on the clinical symptoms, curative, and side effects. The available onset medical data (seizure characteristics, AEDs utilization, and electroencephalogram/neuroimaging findings) were recorded. The electroencephalogram and neuroimaging findings were recorded in the acute phase of the disease.

Definitions

The chronic stage of AE was defined by 3 months after the onset of AE symptoms. SE was defined as continuous seizure activity lasting >5 min or recurrent seizures without regaining consciousness between seizures for >5 min (10). Refractory seizure was defined as an uncontrolled seizure after treatment by more than three standard therapeutic schedules (11). Seizure remission was defined as having no seizure for at least 1 year after the last time when AEDs were used (12). Seizure with focal characteristics was defined as a partial seizure or a patient with seizure and hemiplegia or hemianesthesia.

Outcome Assessment and Grouping

AEDs utilization and seizure outcomes were assessed through outpatient services and/or telephone interview. AEDs utilization in the chronic stage (time of continuation/withdrawal) and outcomes (refractory, relapse, or remission) data were collected on patients. Before evaluating the outcomes, the patients who discontinued AEDs were observed for at least 1 year after the last AEDs use.

Patients who withdraw AEDs were divided into two groups based on the duration of AEDs use. The early withdrawal (EW) group had AEDs withdrawn within 3 months, and the late withdrawal (LW) group had AEDs withdrawn after 3 months. Outcomes were assessed based on seizure remission rate and the modified Rankin Scale (mRS) (13).

Statistical Analysis

Data analysis was performed using IBM SPSS Statistics 22. The skewness and kurtosis coefficients were used to evaluate whether the quantitative data fit a normal distribution. Data were regarded as a normal distribution if the skewness and kurtosis coefficients <1. For the data that did not fit this criterion, we used the Mann–Whitney test to evaluate significance. Other data was compared using a *t*-test or a Fisher's exact test. The factors affecting the outcomes were assessed through Spearman analysis.

RESULTS

We identified 83 patients with AE. **Figures 1, 2** show a summary of these patients. In the charts reviewed, 5 patients were lost and 3 patients died of severe pneumonia. As a result, 75 patients were enrolled to follow-up. Among the 75 patients, 12 continued taking AEDs, 15 were not given any AEDs, and 37 patients who withdrew from AEDs were followed up for at least 1 year (**Figure 1**). The group with AEDs withdrawal

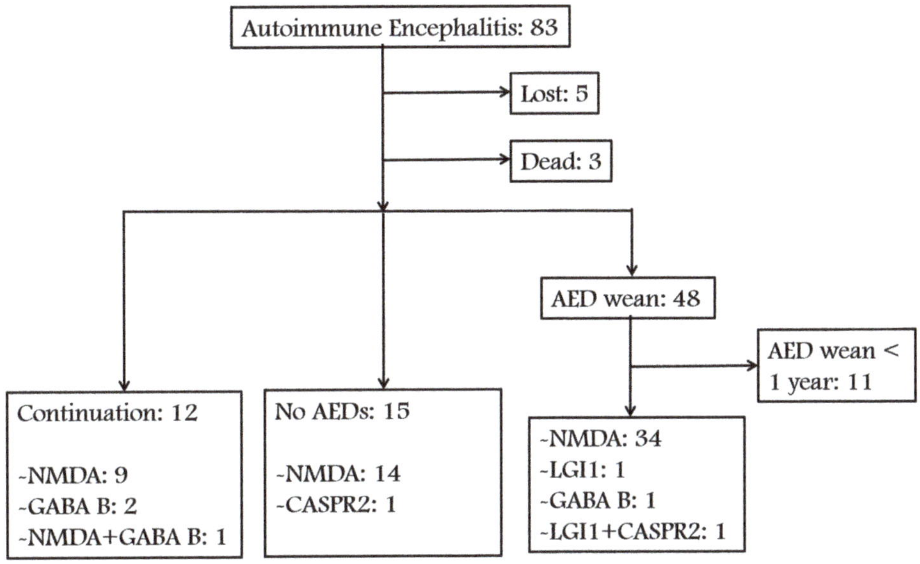

FIGURE 1 | Flow diagram of patient inclusion and grouping.

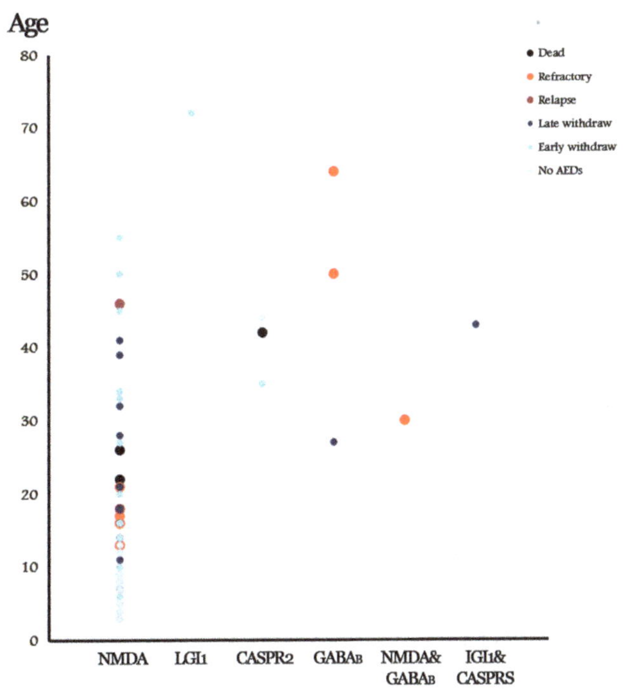

FIGURE 2 | Summary of the presenting patients and outcomes in accordance with the involved antibodies. No AEDs, No AED was given and no relapse was reported. Early withdrawal (EW), AEDs weaned within 3 months and no relapse was reported. Late withdrawal (LW), AEDs weaned after 3 months and no relapse was reported.

included 34 patients with anti-NMDAR encephalitis, 1 with anti-LGI1 encephalitis, 1 with anti-GABA$_B$R encephalitis, and 1 patient presented coexisting antibodies of anti-LGI1 and CASPR2 (**Figure 1**).

Anti-NMDAR Encephalitis

Among the patients with anti-NMDAR encephalitis, 14 were not given any AEDs, in which 7 suffered from one-time seizure attack at the onset of the encephalitis. Compared to the patients with AEDs, the majority of this group was considerably young (6.8 ± 3.26, $P = 0.004$, **Table 1**) and less likely to have repetitive seizures ($P = 0.038$, **Table 1**). The median duration of follow up was 20 months (range: 14–36 months), and no relapse was reported. Furthermore, 12 patients (85.7%) had good outcomes with a 0 mRS score; the remaining 2 patients presented with cognitive dysfunction.

Among the 34 patients (20 men and 14 women, 23 in EW and 11 in LW) who were discontinued from AEDs, 7 patients (20.6%) did not report seizure, and 5 patients (14.7%) reported a one-time seizure at the onset. Two patients in the EW group reported hemianesthesia before presenting seizures. The occurrence of SE was 32.4% in total. Eighteen patients had an magnetic resonance imaging (MRI) scan and abnormalities were found in 33.3% of the patients, including 4 patients with white matter changes and 2 patients with cortical mass (**Table 1**). The patterns of AEDs selection and discontinuation were variable (**Figure 3B**). Monotherapy was the most common selection, with 69.5% in the EW group and 63.9% in the LW group. At the early stage, carbamazepine ($n = 11$) and oxcarbazepine ($n = 16$) were the most chosen AEDs. Valproic acid was among the most commonly continued therapies over the course of follow-up (**Figure 3B**). Seven patients without seizure were treated with AEDs upon onset. Five of these discontinued AEDs within 1 month, and the remaining 2 patients underwent LW because of frequent subclinical discharge.

The patients' data were compared between the EW and LW groups (**Table 1**). No statistically significant difference was observed between the two groups in terms of age ($P = 0.935$), sex ($P = 0.458$), seizure characteristics ($P = 0.359$), antibody

TABLE 1 | Clinical characteristics and outcomes of patients with anti-NMDA encephalitis.

	No AEDs (14 patients)	Early withdraw (23 patients)	Late withdraw (11 patients)	P1	P2
Sex (male/female)	7/7	15/8	5/6	0.474	0.458
Age (Ave ± SD)	6.8 ± 3.26	21.0 ± 16.19	21.4 ± 11.89	0.004	0.935
Seizure frequency				0.038	0.359
None	4	5	2		
Once	7	2	3		
Repeated	3	16	6		
Seizure with focal characters	0	2	0	0.322	0.313
Status epilepticus(Yes/No)	0/14	6/17	5/6	0.024	0.259
Antibody titer				0.129	0.727
1:10	6	3	1		
1:32	7	19	10		
1:100	1	1	0		
MRI abnormalities				0.400	0.329
None	4	6	6		
White matter	3	3	1		
Cortex	3	2	0		
Anti-epileptic drugs				–	0.934
1 kind	–	16	7		
2 kinds	–	5	3		
3 or more kinds	–	2	1		
Followed up					
Median duration (months)	20 (14–36)	36 (15–50)	32 (17–62)		
Relapse	–	2/21	0/11	–	0.313
mRS score (≤1/>1)	12/2	22/1	9/2	0.398	0.239

AED, Antiepileptic drug. P1, P-value among No AED, Early withdraw, and late withdraw group. P2, P-value between Early withdraw, and late withdraw group.

titers ($P = 0.727$), SE ($P = 0.259$), MRI findings ($P = 0.329$), or AEDs selection ($P = 0.934$). The medium durations of follow up were 36 months (range: 15–50 months) and 32 months (range: 17–62 months) for the EW and LW groups, respectively. 2 patients in the EW group relapsed in the first month after drug discontinuation. No remarkable difference in the percentage of relapse was observed between the two groups.

Detail of patients with anti-NMDAR encephalitis was presented in **Supplementary File 1**.

Other AEs

A 44-year-old woman who was diagnosed with anti-CASPR2 encephalitis presented lethargy and headache without seizure at the onset. She did not take any AEDs. No relapse was reported during her 16-month follow up. A 72-year-old man with anti-LGI1 encephalitis and a 35-year-old woman with anti-GABA$_B$R encephalitis presented frequent seizures at onset and underwent an AED withdrawal 3 and 6 months later, respectively. No relapse was reported during their 1-year follow up. The other two elder patients (50 and 64 years-old, respectively) with anti-GABA$_B$ encephalitis presented refractory seizures (**Figure 2**).

We also reviewed 2 coexisting AE. One is a 30-year-old female who presented with anti-NMDAR and GABA$_B$R encephalitis. She had a seizure 10 years ago before she was diagnosed with AE through CSF detection. Her EEG presented δ brushes with generalized paroxysmal θ activities. The brain MRI was unremarkable. She developed refractory seizures after being treated by oxcarbazepine, carbamazepine, and clonazepam. The other patient was a 43-year-old woman with LGI1 and CASPR2 antibodies. She presented repeated generalized tonic-clonic seizure and paroxysmal speech dysfunction. Bilateral paracentral lesion was found in the MRI scan. She was given levetiracetam and valproic acid. The AEDs were withdrawn 2 years later, and no relapse was reported during her 1-year follow up (**Figure 2**).

Risk Factors

Among the 12 patients who remained on AEDs, 9 patients presented refractory seizure, including 6 patients with anti-NMDAR encephalitis, 2 patients with anti-GABA$_B$R encephalitis, and 1 patient with anti-NMDAR and GABA$_B$R encephalitis (**Figure 2**). Among patients with anti-NMDAR encephalitis, refractory seizures occurred more often in the patients younger than 30 years of age (**Figure 2**), and who presented repetitive seizures and SE, moreover, 4 patients (66%) showed cortical abnormalities on the MRI scan.

By combining the data of the 2 relapse cases, we evaluated the risk factors that contributed to the worse outcomes of anti-NMDAR encephalitis. The patients with relapse or refractory seizure were more likely to be accompanied with cortical lesions on MRI ($P = 0.028$) and SE ($P = 0.004$) than those who reached seizure remission (**Table 2**). Moreover, the seizures with

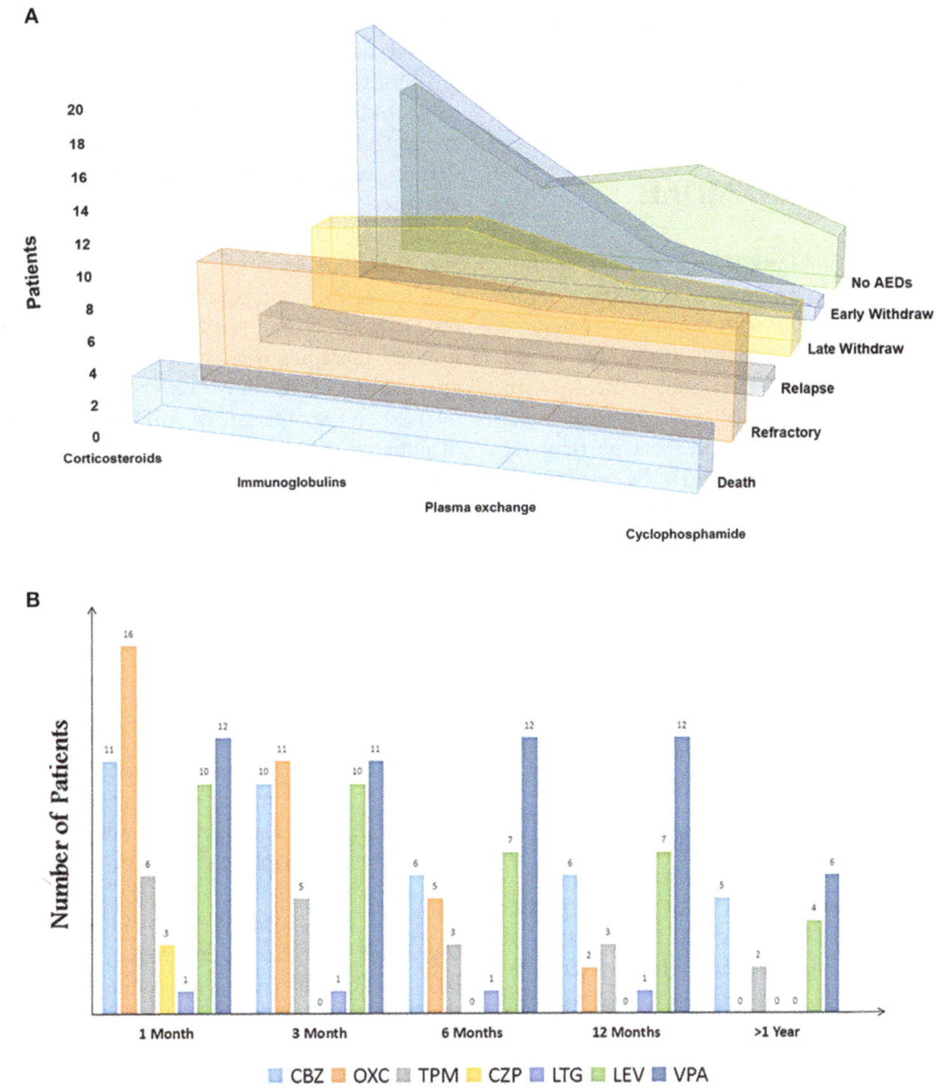

FIGURE 3 | (A) Immunotherapies of patients with autoimmune encephalitis (Sort by outcomes). **(B)** Clinical patterns of AED discontinuation of patients with anti-NMDA encephalitis. CBZ, carbamazepine; OXC, oxcarbazepine; TPM, topiramate; CZP, clonazepam; LTG, lamotrigine; LEV, levetiracetam; VPA, valproate.

TABLE 2 | Spearman analysis of factors associated with outcomes.

	Refractory Seizure/P	Relapse/P	Both/P
Sex	0.571	0.859	0.516
Age	0.528	0.116	0.259
Antibody titers	0.640	0.590	0.555
Seizure with focal characters	<0.001	0.769	0.099
Status epilepticus	<0.001	0.415	0.004
MRI abnormalities	0.010	0.961	0.028

focal characteristics ($P < 0.001$), SE ($P < 0.001$), and MRI abnormalities ($P = 0.010$) were significantly associated with refractory seizure (**Table 2**). For other kinds of AEs, we found 3 patients with anti-GABA$_B$R encephalitis (75% in all, including 1 patient with concomitant disease) developed refractory seizure; this number is much higher than those of others.

DISCUSSIONS

Parts of AE have been linked to cell surface antigens, which included voltage-gated potassium channel (VGPC, e.g., LGI1 and CASPR2), NMDAR, and GABA$_B$R (14). To evaluate the AEDs utilization associated with AE, we focused on seizure in a cohort of patients with anti-NMDAR, anti-GABA$_B$R, anti-LGI1, and CASPR2 encephalitis. This study demonstrated low recurrence rates in young patients with AE who experienced first unprovoked seizures and highlighted an overall remission rate of 94% after the patients discontinued AEDs therapy. No difference was noted between the EW ($\leq$3 months) and LW (>3 months) of AEDs. Moreover, a higher number of patients with anti-$GABA_BR$ antibody, SE, cortical abnormalities, and focal neurological dysfunction experienced refractory seizure or seizure relapses compared to those who did not.

Seizure Remission in Anti-NMDAR Encephalitis

Since 2005, the characteristics and long-term outcomes of anti-NMDAR encephalitis have aroused public attention due to the high incidence in young patients with serious neurological dysfunctions (15). According to a previous study, we found that the probable predicted factors for poor outcomes in the acute phase included older age, altered consciousness, and SE, and the process of terminating SE was particularly important for anti-NMDAR encephalitis (5). By evaluating patients through the mRS score, the other multi-institutional study which included clinical data from 577 patients with anti-NMDAR antibodies observed that 81% of the patients responded to immunotherapy (8). Seizure occurs as a prominent feature in AE (16), whether long-term AEDs are necessary after patients achieving good outcomes has not been established (14, 16).

AEDs withdrawal after a successful seizure control may prevent adverse side effects and excessive cost. However, the studies which have evaluated the safety of AEDs weaning in patients with anti-NMDAR encephalitis are rare. One study demonstrated that no difference in seizure recurrence between 1 and 2 years of AEDs therapy in children with viral encephalitis (17), and the relative risk factors might have included EEG abnormalities or HIV infection (18). However, the duration of AEDs in anti-NMDAR encephalitis tended to be shorter (19). Among the 34 enrolled patients with AEDs withdrawal, only 5.8% suffered from relapse during the follow up. Moreover, no difference was found between the EW (≤3 months) and LW (>3 months) groups, which is consistent with that of a previous study (16).

Information regarding AEDs use in adolescents and adults with anti-NMDAR encephalitis has been reported previously, but data from younger children remain limited (16). In the present study, we enrolled 14 young patients with average age of 6.8 (range: 3–12 years). Compared with the older age group, the young group was more likely be seizure free during the long-term follow-up without AEDs, even if they suffered one-time seizure attacks at the onset. The key treatment decisions after the first unprovoked seizure are a controversial issue in children (20, 21). In some epilepsy syndromes, such as in benign childhood epilepsy with centrotemporal spikes or childhood absence epilepsy, remission is a regular feature of the natural history, whereas juvenile myoclonic epilepsy or other symptomatic epilepsies have long been considered to present in AEDs continuation (22). By using the statistical methods for survival analysis, one study indicated that the cumulative risk of repetitive seizure in children was 29% in the first year and elevated to 45% within the 10-year follow up (23). However, the factors associated with recurrences after the first seizure are complex. The probable risk factors may include age (24) and etiology (25). For anti-NMDA encephalitis, our data indicated that seizure in young patients tended to be self-limited. Moreover, some scholars indicate that a cognitive comorbidity likely accompany with the initial seizure if AEDs are not used (26). However, evaluation of mRS score revealed that the majority of children in this group presented normal daily activities.

Although our data supports that seizure remission is common and that long-term use of AEDs may not be necessary, the significance of immunotherapy cannot be ignored to control the seizure. Numerous studies demonstrated that it is the immunotherapies that control the symptoms in anti-NMDAR encephalitis (5, 8, 9). Moreover, one retrospective study which focused on the outcome of AEDs alone in controlling the seizure of patients with anti-VGPC-complex antibodies indicated that only 23.5% of patients became seizure free compared with 61.5% of patients with immunotherapy (14).

Seizure Remission in Anti-GABABR, LGI1, and CASPR2 Encephalitis

Anti-$GABA_BR$, LGI1, and CASPR2 antibodies have been recently detected in patients with limbic encephalitis (27). Seizures are frequently reported in limbic encephalitis, but autonomic and psychiatric symptoms are more highlighted. In these antibody-mediated seizures, remission rate is variable, and may be related to complications, immunotherapy, and ICU management (7).

Although rare, seizure with additional auto-antibodies may be a other probable risk factor. LGI1 and CASPR2 are the extracellular domains of VGPC. The coexistence of anti-LGI1 and anti-CASPR2 encephalitis may contribute to seizure, cognitive disturbance, movement disorders, and pain (7). Besides AEDs use, the empirical approach to seizure control is corticosteroid treatment (28, 29). A $GABA_BR$ antibody is rarely accompanied with other antibodies in a same patient, and a probable reason may involve different genetic predispositions (30, 31). In our study, the presented patients developed refractory seizure and severe cognitive dysfunction. One possible mechanism of AEDs resistance may be associated with different interaction sites, as anti-NMDAR antibodies have been suggested to decrease the synaptic levels of receptors, whereas the anti-$GABA_BR$ antibody would further alter the synaptic function (32).

Risk Factors for Refractory Seizure and Seizure Relapse

As AEDs are supposedly unnecessary to seizure outcomes in AE after appropriate immunotherapy, we evaluate the other probable independent risk factors that contribute to refractory seizure and seizure relapse. In addition to involving the anti-$GABA_BR$ antibody, our result shows that patients with SE, cortical abnormalities in MRI, and focal neurological dysfunction are more likely to develop worse outcomes than those who did not accompany these findings. SE has been proven to be an independent risk factor in major types of epilepsy (33, 34). The complications of SE, such as severe pneumonia and ICU admission, have also contributed to poor outcomes (5). Cortical abnormalities seem positively correlate with refractory seizure. By using structural MRI scans, one study demonstrated a strong association between incomplete recovery and superficial white matter lesions (35). This observation indicates that the injured connection between adjacent cortices may play a crucial role in seizure control after AE.

LIMITATIONS

This study has some limitations. First, we tried to discuss the risk factors of seizure outcomes for AE after appropriate immunotherapy. However, as antibodies were not measured at later time points, the direct relationship between persistent antibody levels and seizure outcomes remained unclear. A previous study presented that the neurological recovery accompanied with reduced antibody titer (15), while the correlation between antibody titer and refractory seizure showed unremarkable in our study. One probability which caused the difference might involve the time when antibody was measured. Though the seizure outcomes were assessed based on the data of outpatients, the patients who developed refractory seizure might have persistent higher titer level than those who did not. Second, as the relapse rate was altered with the follow-up period (23), long follow-up times are necessary. However, 54–100% of seizures after AE occurred within the first year, and new-onset seizure after 1 year of follow up was rare (36–38). Third, the results were limited because of the relatively small cohort. Combined with the previous data (16), a probable correlation between seizure remission and AED utilization was noted, and further trials and meta-analysis are needed to confirm these results.

CONCLUSION

Patients with AE have a high rate of seizure remission after proper immunotherapies. The long-term use of AEDs appears not be necessary to control their seizures. Compared with adults, young patients are more likely to become seizure free without AEDs. The risk factors that contribute to refractory seizure or seizure relapse may include anti-$GABA_BR$ encephalitis, SE, and cortical abnormalities.

AUTHOR CONTRIBUTIONS

QH is the first author of this manuscript. YuaW is the corresponding author of this manuscript, they contributed to the study design, data collection and analysis, and draft writing of this work. MM, XW, and YL have revised and improved the manuscript. HQ and YueW contributed in the data collection and figures. All authors have seen and agreed on the finally submitted version of the manuscript.

ACKNOWLEDGMENTS

This work was supported by the National Natural Science Foundation of China Grants (No. 81760242), Natural Science Foundation of Guangxi Grants (No. 2017GXNSFAA198047), and China Association Against Epilepsy-UCB Science Foundation (No. 2017003).

REFERENCES

1. Gaspard N. Autoimmune epilepsy. *Continuum* (2016) 22:227–45. doi: 10.1212/CON.0000000000000272
2. Holz K, Prinz M, Brendecke SM, Holscher A, Deng F, Mitrucker HW, et al. Differing outcome of experimental autoimmune encephalitis in macrophage/neutrophil- and T cell-specific gp130-deficient mice. *Front Immunol.* (2018) 9:836. doi: 10.3389/fimmu.2018.00836
3. Graus F, Titulaer MJ, Balu R, Benseler S, Bien CG, Cellucci T, et al. A clinical approach to diagnosis of autoimmune encephalitis. *Lancet Neurol.* (2016) 15:391–404. doi: 10.1016/S1474-4422(15)00401-9
4. Irani SR, Bera K, Waters P, Zuliani L, Maxwell S, Zandi MS, et al. N-methyl-D-aspartate antibody encephalitis: temporal progression of clinical and paraclinical observations in a predominantly non-paraneoplastic disorder of both sexes. *Brain* (2010) 133 (Pt 6):1655–67. doi: 10.1093/brain/awq113
5. Huang Q, Wu Y, Qin R, Wei X, Ma M. Clinical characteristics and outcomes between children and adults with anti-N-Methyl-D-Aspartate receptor encephalitis. *J Neurol.* (2016) 263:2446–55. doi: 10.1007/s00415-016-8282-1
6. Troscher AR, Klang A, French M, Quemada-Garrido L, Kneissl SM, Bien CG, et al. Selective limbic blood-brain barrier breakdown in a feline model of limbic encephalitis with LGI1 antibodies. *Front Immunol.* (2017) 8:1364. doi: 10.3389/fimmu.2017.01364
7. Binks SNM, Klein CJ, Waters P, Pittock SJ, Irani SR. LGI1, CASPR2 and related antibodies: a molecular evolution of the phenotypes. *J Neurol Neurosurg Psychiatr.* (2018) 89:526–34. doi: 10.1136/jnnp-2017-315720
8. Titulaer MJ, McCracken L, Gabilondo I, Armangue T, Glaser C, Iizuka T, et al. Treatment and prognostic factors for long-term outcome in patients with anti-NMDA receptor encephalitis: an observational cohort study. *Lancet Neurol.* (2013) 12:157–65. doi: 10.1016/S1474-4422(12)70310-1
9. Zekeridou A, Karantoni E, Viaccoz A, Ducray F, Gitiaux C, Villega F, et al. Treatment and outcome of children and adolescents with N-methyl-D-aspartate receptor encephalitis. *J Neurol.* (2015) 262:1859–66. doi: 10.1007/s00415-015-7781-9
10. Sakellariou DF, Kostopoulos GK, Richardson MP, Koutroumanidis M. Topography of generalized periodic epileptiform discharges in postanoxic nonconvulsive status epilepticus. *Epilepsia Open* (2017) 2:472–5. doi: 10.1002/epi4.12073
11. Cooper YA, Pianka ST, Alotaibi NM, Babayan D, Salavati B, Weil AG, et al. Repetitive transcranial magnetic stimulation for the treatment of drug-resistant epilepsy: a systematic review and individual participant data meta-analysis of real-world evidence. *Epilepsia Open* (2018) 3:55–65. doi: 10.1002/epi4.12092
12. Yu P, Zhou D, Liao W, Wang X, Wang Y, Wang T, et al. An investigation of the characteristics of outpatients with epilepsy and antiepileptic drug utilization in a multicenter cross-sectional study in China. *Epilepsy Behav.* (2017) 69:126–32. doi: 10.1016/j.yebeh.2016.09.021
13. Saver JL, Filip B, Hamilton S, Yanes A, Craig S, Cho M, et al. Improving the reliability of stroke disability grading in clinical trials and clinical practice: the Rankin Focused Assessment (RFA). *Stroke* (2010) 41:992–5. doi: 10.1161/STROKEAHA.109.571364

14. Feyissa AM, Lopez Chiriboga AS, Britton JW. Antiepileptic drug therapy in patients with autoimmune epilepsy. *Neurol Neuroimmunol Neuroinflamm.* (2017) 4:e353. doi: 10.1212/NXI.0000000000000353
15. Dalmau J, Gleichman AJ, Hughes EG, Rossi JE, Peng X, Lai M, et al. Anti-NMDA-receptor encephalitis: case series and analysis of the effects of antibodies. *Lancet Neurol.* (2008) 7:1091–8. doi: 10.1016/S1474-4422(08)70224-2
16. Liu X, Yan B, Wang R, Li C, Chen C, Zhou D, et al. Seizure outcomes in patients with anti-NMDAR encephalitis: a follow-up study. *Epilepsia* (2017) 58:2104–11. doi: 10.1111/epi.13929
17. Singhi PD, Dinakaran J, Khandelwal N, Singhi SC. One vs. two years of anti-epileptic therapy in children with single small enhancing CT lesions. *J Trop Pediatr.* (2003) 49:274–8. doi: 10.1093/tropej/49.5.274
18. Singhi P. Infectious causes of seizures and epilepsy in the developing world. *Dev Med Child Neurol.* (2011) 53:600–9. doi: 10.1111/j.1469-8749.2011.03928.x
19. Miya K, Takahashi Y, Mori H. Anti-NMDAR autoimmune encephalitis. *Brain Dev.* (2014) 36:645–52. doi: 10.1016/j.braindev.2013.10.005
20. Beghi E, Ciccone A. Recurrence after a first unprovoked seizure. Is it still a controversial issue? First Seizure Trial Group (first). *Seizure* (1993) 2:5–10. doi: 10.1016/S1059-1311(05)80096-2
21. Wendt WL, Dang LT, Rogers AJ. What happens next? Recurrence rates for first unprovoked seizures in children. *Acad Emerg Med.* (2018) 25:362–4. doi: 10.1111/acem.13374
22. Wolf P. Remission of epilepsy as a function of time. *Epilepsy Behav.* (2016) 61:46–50. doi: 10.1016/j.yebeh.2016.04.043
23. Shinnar S, Berg AT, O'Dell C, Newstein D, Moshe SL, Hauser WA. Predictors of multiple seizures in a cohort of children prospectively followed from the time of their first unprovoked seizure. *Ann Neurol.* (2000) 48:140–7. doi: 10.1002/1531-8249(200008)48:2<140::aid-ana2>3.0.co;2-y
24. Goldberg LR, Kernie CG, Lillis K, Bennett J, Conners G, Macias CG, et al. Early recurrence of first unprovoked seizures in children. *Acad Emerg Med.* (2018) 25:275–82. doi: 10.1111/acem.13341
25. Mahamud Z, Burman J, Zelano J. Risk of epilepsy after a single seizure in multiple sclerosis. *Eur J Neurol.* (2018) 25:854–60. doi: 10.1111/ene.13618
26. Jason EA, Tomson T, Carlsson S, Tedroff K, Amark P. Neurodevelopmental comorbidities and seizure control 24 months after a first unprovoked seizure in children. *Epilepsy Res.* (2018) 143:33–40. doi: 10.1016/j.eplepsyres.2018.03.015
27. Boronat A, Sabater L, Saiz A, Dalmau J, Graus F. GABA(B) receptor antibodies in limbic encephalitis and anti-GAD-associated neurologic disorders. *Neurology* (2011) 76:795–800. doi: 10.1212/WNL.0b013e31820e7b8d
28. Irani SR, Michell AW, Lang B, Pettingill P, Waters P, Johnson MR, et al. Faciobrachial dystonic seizures precede Lgi1 antibody limbic encephalitis. *Ann Neurol.* (2011) 69:892–900. doi: 10.1002/ana.22307
29. Irani SR, Stagg CJ, Schott JM, Rosenthal CR, Schneider SA, Pettingill P, et al. Faciobrachial dystonic seizures: the influence of immunotherapy on seizure control and prevention of cognitive impairment in a broadening phenotype. *Brain* (2013) 136 (Pt 10):3151–62. doi: 10.1093/brain/awt212
30. Mueller SH, Farber A, Pruss H, Melzer N, Golombeck KS, Kumpfel T, et al. Genetic predisposition in anti-LGI1 and anti-NMDA receptor encephalitis. *Ann Neurol.* (2018) 83:863–9. doi: 10.1002/ana.25216
31. Petit-Pedrol M, Armangue T, Peng X, Bataller L, Cellucci T, Davis R, et al. Encephalitis with refractory seizures, status epilepticus, and antibodies to the GABAA receptor: a case series, characterisation of the antigen, and analysis of the effects of antibodies. *Lancet Neurol.* (2014) 13:276–86. doi: 10.1016/S1474-4422(13)70299-0
32. Hughes EG, Peng X, Gleichman AJ, Lai M, Zhou L, Tsou R, et al. Cellular and synaptic mechanisms of anti-NMDA receptor encephalitis. *J Neurosci.* (2010) 30:5866–75. doi: 10.1523/JNEUROSCI.0167-10.2010
33. Bleck TP. Status epilepticus and the use of continuous EEG monitoring in the intensive care unit. *Continuum* (2012) 18:560–78. doi: 10.1212/01.CON.0000415428.61277.90
34. Chen W, Su Y, Jiang M, Liu G, Tian F, Ren G. Status epilepticus associated with acute encephalitis: long-term follow-up of functional and cognitive outcomes in 72 patients. *Eur J Neurol.* (2018) 25:1228–34. doi: 10.1111/ene.13678
35. Phillips OR, Joshi SH, Narr KL, Shattuck DW, Singh M, Di Paola M, et al. Superficial white matter damage in anti-NMDA receptor encephalitis. *J Neurol Neurosurg Psychiatr.* (2018) 89:518–25. doi: 10.1136/jnnp-2017-316822
36. Appenzeller S, Cendes F, Costallat LT. Epileptic seizures in systemic lupus erythematosus. *Neurology* (2004) 63:1808–12. doi: 10.1212/01.WNL.0000144178.32208.4F
37. Omori N, Narai H, Tanaka T, Tanaka S, Yamadori I, Ichimura K, et al. Epstein-Barr virus-associated T/NK cell-type central nervous system lymphoma which manifested as a post-transplantation lymphoproliferative disorder in a renal transplant recipient. *J Neurooncol.* (2008) 87:189–91. doi: 10.1007/s11060-007-9504-2
38. Kishitani T, Matsunaga A, Ikawa M, Hayashi K, Yamamura O, Hamano T, et al. Limbic encephalitis associated with anti-NH2-terminal of alpha-enolase antibodies: a clinical subtype of Hashimoto encephalopathy. *Medicine* (2017) 96:e6181. doi: 10.1097/MD.0000000000006181

2

Steroid Transport, Local Synthesis and Signaling within the Brain: Roles in Neurogenesis, Neuroprotection and Sexual Behaviors

Nicolas Diotel[1], Thierry D. Charlier[2], Christian Lefebvre d'Hellencourt[1], David Couret[1,3], Vance L. Trudeau[4], Joel C. Nicolau[2], Olivier Meilhac[1,3], Olivier Kah[2] and Elisabeth Pellegrini[2*]*

[1] Université de La Réunion, Institut National de la Santé et de la Recherche Médicale, UMR 1188, Diabète athérothrombose Thérapies Réunion Océan Indien, Saint-Denis de La Réunion, France, [2] Univ Rennes, Inserm, EHESP, Irset (Institut de recherche en santé, environnement et travail) - UMR_S 1085, Rennes, France, [3] CHU de La Réunion, Saint-Denis, France, [4] Department of Biology, University of Ottawa, Ottawa, ON, Canada

***Correspondence:**
Nicolas Diotel
nicolas.diotel@univ-reunion.fr
Elisabeth Pellegrini
elisabeth.pellegrini@univ-rennes1.fr

Sex steroid hormones are synthesized from cholesterol and exert pleiotropic effects notably in the central nervous system. Pioneering studies from Baulieu and colleagues have suggested that steroids are also locally-synthesized in the brain. Such steroids, called neurosteroids, can rapidly modulate neuronal excitability and functions, brain plasticity, and behavior. Accumulating data obtained on a wide variety of species demonstrate that neurosteroidogenesis is an evolutionary conserved feature across fish, birds, and mammals. In this review, we will first document neurosteroidogenesis and steroid signaling for estrogens, progestagens, and androgens in the brain of teleost fish, birds, and mammals. We will next consider the effects of sex steroids in homeostatic and regenerative neurogenesis, in neuroprotection, and in sexual behaviors. In a last part, we will discuss the transport of steroids and lipoproteins from the periphery within the brain (and vice-versa) and document their effects on the blood-brain barrier (BBB) permeability and on neuroprotection. We will emphasize the potential interaction between lipoproteins and sex steroids, addressing the beneficial effects of steroids and lipoproteins, particularly HDL-cholesterol, against the breakdown of the BBB reported to occur during brain ischemic stroke. We will consequently highlight the potential anti-inflammatory, anti-oxidant, and neuroprotective properties of sex steroid and lipoproteins, these latest improving cholesterol and steroid ester transport within the brain after insults.

Keywords: aromatase, cholesterol, blood-brain barrier, estrogens, HDL, lipoproteins, stroke, progestins

INTRODUCTION

Steroid hormones display important physiological functions and exert pleiotropic effects on many target organs including among others the gonads, the liver, and the nervous system. Neurosteroids are produced in the central nervous system (CNS), either via *de novo* synthesis from cholesterol or from local metabolism of steroid intermediate produced in the periphery. The shift from systemic to local synthesis and regulation of steroid action within target tissues, such as the brain, was referred to "Balkanization" of the endocrine system, and could allow the tissue to autonomously synthesize and modulate local steroid signaling (Schmidt et al., 2008). Neurosteroids and peripherally produced steroids have pleiotropic effects and can modulate both brain homeostasis and cerebral functions. The aim of the present review is to summarize the current knowledge regarding the activity and the expression of the steroidogenic enzymes and the targets of steroids, produced in the periphery as well as locally in the brain. We will further consider the roles of androgens, estrogens, and progestagens on physiology and behavior, focusing our discussion on constitutive and regenerative neurogenesis, notably in stroke conditions, as well as the impact of these locally-produced sex steroids on sexual behavior. These points will be discussed from studies performed in fish, birds, and mammals from a comparative point of view. Furthermore, we will discuss the transport of peripheral steroids through the blood-brain barrier (BBB) and their effects on its permeability. We will emphasize the role of this transport by lipoproteins in the functioning of the BBB and during CNS insults, raising the question of the potential roles of cholesterol/steroid transport in neuroprotection and reactive neurogenesis.

NEUROSTEROIDOGENESIS IN THE BRAIN: AN OVERVIEW IN FISH, BIRDS, AND MAMMALS

Steroidogenesis

Steroidogenesis is the enzymatic process by which cholesterol is converted to biologically active steroid hormones. The steroidogenic acute regulatory protein (StAR), and translocator protein (TSPO), in a complex with various proteins including VDAC and ATAD3A, are involved in the transport of cholesterol to the inner membrane of the mitochondria. The first and rate-limiting enzymatic step of the steroidogenic process is the conversion of cholesterol into pregnenolone by P450 side chain cleavage ($P450_{SCC}$; CYP11A1). As shown in the steroidogenic pathway illustrated in **Figure 1**, pregnenolone can subsequently be converted into progesterone (P) by 3-beta-hydroxysteroid dehydrogenase (3β-HSD) or into 17-hydroxypregnenolone by 17-alpha-hydroxylase/17,20 lyase (CYP17). Then, CYP17 can convert progesterone into 17-hydroxyprogesterone, while 3β-HSD can convert 17-hydroxypregnenolone into 17-hydroxyprogesterone. In a next step, 17-hydroxypregnenolone and 17-hydroxyprogesterone can be converted by CYP17 into dehydroepiandrosterone (DHEA) and androstenedione, respectively. In turn, the activity of different 17β-HSD enzymes catalyzes the synthesis of androstenediol from DHEA and testosterone (T) from androstenedione. Aromatase converts androstenedione and testosterone into estrone (E1) and estradiol (E2), respectively, while 5α-reductase converts testosterone into 5α-dihydrotestosterone (DHT). Considering glucocorticoids, the synthesis of 11-deoxycortisol and 11-deoxycorticosterone from 17-hydroxyprogesterone and progesterone, respectively, are catalyzed by 21-hydroxylase (CYP21A2), followed by the P450C11 (Cyp11, cytochrome P450 11β-hydroxylase B1 and/or B2) activity leading to the synthesis of cortisol and corticosterone. Cortisone can also be converted into cortisol by 11β-HSD.

Steroidogenic Activities in the Brains of Fish

In the 80s, pioneering studies performed in the goldfish (*Carassius auratus*) and the toadfish (*Opsanus tau*) documented very high brain aromatase and 5α-reductase activities (Pasmanik and Callard, 1985, 1988). High aromatase expression and activity in the brain is a common feature of teleost fish (Kah et al., 2009; Diotel et al., 2010), as reported in the African catfish (*Clarias gariepinus*) (Timmers and Lambert, 1987), the Atlantic Salmon (*Salmo salar*) (Andersson et al., 1988), the three-spined stickleback (*Gasterosteus aculeatus*) (Borg et al., 1989), the European sea bass (*Dicentrarchus labrax*) (Gonzalez and Piferrer, 2003), and the zebrafish (*Danio rerio*) (Goto-Kazeto et al., 2004; Diotel et al., 2011b). The high aromatase activity in the brain of fish is due to the sustained expression of the *cyp19a1b* gene coding for the Cyp19a1b/Aromatase B protein (AroB), while the *cyp19a1a* isoform coding for Cyp19a1a/Aromatase A protein is mainly expressed in gonads. These two isoforms likely resulted from a third round of genomic duplication event occurring ~320–350 million years ago in fish (Ravi and Venkatesh, 2008).

Biochemical studies using RP-HPLC analysis showed that the brains of adult zebrafish is able to convert [^{3}H]-pregnenolone into [^{3}H]-progesterone, documenting subsequently 3β-HSD activity in the brain of this teleost. These data were reinforced by the absence of progesterone synthesis following treatment with trilostane, a specific inhibitor of 3β-HSD (Sakamoto et al., 2001a). Ten years later, using similar methods, it was shown that the adult zebrafish brain can convert [^{3}H]-pregnenolone into a wide variety of radiolabeled steroids including 17OH-pregnenolone, progesterone (P), and tetrahydro-P, DHEA, androstenedione, testosterone (T), dihydrotestosterone (DHT), 17β-estradiol (17β-E2), and also estrone (E1) (Diotel et al., 2011b). Expression and activity studies in the brain of adult zebrafish were documented for 3α-Hsd, 3β-Hsd, 17β-Hsd, Cyp17, AroB, and 5α-reductase (Diotel et al., 2011b). The recent reanalysis of the RP-HPLC profiles previously reported by Diotel et al. (2011a) indicated that [^{3}H]-pregnenolone can also be converted into cortisol and tetrahydrodeoxycorticosterone (THDOC), further highlighting Cyp21A2 and Cyp11C1 activities within the brain of adult zebrafish (Weger et al., accepted).

Taken together, these data demonstrate that the brain of adult fish is able to *de novo* synthesize a wide variety of steroids from pregnenolone, suggesting that the substrates available for steroidogenesis can originate from local synthesis within the brain, and also from the conversion of peripherally produced precursors.

Steroidogenic Enzyme Expression in the Brains of Fish

The first attempts to localize aromatase-expressing cells in the brain of fish were performed in goldfish using antibodies raised against human placental aromatase (Gelinas and Callard,

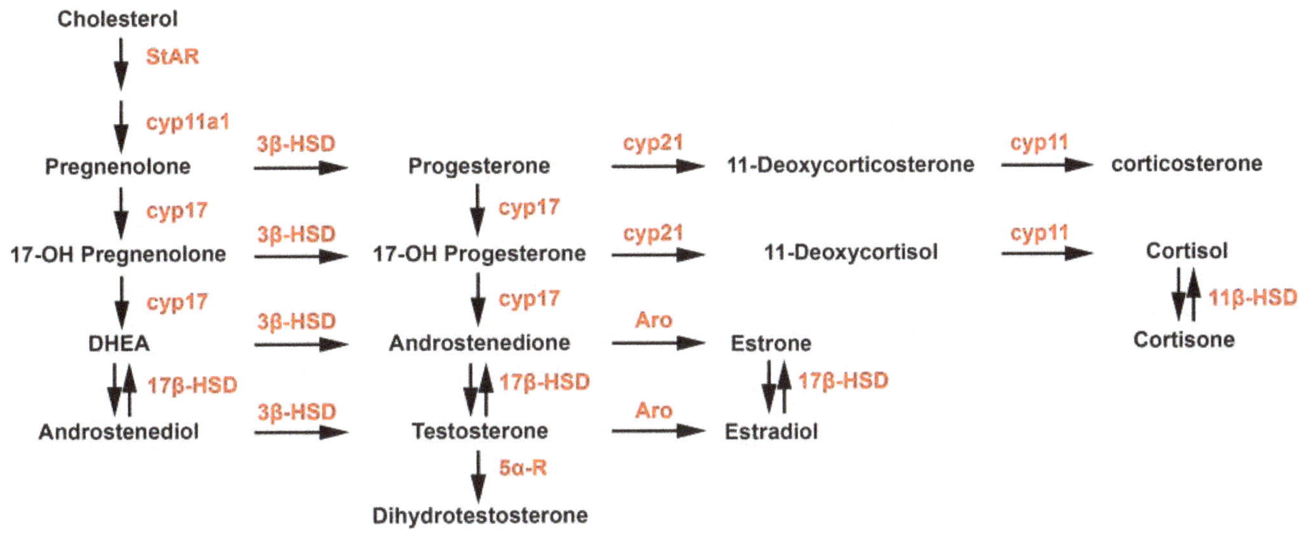

FIGURE 1 | Biosynthetic pathways of neurosteroid synthesis. Cyp11a1, cytochrome P450 family 11 subfamily A member 1 (P450scc), cytochrome P450 side-chain cleavage; Cyp17, cytochrome P450 17α-hydroxylase/C17, 20-lyase; Aro, aromatase; 3β-HSD, 3β-hydroxysteroid dehydrogenase D5–D4 isomerase; 5α-R, 5α-reductase; 17β-HSD, 17β-hydroxysteroid dehydrogenase; Cyp21, cytochrome P450 21 hydroxylase; Cyp11, cytochrome P450 11β-hydroxylase B1 and/or B2. StAR, steroidogenic acute regulatory protein.

1997). In this work, neuron-like cells were labeled in the olfactory bulb, the telencephalon, the preoptic area, and the hypothalamus. However, *cyp19a1b in situ* hybridization and double immunohistochemistry using specific AroB antibodies and glial (GFAP, S100β, and BLBP) or neuronal markers (HuC/D or NeuN) clearly demonstrated the exclusive glial nature of $AroB^+$ cells in others teleost species (Forlano et al., 2001; Goto-Kazeto et al., 2004; Forlano and Bass, 2005; Strobl-Mazzulla et al., 2005; Pellegrini et al., 2007; Mouriec et al., 2008; Tong et al., 2009; März et al., 2010; Coumailleau et al., 2015; Diotel et al., 2016). These data were further reinforced by the development of a *cyp19a1b*-GFP transgenic zebrafish line, showing the exclusive GFP co-expression with glial markers (Tong et al., 2009). Interestingly, $AroB^+$ cells correspond to radial glial cells (RGCs), a particular type of cells with a characteristic morphology. Radial glial cells display a soma localized in the vicinity of the ventricular layer and exhibit two cytoplasmic processes, a short one extending to the ventricle and a longer one running through the brain parenchyma toward the pial surface. In mammals, RGCs behave as neural stem cells (NSCs) during embryonic development and transform into astrocytes at the perinatal stage (Noctor et al., 2001; Weissman et al., 2003; Kriegstein and Alvarez-Buylla, 2009). In fish, they persist during adulthood and maintain neural progenitor properties (Adolf et al., 2006; Pellegrini et al., 2007, 2013, 2015; Tong et al., 2009; März et al., 2010; Rothenaigner et al., 2011; Kizil et al., 2012; Diotel et al., 2016).

Other studies performed in zebrafish documented the expression of 3β-Hsd in neuronal soma and fibers throughout the brain (i.e., dorsal telencephalon, thalamus, preoptic area, paraventricular organ), the cerebellum and the spinal cord (Sakamoto et al., 2001a). In the African lungfish (*Protopterus annectens*), 3β-Hsd was also shown to be expressed in neurons while 5α-reductase was detected in both glia and neurons (Mathieu et al., 2001). Furthermore, numerous experiments documented the expression of the steroidogenic enzymes (*P450scc, 3β-hsd, cyp17,* and *cyp19a1b*) in the brains of fish including the Tongue sole (*Cynoglossus semilaevis*) and the Black porgy (*Acanthopagrus schlegeli*) (Tomy et al., 2007; Chen et al., 2010b). In adult zebrafish, *in situ* hybridization experiments indicate that there is a wide and overlapping distribution of *P450scc, 3β-hsd, cyp17,* and *cyp19a1b* throughout the brain particularly in the telencephalon, the preoptic area, the hypothalamus, and the cerebellum (Diotel et al., 2011b). The distributions of *P450scc, 3β-hsd,* and *cyp17* suggest a potential expression in neurons as well as in neural progenitors, as shown by co-expression with AroB, a RGC marker. From 2011 until now, new isoforms for these steroidogenic enzymes have been identified: *3-βhsd1, 3-βhsd2, cyp11a1, cyp11a2, cyp17a1,* and *cyp17a2.* Recent work confirmed the sites of expression of these steroidogenic enzymes in the brain of adult zebrafish and further described the distribution of their respective isoforms (Weger et al., accepted). It appears that all these steroidogenic enzymes display overlapping distributions. In addition, expression of *cyp21a2, cyp11c1,* and *fdx1/fdx1b* (co-factors of glucocorticoid synthesis) was recently described in adult zebrafish brain (Weger et al., accepted), and patterns appeared similar to other steroidogenic enzymes. Furthermore, isolation and culture of goldfish RGCs was performed (Xing et al., 2014), and deep RNA sequencing of these RGCs indicates expression of steroidogenic acute regulatory protein (*star*), *cyp11a1, cyp17a1, fdx1, hsd17b10* in addition to *cyp19a1b* and *5α-reductase* (Da Fonte et al., 2017). Proteomic analyses also revealed the production of 20β-Hsd (Xing et al., 2016).

Altogether, these studies suggest that the brains of adult fish widely express the biologically active steroidogenic enzymes leading to sex steroid synthesis. They also suggest that RGCs in fish may be capable of *de novo* steroid production from cholesterol and could be consequently envisioned as true steroidogenic cells (**Figure 2A**).

Steroidogenic Enzyme Activities and Expression in the Brains of Birds

Birds are excellent models for understanding the impact of peripherally and locally produced steroids on brain functions, including behavior. Pioneering studies from the groups of Tsutsui and Schlinger have shown that the brains of the quail (*Coturnix japonica*) and zebra finch (*Taeniopygia guttata*) are capable of *de novo* steroidogenesis. They showed that the avian brain expresses the active P450scc, 3β-HSD, CYP17, 17β-HSD, and aromatase enzymes, leading to the production of a wide variety of neurosteroids including pregnenolone, progesterone, androstenedione, testosterone, and estradiol from cholesterol (Tsutsui and Yamazaki, 1995; Tsutsui et al., 1999, 2006, 2009; Matsunaga et al., 2001; London et al., 2006, 2009; London and Schlinger, 2007; Tsutsui, 2011; Schlinger and Remage-Healey, 2012). Western-Blot and immunohistochemistry experiments allow the detection of P450scc immunoreactive neurons through the preoptic area, the thalamus, the hypothalamus, and the cerebellum in Purkinje cells (Tsutsui, 2011). 3β-HSD expression was highlighted based on enzymatic activity in the brain of the adult quail, with a strong presence in the telencephalon and the diencephalon and a lower one in the mesencephalon (Ukena et al., 1999). In quail, *Cyp17* gene expression is detected in the preoptic area, the thalamus, the hypothalamus, and the optic tectum as well as in Purkinje cells (Matsunaga et al., 2001).

Aromatase expression was thoroughly studied in several brain regions particularly, in the hypothalamus and the preoptic area in quail (Balthazart and Foidart, 1993; Balthazart et al., 1996; Balthazart and Ball, 1998; Tsutsui, 2011) and in the telencephalon in zebra finches (Schlinger, 1997). Interestingly, data showed overlapping distribution of *StAR*, *CYP11A1*, *3β-HSD*, and *CYP17 mRNA* in the ventricular proliferative zone of the avian brain during support (London and Schlinger, 2007), suggesting potential roles of neurosteroids in neurogenesis and CNS development. It should be noted that 3β-HSD is also present throughout the telencephalon in adult song birds (Soma et al., 2004; Schlinger et al., 2008). Furthermore, aromatase expression was also studied throughout the avian brain during support and *de novo* expression was documented in RGCs following brain injury in adult birds (Peterson et al., 2004). These data surface a potential role of aromatase and estrogen synthesis in neuroprotection and brain repair mechanisms.

These different studies highlight the capacity of the avian brain to synthesize its own steroids and suggest key roles of neurosteroids in reproductive behavior and neurogenesis.

Steroidogenic Enzyme Activities and Expression in the Brains of Mammals

$P450_{scc}$ gene expression was detected in numerous brain regions of the rodent (i.e., cerebral cortex) and human brain (i.e., cerebral cortex, olfactory bulbs, hippocampus, cerebellum) (Pelletier, 2010). Cells immunoreactive for $P450_{scc}$ were observed in the white matter, the pyramidal and granular neurons of the developing and adult hippocampus (a brain region known for maintaining active neurogenesis during adulthood), and also in Purkinje cells from the cerebellum (Le Goascogne et al., 1987; Tsutsui and Ukena, 1999; Kimoto et al., 2001).

In the 80s, 3β-HSD activity was reported in rat brain homogenates through the conversion of pregnenolone into progesterone (Weidenfeld et al., 1980). More generally, 3β-HSD gene and protein expressions were documented in primary cultures of rodent oligodendrocytes and neurons, and distributed especially in the olfactory bulbs, the thalamus, the cerebral cortex, the hypothalamus, and the cerebellum (Dupont et al., 1994; Guennoun et al., 1995; Meffre et al., 2007; Pelletier, 2010). In humans, *3β-HSD* gene expression was detected in neuronal, astroglial, and oligodendrocyte cell lines (Brown et al., 2000) and had a similar distribution compared to rodents, notably in the thalamus, the hippocampus, and the cerebellum (Yu et al., 2002).

The presence of Cyp17 in the mammalian central nervous system (CNS) is currently not clear. Indeed, some work suggested the absence of *Cyp17* gene expression while other studies reported *Cyp17* gene expression in the cerebellum and the brainstem of rat, and showed Cyp17 immuno-positive cells in the hippocampus, the hypothalamus, and in the Purkinje cells (Mellon and Deschepper, 1993; Strömstedt and Waterman, 1995; Hojo et al., 2004; Pelletier, 2010). During development, the expression of *Cyp17* in the rat brain is present but decreases postnatally (Compagnone and Mellon, 2000). Hence, the question of Cyp17 expression and activity in the mammalian brain remains open.

In rodents, aromatase expression (mRNA and protein) and activity were documented in numerous brain regions including the cerebral cortex, the preoptic nucleus, the hypothalamus as well as the hippocampus; in humans, it was also detected in the pons, the thalamus, the hypothalamus, and the hippocampus (Lephart et al., 1992; Lephart, 1996; Sasano et al., 1998; Garcia-Segura et al., 2003; Hojo et al., 2004; Yague et al., 2006; Pelletier, 2010). In rodents, aromatase expression was mainly detected in neurons and not in glial cells, except following brain injury that results in a *de novo* aromatase expression by astrocytes, suggesting a role of estrogens in neuroprotection (Garcia-Segura et al., 1999; Azcoitia et al., 2001; Garcia-Segura, 2008). In contrast to rodents, in some primates including humans, the estrogen-synthesizing enzyme expression was also reported in some subpopulations of astrocytes in addition to neurons (Yague et al., 2006; Roselli, 2007). As reviewed by Pelletier (2010), numerous studies demonstrate aromatase activity in the brain of mammals including primates.

Consequently, *de novo* steroid synthesis occurs in the brains of mammals (**Figure 2B**). Neurosteroidogenesis is active in

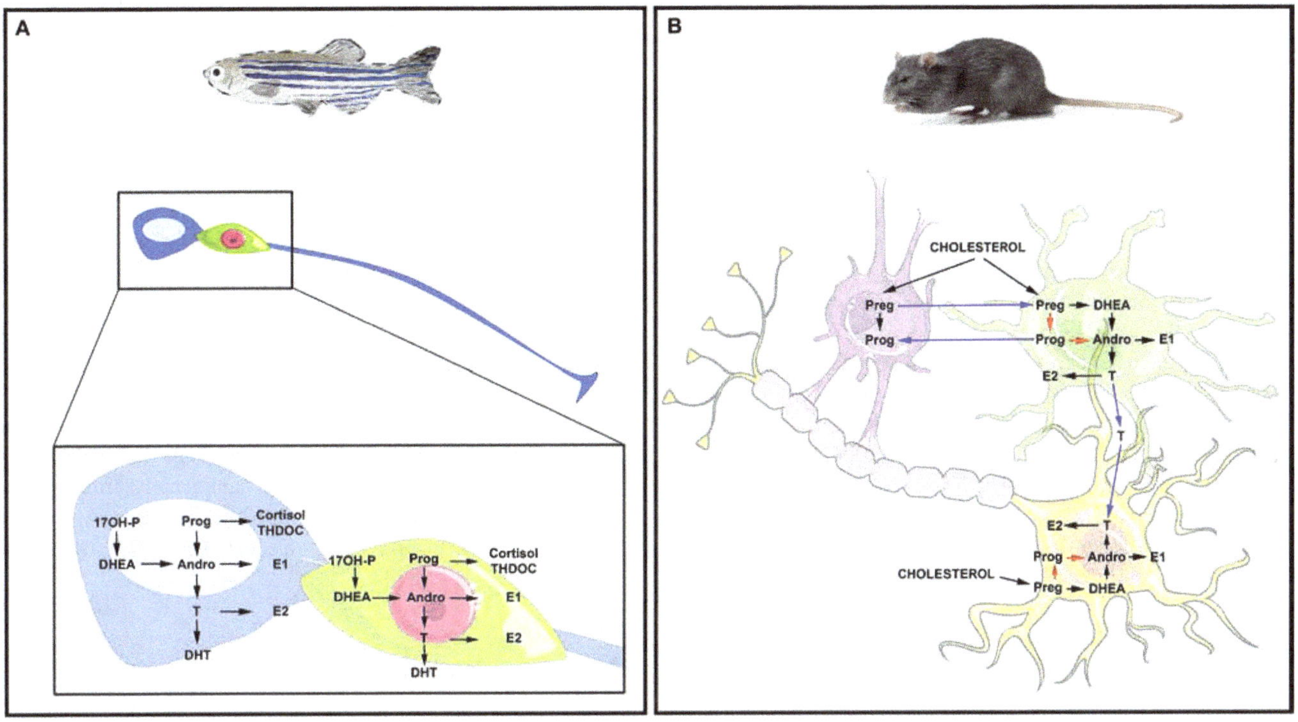

FIGURE 2 | Steroidogenesis in the brain of fish and mammals. **(A)** Steroidogenesis in the brain of adult fish. The blue cell corresponds to a radial glia cell acting as neural stem cell, while the green cell corresponds to a neuron. Data obtained by *in situ* hybridization, RNA sequencing and/or proteomics show neuronal and radial glial expression of steroidogenic enzymes involved in the synthesis of 17OH-Pregnenolone (17OH-P), Progesterone (P), dehydroepiandrosterone (DHEA), Androstenedione (Andro), Estrone (E1), 17β-estradiol (17β-E2, called here E2), testosterone (T) and dihydro-testosterone (DHT), cortisol and THDOC (tetrahydrodeoxycorticosterone). **(B)** Steroidogenesis in the brain of rat. The purple cell corresponds to an oligodendrocyte that participates in the myelin sheath genesis of axons; the green cell is an astrocyte and the yellow one is a neuron whose axon is myelinated by the oligodendrocyte. This schematic view adapted from Zwain and Yen (1999) highlights potential interaction of oligodendrocytes, astrocytes, and neurons in neurosteroidogenesis. The main steroidogenic pathway is shown by black arrows, the minor ones by red arrows and the suggested ones by blue arrows referring to the work of Zwain and Yen (1999). Note that arrows do not necessarily document the direct conversion of the one steroid into another, but can include several enzymatic processes.

numerous regions including the hippocampus, known for maintaining an intense neurogenic activity during adulthood. Interestingly, this region was shown to synthesize 17β-E2 from pregnenolone (Hojo et al., 2004), reinforcing the idea that steroids could impact neurogenesis.

In conclusion, neurosteroidogenesis appears to be a conserved process well-documented in fish, birds and mammals (**Figure 2**). It occurs in numerous evolutionary conserved regions such as the telencephalon, the diencephalon (i.e., preoptic area and hypothalamus), and also the cerebellum. This sustained synthesis of steroids may regulate several brain functions and participate to brain homeostasis, neurotransmission, neurogenesis, and brain plasticity by targeting different cell types.

STEROID SIGNALING IN THE BRAIN: FOCUS ON THE BRAINS OF FISH, BIRDS, AND MAMMALS

Peripherally and locally produced steroids can target different brain regions and cell-types expressing their respective and specific receptors. Here, we will describe the main sites of expression of steroid receptors, with a special focus on estrogen, progesterone, and androgen receptors. We will first discuss receptor distributions in the brain of fish and birds before highlighting the situation in mammals.

Expression of Nuclear and Membrane-Associated Steroid Receptors in the Brains of Fish

Nuclear Estrogen Receptors (ER)

Unique among vertebrates, fish have three nuclear estrogen receptors resulting from an ancient genome duplication: one ERα and two ERβ. The ERα and ERβ probably arose from a first duplication event prior the emergence of ray-finned species. A second duplication led to the emergence of two *ERβ* and *ERα* genes but the second copy of the *ERα* probably disappeared (Thornton, 2001; Bardet et al., 2002; Nagler et al., 2007).

Nuclear estrogen receptors genes [*ERα* (*esr1*), *ERβ1* (*esr2b*), and *ERβ2* (*esr2a*)] were identified in many teleost species, including the rainbow trout (*Oncorhynchus mykiss*), tilapia (*Oreochromis niloticus*), medaka (*Oryzias latipes*), goldfish, and zebrafish among others (Pakdel et al., 1990; Tan et al., 1995;

Muñoz-Cueto et al., 1999; Tchoudakova et al., 1999; Xia et al., 1999; Hawkins et al., 2000; Kawahara et al., 2000; Ma et al., 2000; Socorro et al., 2000; Bardet et al., 2002; Lassiter et al., 2002; Menuet et al., 2002; Andreassen et al., 2003; Choi and Habibi, 2003; Halm et al., 2004; Sabo-Attwood et al., 2004; Filby and Tyler, 2005; Forlano et al., 2005; Nagler et al., 2007; Strobl-Mazzulla et al., 2008; Chakraborty et al., 2011; Zhang et al., 2012; Katsu et al., 2013).

Most studies carried out so far reported the presence of *esr* transcripts in the brain of adult fish. *In situ* hybridization and immunohistochemistry experiments used to localize ER-expressing cells in the brain revealed distinct but partly overlapping patterns of expression in many fish species including medaka, Atlantic croaker (*Micropogonias undulatus*), pejerrey (*Odontesthes argentinensis*), trout and zebrafish (Salbert et al., 1991; Anglade et al., 1994; Hawkins et al., 2000, 2005; Menuet et al., 2002; Pellegrini et al., 2005; Nagler et al., 2007; Strobl-Mazzulla et al., 2008; Zempo et al., 2013; Coumailleau et al., 2015). In general, transcripts for ERs have a broad distribution and were detected in many brain regions known to regulate sexual, reproductive, social behaviors, and sensory-motor activities such as the telencephalon, the preoptic area, the hypothalamus, and the cerebellum. Additionally, ER transcripts have been reported in cells lining the ventricles, where RGCs are localized, and also in cells localized more deeply in the brain parenchyma. Interestingly, there are clear evidences that ERα is expressed in dopaminergic, GABAergic, kisspeptin- and neuropeptide B-positive neurons in several species (Linard et al., 1996; Anglade et al., 1999; Mitani et al., 2010; Escobar et al., 2013; Zempo et al., 2013; Hiraki et al., 2014). Similarly to rodents, ERs were not reported in neurons expressing gonadotrophin-releasing hormone (Navas et al., 1995).

In midshipman (*Porichthys notatus*), pejerrey, and zebrafish, the pattern of expression of the nuclear estrogen receptors and AroB (Cyp19a1b) are closely related (Forlano et al., 2005; Strobl-Mazzulla et al., 2008; Diotel et al., 2011a). Careful examination of adjacent sections hybridized with *cyp19a1b* and *esr1* riboprobes in trout and zebrafish failed to evidence any co-localization (Menuet et al., 2003, 2005). However, *esr2b* was recently shown to be expressed in AroB-expressing RGCs (Pellegrini et al., 2015), and RT-PCR analysis performed in glial cells enriched cultures from adult trout or goldfish suggested that a weak expression of ERα could not be excluded (Menuet et al., 2003; Xing et al., 2015). A recent study designed to characterize the transcriptome of cultured goldfish RGCs and reported *esr1*, *esr2b*, and *esr2a* expression in these neural progenitors (Da Fonte et al., 2017).

Knowledge about estrogen signaling during early development in fish is very limited and the zebrafish is the only species in which expression of the three ERs during embryogenesis was monitored. Quantitative-PCR experiments established that *esr1*, *esr2a*, and especially *esr2b* mRNA were maternally inherited and expressed in eggs before dropping down to 24 h post-fertilization (hpf) (Bardet et al., 2002; Lassiter et al., 2002; Mouriec et al., 2009; Bondesson et al., 2015). Nuclear estrogen receptor expression then started to increase at 24 h, when the onset of zygotic transcription is activated (Bardet et al., 2002; Lassiter et al., 2002; Mouriec et al., 2009). Whole mount *in situ* hybridization showed that *esr2a* and *esr2b* mRNA were detectable at 48 hpf in the ventral telencephalon and in the presumptive preoptic area as well as in the hypothalamus, in line with what was described in the adult brain (Mouriec et al., 2009). A clear expression for *esr1* is described in these regions but at later stages, between 14 days post-fertilization (dpf) and 21 dpf (Kallivretaki et al., 2007; Mouriec et al., 2009). Using *cyp19a1b*-GFP zebrafish embryos, GFP expression was shown to be inducible in RGCs at 24 h after 17β-E2 treatment, an effect blocked by the ER antagonist ICI 182,780, indicating that ERs were fully functional in the brain early during development (Mouriec et al., 2009). A morpholino approach confirmed the specific role of *esr2b* in the induction of the *cyp19a1b* gene (Griffin et al., 2013). Temporary disruption of *esr2a* expression in zebrafish with the same technological approach was associated with a developmental defect of sensory hair cells (Froehlicher et al., 2009). Knockdown of both maternally inherited and zygotic *esr2a* was associated with an increase in apoptotic cells particularly in the brain leading to severe brain defects (Celeghin et al., 2011).

Membrane-Associated Estrogen Receptors (mER)

Membrane receptors responding to 17β-E2 stimulation via rapid non-genomic signaling have been characterized in fish. G protein-coupled estrogen receptor 1 (GPER or GPR30) is a member of this receptor family. A partial or full-length *gper* was cloned, characterized, and detected in the brain of adult zebrafish, Atlantic croaker, and goldfish (Pang et al., 2008; Liu et al., 2009; Pang and Thomas, 2009; Mangiamele et al., 2017). In zebrafish, *gper in situ* hybridization on adult brain sections showed a specific pattern of expression in the olfactory bulbs, the telencephalon, the hypothalamus, the optic tectum, the cerebellum, and the medulla oblongata (Liu et al., 2009). In goldfish, *gper* was also expressed in the forebrain and the suprachiasmatic nucleus, the preoptic area, and the optic tectum (Mangiamele et al., 2017). Originally, it was proposed that goldfish RGCs did not express the G-protein coupled estrogen receptor because attempts to amplify a specific cDNA from cultured cells failed (Xing et al., 2015). However, whole RNA sequencing of separate primary cultures of these cells revealed expression of *gper1*, suggesting that some subpopulations of RGCs express the membrane ER (Da Fonte et al., 2017).

The spatiotemporal distribution of *gper* was investigated in zebrafish using PCR. Its expression was observed in the anterior diencephalon, the midbrain and the hindbrain (Jayasinghe and Volz, 2012; Shi et al., 2013). Both *gper* and *esr2b* mRNA are expressed in neuromasts, suggesting a role of estrogens and a close interaction between these receptors in the developmental regulation of this mecanoreceptive organ (Froehlicher et al., 2009). Knock-down of *gper* resulted in morphological defects in the zebrafish brain at 24 hpf (Shi et al., 2013). At 30 hpf, these morphants displayed an increased number of apoptotic cells, and a decreased brain cell proliferation (Shi et al., 2013). A slight reduction in *otx2* gene expression, which is required for sensory organs development and brain function, was also observed in *gper* knock-down zebrafish. Taken together, these data show the potential involvement of both nuclear and membrane-associated estrogen receptors in brain development and functions.

Nuclear Progestin Receptors (PR)

Nuclear progestin receptor (PR) genes have been characterized in a few fish species (Ikeuchi et al., 2002; Morini et al., 2017). In European eel (*Anguilla Anguilla*), two PR genes, *pgr1* and *pgr2*, were differentially expressed in the brain (olfactory bulb, telencephalon, diencephalon, cerebellum) and in the pituitary of immatures males and females (Morini et al., 2017). Two genes were also identified in the Japanese eel (*Anguilla japonica*) but only *pgr2* mRNA was detected in the brain (Ikeuchi et al., 2002). In zebrafish, a single locus encoding PR (Pgr) was identified (Chen et al., 2010a; Hanna et al., 2010). Ontogenic expression analysis determined by PCR during early embryogenesis showed that *pgr* mRNA was not maternally inherited and became detectable in embryos at 8 hpf (Chen et al., 2010a). Immunohistochemistry and *in situ* hybridization revealed a widespread distribution of zebrafish Pgr receptor (protein and mRNA) in the brain especially neuroendocrine regions (olfactory bulbs, preoptic area, telencephalon, thalamus, hypothalamus, optic tectum, torus longitudinalis, valvula cerebelli) (Hanna et al., 2010; Diotel et al., 2011c). It should be noted that Pgr-positive cells were observed along the ventricular cavities and also more deeply in the brain parenchyma. In this work, it was shown that periventricular Pgr-positive cells displayed a stronger staining compared to Pgr-positive cells located deeply in the parenchyma (Hanna et al., 2010; Diotel et al., 2011c). By performing double immunostainings, it was shown that a large portion of Pgr-positive cells located in the cerebral parenchyma correspond to acetylated-tubulin positive neurons (Diotel et al., 2011c). In contrast, immunohistochemistry on *cyp19a1b*-GFP transgenic zebrafish clearly showed Pgr-expressing cells along the ventricle correspond to AroB$^+$ RGCs (Diotel et al., 2011c). These data were confirmed by a transcriptomic analysis showing *pgr* mRNA expression in cultured goldfish RGCs (Da Fonte et al., 2017). Pgr expression is consequently high in the estrogen-synthesizing RGCs. This suggests a relationship between locally-produced estrogens and Pgr expression. Indeed, treatments with the aromatase inhibitor ATD or with 17β-E2 respectively decrease or increase *prg* expression in the brains of adult zebrafish and also in larvae (Diotel et al., 2011c).

Gene knockout using the TALENs strategy allowed to generate zebrafish lines with null Pgr expression to assess the *in vivo* function of this receptor. Unfortunately, all studies performed with these models have focused at the gonadal levels and none of them looked at the effect of Pgr expression disruption in the brain (Zhu et al., 2015; Tang et al., 2016; Wang et al., 2016).

Membrane-Associated Progestin Receptors (mPR)

In mammals, many progestins exert non-genomic effects through rapid activation of intracellular signaling pathways mediated by two groups of membrane progestin receptors: mPRs (belonging to the PARQ family) and PGRMC1 and PGRMC2 (Petersen et al., 2013). However, there are only scarce data on membrane-associated progestin receptors existence and sites of expression in the brain and the pituitary of fish (Thomas, 2008).

The *mPRα* was identified and detected in the brain of adult spotted seatrout (*Cynoscion nebulosus*) (Zhu et al., 2003). It was also recently cloned in medaka but no data about its brain expression are available (Roy et al., 2017). In goldfish, *mPRα*, *mPRβ*, *mPRγ1*, and *mPRγ2* were also detected in the brain (Tokumoto et al., 2006, 2012). Other studies documented the expression of different mPRs and/or PGMRCs in the brain and the pituitary of the European eel (*Anguilla anguilla*), the channel catfish (*Ictalurus punctatus*) and also the rainbow trout (Kazeto et al., 2005; Mourot et al., 2006; Morini et al., 2017). To date, mPRα and mPRβ were the only form to be identified in zebrafish (Zhu et al., 2003). Using specific antibodies for zebrafish mPRα and mPRβ, Hanna and Zhu demonstrated their expression in brain samples (Hanna and Zhu, 2009). Currently, the distributions and functions of mPR in the brain of fish, if any, are completely unknown.

Nuclear Androgen Receptors (AR)

Two *ar* genes (*ar*1 and *ar*2) were isolated and characterized in several fish species including the Japanese eel (*Anguilla japonica*), the rainbow trout, the kelp bass (*Paralabrax clathratus*), the Atlantic croaker, and cichlids (Ikeuchi et al., 1999; Sperry and Thomas, 1999a,b; Takeo and Yamashita, 1999, 2000; Harbott et al., 2007). More recently, only one *ar* isoform was described in the stickleback (Olsson et al., 2005), the wrasse (*Halichoeres trimaculatus*) (Kim et al., 2002), the zebrafish (Jorgensen et al., 2007; de Waal et al., 2008; Gorelick et al., 2008; Hossain et al., 2008), and in the plainfish midshipman (Forlano et al., 2010).

The first immunohistochemistry studies carried out on the brains of adult goldfish with an heterologous antibody revealed AR-positive cells with neuronal appearance in neuroendocrine regions such as the preoptic area and the hypothalamus, as well as in the olfactory bulbs, the telencephalon and the optic tectum (Gelinas and Callard, 1997). More detailed results were obtained in the brain of the plainfin midshipman, a fish that express mating behavior triggered by auditory signal. These data showed mRNA expression in auditory-related nuclei of the telencephalon, hypothalamus, midbrain, and in the vocal prepacemaker and vocal motor nuclei (Forlano et al., 2010). Numerous studies showed AR expression in the brain of fish including among others wrasse and zebrafish (Kim et al., 2002; Harbott et al., 2007; Hossain et al., 2008; Pouso et al., 2010).

In adult zebrafish, *ar* is strongly expressed along the ventricle and within the brain parenchyma of the telencephalon, the preoptic area, and the hypothalamus (Gorelick et al., 2008). In embryos, *ar* trancripts are maternally deposited and expression levels start to increase substantially at 24 hpf (Hossain et al., 2008). The *ar* gene expression is detected at 24 hpf in the olfactory placodes and in the midbrain, at 48 hpf in the medial diencephalon and at 3 dpf in the pineal organ (Gorelick et al., 2008). All neuroanatomical studies undertaken to date show that ARs are expressed in ventricular margins, where RGC are located (Harbott et al., 2007; Gorelick et al., 2008; Forlano et al., 2010; Pouso et al., 2010). Recently, transcriptomic analysis showed the expression of *ar* in goldfish RGCs (Da Fonte et al., 2017).

As mentioned above, it was shown that goldfish RGCs express progesterone receptor (Pgr), androgen receptor (*ar*), estrogen receptor α (*esr1*), estrogen receptor $\beta 1$ (*esr2b*), and estrogen receptor $\beta 2$ (*esr2a*) (Da Fonte et al., 2017). This data supports other reports in zebrafish showing that RGCs express Pgr protein (Diotel et al., 2011c) and observations for the expression of *ar*, *esr1*, *esr2a*, and *esr2b* mRNAs within neurons and/or AroB$^+$ RGCs (Diotel et al., 2011a; Pellegrini et al., 2015). All this suggests that RGCs are both a source and a target of neurosteroids (Diotel et al., 2011a; Pellegrini et al., 2015; Xing et al., 2016), arguing for key roles of steroids in RGC activity.

Expression of Nuclear and Membrane-Associated Steroid Receptors in the Brains of Birds

Nuclear and Membrane-Associated Estrogen Receptors

Early data on the distribution of sex hormone receptors in the brain of birds was extensively reviewed (Gahr, 2001). Similar to mammals, there are two different avian genes coding for ERα and ERβ (Bernard et al., 1999; Jacobs et al., 1999). In birds, ERα is expressed in the brain of all the species studies so far, including members of Apodiformes, Passeriformes, Galliformes, Columbiformes, and Psittaciformes. These ERs are distributed in various brain territories including the telencephalon, the diencephalon, and the rhombencephalon, with more noticeable expression in the preoptic area and the hippocampus (Gahr, 2001). For instance, in the brain of zebra finch, ERα mRNAs was observed in the nidopallium, the arcopallium, the hippocampus, the diencephalon, the midbrain and within the vocal control circuitry (Jacobs et al., 1999). Interestingly, ERα mRNAs expression overlap with that of aromatase (Jacobs et al., 1999). ERβ was first described in the brain of the Japanese quail, the European starling (*Sturnus vulgaris*), and the canary (Bernard et al., 1999; Foidart et al., 1999; Gahr, 2001). In general, ERβ was reported in the preoptic area, the hypothalamus, the thalamus and different midbrain nuclei. In the European starling, *in situ* hybridization experiments allowed the detection of ERβ mRNA in the nidopallium and the preoptic area in a pattern reminiscent of aromatase (Bernard et al., 1999; Axelsson et al., 2007). Consequently, ERα, ERβ and aromatase distributions strongly overlap. As reported in oscine birds, ER labeling was detected in different forebrain regions while it was not found in non-oscine ones, highlighting discrete differences in ER expression in songbird species and families (Gahr, 2001). It should be noted that, while histological studies have focused on the distribution of the nuclear isoforms, numerous functional studies suggest that estrogen receptors act at the level of the membrane, probably via interaction with other receptors such as glutamate receptors (Pawlisch and Remage-Healey, 2015; Seredynski et al., 2015).

Nuclear and Membrane-Associated Progesterone Receptors

Concerning PR expression, most studies in birds have focused on the hypothalamic region, because of the potential role of PR signaling in reproductive and egg-laying behaviors. Similarly to ER and AR, PR expression was investigated and documented by *in situ* hybridization and immunohistochemistry in the preoptic area, the hypothalamus, the thalamus, the hippocampus of the zebra finch, and the hen (Sterling et al., 1987; Lubischer and Arnold, 1990).

Androgen Receptors

The first studies documenting AR distribution in the brain of birds were performed by *in vivo* autoradiography with radio-labeled steroids (Arnold, 1980; Gahr, 2001). In zebra finch, these autoradiographic studies demonstrated the binding of tritiated testosterone in the HVC (used as the proper term, but previously known as hyperstriatum ventrale pars caudalis or and high vocal center), the magnocellular nucleus of the anterior nidopallium, the robust nucleus of the arcoplallium, the nucleus intercollicularis of the midbrain, and the periventricular magnocellular nucleus of the anterior hypothalamus (Arnold, 1980). In the golden-collared manakins (*Manacus vitellinus*), *in situ* hybridization for AR revealed expression in the forebrain, in the nucleus taeniae of the amygdala and in the arcopallium (Fusani et al., 2014). In general, ARs are detected in the hypothalamus, the preoptic area, the midbrain, and hindbrain in all species studied to date.

Taken together, it appears that ER, AR, and PR display almost similar distribution in the avian brain, with higher expression in the preoptic area, hypothalamus, thalamus, and hippocampus.

Expression of Nuclear and Membrane-Associated Steroid Receptor in the Brains of Mammals

Estrogen Receptors

Data concerning ERs mRNA and protein expression mostly originate from rat studies showing a strong expression of ERα and ERβ throughout the brain (Li et al., 1997; Shughrue et al., 1997). *In situ* hybridization and immunohistochemistry experiments revealed that ERα and ERβ are expressed in neurons and glia from many CNS regions including the olfactory bulbs, the preoptic area, the hypothalamus, the zona incerta, the ventral tegmentum as well as the cerebellum in Purkinje cells (Li et al., 1997; Shughrue et al., 1997; Mitra et al., 2003; Frick et al., 2015). Both ERs were also detected in the cerebral cortex and in the hippocampus, with higher ERβ expression compared to ERα (Shughrue et al., 1997). In the brain of mouse, immunohistochemistry against ERβ allows the detection of immunoreactive cells in regions similar to the rat. However, ERα expression appears stronger in the hippocampus and the hypothalamus, and lower in the cerebral cortex and cerebellum (Mitra et al., 2003), suggesting some differences in ER signaling between rat and mouse. Importantly, ERs are widely and strongly expressed in the brain of mouse at postnatal day 7, but their respective expression declines the two following days with different kinetics (Sugiyama et al., 2009). In humans, ERα is detected in the cortex at 9 gestational weeks in proliferating zones and in the cortical plate. Its expression subsequently decreases until birth before increasing gain during adulthood. At 15 gestational weeks, ERβ was also detected in proliferating zones and in the cortical plate with expression persisting in the adult cortex (González et al., 2007). Interestingly, from 15 gestational weeks to adulthood, ERα and ERβ are detected in the hippocampus including the dentate gyrus, known to be a neurogenic region (González et al., 2007). In the same line, ERs have been detected in embryonic/adult NSCs in rodents and humans, suggesting a roles of estrogen signaling in NSC activity (Brännvall et al., 2002; Kishi et al., 2005; Hajszan et al., 2007; Suzuki et al., 2007; Okada et al., 2010). The spatiotemporally regulated expression of ERs in the embryonic brain of mouse and human, notably in the cerebral cortex and the hippocampus, argue in favor of different roles of estradiol during development (González et al., 2007; Sugiyama et al., 2009). Furthermore, a plasma membrane-associated ER (ER-X, GPER, GPR30, GPER1) was identified in the brain, mediating estrogen activation of MAPK/ERK (Toran-Allerand, 2005). This receptor is functionally distinct from ERα and ERβ and is up-regulated in the adult brain after ischemic stroke (Toran-Allerand et al., 2002). Its expression in the hippocampus is likely to play a role in synaptic plasticity (Waters et al., 2015).

Progesterone Receptors

In mammals, progesterone receptors include the classic nuclear PRA and PRB receptors, splice variants, and membrane-associated receptors mPR (mPRα, mPRβ, and mPRγ) (Brinton et al., 2008). Nuclear PRs are expressed through the brain in neurons and glial cells of the hippocampus, the cortex and the hypothalamus (Hagihara et al., 1992a,b; Brinton et al., 2008), and their expression is up-regulated by estrogens in a region specific manner (Guerra-Araiza et al., 2003). Among the three mPR subtypes described, mPRα is the best characterized pharmacologically. *In situ* hybridization and immunohistochemistry experiments have shown a wide mPRα neuronal expression in the olfactory bulbs, the cortex, the hypothalamus, the hippocampus, and the cerebellum (Meffre et al., 2013). Very interestingly, after traumatic brain injury, mPRα is *de novo* expressed in microglia, astrocytes and oligodendrocytes, highlighting a potential role of this receptor in inflammation and brain repair mechanisms (Meffre et al., 2013). In rat, mPRβ-expressing neurons are detected in the forebrain and the midbrain (Zuloaga et al., 2012). In human, mPR mRNAs are distributed in the forebrain, the hypothalamus and also the hippocampus (Pang et al., 2013).

Androgen Receptors

In adult rodents, AR mRNA and protein are detected in neurons and glia of the medial amygdala, the preoptic area, the hypothalamus, the cerebellum, and the dentate gyrus of the hippocampus (Commins and Yahr, 1985; Sar et al., 1990; Hajszan et al., 2007; Feng et al., 2010; Pelletier, 2010; Mhaouty-Kodja, 2017). Interestingly, AR protein level is correlated with circulating levels of estradiol and testosterone across the estrous cycle, suggesting an estrogenic regulation of its expression (Feng et al., 2010).

To conclude, across vertebrate species, the distribution of ER, PR, and AR in the brain are evolutionary conserved, especially in the hypothalamus, the preoptic area, and some striatal regions. They are also expressed in neurogenic brain regions, arguing in favor of a role sex steroids in the regulation of NSC activity, neuronal differentiation, and cell survival.

ROLE OF STEROIDS IN THE BRAINS OF FISH, MAMMALS, AND BIRDS

In this third part, we will discuss the action of estrogens, progestagens and androgens on constitutive neurogenesis and their effects on CNS following insults such as stroke and traumatic brain injury, with a focus on the impact of sex on brain injury. Then, we will discuss the impact of neurosteroids on behavior in fish, birds, and rodents, focusing only on sexual behavior.

Constitutive and Regenerative Neurogenesis

The actions of steroids in the brain are complex and depend of many factors such as the strain, the species, the timing, the concentration, and the rhythm of secretion, as well as the regions studied (Duarte-Guterman et al., 2015; Heberden, 2017). Sex steroids are well-documented for impacting neuronal plasticity including synaptogenesis/spinogenesis such as shown for estrogens (Fester et al., 2012; Brandt et al., 2013; Sellers et al., 2015; Sager et al., 2017), progesterone (Sakamoto et al., 2001b, 2002; Zhao et al., 2011), and testosterone (Manolides and Baloyannis, 1984; Devoogd et al., 1985). They have been also well-characterized for their role on learning/memory processes (Frye and Walf, 2008, 2010; Frye et al., 2008; Phan et al., 2012; Celec et al., 2015; Frick et al., 2015). In addition, estrogens, progestins, and androgens display neuroprotective effects through genomic and non-genomic mechanisms (López-Rodríguez et al., 2015). These neuroprotective effects involved the upregulation of anti-apoptotic factors (i.e., Bcl2) and antioxidant enzymes (i.e., SOD and GPx), as well as the down-regulation of pro-inflammatory cytokines (López-Rodríguez et al., 2015). Due to limited space and to avoid redundancy with recently published reviews (Shahrokhi et al., 2012; Heberden, 2017; McEwen and Milner, 2017), we will mainly focus on the roles of these sex steroids on neurogenesis under homeostatic and regenerative conditions (i.e., stroke, traumatic brain injury).

Effects of Estrogens

In the brain, estrogens modulate synaptic plasticity, NSC proliferation, newborn neuron migration, differentiation, and survival, as well as neuroprotection (McEwen and Woolley, 1994; McEwen et al., 1995; Azcoitia et al., 2001; McCullough et al., 2003; Murashov et al., 2004; Mukai et al., 2010; Frick et al., 2015).

For instance, 17β-E2 treatment of rat embryonic NSCs increases cell proliferation and neuronal differentiation (Brännvall et al., 2002), and promotes human embryonic NSC differentiation into dopaminergic neurons (Kishi et al., 2005). In addition, ERβ knock-out mice display a thinner cortex at E18.5 due to defects in neuronal migration and increased cell-death arguing for a role of ERβ in newborn neuronal differentiation and survival during the late phase of corticogenesis (Wang et al., 2003).

During adulthood, rat hippocampal cell genesis in female is modulated by ovarian hormone levels and is higher during pro-estrus, when 17β-E2 concentration is elevated (Tanapat et al., 1999, 2005). In the same line of evidence, ovariectomy leads to decreased hippocampal proliferation that is restored by 17β-E2 treatments through ER dependent mechanism as demonstrated by the use of specific ER agonists (Mazzucco et al., 2006). The impact of other estrogens such as estradiol-benzoate, 17α-E2, and estrone have been shown to also increase cell proliferation in ovariectomized rats suggesting that the positive neurogenic effects of estrogens are a general feature of female sex hormones (Frick et al., 2015). In meadow voles (*Microtus pennsylvanicus*), the reproductive status also influences dentate gyrus cell proliferation and/or surviving (higher in inactive females; higher in active males) (Ormerod and Galea, 2001, 2003). However, hippocampal cell proliferation in squirrels (*Sciurus carolinensis*) was not shown to be sexually dimorphic and to be modulated across the reproductive cycle (Lavenex et al., 2000). Furthermore, in striking contrast with most studies, an acute 17β-E2 treatment decreases cell proliferation in the subventricular zone (SVZ) and leads to a decrease in newborn cells in the olfactory bulbs (Brock et al., 2010). In addition, chronic 17β-E2 treatments in zebrafish impair NSC proliferation, cell survival, and the newborn cell migration (Diotel et al., 2013).

Estrogens also display neuroprotective properties and promote neural regeneration following traumatic brain injury and cerebral ischemia by decreasing apoptotic signaling, neuroinflammation, and oxidatative stress and by normalizing glutamate concentrations (Petrone et al., 2015). These neuroprotective effects of estrogens on brain ischemia have been well-established in ovariectomized rodents, and result in a significang decrease in the size of the lesion and in the infarct volume (Gibson et al., 2006; Petrone et al., 2015).

Effects of Progesterone and Allopregnenolone

In the brain, progesterone is known to regulate spinogenesis, synaptogenesis, neuronal survival, and dendritic growth (McEwen and Woolley, 1994; Brinton et al., 2008; Tsutsui, 2008; Zhang et al., 2010; Rossetti et al., 2016). Following cerebral ischemia in rat, progesterone promotes neurogenesis in the SVZ of the lateral ventricles and favors cell survival in the peri-infarct region several days post-stroke (Jiang et al., 2016). Interestingly, numerous studies documented estrogen and progesterone effects on learning and memory across the estrous cycle as reviewed in Duarte-Guterman et al. (2015). Allopregnanolone, a progesterone metabolite considered as one of the most important neuroactive steroid in the CNS, also plays key roles by increasing neurogenesis, neuronal cell survival, and by reducing cell-death in the hippocampus and the midbrain (Charalampopoulos et al., 2008; Zhang et al., 2015; Rossetti et al., 2016). It also exerts major neuroprotective roles in neurodegenerative diseases (Rossetti et al., 2016).

Effects of Androgens

Concerning androgens, a pioneer study in songbird suggested that testosterone could favor neurogenesis (Louissaint et al., 2002), further corroborated by mice castration studies resulting in decreased hippocampal neurogenesis (Spritzer and Galea, 2007; Heberden, 2017). In songbirds, androgens and estrogens are well-known to induce seasonal-like growth of song nuclei in the adult (Tramontin et al., 2003; Balthazart and Ball, 2016). Additional experiments in rodents document the positive effect of testosterone on SVZ cell proliferation (Tramontin et al., 2003; Farinetti et al., 2015; Balthazart and Ball, 2016), and those of testosterone and dihydrotestosterone on newborn neuron survival (Spritzer and Galea, 2007). In the same line, testosterone increases neurogenesis in wild-type males but not in androgen-insensitive ones (Hamson et al., 2013). This effect is blocked by AR antagonist (flutamide), demonstrating that androgens act through AR and not through ER after conversion into estrogens (Hamson et al., 2013). However, the reality appears more complex as treatment with nandrolone, a synthetic androgen, decreases hippocampal neurogenesis in male and female (Brännvall et al., 2005). Experiments performed in post-ischemic mice established that endogenous androgens do not alter injury-induced neurogenesis, while supra-physiological levels of testosterone and dihydrotestosterone strongly inhibits post-stroke neurogenesis in the dentate gyrus, reducing brain repair (Zhang et al., 2014).

Sex Difference after Brain Injuries

Interestingly, clinical and experimental findings are abundant and highlight important sex differences after stroke (Roof and Hall, 2000; Girijala et al., 2017). Clinical studies showed that aging women display worse outcomes following ischemic stroke than men, and higher mortality after hemorrhagic stroke (Sohrabji, 2015). In addition, ischemic stroke model in rodents document that young female have smaller infarcted area than young males (Alkayed et al., 1998), and also exhibit less severe stroke consequences during pro-estrus (high 17β-E2 concentration) than during metestrus (low 17β-E2 concentration) (Liao et al., 2001). However, these studies only correlate between levels of 17β-E2 and stroke severity without taking into consideration other steroid hormone such as progesterone. During aging, mortality is higher in female than in male, and in the case of hemorrhagic stroke, males display greater bleeding and mortality (Sohrabji, 2015). It was also shown that estrogen treatments improve outcomes in young females and males after ischemic and hemorrhagic stroke, while their effects are controversial on aging females during ischemia (Sohrabji, 2015). Other clinical and experimental findings also document the impact of gender and of sex steroids on other CNS insults. For instance, after traumatic brain injury, men displayed greater levels of injury severity as indicated by the Glasgow Coma Scale score, but such an effect is not always found (Slewa-Younan et al., 2004; Davis et al., 2006). Taken together, these data argue in favor of an impact of sex and circulating steroids on the consequences of CNS insults.

In conclusion, sex steroids, peripherally or centrally produced, exert numerous actions on constitutive and regenerative neurogenesis, on brain plasticity, learning, and behaviors (**Figure 3**). For more details on sex hormone modulation of hippocampal neurogenesis, see (Galea et al., 2006; Frick et al., 2015).

Sexual Behavior

As introduced earlier, sex steroids module in a wide array of behaviors, including aggression, parental behavior, sexual behavior, but also more cognitive aspects, including attention and visual and verbal memory. Although original studies investigated the role of gonadally-produced steroids, it is now clear that the local synthesis of these steroids directly in the central nervous system play a significant role as well. The shift from systemic to local synthesis and regulation of steroid action within target tissues, such as the brain, was called "Balkanization" of the endocrine system (Schmidt et al., 2008). This process would allow the brain to produce specific steroids required for the activation of defined behavior, while leaving other tissues unaffected. The central synthesis of estrogens in the male brain is probably the best example, as high peripheral production of these steroids would have major feminizing effects. Amongst the many behavioral effects of steroids, we chose to discuss in more detail the steroid-dependent modulation of sexual behavior. Indeed, the neuroanatomy and physiology underlying this reproductive behavior have been under study for decades, and sexual behavior provide an excellent model to further investigate the respective role of locally- vs. peripherally- produced sex steroids.

Importance of Neuroestrogens

The role for aromatase on male sexual behavior was hypothesized over 50 years ago (Clemens, 2013; Södersten, 2013) and a very large number of studies using pharmacological tools have demonstrated that testosterone action on male sexual behavior in various species requires its aromatization in the brain (Christensen and Clemens, 1975; Beyer et al., 1976; Morali et al., 1977; Balthazart and Foidart, 1993; Roselli et al., 2003). These observations were further confirmed by the use of various aromatase knock-out mice (Fisher et al., 1998; Honda et al., 1998; Matsumoto et al., 2003; Bakker et al., 2004). Furthermore, the importance of the central production of estrogens was highlighted by stereotaxic experiments affecting estrogen synthesis within the preoptic area. This region is a key brain center involved the control of male sexual behavior in most vertebrate species and, importantly, contains a very high concentration of aromatase, especially in birds (Balthazart et al., 2004; Perkins and Roselli, 2007; McCarthy, 2011). Numerous studies have shown that preoptic aromatase activity is critical for the activation of male sexual differentiation and male sexual behavior. For example, chronic inhibition of aromatase activity by specific inhibitors delivered to the preoptic area results in the complete suppression of copulatory behavior within a few days (Christensen and Clemens, 1975; Watson and Adkins-Regan, 1989a; Balthazart and Surlemont, 1990; Balthazart et al., 1990). In castrates, the male sexual behavior can be restored by the local administration of testosterone as well as estrogens (Christensen and Clemens, 1974; Watson and Adkins-Regan, 1989b). These results indicate that the expression of male sexual behavior is tied to changes in aromatase concentration and activity in the preoptic area (POA). Interestingly, these change in aromatase expression and male sexual behavior are also linked to an important local neuroplasticity (Aste et al., 1993; Panzica et al., 1998; Charlier et al., 2008). It should be noted that most of these effects were taking place after several days of steroid treatment, clearly suggesting direct genomic effects via the activation of nuclear receptors (Panzica et al., 1998; Scordalakes et al., 2002; Balthazart et al., 2004).

In addition to the long-term effects of estrogens, estrogens also display rapid effects on several aspects of male sexual behavior. For example, research in mouse and Japanese quail showed that acute modulation of estrogen concentrations rapidly affect male sexual behavior (Cornil et al., 2006; Taziaux et al., 2007; Seredynski et al., 2013, 2015). Many of these rapid effects require doses of estradiol that surpass systemic estradiol concentrations in the blood, but local estradiol levels could reach high concentrations quickly, because aromatase and other steroidogenic enzymes can be rapidly regulated in the brain (see below) and are enriched in subcellular compartments such as the presynaptic bouton (Peterson et al., 2005; Saldanha et al., 2011; Cornil et al., 2012). These rapid and local effects of steroids have led to the hypothesis that neuroestrogens act as neurotransmitters (Balthazart and Ball, 2006). Moreover, exposure to sexual stimuli will in turn affect aromatase activity in several regions. Indeed, copulation rapidly and significantly reduced aromatase activity in hypothalamic nuclei and in median preoptic nucleus or tuberal hypothalamus isolated using the Palkovits punch technique (Cornil et al., 2005; de Bournonville et al., 2013). Conversely, exposure to stress upregulates aromatase activity within 5 min in a sex- and brain region-dependent manner in quail (Dickens et al., 2011, 2013), but this increase was counteracted by copulation with a female (Dickens et al., 2012). The mechanisms leading to rapid changes of aromatase activity seem to rely on phosphorylation-dephosphorylation processes but the exact mechanisms are far from being understood (Balthazart et al., 2005, 2006; Charlier et al., 2011a).

It should be noted that the measurements of estrogens do not correlate with aromatase activity in most cases and future work should tackle this discrepancy (Charlier et al., 2011b; Dickens et al., 2014; de Bournonville et al., 2017b). Interestingly, central aromatase is not only important for male sexual behavior but was also shown recently to be involved in female sexual behavior in Japanese quail (de Bournonville et al., 2016, 2017a), see also recent discussion in Cornil (2017). The very high concentration of aromatase in birds make them a very suitable model to investigate its function in modulating sexual behavior but it is likely that rapid change in aromatase activity are also important in mammals and fish, as rapid effects of estrogens were demonstrated on sexual motivation in rat and Goldfish (Cross and Roselli, 1999). However, little is known about the behavioral role of aromatase in fish. As stated above, fish in general possess a very wide distribution of aromatase but the presence of high levels of aromatase, androgen, and estrogen receptors, in brain regions involved in the detection and processing of visual stimuli, suggests that visual processes related to reproduction may be influenced by sex steroids (Gelinas and Callard, 1993, 1997). Testosterone is necessary and sufficient for the enhancement of male approach responses toward a female stimulus to occur and androgen treatments in female goldfish also induce selective approach responses toward female visual stimuli (Thompson et al., 2004). Injections of 17β-E2 had the same behavioral effect

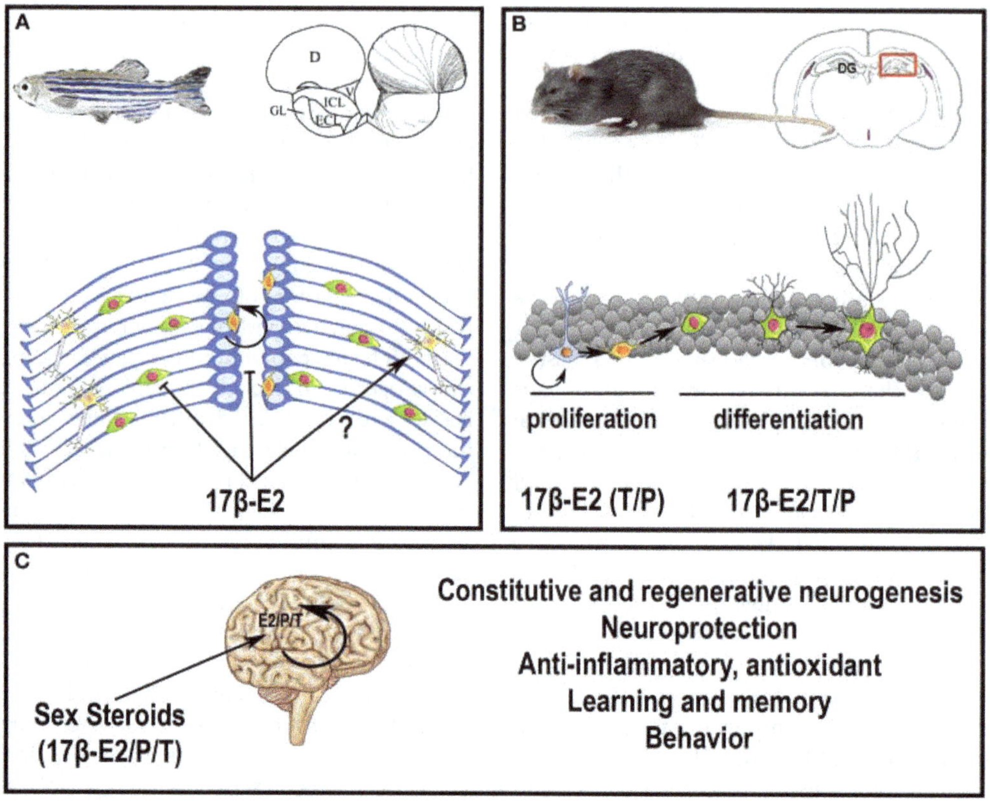

FIGURE 3 | Potential roles of steroids in the brain. **(A)** Effects of 17β-estradiol on neurogenesis in adult zebrafish. At the top, the scheme represents a zebrafish and a transversal brain section through the olfactory bulbs, taken from Menuet et al. (2005). The lines on the right hemisphere correspond to radial glial cells, that behave as neural stem cells. At the bottom, the scheme illustrates neurogenesis events occurring on the zebrafish brain. Radial glial cells (blue) give rise to new neurons (green) that migrate and differentiate into mature and functional neurons (yellow). The orange cells close to the ventricle vicinity are further committed progenitors. It was shown that 17β-estradiol impairs neural progenitor proliferation and new born cell migration; the data obtained for neural differentiation and survival are not clear (Diotel et al., 2013; Pellegrini et al., 2015). **(B)** Effects of sex steroids on neurogenesis in adult rodents. At the top, the scheme represents a rodent and a transversal brain section through the dentate gyrus (DG) of the hippocampus (framed box), where neurogenesis is maintained during adulthood. At the bottom, the scheme illustrates neurogenesis events occurring in the granular cell layer of the dentate gyrus. Radial glial cells (blue light) give rise to neural progenitors (orange) that give birth to new neurons (green with a small neuritic arborescence) that migrate and differentiate into mature and functional neurons (green with a huge neuritic arborescence). In general, 17β-estradiol (17β-E2) favors neural stem cell/progenitor proliferation; to a lesser extent, testosterone (T) and progesterone (P) also exert positive role on proliferation; 17β-estradiol, testosterone and progesterone also promote neuronal migration and differentiation (Heberden, 2017). In addition, these three sex steroids promote new born cell survival in constitutive and regenerative neurogenesis. Note, that the effects of sex steroids on neurogenesis could be dependent of the timing, the concentration, the rhythm of exposure and the regions targeted. For instance, estradiol treatment has been shown to decrease neurogenesis in the SVZ (Brock et al., 2010). **(C)** Peripheral steroids and neurosteroids impact brain functions and homeostasis, by modulating neurogenesis under homeostatic and regenerative conditions, by promoting neuroprotection, learning, and memory, and by exerting anti-inflammatory and antioxidant properties. They also modulate sexual behavior.

as testosterone, and pretreatment with the aromatase inhibitor (fadrozole) 15 min prior to testosterone injections significantly reduced the male's ability to detect and/or orient toward potential mates. Local 17β-E2 synthesis in neural pathways involved in visual processing could therefore sensitize the males to some visual features of females and modulate orientation responses in the context of reproduction (Lord et al., 2009).

Importance of Neuroprogestins: Neuroprogesterone

In most species, the synchrony between ovulation and female sexual behavior is obviously fundamental for efficient reproductive output. Both processes require a sequential elevation of estradiol and progesterone (Mahesh and Brann, 1998; Stephens et al., 2015). Although preliminary observations suggested that progesterone originating from the periphery (Buckingham et al., 1978; Putnam et al., 1991; Mahesh and Brann, 1992), ovariectomized and adrenalectomized rats continue to produce a LH surge in response to estradiol priming, suggesting a role for the central production of progesterone (Ferin et al., 1969; Micevych et al., 2003). This central production of neuroprogesterone is linked to astrocytic activity as astrocytes possess transport proteins (TSPO, StAR) and steroidogenic enzymes (P450ssc, 3βHSD, etc.) required to transform cholesterol into progesterone. Importantly, the synthesis of progesterone in female hypothalamic astrocytes is regulated by estradiol. This estradiol, from gonadal origin will likely affect the transcription and/or activity of multiple transporters and enzymes, including StAR, TSPO, P450ssc, and 3β-HSD, as observed *in vitro* and *in vivo* (Sinchak et al., 2003; Soma et al., 2005; Micevych et al., 2007; Micevych and Sinchak, 2008a; Kuo et al., 2010; Chen et al., 2014). To our knowledge, the role of neuroprogesterone on the display of sexual behavior is currently not known, although the very fast effect of progesterone receptor antisense oligonucleotides on lordosis behavior could suggest a local synthesis of progesterone (Mani et al., 1994). Although the role of neuroprogesterone on female sexual behavior has not been extensively studied, the function of its metabolite allopregnanolone has been investigated in more detail (Frye, 2011).

Importance of Neuroprogestins: Allopregnanolone

Allopregnanolone, also known as 3α-hydroxy-5α-pregnan-20-one (3α,5α-THP), is a neurosteroid produced in several regions of the central nervous system by local conversion of progesterone via 5α-reductase. After paced mating 3α,5α-THP rapidly increases in the midbrain ventral tegmental area (VTA), a dopaminergic region involved in reproductive behaviors of female rodents. The rapidity of the rise in midbrain 3α,5α-THP levels, and independence of ovaries and/or adrenals as sources of steroids, suggest that biosynthesis underlies mating-induced increases (Frye and Vongher, 1999). Paced mating also increases 3α,5α-THP concentrations in other structures of the mesocorticolimbic circuit, such as hippocampus, and cortex (Frye et al., 2013). Central infusions with an inhibitor of TSPO (PK-11195), or with an inhibitor of 3α-HSD within the midbrain VTA significantly attenuated 3α,5α-THP levels of pro-estrus rats and led to a significant reduction in sexual behavior (Frye and Paris, 2011). In order to assess whether central 3α,5α-THP is necessary and sufficient for these effects, pro-estrus rats were infused with 3α,5α-THP subsequent to inhibitor infusions and results indicated a reinstatement of sexual behavior (Frye and Paris, 2011). In hamsters, infusions of a TSPO agonist, to the VTA increased sexual responsiveness and lordosis of cycling, estradiol and progesterone-primed hamsters, compared to vehicle. In contrast, and similarly to what was observed in rat, the TSPO antagonist (PK-11195) injection to the VTA attenuated sexual responsiveness of naturally receptive or estradiol benzoate (EB) + progesterone -primed hamsters compared to vehicle. In parallel, these treatments respectively led to increased and decreased midbrain levels of allopregnenolone (Petralia and Frye, 2005). Future work should define in more detail the precise relationship between localized allopregnanolone synthesis and specific sexual behaviors.

Neurosteroid synthesis is pronounced during early development. Numerous steroidogenic enzymes are expressed at very high levels in the developing avian brain (Goodson et al., 2005; Tsutsui et al., 2006; London and Schlinger, 2007). In rodent brain, most steroidogenic enzymes are typically expressed at much lower levels compared to fish and birds and thus more difficult to quantify but the developmental expression pattern was described for a few steroidogenic enzymes. For example, in rats, brain expression of P450c17, the enzyme responsible for the transformation of pregnenolone to DHEA, is elevated in the embryo and decreases postnatally (Compagnone and Mellon, 2000). Brain 3β-HSD mRNA in rodents is highest during early development (Ibanez et al., 2003). Although steroids from gonadal origin are known to be a significant parameter in sex differentiation in bird, neurosteroids may regulate sexual differentiation in songbird species. In nestling European starlings, neural metabolism of DHEA and 17β-E2 can be greater in males than females at specific ages (Chin et al., 2008; Shah et al., 2011). In zebra finches, 17β-E2 synthesized *de novo* in cultured male brain slices triggers development of an important projection in the song control circuit (Holloway and Clayton, 2001). Female brain slices developed this projection only when co-cultured with male slices, suggesting a sex difference in neural 17β-E2 synthesis during development (Holloway and Clayton, 2001; Schlinger et al., 2001). Progesterone is also synthesized in the brain during development (Zwain and Yen, 1999; Micevych and Sinchak, 2008a,b) and promotes myelination (Koenig et al., 1995; Schumacher et al., 2007).

STEROIDS AND LIPOPROTEINS: FROM PERIPHERY TO THE BRAIN

Transport and Actions of Steroids on the Blood-Brain Barrier

Although neurosteroids play key roles on brain functions, peripheral steroid hormones have the main effects on the CNS, either by crossing the BBB or by targeting the BBB cells, which in turn impact the brain parenchyma by modulating inflammatory and oxidative signals. Some of these possibilities were recently discussed in a review for other hormones called adipokines (Parimisetty et al., 2016). In this part, we will first describe the structure of the BBB in fish, birds, and mammals, then document the transport of steroid through the BBB before discussing the potential roles of steroids on the BBB.

Blood-Brain Barrier in Fish, Bird, and Mammals

The BBB is a specialized layer of cells that controls molecular trafficking between blood and brain, and contributes to the regulation (homeostasis) of the brain microenvironment. In mammalian species, BBB is composed of adjacent endothelial cells bound to each other by tight junctions whose major components are transmembrane and cytoplasmic anchoring protein such as occludin, claudin, and zona occludens (ZO-1). To complete the barrier, endothelial cells are wrapped by pericytes and surrounded by astrocytic cytoplasmic processes called end-feet. This cellular association is important for proper brain homeostasis, neuronal activity but also for protecting nervous tissue pathogens and harmful molecules transported by blood flow. The BBB, by separating the peripheral blood circulation from the brain parenchyma, filters the entrance of many molecules but also the removal of molecules from the brain (Banks, 2012).

Very few studies have focused on anatomical and functional organization of the BBB in birds and fish. Electron microscopy performed in adult and embryonic brains of quail and chicken showed that cerebral endothelial cells of both species are bound by tight junctions and that BBB is probably functional very early during embryonic development (Wakai and Hirokawa, 1978;

Stewart and Wiley, 1981; Roncali et al., 1986). In embryonic chick, aquaporin 4, a molecular water channels identified in mammalian BBB, was described in astroglia (Nico et al., 2001). In zebrafish, anatomical analysis and transmission electron microscopy revealed that adult endothelial cells display physical barrier properties and express Claudin-5 and ZO-1 proteins (Jeong et al., 2008; Eliceiri et al., 2011; Li et al., 2017). Complete maturation of the zebrafish BBB occurs between 3 and 10 days when expression of Claudin-5 and ZO-1 proteins are detected in cerebral endothelial vascular cells (Jeong et al., 2008; Eliceiri et al., 2011; Fleming et al., 2013; Li et al., 2017). Although some studies have highlighted the presence of stellate astrocytes in some fish (Kawai et al., 2001; Alunni et al., 2005; Strobl-Mazzulla et al., 2010), immunohistochemistry against GFAP or S100β protein has generally failed to demonstrate the presence of star-shaped cells resembling mammalian astrocytes in brain of many fish, including trout, carp, and zebrafish (Arochena et al., 2004; Pellegrini et al., 2005; Grupp et al., 2010; März et al., 2010). These findings raise the possibility that specialized functions of mammalian astrocytes could be supported by the GFAP, BLBP, and S100β-positive RGCs that remains numerous in adults. RNA sequencing analysis performed on goldfish RGC revealed the presence of many receptors and signaling molecules known to be expressed by astrocytes in mammals, a finding that strongly suggests that RGCs share functional similarities with mammalian astrocytes (Grupp et al., 2010; Fleming et al., 2013; Da Fonte et al., 2017). Very interestingly, in the zebrafish brain, blood vessels are wrapped by $AroB^+$ processes, in a way similar to astrocytic end-feet in mammals, further reinforcing the idea that RGCs in fish perform some, if not all, functions of astrocytes (**Figures 4A,B**).

Steroid Transport through the Blood-Brain Barrier

Steroid hormones are lipophilic and thus may cross the BBB by simple diffusion (Witt and Sandoval, 2014). Hormones can also enter the brain via specific transporters (Banks, 2012). In mammals, the transporters that help the passage from the blood circulation to the brain parenchyma are named influx transporters and include organic anion transporting polypeptides (OATPs), proton-coupled monocarboxylate transporters (MCTs), and peptide transporter. In the case of simple diffusion through the BBB, steroid concentrations will tend to equilibrate between the plasma and the brain. However, most steroid hormones are transported in the blood by albumin, sex hormone-binding globulin, or by corticosteroid-binding globulin, changing their availability and the possibility of passive diffusion through the BBB, as shown in most vertebrates, including fish, birds, and mammals (Hammond, 2011, 2016; Rosner, 2015). In rats, radiolabeled steroids (i.e., progesterone, testosterone, estradiol and corticosterone, and cortisol), intravenously injected have been shown to diffuse through the BBB, but this diffusion was significantly slowed down by the presence of binding globulin (Pardridge and Mietus, 1979).In addition, one must take into account that the concentration of carrier proteins may be different in the peripheral circulation vs. the cerebrospinal fluid (CSF). For example, the albumin concentration is one hundred time less important in the CSF than in the plasma in humans (Alafuzoff et al., 1983), potentially modulating availability and stability of the steroids.

In addition, hormones may be transported back into the blood circulation by efflux transporters. In mammals, these transporters, belonging to the ABC (ATP Binding Cassette) family, play a key role in brain homeostasis and mediate active efflux of many potential toxicants including lipophilic compounds. They include the P-glycoprotein, also known as

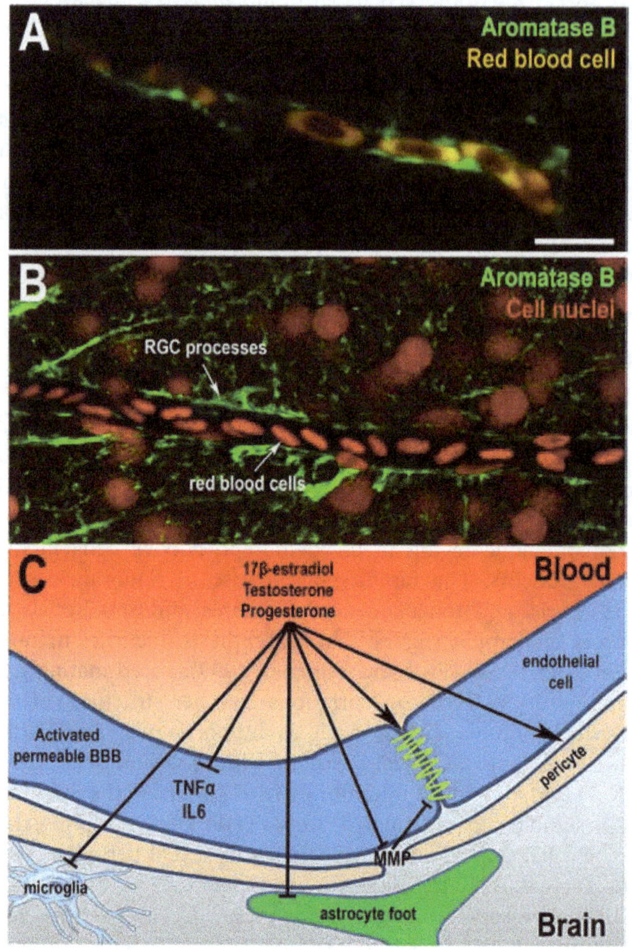

FIGURE 4 | Sex hormones restore blood-brain barrier physiology and integrity. **(A,B)** Aromatase B immunohistochemistry (green) on zebrafish brain highlights that radial glial processes envelop blood vessels as shown by the auto-fluorescence of red blood cells **(A)** or by nuclear staining **(B)**. These data suggest that radial glial cells could endorse the role of astrocytes in the establishment of the BBB, given the absence of astrocytic cell-type in the brain of fish. It also raises the question of the potential role of locally-produced estrogens on the BBB physiology. Scale bar: 7 μm. **(C)** Sex steroids (17β-E2, progesterone, and testosterone) display direct and indirect effects on the BBB through the restauration of thigh junctions, the inhibition of inflammatory cytokine expression and metalloproteinases production, the regulation of pericytes contraction, and consequently the modulation of cerebral blood flow. They also limit reactive gliosis through the inhibition of glial activation under pathological conditions (astrocytes and microglia). Sex steroids participate in the maintenance of a functional BBB, reducing neuroinflammation and promoting neuroprotection.

MDR1, ABCB1), multidrug resistance-associated protein, and breast cancer-related protein (Witt and Sandoval, 2014). Organic ion transporting polypeptides (OATPs) and the organic ion transporters, which belong to the solute-linked carrier (SLC) class, could be involved in uptake and/or efflux (Kusuhara and Sugiyama, 2005). For example, metabolites of estrogens can be transported back in the blood circulation from the brain such as demonstrated in male rats (Sugiyama et al., 2001). The same was also shown in rats for the neuroactive androgenic steroid dehydroepiandrosterone sulfate (DHEAS) that is transported back through a member of the SLC class (Asaba et al., 2000). However, the role of efflux transporter in the regulation of the concentration of steroids in the brain is not well-known and remains controversial.

Effects of Steroids on the Blood-Brain Barrier

Steroids could act directly or indirectly on the BBB, notably by binding to receptors present in the cells composing the BBB. The effects of glucocorticoids on the BBB are well-described and notably include decrease in inflammation (cytokines, chemokines, metalloproteinases) and increase in protective or reparative effects on tight junctions (Witt and Sandoval, 2014). Sex steroids were also shown to exert protective effects on the BBB, using microvessel endothelial bEnd.3 cells (Na et al., 2015). Considering estrogens, treatment with 17β-E2 restores the BBB integrity and its permeability in a model of stroke or in a lipopolysaccharides-induced inflammation in rodents (Maggioli et al., 2016; Xiao et al., 2017). Of interest, the BBB permeability is increased when circulating estrogens decrease with aging (Bake and Sohrabji, 2004). With respect to androgens, when gonadal testosterone is depleted from the body, glial cells (microglia and astrocytes) are activated and BBB permeability and inflammation are increased. Testosterone treatments restore these parameters (Atallah et al., 2017). Finally, it also seems that progesterone exerts positive effects on the BBB physiology after stroke and TBI (Ishrat et al., 2010; Si et al., 2014). The effects (direct and indirect) of steroids on the BBB is described in **Figure 4C**.

Interestingly, it was also demonstrated that sex steroids (17β-E2, testosterone, and progesterone) regulate both cerebrovascular tone, endothelial function, oxidative stress, and inflammation as well as brain functions under normal and/or pathological conditions (i.e., middle cerebral artery occlusion: MCAO) (Krause et al., 2011; Gonzales, 2013; Si et al., 2014).

Lipoproteins in the Brain

Lipid metabolism, high density lipoprotein (HDL)-, and low density lipoprotein (LDL)-cholesterol were studied in a wide variety of groups including rodents, lagomorph, birds, and fish (Liu and Wu, 2004). Lipoprotein metabolism, HDL-, and LDL-cholesterol in zebrafish appear similar to humans, making zebrafish an appropriate model for studying lipoproteins, given that zebrafish express the main set of lipid transporters, apolipoproteins, and enzymes involved in lipoprotein metabolism (Fang et al., 2014). However, to our knowledge, except in rodents, not much is known concerning the effects of HDL-cholesterol in the transport of steroids, in the maintenance of the BBB integrity and in neuroprotection. We consequently emphasize these points in this last part.

The brain is a cholesterol-rich organ, accounting for about 25% of the total amount present in humans. In the CNS, cholesterol is mainly synthesized by astrocytes, oligodendrocytes, microglia and to a lesser extent by neurons, where it is essentially present in its unesterified form (Björkhem and Meaney, 2004; Dietschy and Turley, 2004; Zhang and Liu, 2015). Brain cholesterol is involved in myelin sheath genesis, in synaptogenesis, and neurotransmission as well as in neurosteroidogenesis (Mauch et al., 2001; Do Rego et al., 2009; Linetti et al., 2010; Liu et al., 2010; Zhang and Liu, 2015). In adults, sterols are excreted from the brain to the plasma, and cholesterol is converted into 24S-hydroxycholesterol, which is more soluble and may diffuse across the BBB to reach the plasma where it is metabolized to bile acids after being picked up by circulating lipoproteins (Quan et al., 2003; Mahley, 2016). Almost no cholesterol enters the brain from the peripheral circulation. However, small high density lipoprotein (HDL) particles may cross the BBB and transport cholesterol within the brain (Ladu et al., 2000; Koch et al., 2001).

Spherical lipoproteins similar to HDLs have been isolated from the CSF. They are composed of ApoE and ApoJ for the largest ones whereas smaller particles contain ApoAI and ApoAII. Astrocytes are the main producers of both ApoE (with microglial cells) and ApoJ (with neurons and ependymal cells) (Vance and Hayashi, 2010). Different isoforms of ApoE have been described in brain HDL particles (ApoE2, ApoE3, and ApoE4). ApoE is the main cholesterol carrier in the brain and is associated with Alzheimer's disease and other neurodegenerative disorders (Liu et al., 2013). Interestingly, cultured neurons and astrocytes expressing the ApoE4 isoforms display a reduced secretion of cholesterol and phospholipids, as well as a blunted lipid-binding capacity (Mahley, 2016). In addition, estrogens were shown to promote ApoE expression in microglia and astrocytes (Stone et al., 1997). Other brain apolipoproteins (i.e., ApoA-I, Apo-J, and Apo-D) may participate in cholesterol distribution via different receptors including LDL receptor, ABC (ATP-binding cassette receptor) -A1 and -A2 transporters, LDL Receptor-related protein), VLDL receptor, ApoE receptor 2, and megalin (Herz and Bock, 2002; Björkhem and Meaney, 2004).

In pathological conditions that lead to BBB loss of integrity, such as ischemic stroke, exogenous lipoproteins may enter the cerebral parenchyma and produce different effects. Functional HDL particles (HDLs displaying anti-inflammatory and antioxidant properties, see **Figure 5A**) are taken up by endothelial cells of the BBB in a thrombo-embolic stroke model of rat. Injection of fluorescent lipoproteins post-stroke are taken up by endothelial cells and astrocytes, but not by neurons (Lapergue et al., 2010). In this model and in the MCAO (middle-cerebral artery occlusion), one intravenous injection of HDLs isolated from healthy subjects reduced the mortality, the infarct volume and the hemorrhagic transformation associated with rtPA (recombinant tissue plasminogen activator) treatment (Lapergue et al., 2013). It is not known whether the cholesterol or steroids contained within these HDL particles are involved in the protective effects. It is indeed possible that either ester of steroids or cholesterol delivery for local steroid synthesis could participate in neurogenesis and post-stroke remodeling. In this line, there is no study showing any beneficial effect of reconstituted HDL particles in CNS disorders. Noteworthy, these HDLs are composed of ApoA-I and phospholipids, but are devoid of cholesterol (Darabi et al., 2016). Ortiz-Munoz et al. recently demonstrated that at the acute phase of stroke, HDL particles are dysfunctional (HDLs displaying defective anti-inflammatory and antioxidant properties) and larger than in controls (Ortiz-Muñoz et al., 2016). These qualitative abnormalities blunted their ability to protect the BBB during acute brain injury. In fact, in addition to their action on reverse transport of cholesterol, HDLs also display anti-oxidant, anti-inflammatory, and anti-protease activities (Tran-Dinh et al., 2013). These pleiotropic effects could be due to different proteins associated with HDL particles such as paraoxonase-1 (PON-1), but also to the lipids that they transport, and to steroids. In type 2 diabetes mellitus conditions (T2DM), HDL anti-inflammatory capacity is impaired due to decreased PON-1 activity (Ebtehaj et al., 2017). Another study investigated the association between plasma cholesterol/lipoproteins and BBB permeability in a condition of CNS inflammation such as multiple sclerosis (Fellows et al., 2015). HDL-Cholesterol was associated with lower levels of BBB injury and low CSF total protein concentration. The authors suggest that the BBB structural integrity is associated with plasma membrane subdomains involved in cholesterol homeostasis. HDL particles are larger in stroke patients than in controls and they display a reduced protective effect for the BBB (Ortiz-Muñoz et al., 2016). Small HDL particles enter the CNS via SR-B1-mediated uptake and transcytosis (Balazs et al., 2004; Vitali et al., 2014). Morphological abnormality of HDLs in brain injury condition like stroke could be responsible for their reduced capacity to cross the blood-cerebrospinal fluid barrier. HDL supplementation could represent an interesting and innovative protective therapy for brain injury.

Interestingly, Leszczynski and Schafer (1991) demonstrated the interaction between lipoproteins and steroid hormones (androstenediol, 17β-E2, DHEA, DHT, pregnenolone, and progesterone), highlighting a new pathway in steroid hormone processing in plasma and/or steroid hormone delivery to cells (Leszczynski and Schafer, 1991). Other reports also suggest that 17β-E2 could be incorporated into HDL particles by lecithin:cholesterol acyltransferase under the form of 17β-E2 ester, that could be in turn transferred into LDL particles by cholesteryl ester transfer protein LDL particles as reviewed in Tikkanen et al. (2002) and Höckerstedt et al. (2004). The **Figure 5B** illustrates such a transport of 17β-E2 ester in HDLs and LDLs. These data would argue in favor of potential antioxidant, anti-inflammatory, and neuroprotective effects of HDLs implying cholesterol and other steroids (or their esterified forms) associated to lipoprotein particles. Indeed, estrogen derivatives with an unsubstituted A-ring phenolic hydroxyl group confers stronger antioxidant protection to LDL and HDL (Badeau et al., 2005). Such data could suggest a potential therapeutic use of HDL particles in order to improve their neuroprotective properties through their enrichment with steroids.

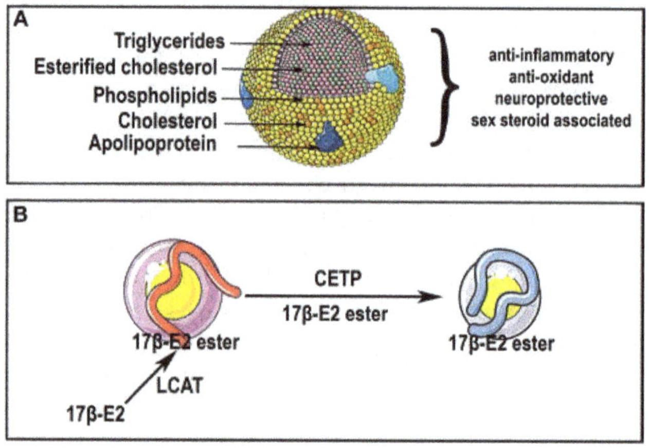

FIGURE 5 | HDL particles and sex steroids. **(A)** Lipoprotein particles display a central core containing cholesterol, cholesterol esters and triglycerides, that is enveloped by free cholesterol, phospholipids, and apolipoproteins. HDL particles display pleiotropic effects partly supported by their anti-inflammatory, anti-oxidant and neuroprotective properties. HDLs have been shown to display metabolic interaction with sex steroids (i.e., androstenediol, estradiol, DHEA, dihydrotestosterone, pregnenolone, and progesterone). **(B)** As suggested by Tikkanen et al. (2002), 17β-E2 could be esterified with fatty acids by lecithin:cholesterol acyltransferase (LCAT) in HDL. Esterified 17β-E2 could be subsequently transferred from HDLs to LDLs by cholesteryl ester transfer protein (CETP). Thus, HDL particles could be a source of cholesterol and steroids in the brain notably after CNS insults, and could be used as a carrier for improving steroids delivery in therapeutically approaches.

CONCLUSION

In this review, we reported that the brains of fish, birds, and mammals are able to *de novo* synthesize a wide variety of sex steroids demonstrating that neurosteroidogenesis is an evolutionary conserved feature shared by common ancestors. We also emphasize that neurogenic regions are closely related to neurosteroid production. In particular, RGCs, acting as neural progenitors in the brain of adult fish, strongly express Aromatase B and some other steroidogenic enzymes, suggesting that RGCs are true steroidogenic cells. Such an expression of aromatase in RGCs is not restricted to fish as it was also observed in mammals during embryonic development (Martínez-Cerdeño et al., 2006) and in birds after mechanical lesion of the brain (Peterson et al., 2001).

Peripheral, we also highlighted the fact that the brains of fish, birds, and mammals are targeted by peripheral and locally-produced steroids namely estrogens, progestins, and androgens. It appears that nuclear and membrane-associated sex steroid receptors are widely expressed in the brains of vertebrates particularly in neuroendocrine regions (i.e., preoptic area and hypothalamus) as well as in neurogenic niches and neural progenitors, suggesting key roles of steroids in sexual behaviors and neurogenesis. Indeed, we notably depicted the roles of estrogens, progestins and androgens in constitutive and regenerative neurogenesis and in sexual behaviors. Due to their anti-inflammatory, antioxidant, and anti-apoptotic properties, sex steroids also exert neuroprotective properties in the brain, particularly after CNS insults such as stroke and traumatic brain injury. However, the effects of steroids are not trivial to study and understand given that their actions are largely dependent on numerous variables (i.e., the timing, the concentration, the rhythm of exposure,...).

Peripheral steroids may diffuse or cross the BBB through transporters, raising the question of the respective roles of peripherally vs. centrally-produced steroids in brain homeostasis and functions. Peripheral sex steroid and neurosteroids can also act on the BBB permeability by modulating inflammatory and oxidative signals and consequently regulate brain homeostasis.

Of interest, in this review, we also discussed the potential hypothesis that the protective effects of HDL particles on stroke could be partly attributed to their interactions with sex-steroids. Thus, we raised the question of the contribution of cholesterol and sex-steroids transported by lipoproteins in the neuroprotection at the acute phase of stroke. Steroids are considered as good therapeutic candidates for CNS insults (i.e., stroke, traumatic brain injury), aging, and neurodegenerative diseases. It opens a door for therapeutic research through the use of steroids alone, in cocktail, or transported to the injured site by HDLs.

AUTHOR CONTRIBUTIONS

ND and EP designed the manuscript and supervised the work. ND, EP, TC, OM, CL, DC, VT, JN, and OK participated in the writing of the review. ND and CL made the figures.

FUNDING

This work was supported by grants from La Réunion University (Bonus Qualité Recherche, Dispositifs incitatifs), Conseil Régional de La Réunion, European Union (CPER/FEDER), Philancia association and Fondation de France (for UMR1188 DéTROI), as well as by grants from the Region Bretagne (SAD) and Rennes Metropole (awarded to TC).

REFERENCES

1. Adolf, B., Chapouton, P., Lam, C. S., Topp, S., Tannhäuser, B., Strähle, U., et al. (2006). Conserved and acquired features of adult neurogenesis in the zebrafish telencephalon. *Dev. Biol.* 295, 278–293. doi: 10.1016/j.ydbio.2006.03.023
2. Alafuzoff, I., Adolfsson, R., Bucht, G., and Winblad, B. (1983). Albumin and immunoglobulin in plasma and cerebrospinal fluid, and blood- cerebrospinal fluid barrier function in patients with dementia of Alzheimer type and multi-infarct dementia. *J. Neurol. Sci.* 60, 465–472. doi: 10.1016/0022-510X(83)90157-0
3. Alkayed, N. J., Harukuni, I., Kimes, A. S., London, E. D., Traystman, R. J., and Hurn, P. D. (1998). Gender-linked brain injury in experimental stroke. Stroke 29, 159–165: discussion 166.
4. Alunni, A., Vaccari, S., Torcia, S., Meomartini, M. E., Nicotra, A., and Alfei,
5. L. (2005). Characterization of glial fibrillary acidic protein and astroglial architecture in the brain of a continuously growing fish, the rainbow trout. *Eur. J. Histochem.* 49, 157–166.
6. Andersson, E., Borg, B., and Lambert, J. G. (1988). Aromatase activity in brain and pituitary of immature and mature Atlantic salmon (*Salmo salar* L.) parr. *Gen. Comp. Endocrinol.* 72, 394–401. doi: 10.1016/0016-6480(88) 90161-X
7. Andreassen, T. K., Skjoedt, K., Anglade, I., Kah, O., and Korsgaard, B. (2003). Molecular cloning, characterisation, and tissue distribution of oestrogen receptor alpha in eelpout (*Zoarces viviparus*). *Gen. Comp. Endocrinol.* 132, 356–368. doi: 10.1016/S0016-6480(03)00101-1
8. Anglade, I., Mazurais, D., Douard, V., Le Jossic-Corcos, C., Mañanos, E. L., Michel, D., et al. (1999). Distribution of glutamic acid decarboxylase mRNA in the forebrain of the rainbow trout as studied by *in situ* hybridization. *J. Comp. Neurol.* 410, 277–289. doi: 10.1002/(SICI)1096-9861(19990726)410:2<277::AID-CNE9>3.0.CO;2-V
9. Anglade, I., Pakdel, F., Bailhache, T., Petit, F., Salbert, G., Jego, P., et al. (1994). Distribution of estrogen receptor-immunoreactive cells in the brain of the rainbow trout (*Oncorhynchus mykiss*). *J. Neuroendocrinol.* 6, 573–583. doi: 10.1111/j.1365-2826.1994.tb00621.x
10. Arnold, A. P. (1980). Quantitative analysis of sex differences in hormone accumulation in the zebra finch brain: methodological and theoretical issues. *J. Comp. Neurol.* 189, 421–436. doi: 10.1002/cne.901890302
11. Arochena, M., Anadón, R., and Diaz-Regueira, S. M. (2004). Development of vimentin and glial fibrillary acidic protein immunoreactivities in the brain of gray mullet (*Chelon labrosus*), an advanced teleost. *J. Comp. Neurol.* 469, 413–436. doi: 10.1002/cne.11021
12. Asaba, H., Hosoya, K., Takanaga, H., Ohtsuki, S., Tamura, E., Takizawa, T., et al. (2000). Blood-brain barrier is involved in the efflux transport of a neuroactive steroid, dehydroepiandrosterone sulfate, via organic anion transporting polypeptide 2. *J. Neurochem.* 75, 1907–1916. doi: 10.1046/j.1471-4159.2000.0751907.x
13. Aste, N., Panzica, G. C., Aimar, P., Viglietti-Panzica, C., Foidart, A., and Balthazart, J. (1993). Implication of testosterone metabolism in the control of the sexually dimorphic nucleus of the quail preoptic area. *Brain Res. Bull.* 31, 601–611. doi:10.1016/0361-9230(93)90129-Y
14. Atallah, A., Mhaouty-Kodja, S., and Grange-Messent, V. (2017). Chronic depletion of gonadal testosterone leads to blood-brain barrier dysfunction and inflammation in male mice. *J. Cereb. Blood Flow Metab.* 37, 3161–3175. doi: 10.1177/0271678X16683961
15. Axelsson, J., Mattsson, A., Brunström, B., and Halldin, K. (2007). Expression of estrogen receptor-alpha and -beta mRNA in the brain of Japanese quail embryos. *Dev. Neurobiol.* 67, 1742–1750. doi: 10.1002/dneu.20544
16. Azcoitia, I., Sierra, A., Veiga, S., Honda, S., Harada, N., and Garcia-Segura, L. M. (2001). Brain aromatase is neuroprotective. *J. Neurobiol.* 47, 318–329. doi: 10.1002/neu.1038
17. Badeau, M., Adlercreutz, H., Kaihovaara, P., and Tikkanen, M. J. (2005). Estrogen A-ring structure and antioxidative effect on lipoproteins. *J. Steroid Biochem. Mol. Biol.* 96, 271–278. doi: 10.1016/j.jsbmb.2005.04.034
18. Bake, S., and Sohrabji, F. (2004). 17beta-estradiol differentially regulates blood-brain barrier permeability in young and aging female rats. *Endocrinology* 145, 5471–5475. doi: 10.1210/en.2004-0984
19. Bakker, J., Honda, S., Harada, N., and Balthazart, J. (2004). Restoration of male sexual behavior by adult exogenous estrogens in male aromatase knockout mice. *Horm. Behav.* 46, 1–10. doi: 10.1016/j.yhbeh.2004.02.003
20. Balazs, Z., Panzenboeck, U., Hammer, A., Sovic, A., Quehenberger, O., Malle, E., et al. (2004). Uptake and transport of high-density lipoprotein (HDL) and HDL-associated alpha-tocopherol by an *in vitro* blood-brain barrier model. *J. Neurochem.* 89, 939–950. doi: 10.1111/j.1471-4159.2004.02373.x
21. Balthazart, J., Absil, P., Foidart, A., Houbart, M., Harada, N., and Ball, G. F. (1996). Distribution of aromatase-immunoreactive cells in the forebrain of zebra finches (*Taeniopygia guttata*): implications for the neural action of steroids and nuclear definition in the avian hypothalamus. *J. Neurobiol.* 31, 129–148. doi: 10.1002/(SICI)1097-4695(199610)31:2>129::AID-NEU1>3.0. CO;2-D
22. Balthazart, J., and Ball, G. F. (1998). New insights into the regulation and function of brain estrogen synthase (aromatase). *Trends Neurosci.* 21, 243–249. doi:10.1016/S0166-2236(97)01221-6
23. Balthazart, J., and Ball, G. F. (2006). Is brain estradiol a hormone or a neurotransmitter? *Trends Neurosci.* 29, 241–249. doi: 10.1016/j.tins.2006.03.004

24. Balthazart, J., and Ball, G. F. (2016). Endocrine and social regulation of adult neurogenesis in songbirds. *Front. Neuroendocrinol.* 41, 3–22. doi: 10.1016/j.yfrne.2016.03.003
25. Balthazart, J., and Foidart, A. (1993). Brain aromatase and the control of male sexual behavior. *J. Steroid Biochem. Mol. Biol.* 44, 521–540. doi: 10.1016/0960-0760(93)90256-V
26. Balthazart, J., and Surlemont, C. (1990). Androgen and estrogen action in the preoptic area and activation of copulatory behavior in quail. *Physiol. Behav.* 48, 599–609. doi: 10.1016/0031-9384(90)90198-D
27. Balthazart, J., Baillien, M., and Ball, G. F. (2005). Interactions between kinases and phosphatases in the rapid control of brain aromatase. *J. Neuroendocrinol.* 17, 553–559. doi: 10.1111/j.1365-2826.2005.01344.x
28. Balthazart, J., Baillien, M., and Ball, G. F. (2006). Rapid control of brain aromatase activity by glutamatergic inputs. *Endocrinology* 147, 359–366. doi: 10.1210/en.2005-0845
29. Balthazart, J., Baillien, M., Cornil, C. A., and Ball, G. F. (2004). Preoptic aromatase modulates male sexual behavior: slow and fast mechanisms of action. *Physiol. Behav.* 83, 247–270. doi: 10.1016/j.physbeh.2004.08.025
30. Balthazart, J., Evrard, L., and Surlemont, C. (1990). Effects of the nonsteroidal inhibitor R76713 on testosterone-induced sexual behavior in the Japanese quail (*Coturnix coturnix japonica*). *Horm. Behav.* 24, 510–531. doi: 10.1016/0018-506X(90)90039-Z
31. Banks, W. A. (2012). Brain meets body: the blood-brain barrier as an endocrine interface. *Endocrinology* 153, 4111–4119. doi: 10.1210/en.2012-1435
32. Bardet, P. L., Horard, B., Robinson-Rechavi, M., Laudet, V., and Vanacker, J. M. (2002). Characterization of oestrogen receptors in zebrafish (*Danio rerio*). *J. Mol. Endocrinol.* 28, 153–163. doi: 10.1677/jme.0.0280153
33. Bernard, D. J., Bentley, G. E., Balthazart, J., Turek, F. W., and Ball, G. F. (1999). Androgen receptor, estrogen receptor alpha, and estrogen receptor beta show distinct patterns of expression in forebrain song control nuclei of European starlings. *Endocrinology* 140, 4633–4643. doi: 10.1210/endo.140.10.7024
34. Beyer, C., Moralí, G., Naftolin, F., Larsson, K., and Pérez-Palacios, G. (1976). Effect of some antiestrogens and aromatase inhibitors on androgen induced sexual behavior in castrated male rats. *Horm. Behav.* 7, 353–363. doi: 10.1016/0018-506X(76)90040-4
35. Björkhem, I., and Meaney, S. (2004). Brain cholesterol: long secret life behind a barrier. *Arterioscler. Thromb. Vasc. Biol.* 24, 806–815. doi: 10.1161/01.ATV.0000120374.59826.1b
36. Bondesson, M., Hao, R., Lin, C. Y., Williams, C., and Gustafsson, J. Å. (2015). Estrogen receptor signaling during vertebrate development. *Biochim. Biophys. Acta* 1849, 142–151. doi: 10.1016/j.bbagrm.2014.06.005
37. Borg, B., Andersson, E., Mayer, I., and Lambert, J. G. (1989). Aromatase activity in the brain of the three-spined stickleback, *Gasterosteus aculeatus*. III. Effects of castration under different conditions and of replacement with different androgens. *Exp. Biol.* 48, 149–152.
38. Brandt, N., Vierk, R., and Rune, G. M. (2013). Sexual dimorphism in estrogen- induced synaptogenesis in the adult hippocampus. *Int. J. Dev. Biol.* 57, 351–356. doi: 10.1387/ijdb.120217gr
39. Brännvall, K., Bogdanovic, N., Korhonen, L., and Lindholm, D. (2005). 19-Nortestosterone influences neural stem cell proliferation and neurogenesis in the rat brain. *Eur. J. Neurosci.* 21, 871–878. doi: 10.1111/j.1460-9568.2005.03942.x
40. Brännvall, K., Korhonen, L., and Lindholm, D. (2002). Estrogen-receptor-dependent regulation of neural stem cell proliferation and differentiation. *Mol. Cell. Neurosci.* 21, 512–520. doi: 10.1006/mcne.2002.1194
41. Brinton, R. D., Thompson, R. F., Foy, M. R., Baudry, M., Wang, J., Finch, C. E., et al. (2008). Progesterone receptors: form and function in brain. *Front. Neuroendocrinol.* 29, 313–339. doi: 10.1016/j.yfrne.2008.02.001
42. Brock, O., Keller, M., Veyrac, A., Douhard, Q., and Bakker, J. (2010). Short term treatment with estradiol decreases the rate of newly generated cells in the subventricular zone and main olfactory bulb of adult female mice. *Neuroscience* 166, 368–376. doi: 10.1016/j.neuroscience.2009.12.050
43. Brown, R. C., Cascio, C., and Papadopoulos, V. (2000). Pathways of neurosteroid biosynthesis in cell lines from human brain: regulation of dehydroepiandrosterone formation by oxidative stress and beta-amyloid peptide. *J. Neurochem.* 74, 847–859. doi: 10.1046/j.1471-4159.2000.740847.x
44. Buckingham, J. C., Döhler, K. D., and Wilson, C. A. (1978). Activity of the pituitary-adrenocortical system and thyroid gland during the oestrous cycle of the rat. *J. Endocrinol.* 78, 359–366. doi: 10.1677/joe.0.0780359
45. Celec, P., Ostatníková, D., and Hodosy, J. (2015). On the effects of testosterone on brain behavioral functions. *Front. Neurosci.* 9:12. doi: 10.3389/fnins.2015.00012
Celeghin, A., Benato, F., Pikulkaew, S., Rabbane, M. G., Colombo, L., and Dalla Valle, L. (2011). The knockdown of the maternal estrogen receptor 2a (esr2a) mRNA affects embryo transcript contents and larval development in zebrafish. *Gen. Comp. Endocrinol.* 172, 120–129. doi: 10.1016/j.ygcen.2010.12.020
Chakraborty, T., Shibata, Y., Zhou, L. Y., Katsu, Y., Iguchi, T., and Nagahama, Y.
46. (2011). Differential expression of three estrogen receptor subtype mRNAs in gonads and liver from embryos to adults of the medaka, *Oryzias latipes*. *Mol. Cell. Endocrinol.* 333, 47–54. doi: 10.1016/j.mce.2010.12.002
47. Charalampopoulos, I., Remboutsika, E., Margioris, A. N., and Gravanis, A. (2008). Neurosteroids as modulators of neurogenesis and neuronal survival. *Trends Endocrinol. Metab.* 19, 300–307. doi: 10.1016/j.tem.2008.07.004.
48. Charlier, T. D., Ball, G. F., and Balthazart, J. (2008). Rapid action on neuroplasticity precedes behavioral activation by testosterone. *Horm. Behav.* 54, 488–495. doi: 10.1016/j.yhbeh.2008.03.001
49. Charlier, T. D., Harada, N., Balthazart, J., and Cornil, C. A. (2011a). Human and quail aromatase activity is rapidly and reversibly inhibited by phosphorylating conditions. *Endocrinology* 152, 4199–4210. doi: 10.1210/en.2011-0119
50. Charlier, T. D., Newman, A. E., Heimovics, S. A., Po, K. W., Saldanha, C. J., and Soma, K. K. (2011b). Rapid effects of aggressive interactions on aromatase activity and oestradiol in discrete brain regions of wild male white-crowned sparrows. *J. Neuroendocrinol.* 23, 742–753. doi: 10.1111/j.1365-2826.2011.02170.x
51. Chen, C. F., Wen, H. S., Wang, Z. P., He, F., Zhang, J. R., Chen, X. Y., et al. (2010b). Cloning and expression of P450c17-I (17alpha-hydroxylase/17,20-lyase) in brain and ovary during gonad development in *Cynoglossus semilaevis*. *Fish Physiol. Biochem.* 36, 1001–1012. doi: 10.1007/s10695-009-9378-7
52. Chen, C., Kuo, J., Wong, A., and Micevych, P. (2014). Estradiol modulates translocator protein (TSPO) and steroid acute regulatory protein (StAR) via protein kinase A (PKA) signaling in hypothalamic astrocytes. *Endocrinology* 155, 2976–2985. doi: 10.1210/en.2013-1844
53. Chen, S. X., Bogerd, J., García-López, A., de Jonge, H., de Waal, P. P., Hong, W. S., et al. (2010a). Molecular cloning and functional characterization of a zebrafish nuclear progesterone receptor. *Biol. Reprod.* 82, 171–181. doi: 10.1095/biolreprod.109.077644
54. Chin, E. H., Shah, A. H., Schmidt, K. L., Sheldon, L. D., Love, O. P., and Soma, K. K. (2008). Sex differences in DHEA and estradiol during development in a wild songbird: Jugular versus brachial plasma. *Horm. Behav.* 54, 194–202. doi: 10.1016/j.yhbeh.2008.02.014
55. Choi, C. Y., and Habibi, H. R. (2003). Molecular cloning of estrogen receptor alpha and expression pattern of estrogen receptor subtypes in male and female goldfish. *Mol. Cell. Endocrinol.* 204, 169–177. doi: 10.1016/S0303-7207(02)00182-X
56. Christensen, L. W., and Clemens, L. G. (1974). Intrahypothalamic implants of testosterone or estradiol and resumption of masculine sexual behavior in long-term castrated male rats. *Endocrinology* 95, 984–990. doi: 10.1210/endo-95-4-984
57. Christensen, L. W., and Clemens, L. G. (1975). Blockade of testosterone-induced mounting behavior in the male rat with intracranial application of the aromatization inhibitor, androst-1,4,6,-triene-3,17-dione. *Endocrinology* 97, 1545–1551. doi: 10.1210/endo-97-6-1545
58. Clemens, L. G. (2013). "The aromatization hypothesis, 1970–1990," in *Brain Aromatase, Estrogens, and Behavior*, eds J. Balthazart and G. F. Ball (New York, NY; Oxford UP), 155–168.
59. Commins, D., and Yahr, P. (1985). Autoradiographic localization of estrogen and androgen receptors in the sexually dimorphic area and other regions of the gerbil brain. *J. Comp. Neurol.* 231, 473–489. doi: 10.1002/cne.902310406
60. Compagnone, N. A., and Mellon, S. H. (2000). Neurosteroids: biosynthesis and function of these novel neuromodulators. *Front. Neuroendocrinol.* 21, 1–56. doi: 10.1006/frne.1999.0188
61. Cornil, C. A.(2017). On the role of brain aromatase in females: why are estrogens produced locally when they are available systemically? *J. Comp. Physiol. A Neuroethol. Sens. Neural Behav. Physiol.* 204, 31–49. doi: 10.1007/s00359-017-1224-2
62. Cornil, C. A., Dalla, C., Papadopoulou-Daifoti, Z., Baillien, M., Dejace, C., Ball, G. F., et al. (2005). Rapid decreases in preoptic aromatase activity and brain monoamine concentrations after engaging in male sexual behavior. *Endocrinology* 146, 3809–3820. doi: 10.1210/en.2005-0441
63. Cornil, C. A., Leung, C. H., Pletcher, E. R., Naranjo, K. C., Blauman, S. J.,

and Saldanha, C. J. (2012). Acute and specific modulation of presynaptic aromatization in the vertebrate brain. *Endocrinology* 153, 2562–2567. doi: 10.1210/en.2011-2159

64. Cornil, C. A., Taziaux, M., Baillien, M., Ball, G. F., and Balthazart, J. (2006). Rapid effects of aromatase inhibition on male reproductive behaviors in Japanese quail. *Horm. Behav.* 49, 45–67. doi: 10.1016/j.yhbeh.2005.05.003
65. Coumailleau, P., Pellegrini, E., Adrio, F., Diotel, N., Cano-Nicolau, J., Nasri, A., et al. (2015). Aromatase, estrogen receptors and brain development in fish and amphibians. *Biochim. Biophys. Acta* 1849, 152–162. doi:10.1016/j.bbagrm.2014.07.002
66. Cross, E., and Roselli, C. E. (1999). 17beta-estradiol rapidly facilitates chemoinvestigation and mounting in castrated male rats. *Am. J. Physiol.* 276, R1346–R1350.
67. Da Fonte, D. F., Martyniuk, C. J., Xing, L., Pelin, A., Corradi, N., Hu, W., et al. (2017). Secretoneurin A regulates neurogenic and inflammatory transcriptional networks in goldfish (*Carassius auratus*) radial glia. *Sci. Rep.* 7:14930. doi: 10.1038/s41598-017-14930-8
68. Darabi, M., Guillas-Baudouin, I., Le Goff, W., Chapman, M. J., and Kontush, A. (2016). Therapeutic applications of reconstituted HDL: when structure meets function. *Pharmacol. Ther.* 157, 28–42. doi: 10.1016/j.pharmthera.2015.10.010
Davis, D. P., Douglas, D. J., Smith, W., Sise, M. J., Vilke, G. M., Holbrook, T. L., et al. (2006). Traumatic brain injury outcomes in pre- and post-menopausal females versus age-matched males. *J. Neurotrauma* 23, 140–148. doi:10.1089/neu.2006.23.140
69. de Bournonville, C., Ball, G. F., Balthazart, J., and Cornil, C. A. (2017a). Rapid changes in brain aromatase activity in the female quail brain following expression of sexual behavior. *J. Neuroendocrinol.* 29:e12542. doi: 10.1111/jne.12542
70. de Bournonville, C., Balthazart, J., Ball, G. F., and Cornil, C. A. (2016). Non-ovarian aromatization is required to activate female sexual motivation in testosterone-treated ovariectomized quail. *Horm. Behav.* 83, 45–59. doi: 10.1016/j.yhbeh.2016.05.011
71. de Bournonville, C., Dickens, M. J., Ball, G. F., Balthazart, J., and Cornil, C. A. (2013). Dynamic changes in brain aromatase activity following sexual interactions in males: where, when and why? *Psychoneuroendocrinology* 38, 789–799. doi: 10.1016/j.psyneuen.2012.09.001
72. de Bournonville, C., Smolders, I., Van Eeckhaut, A., Ball, G. F., Balthazart, J., and Cornil, C. A. (2017b). Glutamate released in the preoptic area during sexual behavior controls local estrogen synthesis in male quail. *Psychoneuroendocrinology* 79, 49–58. doi: 10.1016/j.psyneuen.2017.02.002
73. de Waal, P. P., Wang, D. S., Nijenhuis, W. A., Schulz, R. W., and Bogerd, J. (2008). Functional characterization and expression analysis of the androgen receptor in zebrafish (*Danio rerio*) testis. *Reproduction* 136, 225–234. doi: 10.1530/REP-08-0055
74. Devoogd, T. J., Nixdorf, B., and Nottebohm, F. (1985). Synaptogenesis and changes in synaptic morphology related to acquisition of a new behavior. *Brain Res.* 329, 304–308. doi: 10.1016/0006-8993(85)90539-6
75. Dickens, M. J., Balthazart, J., and Cornil, C. A. (2012). Brain aromatase and circulating corticosterone are rapidly regulated by combined acute stress and sexual interaction in a sex-specific manner. *J. Neuroendocrinol.* 24, 1322–1334. doi:10.1111/j.1365-2826.2012.02340.x
76. Dickens, M. J., Cornil, C. A., and Balthazart, J. (2011). Acute stress differentially affects aromatase activity in specific brain nuclei of adult male and female quail. *Endocrinology* 152, 4242–4251. doi: 10.1210/en.2011-1341
77. Dickens, M. J., Cornil, C. A., and Balthazart, J. (2013). Neurochemical control of rapid stress-induced changes in brain aromatase activity. *J. Neuroendocrinol.* 25, 329–339. doi: 10.1111/jne.12012
78. Dickens, M. J., de Bournonville, C., Balthazart, J., and Cornil, C. A. (2014). Relationships between rapid changes in local aromatase activity and estradiol concentrations in male and female quail brain. *Horm. Behav.* 65, 154–164. doi:10.1016/j.yhbeh.2013.12.011
79. Dietschy, J. M., and Turley, S. D. (2004). Thematic review series: brain Lipids. Cholesterol Metabolism in the central nervous system during early development and in the mature animal. *J. Lipid Res.* 45, 1375–1397. doi: 10.1194/jlr.R400004-JLR200
80. Diotel, N., Do Rego, J. L., Anglade, I., Vaillant, C., Pellegrini, E., Gueguen, M. M., et al. (2011b). Activity and expression of steroidogenic enzymes in the brain of adult zebrafish. *Eur. J. Neurosci.* 34, 45–56. doi: 10.1111/j.1460-9568.2011.07731.x
81. Diotel, N., Do Rego, J. L., Anglade, I., Vaillant, C., Pellegrini, E., Vaudry, H., et al. (2011a). The brain of teleost fish, a source, and a target of sexual steroids. *Front. Neurosci.* 5:137. doi: 10.3389/fnins.2011.00137
82. Diotel, N., Le Page, Y., Mouriec, K., Tong, S. K., Pellegrini, E., Vaillant, C., et al. (2010). Aromatase in the brain of teleost fish: expression, regulation and putative functions. *Front. Neuroendocrinol.* 31, 172–192. doi: 10.1016/j.yfrne.2010.01.003
83. Diotel, N., Servili, A., Gueguen, M. M., Mironov, S., Pellegrini, E., Vaillant, C., et al. (2011c). Nuclear progesterone receptors are up-regulated by estrogens in neurons and radial glial progenitors in the brain of zebrafish. *PLoS ONE* 6:e28375. doi: 10.1371/journal.pone.0028375
84. Diotel, N., Vaillant, C., Gabbero, C., Mironov, S., Fostier, A., Gueguen, M. M., et al. (2013). Effects of estradiol in adult neurogenesis and brain repair in zebrafish. *Horm. Behav.* 63, 193–207. doi: 10.1016/j.yhbeh.2012.04.003
85. Diotel, N., Vaillant, C., Kah, O., and Pellegrini, E. (2016). Mapping of brain lipid binding protein (Blbp) in the brain of adult zebrafish, co-expression with aromatase B and links with proliferation. *Gene Expr. Patterns* 20, 42–54. doi:10.1016/j.gep.2015.11.003
86. Do Rego, J. L., Seong, J. Y., Burel, D., Leprince, J., Luu-The, V., Tsutsui, K., et al. (2009). Neurosteroid biosynthesis: enzymatic pathways and neuroendocrine regulation by neurotransmitters and neuropeptides. *Front. Neuroendocrinol.* 30, 259–301. doi: 10.1016/j.yfrne.2009.05.006
87. Duarte-Guterman, P., Yagi, S., Chow, C., and Galea, L. A. (2015). Hippocampal learning, memory, and neurogenesis: effects of sex and estrogens across the lifespan in adults. *Horm. Behav.* 74, 37–52. doi: 10.1016/j.yhbeh.2015.05.024
88. Dupont, E., Simard, J., Luu-The, V., Labrie, F., and Pelletier, G. (1994). Localization of 3 beta-hydroxysteroid dehydrogenase in rat brain as studied by *in situ* hybridization. *Mol. Cell. Neurosci.* 5, 119–123. doi: 10.1006/mcne.1994.1014
89. Ebtehaj, S., Gruppen, E. G., Parvizi, M. U., Tietge, U. J. F., and Dullaart, R. P. F. (2017). The anti-inflammatory function of HDL is impaired in type 2 diabetes: role of hyperglycemia, paraoxonase-1 and low grade inflammation. *Cardiovasc. Diabetol.* 16, 132. doi: 10.1186/s12933-017-0613-8
90. Eliceiri, B. P., Gonzalez, A. M., and Baird, A. (2011). Zebrafish model of the blood- brain barrier: morphological and permeability studies. *Methods Mol. Biol.* 686, 371–378. doi: 10.1007/978-1-60761-938-3_18
91. Escobar, S., Felip, A., Gueguen, M. M., Zanuy, S., Carrillo, M., Kah, O., et al. (2013). Expression of kisspeptins in the brain and pituitary of the European sea bass (*Dicentrarchus labrax*). *J. Comp. Neurol.* 521, 933–948. doi: 10.1002/cne. 23211
92. Fang, L., Liu, C., and Miller, Y. I. (2014). Zebrafish models of dyslipidemia: relevance to atherosclerosis and angiogenesis. *Trans. Res.* 163, 99–108. doi: 10.1016/j.trsl.2013.09.004
93. Farinetti, A., Tomasi, S., Foglio, B., Ferraris, A., Ponti, G., Gotti, S., et al. (2015). Testosterone and estradiol differentially affect cell proliferation in the subventricular zone of young adult gonadectomized male and female rats. *Neuroscience* 286, 162–170. doi: 10.1016/j.neuroscience.2014.11.050
94. Fellows, K., Uher, T., Browne, R. W., Weinstock-Guttman, B., Horakova, D., Posova, H., et al. (2015). Protective associations of HDL with blood-brain barrier injury in multiple sclerosis patients. *J. Lipid Res.* 56, 2010–2018. doi: 10.1194/jlr.M060970
95. Feng, Y., Weijdegård, B., Wang, T., Egecioglu, E., Fernandez-Rodriguez, J., Huhtaniemi, I., et al. (2010). Spatiotemporal expression of androgen receptors in the female rat brain during the oestrous cycle and the impact of exogenous androgen administration: a comparison with gonadally intact males. *Mol. Cell. Endocrinol.* 321, 161–174. doi: 10.1016/j.mce.2010.02.029
96. Ferin, M., Tempone, A., Zimmering, P. E., and Van de Wiele, R.L. (1969). Effect of antibodies to 17beta-estradiol and progesterone on the estrous cycle of the rat. *Endocrinology* 85, 1070–1078. doi: 10.1210/endo-85-6-1070
97. Fester, L., Prange-Kiel, J., Zhou, L., Blittersdorf, B. V., Bohm, J., Jarry, H., et al. (2012). Estrogen-regulated synaptogenesis in the hippocampus: sexual dimorphism *in vivo* but not *in vitro*. *J. Steroid Biochem. Mol. Biol.* 131, 24–29. doi: 10.1016/j.jsbmb.2011.11.010
98. Filby, A. L., and Tyler, C. R. (2005). Molecular characterization of estrogen receptors 1, 2a, and 2b and their tissue and ontogenic expression profiles in fathead minnow (*Pimephales promelas*). *Biol. Reprod.* 73, 648–662. doi: 10.1095/biolreprod.105.039701
99. Fisher, C. R., Graves, K. H., Parlow, A. F., and Simpson, E. R. (1998). Characterization of mice deficient in aromatase (ArKO) because of targeted disruption of the cyp19 gene. *Proc. Natl. Acad. Sci. U.S.A.* 95, 6965–6970. doi: 10.1073/pnas.95.12.6965

100. Fleming, A., Diekmann, H., and Goldsmith, P. (2013). Functional characterisation of the maturation of the blood-brain barrier in larval zebrafish. *PLoS ONE* 8:e77548. doi: 10.1371/journal.pone.0077548
101. Foidart, A., Lakaye, B., Grisar, T., Ball, G. F., and Balthazart, J. (1999). Estrogen receptor-beta in quail: cloning, tissue expression and neuroanatomical distribution. *J. Neurobiol.* 40, 327–342. doi: 10.1002/(SICI)1097-4695(19990905)40:3<327::AID-NEU5>3.0.CO;2-L
102. Forlano, P. M., and Bass, A. H. (2005). Seasonal plasticity of brain aromatase mRNA expression in glia: divergence across sex and vocal phenotypes. *J. Neurobiol.* 65, 37–49. doi: 10.1002/neu.20179
103. Forlano, P. M., Deitcher, D. L., and Bass, A. H. (2005). Distribution of estrogen receptor alpha mRNA in the brain and inner ear of a vocal fish with comparisons to sites of aromatase expression. *J. Comp. Neurol.* 483, 91–113. doi: 10.1002/cne.20397
104. Forlano, P. M., Deitcher, D. L., Myers, D. A., and Bass, A. H. (2001). Anatomical distribution and cellular basis for high levels of aromatase activity in the brain of teleost fish: aromatase enzyme and mRNA expression identify glia as source. *J. Neurosci.* 21, 8943–8955.
105. Forlano, P. M., Marchaterre, M., Deitcher, D. L., and Bass, A. H. (2010). Distribution of androgen receptor mRNA expression in vocal, auditory, and neuroendocrine circuits in a teleost fish. *J. Comp. Neurol.* 518, 493–512. doi: 10.1002/cne.22233
106. Frick, K. M., Kim, J., Tuscher, J. J., and Fortress, A. M. (2015). Sex steroid hormones matter for learning and memory: estrogenic regulation of hippocampal function in male and female rodents. *Learn. Mem.* 22, 472–493. doi: 10.1101/lm.037267.114
107. Froehlicher, M., Liedtke, A., Groh, K., López-Schier, H., Neuhauss, S. C., Segner, H., et al. (2009). Estrogen receptor subtype beta2 is involved in neuromast development in zebrafish (*Danio rerio*) larvae. *Dev. Biol.* 330, 32–43. doi: 10.1016/j.ydbio.2009.03.005
108. Frye, C. A. (2011). Novel substrates for, and sources of, progestogens for reproduction. *J. Neuroendocrinol.* 23, 961–973. doi: 10.1111/j.1365-2826.2011.02180.x
109. Frye, C. A., and Paris, J. J. (2011). Progesterone turnover to its 5alpha-reduced metabolites in the ventral tegmental area of the midbrain is essential for initiating social and affective behavior and progesterone metabolism in female rats. *J. Endocrinol. Invest.* 34, e188–e199. doi: 10.3275/7334
110. Frye, C. A., and Vongher, J. M. (1999). 3alpha,5alpha-THP in the midbrain ventral tegmental area of rats and hamsters is increased in exogenous hormonal states associated with estrous cyclicity and sexual receptivity. *J. Endocrinol. Invest.* 22, 455–464. doi: 10.1007/BF03343590
111. Frye, C. A., and Walf, A. A. (2008). Progesterone enhances performance of aged mice in cortical or hippocampal tasks. *Neurosci. Lett.* 437, 116–120. doi: 10.1016/j.neulet.2008.04.004
112. Frye, C. A., and Walf, A. A. (2010). Progesterone enhances learning and memory of aged wildtype and progestin receptor knockout mice. *Neurosci. Lett.* 472, 38–42. doi: 10.1016/j.neulet.2010.01.051
113. Frye, C. A., Edinger, K., and Sumida, K. (2008). Androgen administration to aged male mice increases anti-anxiety behavior and enhances cognitive performance. *Neuropsychopharmacology* 33, 1049–1061. doi: 10.1038/sj.npp.1301498
114. Frye, C. A., Koonce, C. J., Walf, A. A., and Rusconi, J. C. (2013). Motivated behaviors and levels of 3alpha,5alpha-THP in the midbrain are attenuated by knocking down expression of pregnane xenobiotic receptor in the midbrain ventral tegmental area of proestrous rats. *J. Sex. Med.* 10, 1692–1706. doi: 10.1111/jsm.12173
115. Fusani, L., Donaldson, Z., London, S. E., Fuxjager, M. J., and Schlinger, B. A. (2014). Expression of androgen receptor in the brain of a sub-oscine bird with an elaborate courtship display. *Neurosci. Lett.* 578, 61–65. doi: 10.1016/j.neulet.2014.06.028
116. Gahr, M. (2001). Distribution of sex steroid hormone receptors in the avian brain: functional implications for neural sex differences and sexual behaviors. *Microsc. Res. Tech.* 55, 1–11. doi: 10.1002/jemt.1151
117. Galea, L. A., Spritzer, M. D., Barker, J. M., and Pawluski, J. L. (2006). Gonadal hormone modulation of hippocampal neurogenesis in the adult. *Hippocampus* 16, 225–232. doi: 10.1002/hipo.20154
118. Garcia-Segura, L. M. (2008). Aromatase in the brain: not just for reproduction anymore. *J. Neuroendocrinol.* 20, 705–712. doi: 10.1111/j.1365-2826.2008.01713.x
119. Garcia-Segura, L. M., Veiga, S., Sierra, A., Melcangi, R. C., and Azcoitia, I. (2003). Aromatase: a neuroprotective enzyme. *Prog. Neurobiol.* 71, 31–41. doi: 10.1016/j.pneurobio.2003.09.005
120. Garcia-Segura, L. M., Wozniak, A., Azcoitia, I., Rodriguez, J. R., Hutchison, R. E. and Hutchison, J. B. (1999). Aromatase expression by astrocytes after brain injury: implications for local estrogen formation in brain repair. *Neuroscience* 89, 567–578. doi: 10.1016/S0306-4522(98)00340-6
121. Gelinas, D., and Callard, G. V. (1993). Immunocytochemical and biochemical evidence for aromatase in neurons of the retina, optic tectum and retinotectal pathways in goldfish. *J. Neuroendocrinol.* 5, 635–641. doi: 10.1111/j.1365-2826.1993.tb00533.x
122. Gelinas, D., and Callard, G. V. (1997). Immunolocalization of aromatase- and androgen receptor-positive neurons in the goldfish brain. *Gen. Comp. Endocrinol.* 106, 155–168. doi: 10.1006/gcen.1997.6891
123. Gibson, C. L., Gray, L. J., Murphy, S. P., and Bath, P. M. (2006). Estrogens and experimental ischemic stroke: a systematic review. *J. Cereb. Blood Flow Metab.* 26, 1103–1113. doi: 10.1038/sj.jcbfm.9600270
124. Girijala, R. L., Sohrabji, F., and Bush, R. L. (2017). Sex differences in stroke: review of current knowledge and evidence. *Vasc. Med.* 22, 135–145. doi: 10.1177/1358863X16668263
125. Gonzales, R. J. (2013). Androgens and the cerebrovasculature: modulation of vascular function during normal and pathophysiological conditions. *Pflugers Archiv.* 465, 627–642. doi: 10.1007/s00424-013-1267-3
126. Gonzalez, A., and Piferrer, F. (2003). Aromatase activity in the European sea bass (*Dicentrarchus labrax* L.) brain. Distribution and changes in relation to age, sex, and the annual reproductive cycle. *Gen. Comp. Endocrinol.* 132, 223–230. doi: 10.1016/S0016-6480(03)00086-8
127. González, M., Cabrera-Socorro, A., Pérez-García, C. G., Fraser, J. D., López, F. J., Alonso, R., et al. (2007). Distribution patterns of estrogen receptor alpha and beta in the human cortex and hippocampus during development and adulthood. *J. Comp. Neurol.* 503, 790–802. doi: 10.1002/cne.21419
128. Goodson, J. L., Saldanha, C. J., Hahn, T. P., and Soma, K. K. (2005). Recent advances in behavioral neuroendocrinology: insights from studies on birds. *Horm. Behav.* 48, 461–473. doi: 10.1016/j.yhbeh.2005.04.005
129. Gorelick, D. A., Watson, W., and Halpern, M. E. (2008). Androgen receptor gene expression in the developing and adult zebrafish brain. *Dev. Dyn.* 237, 2987–2995. doi: 10.1002/dvdy.21700
130. Goto-Kazeto, R., Kight, K. E., Zohar, Y., Place, A. R., and Trant, J. M. (2004). Localization and expression of aromatase mRNA in adult zebrafish. *Gen. Comp. Endocrinol.* 139, 72–84. doi: 10.1016/j.ygcen.2004.07.003
131. Griffin, L. B., January, K. E., Ho, K. W., Cotter, K. A., and Callard, G. V. (2013). Morpholino-mediated knockdown of ERalpha, ERbetaa, and ERbetab mRNAs in zebrafish (*Danio rerio*) embryos reveals differential regulation of estrogen-inducible genes. *Endocrinology* 154, 4158–4169. doi: 10.1210/en.2013-1446
132. Grupp, L., Wolburg, H., and Mack, A. F. (2010). Astroglial structures in the zebrafish brain. *J. Comp. Neurol.* 518, 4277–4287. doi: 10.1002/cne.22481
133. Guennoun, R., Fiddes, R. J., Gouézou, M., Lombès, M., and Baulieu,E. E. (1995). A key enzyme in the biosynthesis of neurosteroids, 3 beta-hydroxysteroid dehydrogenase/delta 5-delta 4-isomerase (3 beta-HSD), is expressed in rat brain. *Brain Res. Mol. Brain Res.* 30, 287–300. doi: 10.1016/0169-328X(95)00016-L
134. Guerra-Araiza, C., Villamar-Cruz, O., González-Arenas, A., Chavira, R., and Camacho-Arroyo, I. (2003). Changes in progesterone receptor isoforms content in the rat brain during the oestrous cycle and after oestradiol and progesterone treatments. *J. Neuroendocrinol.* 15, 984–990. doi: 10.1046/j.1365-2826.2003.01088.x
135. Hagihara, K., Hirata, S., Osada, T., Hirai, M., and Kato, J. (1992a). Distribution of cells containing progesterone receptor mRNA in the female rat di- and telencephalon: an *in situ* hybridization study. *Brain Res. Mol. Brain Res.* 14, 239–249. doi: 10.1016/0169-328X(92)90179-F
136. Hagihara, K., Hirata, S., Osada, T., Hirai, M., and Kato, J. (1992b). Expression of progesterone receptor in the neonatal rat brain cortex: detection of its mRNA using reverse transcription-polymerase chain reaction. *J. Steroid Biochem. Mol. Biol.* 41, 637–640. doi: 10.1016/0960-0760(92)90396-Z
137. Hajszan, T., Milner, T. A., and Leranth, C. (2007). Sex steroids and the dentate gyrus. *Prog. Brain Res.* 163, 399–415. doi: 10.1016/S0079-6123(07)63023-4
138. Halm, S., Martínez-Rodríguez, G., Rodríguez, L., Prat, F., Mylonas, C. C., Carrillo, M., et al. (2004). Cloning, characterisation, and expression of three oestrogen receptors (ERalpha, ERbetal and ERbeta2) in the European sea bass, *Dicentrarchus labrax*. *Mol. Cell. Endocrinol.* 223, 63–75. doi: 10.1016/j.mce.2004.05.009

139. Hammond, G. L. (2011). Diverse roles for sex hormone-binding globulin in reproduction. *Biol. Reprod.* 85, 431–441. doi: 10.1095/biolreprod.111.092593

140. Hammond, G. L. (2016). Plasma steroid-binding proteins: primary gatekeepers of steroid hormone action. *J. Endocrinol.* 230, R13–R25. doi: 10.1530/JOE-16-0070

141. Hamson, D. K., Wainwright, S. R., Taylor, J. R., Jones, B. A., Watson, N. V., and Galea, L. A. (2013). Androgens increase survival of adult-born neurons in the dentate gyrus by an androgen receptor-dependent mechanism in male rats. *Endocrinology* 154, 3294–3304. doi: 10.1210/en.2013-1129

142. Hanna, R. N., and Zhu, Y. (2009). Expression of membrane progestin receptors in zebrafish (*Danio rerio*) oocytes, testis and pituitary. *Gen. Comp. Endocrinol.* 161, 153–157. doi: 10.1016/j.ygcen.2008.10.006

143. Hanna, R. N., Daly, S. C., Pang, Y., Anglade, I., Kah, O., Thomas, P., et al. (2010). Characterization and expression of the nuclear progestin receptor in zebrafish gonads and brain. *Biol. Reprod.* 82, 112–122. doi: 10.1095/biolreprod.109.078527

144. Harbott, L. K., Burmeister, S. S., White, R. B., Vagell, M., and Fernald, R. D. (2007). Androgen receptors in a cichlid fish, *Astatotilapia burtoni*: structure, localization, and expression levels. *J. Comp. Neurol.* 504, 57–73. doi: 10.1002/cne.21435

145. Hawkins, M. B., Godwin, J., Crews, D., and Thomas, P. (2005). The distributions of the duplicate oestrogen receptors ER-beta a and ER-beta b in the forebrain of the Atlantic croaker (*Micropogonias undulatus*): evidence for subfunctionalization after gene duplication. *Proc. Biol. Sci.* 272, 633–641. doi: 10.1098/rspb.2004.3008

146. Hawkins, M. B., Thornton, J. W., Crews, D., Skipper, J. K., Dotte, A., and Thomas, P. (2000). Identification of a third distinct estrogen receptor and reclassification of estrogen receptors in teleosts. *Proc. Natl. Acad. Sci. U.S.A.* 97, 10751–10756. doi: 10.1073/pnas.97.20.10751

147. Heberden, C. (2017). Sex steroids and neurogenesis. *Biochem. Pharmacol.* 141, 56–62. doi: 10.1016/j.bcp.2017.05.019

148. Herz, J., and Bock, H. H. (2002). Lipoprotein receptors in the nervous system. *Annu. Rev. Biochem.* 71, 405–434. doi: 10.1146/annurev.biochem.71.110601.135342

149. Hiraki, T., Nakasone, K., Hosono, K., Kawabata, Y., Nagahama, Y., and Okubo, K. (2014). Neuropeptide B is female-specifically expressed in the telencephalic and preoptic nuclei of the medaka brain. *Endocrinology* 155, 1021–1032. doi: 10.1210/en.2013-1806

150. Höckerstedt, A., Jauhiainen, M., and Tikkanen, M. J. (2004). Lecithin/cholesterol acyltransferase induces estradiol esterification in high-density lipoprotein, increasing its antioxidant potential. *J. Clin. Endocrinol. Metab.* 89, 5088–5093. doi: 10.1210/jc.2004-0141

151. Hojo, Y., Hattori, T. A., Enami, T., Furukawa, A., Suzuki, K., Ishii, H. T., et al. (2004). Adult male rat hippocampus synthesizes estradiol from pregnenolone by cytochromes P45017alpha and P450 aromatase localized in neurons. *Proc. Natl. Acad. Sci. U.S.A.* 101, 865–870. doi: 10.1073/pnas.2630225100

152. Holloway, C. C., and Clayton, D. F. (2001). Estrogen synthesis in the male brain triggers development of the avian song control pathway *in vitro*. *Nat. Neurosci.* 4, 170–175. doi: 10.1038/84001

153. Honda, S., Harada, N., Ito, S., Takagi, Y., and Maeda, S. (1998). Disruption of sexual behavior in male aromatase-deficient mice lacking exons 1 and 2 of the cyp19 gene. *Biochem. Biophys. Res. Commun.* 252, 445–449. doi: 10.1006/bbrc.1998.9672

154. Hossain, M. S., Larsson, A., Scherbak, N., Olsson, P. E., and Orban, L. (2008). Zebrafish androgen receptor: isolation, molecular, and biochemical characterization. *Biol. Reprod.* 78, 361–369. doi: 10.1095/biolreprod.107.062018

Ibanez, C., Guennoun, R., Liere, P., Eychenne, B., Pianos, A., El-Etr, M., et al. (2003). Developmental expression of genes involved in neurosteroidogenesis: 3beta-hydroxysteroid dehydrogenase/delta5-delta4 isomerase in the rat brain. *Endocrinology* 144, 2902–2911. doi: 10.1210/en.2002-0073

155. Ikeuchi, T., Todo, T., Kobayashi, T., and Nagahama, Y. (1999). cDNA cloning of a novel androgen receptor subtype. *J. Biol. Chem.* 274, 25205–25209. doi: 10.1074/jbc.274.36.25205

156. Ikeuchi, T., Todo, T., Kobayashi, T., and Nagahama, Y. (2002). A novel progestogen receptor subtype in the Japanese eel, *Anguilla japonica*. *FEBS Lett.* 510, 77–82. doi: 10.1016/S0014-5793(01)03220-3

157. Ishrat, T., Sayeed, I., Atif, F., Hua, F., and Stein, D. G. (2010). Progesterone and allopregnanolone attenuate blood-brain barrier dysfunction following permanent focal ischemia by regulating the expression of matrix metalloproteinases. *Exp. Neurol.* 226, 183–190. doi: 10.1016/j.expneurol.2010.08.023

158. Jacobs, E. C., Arnold, A. P., and Campagnoni, A. T. (1999). Developmental regulation of the distribution of aromatase- and estrogen-receptor- mRNA-expressing cells in the zebra finch brain. *Dev. Neurosci.* 21, 453–472. doi: 10.1159/000017413

159. Jayasinghe, B. S., and Volz, D. C. (2012). Aberrant ligand-induced activation of G protein-coupled estrogen receptor 1 (GPER) results in developmental malformations during vertebrate embryogenesis. *Toxicol. Sci.* 125, 262–273. doi: 10.1093/toxsci/kfr269

160. Jeong, J. Y., Kwon, H. B., Ahn, J. C., Kang, D., Kwon, S. H., Park, J. A., et al. (2008). Functional and developmental analysis of the blood-brain barrier in zebrafish. *Brain Res. Bull.* 75, 619–628. doi: 10.1016/j.brainresbull.2007.10.043

161. Jiang, C., Zuo, F., Wang, Y., Lu, H., Yang, Q., and Wang, J. (2016). Progesterone changes VEGF and BDNF expression and promotes neurogenesis after ischemic stroke. *Mol. Neurobiol.* 54, 571–581. doi: 10.1007/s12035-015-9651-y

Jorgensen, A., Andersen, O., Bjerregaard, P., and Rasmussen, L. J. (2007). Identification and characterisation of an androgen receptor from zebrafish *Danio rerio*. *Comp. Biochem. Physiol. C. Toxicol. Pharmacol.* 146, 561–568. doi: 10.1016/j.cbpc.2007.07.002

162. Kah, O., Pellegrini, E., Mouriec, K., Diotel, N., Anglade, I., Vaillant, C., et al. (2009). [Oestrogens and neurogenesis: new functions for an old hormone. Lessons from the zebrafish.]. *J. Soc. Biol,* 203, 29–38. doi: 10.1051/jbio:2009007

163. Kallivretaki, E., Eggen, R. I., Neuhauss, S. C., Kah, O., and Segner, H. (2007). The zebrafish, brain-specific, aromatase cyp19a2 is neither expressed nor distributed in a sexually dimorphic manner during sexual differentiation. *Dev. Dyn.* 236, 3155–3166. doi: 10.1002/dvdy.21344

164. Katsu, Y., Lange, A., Miyagawa, S., Urushitani, H., Tatarazako, N., Kawashima, Y., et al. (2013). Cloning, expression and functional characterization of carp, *Cyprinus carpio*, estrogen receptors and their differential activations by estrogens. *J. Appl. Toxicol.* 33, 41–49. doi: 10.1002/jat.170

165. Kawahara, T., Okada, H., and Yamashita, I. (2000). Cloning and expression of genomic and complementary DNAs Encoding an estrogen receptor in the medaka fish, *Oryzias latipes*. *Zool. Sci.* 17, 643–649. doi: 10.2108/zsj.17.643

166. Kawai, H., Arata, N., and Nakayasu, H. (2001). Three-dimensional distribution of astrocytes in zebrafish spinal cord. *Glia* 36, 406–413. doi: 10.1002/glia.1126

167. Kazeto, Y., Goto-Kazeto, R., Thomas, P., and Trant, J. M. (2005). Molecular characterization of three forms of putative membrane-bound progestin receptors and their tissue-distribution in channel catfish, *Ictalurus punctatus*. *J. Mol. Endocrinol.* 34, 781–791. doi: 10.1677/jme.1.01721

168. Kim, S. J., Ogasawara, K., Park, J. G., Takemura, A., and Nakamura, M. (2002). Sequence and expression of androgen receptor and estrogen receptor gene in the sex types of protogynous wrasse, *Halichoeres trimaculatus*. *Gen. Comp. Endocrinol.* 127, 165–173. doi: 10.1016/S0016-6480(02)00020-5

169. Kimoto, T., Tsurugizawa, T., Ohta, Y., Makino, J., Tamura, H., Hojo, Y., et al. (2001). Neurosteroid synthesis by cytochrome p450-containing systems localized in the rat brain hippocampal neurons: N-methyl-D- aspartate and calcium-dependent synthesis. *Endocrinology* 142, 3578–3589. doi: 10.1210/endo.142.8.8327

170. Kishi, Y., Takahashi, J., Koyanagi, M., Morizane, A., Okamoto, Y., Horiguchi, S., et al. (2005). Estrogen promotes differentiation and survival of dopaminergic neurons derived from human neural stem cells. *J. Neurosci. Res.* 79, 279–286. doi: 10.1002/jnr.20362

171. Kizil, C., Kaslin, J., Kroehne, V., and Brand, M. (2012). Adult neurogenesis and brain regeneration in zebrafish. *Dev. Neurobiol.* 72, 429–461. doi: 10.1002/dneu.20918

172. Koch, S., Donarski, N., Goetze, K., Kreckel, M., Stuerenburg, H. J., Buhmann, C., et al. (2001). Characterization of four lipoprotein classes in human cerebrospinal fluid. *J. Lipid Res.* 42 1143–1151.

173. Koenig, H. L., Schumacher, M., Ferzaz, B., Thi, A. N., Ressouches, A., Guennoun, R., et al. (1995). Progesterone synthesis and myelin formation by Schwann cells. *Science* 268, 1500–1503. doi: 10.1126/science.7770777

174. Krause, D. N., Duckles, S. P., and Gonzales, R. J. (2011). Local oestrogenic/androgenic balance in the cerebral vasculature. *Acta Physiol.* 203, 181–186. doi: 10.1111/j.1748-1716.2011.02323.x

175. Kriegstein, A., and Alvarez-Buylla, A. (2009). The glial nature of embryonic and adult neural stem cells. *Annu. Rev. Neurosci.* 32, 149–184. doi: 10.1146/annurev.neuro.051508.135600

176. Kuo, J., Hamid, N., Bondar, G., Prossnitz, E. R., and Micevych, P. (2010).

Membrane estrogen receptors stimulate intracellular calcium release and progesterone synthesis in hypothalamic astrocytes. *J. Neurosci.* 30, 12950–12957. doi: 10.1523/JNEUROSCI.1158-10.2010

177. Kusuhara, H., and Sugiyama, Y. (2005). Active efflux across the blood-brain barrier: role of the solute carrier family. *NeuroRx* 2, 73–85. doi: 10.1602/neurorx.2.1.73
178. Ladu, M. J., Reardon, C., Van Eldik, L., Fagan, A. M., Bu, G., Holtzman, D., et al. (2000). Lipoproteins in the central nervous system. *Ann. N. Y. Acad. Sci.* 903, 167–175. doi: 10.1111/j.1749-6632.2000.tb06365.x
179. Lapergue, B., Dang, B. Q., Desilles, J. P., Ortiz-Munoz, G., Delbosc, S., Loyau, S., et al. (2013). High-density lipoprotein-based therapy reduces the hemorrhagic complications associated with tissue plasminogen activator treatment in experimental stroke. *Stroke* 44, 699–707. doi: 10.1161/STROKEAHA.112.667832
180. Lapergue, B., Moreno, J. A., Dang, B. Q., Coutard, M., Delbosc, S., Raphaeli, G., et al. (2010). Protective effect of high-density lipoprotein-based therapy in a model of embolic stroke. *Stroke* 41, 1536–1542. doi: 10.1161/STROKEAHA.110.581512
181. Lassiter, C. S., Kelley, B., and Linney, E. (2002). Genomic structure and embryonic expression of estrogen receptor beta a (ERbetaa) in zebrafish (*Danio rerio*). *Gene* 299, 141–151. doi: 10.1016/S0378-1119(02)01050-8
182. Lavenex, P., Steele, M. A., and Jacobs, L. F. (2000). The seasonal pattern of cell proliferation and neuron number in the dentate gyrus of wild adult eastern grey squirrels. *Eur. J. Neurosci.* 12, 643–648. doi: 10.1046/j.1460-9568.2000.00949.x
183. Le Goascogne, C., Robel, P., Gouézou, M., Sananès, N., Baulieu, E. E., and Waterman, M. (1987). Neurosteroids: cytochrome P-450scc in rat brain. *Science* 237, 1212–1215. doi: 10.1126/science.3306919
184. Lephart, E. D. (1996). A review of brain aromatase cytochrome P450. *Brain Res. Brain Res. Rev.* 22, 1–26. doi: 10.1016/0165-0173(96)00002-1
185. Lephart, E. D., Simpson, E. R., McPhaul, M. J., Kilgore, M. W., Wilson, J. D., and Ojeda, S. R. (1992). Brain aromatase cytochrome P-450 messenger RNA levels and enzyme activity during prenatal and perinatal development in the rat. *Brain Res. Mol. Brain Res.* 16, 187–192. doi: 10.1016/0169-328X(92)90224-Y
186. Leszczynski, D. E., and Schafer, R. M. (1991). Metabolic conversion of six steroid hormones by human plasma high-density lipoprotein. *Biochim. Biophys. Acta* 1083, 18–28. doi: 10.1016/0005-2760(91)90120-7
187. Li, X., Schwartz, P. E., and Rissman, E. F. (1997). Distribution of estrogen receptor- beta-like immunoreactivity in rat forebrain. *Neuroendocrinology* 66, 63–67. doi: 10.1159/000127221
188. Li, Y., Chen, T., Miao, X., Yi, X., Wang, X., Zhao, H., et al. (2017). Zebrafish: a promising *in vivo* model for assessing the delivery of natural products, fluorescence dyes and drugs across the blood-brain barrier. *Pharmacol. Res.* 125, 246–257. doi: 10.1016/j.phrs.2017.08.017
189. Liao, S., Chen, W., Kuo, J., and Chen, C. (2001). Association of serum estrogen level and ischemic neuroprotection in female rats. *Neurosci. Lett.* 297, 159–162. doi: 10.1016/S0304-3940(00)01704-3
190. Linard, B., Anglade, I., Corio, M., Navas, J. M., Pakdel, F., Saligaut, C., et al. (1996). Estrogen receptors are expressed in a subset of tyrosine hydroxylase-positive neurons of the anterior preoptic region in the rainbow trout. *Neuroendocrinology* 63, 156–165. doi: 10.1159/000126952
191. Linetti, A., Fratangeli, A., Taverna, E., Valnegri, P., Francolini, M., Cappello, V., et al. (2010). Cholesterol reduction impairs exocytosis of synaptic vesicles. *J. Cell Sci.* 123, 595–605. doi: 10.1242/jcs.060681
192. Liu, C. C., Liu, C. C., Kanekiyo, T., Xu, H., and Bu, G. (2013). Apolipoprotein E and Alzheimer disease: risk, mechanisms and therapy. *Nature reviews. Neurology* 9, 106–118. doi: 10.1038/nrneurol.2012.263
193. Liu, J. P., Tang, Y., Zhou, S., Toh, B. H., McLean, C., and Li, H. (2010). Cholesterol involvement in the pathogenesis of neurodegenerative diseases. *Mol. Cell. Neurosci.* 43, 33–42. doi: 10.1016/j.mcn.2009.07.013
194. Liu, X. M., and Wu, F. H. (2004). [Comparison of animal models of hyperlipidemia]. *Zhong Xi Yi Jie He Xue Bao* 2, 132–134. doi: 10.3736/jcim20040217
195. Liu, X., Zhu, P., Sham, K. W., Yuen, J. M., Xie, C., Zhang, Y., et al. (2009). Identification of a membrane estrogen receptor in zebrafish with homology to mammalian GPER and its high expression in early germ cells of the testis. *Biol. Reprod.* 80, 1253–1261. doi: 10.1095/biolreprod.108.070250
196. London, S. E., and Schlinger, B. A. (2007). Steroidogenic enzymes along the ventricular proliferative zone in the developing songbird brain. *J. Comp. Neurol.* 502, 507–521. doi: 10.1002/cne.21335
197. London, S. E., Monks, D. A., Wade, J., and Schlinger, B. A. (2006). Widespread capacity for steroid synthesis in the avian brain and song system. *Endocrinology* 147, 5975–5987. doi: 10.1210/en.2006-0154
198. London, S. E., Remage-Healey, L., and Schlinger, B. A. (2009). Neurosteroid production in the songbird brain: a re-evaluation of core principles. *Front. Neuroendocrinol.* 30, 302–314. doi: 10.1016/j.yfrne.2009.05.001
199. López-Rodríguez, A. B., Ávila-Rodríguez, M., Vega-Vela, N. E., Capani, F., González, J., García-Segura, L. M., et al. (2015). "Neuroprotection by exogenous estrogenic compounds following traumatic brain injury," in *Estrogen Effects on Traumatic Brain Injury - Mechanisms of Neuroprotection and Repair,* ed
200. A. Duncan Kelli (Amsterdam: Academic Press Elsevier), 73–90.
201. Lord, L. D., Bond, J., and Thompson, R. R. (2009). Rapid steroid influences on visually guided sexual behavior in male goldfish. *Horm. Behav.* 56, 519–526. doi: 10.1016/j.yhbeh.2009.09.002
202. Louissaint, A. Jr., Rao, S., Leventhal, C., and Goldman, S. A. (2002). Coordinated interaction of neurogenesis and angiogenesis in the adult songbird brain. *Neuron* 34, 945–960. doi: 10.1016/S0896-6273(02)00722-5
203. Lubischer, J. L., and Arnold, A. P. (1990). Autoradiographic localization of progestin-concentrating cells in the brain of the zebra finch. *J. Comp. Neurol.* 291, 450–456. doi: 10.1002/cne.902910310
204. Ma, C. H., Dong, K. W., and Yu, K. L. (2000). cDNA cloning and expression of a novel estrogen receptor beta-subtype in goldfish (*Carassius auratus*). *Biochim. Biophys. Acta* 1490, 145–152. doi: 10.1016/S0167-4781(99)00235-3
205. Maggioli, E., McArthur, S., Mauro, C., Kieswich, J., Kusters, D. H., Reutelingsperger, C. P., et al. (2016). Estrogen protects the blood-brain barrier from inflammation-induced disruption and increased lymphocyte trafficking. *Brain Behav. Immun.* 51, 212–222. doi: 10.1016/j.bbi.2015.08.020
206. Mahesh, V. B., and Brann, D. W. (1992). Interaction between ovarian and adrenal steroids in the regulation of gonadotropin secretion. *J. Steroid Biochem. Mol. Biol.* 41, 495–513. doi: 10.1016/0960-0760(92)90375-S
207. Mahesh, V. B., and Brann, D. W. (1998). Regulation of the preovulatory gonadotropin surge by endogenous steroids. *Steroids* 63, 616–629. doi: 10.1016/S0039-128X(98)00075-0
208. Mahley, R. W. (2016). Central nervous system lipoproteins: ApoE and regulation of cholesterol metabolism. *Arterioscler. Thromb. Vasc. Biol.* 36, 1305–1315. doi: 10.1161/ATVBAHA.116.307023
209. Mangiamele, L. A., Gomez, J. R., Curtis, N. J., and Thompson, R. R. (2017). GPER/GPR30, a membrane estrogen receptor, is expressed in the brain and retina of a social fish (*Carassius auratus*) and colocalizes with isotocin. *J. Comp. Neurol.* 525, 252–270. doi: 10.1002/cne.24056
210. Mani, S. K., Blaustein, J. D., Allen, J. M., Law, S. W., O'Malley, B. W., and Clark, J. H. (1994). Inhibition of rat sexual behavior by antisense oligonucleotides to the progesterone receptor. *Endocrinology* 135, 1409–1414. doi: 10.1210/endo.135.4.7925102
211. Manolides, L. S., and Baloyannis, S. J. (1984). Influence of hydrocortisone, progesterone and testosterone on dendritic growth *in vitro*. *Acta Otolaryngol.* 97, 509–522. doi: 10.3109/00016488409132929
212. Martínez-Cerdeño, V., Noctor, S. C., and Kriegstein, A. R. (2006). Estradiol stimulates progenitor cell division in the ventricular and subventricular zones of the embryonic neocortex. *Eur. J. Neurosci.* 24, 3475–3488. doi: 10.1111/j.1460-9568.2006.05239.x
213. März, M., Chapouton, P., Diotel, N., Vaillant, C., Hesl, B., Takamiya, M., et al. (2010). Heterogeneity in progenitor cell subtypes in the ventricular zone of the zebrafish adult telencephalon. *Glia* 58, 870–888. doi: 10.1002/glia.20971
214. Mathieu, M., Mensah-Nyagan, A. G., Vallarino, M., Do-Régo, J. L., Beaujean, D., Vaudry, D., et al. (2001). Immunohistochemical localization of 3 beta-hydroxysteroid dehydrogenase and 5 alpha-reductase in the brain of the African lungfish *Protopterus annectens*. *J. Comp. Neurol.* 438, 123–135. doi: 10.1002/cne.1304
215. Matsumoto, T., Honda, S., and Harada, N. (2003). Alteration in sex-specific behaviors in male mice lacking the aromatase gene. *Neuroendocrinology* 77, 416–424. doi: 10.1159/000071313
216. Matsunaga, M., Ukena, K., and Tsutsui, K. (2001). Expression and localization of cytochrome P450 17 alpha-hydroxylase/c17,20-lyase in the avian brain. *Brain Res.* 899, 112–122. doi: 10.1016/S0006-8993(01)02217-X
217. Mauch, D. H., Nägler, K., Schumacher, S., Göritz, C., Müller, E. C., Otto, A., et al. (2001). CNS synaptogenesis promoted by glia-derived cholesterol. *Science* 294, 1354–1357. doi: 10.1126/science.294.5545.1354
218. Mazzucco, C. A., Lieblich, S. E., Bingham, B. I., Williamson, M. A., Viau, V., and Galea, L. A. (2006). Both estrogen receptor alpha and estrogen receptor

beta agonists enhance cell proliferation in the dentate gyrus of adult female rats. *Neuroscience* 141, 1793–1800. doi: 10.1016/j.neuroscience.2006.05.032

219. McCarthy, M. M. (2011). A lumpers versus splitters approach to sexual differentiation of the brain. *Front. Neuroendocrinol.* 32, 114–123. doi: 10.1016/j.yfrne.2011.01.004
220. McCullough, L. D., Blizzard, K., Simpson, E. R., Oz, O. K., and Hurn, P. D. (2003). Aromatase cytochrome P450 and extragonadal estrogen play a role in ischemic neuroprotection. *J. Neurosci.* 23, 8701–8705.
221. McEwen, B. S., and Milner, T. A. (2017). Understanding the broad influence of sex hormones and sex differences in the brain. *J. Neurosci. Res.* 95, 24–39. doi: 10.1002/jnr.23809
222. McEwen, B. S., and Woolley, C. S. (1994). Estradiol and progesterone regulate neuronal structure and synaptic connectivity in adult as well as developing brain. *Exp. Gerontol.* 29, 431–436. doi: 10.1016/0531-5565(94)90022-1
223. McEwen, B. S., Gould, E., Orchinik, M., Weiland, N. G., and Woolley, C. S. (1995). Oestrogens and the structural and functional plasticity of neurons: implications for memory, ageing and neurodegenerative processes. *Ciba Found Symp,* 191, 52–66: discussion 66–73.
224. Meffre, D., Delespierre, B., Gouézou, M., Schumacher, M., Stein, D. G., and Guennoun, R. (2007). 3beta-Hydroxysteroid dehydrogenase/5-ene-4-ene isomerase mRNA expression in rat brain: effect of pseudopregnancy and traumatic brain injury. *J. Steroid Biochem. Mol. Biol.* 104, 293–300. doi: 10.1016/j.jsbmb.2007.03.003
225. Meffre, D., Labombarda, F., Delespierre, B., Chastre, A., De Nicola, A. F., Stein, D. G., et al. (2013). Distribution of membrane progesterone receptor alpha in the male mouse and rat brain and its regulation after traumatic brain injury. *Neuroscience* 231, 111–124. doi: 10.1016/j.neuroscience.2012.11.039
226. Mellon, S. H., and Deschepper, C. F. (1993). Neurosteroid biosynthesis: genes for adrenal steroidogenic enzymes are expressed in the brain. *Brain Res.* 629, 283–292. doi: 10.1016/0006-8993(93)91332-M
227. Menuet, A., Anglade, I., Le Guevel, R., Pellegrini, E., Pakdel, F., and Kah, O. (2003). Distribution of aromatase mRNA and protein in the brain and pituitary of female rainbow trout: comparison with estrogen receptor alpha. *J. Comp. Neurol.* 462, 180–193. doi: 10.1002/cne.10726
228. Menuet, A., Pellegrini, E., Anglade, I., Blaise, O., Laudet, V., Kah, O., et al. (2002). Molecular characterization of three estrogen receptor forms in zebrafish: binding characteristics, transactivation properties, and tissue distributions. *Biol. Reprod.* 66, 1881–1892. doi: 10.1095/biolreprod66.6.1881
229. Menuet, A., Pellegrini, E., Brion, F., Gueguen, M. M., Anglade, I., Pakdel, F., et al. (2005). Expression and estrogen-dependent regulation of the zebrafish brain aromatase gene. *J. Comp. Neurol.* 485, 304–320. doi: 10.1002/cne.20497
230. Mhaouty-Kodja, S. (2017). Role of the androgen receptor in the central nervous system. *Mol. Cell. Endocrinol.* doi: 10.1016/j.mce.2017.08.001
231. Micevych, P. E., Chaban, V., Ogi, J., Dewing, P., Lu, J. K., and Sinchak, K. (2007). Estradiol stimulates progesterone synthesis in hypothalamic astrocyte cultures. *Endocrinology* 148, 782–789. doi: 10.1210/en.2006-0774
232. Micevych, P., and Sinchak, K. (2008a). Synthesis and function of hypothalamic neuroprogesterone in reproduction. *Endocrinology* 149, 2739–2742. doi: 10.1210/en.2008-0011
233. Micevych, P., and Sinchak, K. (2008b). Estradiol regulation of progesterone synthesis in the brain. *Mol. Cell. Endocrinol.* 290, 44–50. doi: 10.1016/j.mce.2008.04.016
234. Micevych, P., Sinchak, K., Mills, R. H., Tao, L., LaPolt, P., and Lu, J. K. (2003). The luteinizing hormone surge is preceded by an estrogen-induced increase of hypothalamic progesterone in ovariectomized and adrenalectomized rats. *Neuroendocrinology* 78, 29–35. doi: 10.1159/000071703
235. Mitani, Y., Kanda, S., Akazome, Y., Zempo, B., and Oka, Y. (2010). Hypothalamic Kiss1 but not Kiss2 neurons are involved in estrogen feedback in medaka (*Oryzias latipes*). *Endocrinology* 151, 1751–1759. doi: 10.1210/en.2009-1174
236. Mitra, S. W., Hoskin, E., Yudkovitz, J., Pear, L., Wilkinson, H. A., Hayashi, S., et al. (2003). Immunolocalization of estrogen receptor beta in the mouse brain: comparison with estrogen receptor alpha. *Endocrinology* 144, 2055–2067. doi: 10.1210/en.2002-221069
237. Morali, G., Larsson, K., and Beyer, C. (1977). Inhibition of testosterone-induced sexual behavior in the castrated male rat by aromatase blockers. *Horm. Behav.* 9, 203–213. doi: 10.1016/0018-506X(77)90056-3
238. Morini, M., Peñaranda, D. S., Vílchez, M. C., Nourizadeh-Lillabadi, R., Lafont, A. G., Dufour, S., et al. (2017). Nuclear and membrane progestin receptors in the European eel: characterization and expression *in vivo* through spermatogenesis. *Comp. Biochem. Physiol. Part A Mol. Integr. Physiol.* 207, 79–92. doi: 10.1016/j.cbpa.2017.02.009
239. Mouriec, K., Lareyre, J. J., Tong, S. K., Le Page, Y., Vaillant, C., Pellegrini, E., et al. (2009). Early regulation of brain aromatase (cyp19a1b) by estrogen receptors during zebrafish development. *Dev. Dyn.* 238, 2641–2651. doi: 10.1002/dvdy.22069
240. Mouriec, K., Pellegrini, E., Anglade, I., Menuet, A., Adrio, F., Thieulant, M. L., et al. (2008). Synthesis of estrogens in progenitor cells of adult fish brain: evolutive novelty or exaggeration of a more general mechanism implicating estrogens in neurogenesis? *Brain Res. Bull.* 75, 274–280. doi: 10.1016/j.brainresbull.2007.10.030
241. Mourot, B., Nguyen, T., Fostier, A., and Bobe, J. (2006). Two unrelated putative membrane-bound progestin receptors, progesterone membrane receptor component 1 (PGMRC1) and membrane progestin receptor (mPR) beta, are expressed in the rainbow trout oocyte and exhibit similar ovarian expression patterns. *Reprod. Biol. Endocrinol.* 4:6. doi: 10.1186/1477-7827-4-6
242. Mukai, H., Kimoto, T., Hojo, Y., Kawato, S., Murakami, G., Higo, S., et al. (2010). Modulation of synaptic plasticity by brain estrogen in the hippocampus. *Biochim. Biophys. Acta* 1800, 1030–1044. doi: 10.1016/j.bbagen.2009.11.002
243. Muñoz-Cueto, J. A., Burzawa-Gérard, E., Kah, O., Valotaire, Y., and Pakdel, F. (1999). Cloning and sequencing of the gilthead sea bream estrogen receptor cDNA. *DNA Seq.* 10, 75–84.
244. Murashov, A. K., Pak, E. S., Hendricks, W. A., and Tatko, L. M. (2004). 17beta-Estradiol enhances neuronal differentiation of mouse embryonic stem cells. *FEBS Lett.* 569, 165–168. doi: 10.1016/j.febslet.2004.0 5.042
245. Na, W., Lee, J. Y., Kim, W. S., Yune, T. Y., and Ju, B. G. (2015). 17beta-estradiol ameliorates tight junction disruption via repression of MMP transcription. *Mol. Endocrinol.* 29, 1347–1361. doi: 10.1210/ME.2015-1124
246. Nagler, J. J., Cavileer, T., Sullivan, J., Cyr, D. G., and Rexroad, C. III. (2007). The complete nuclear estrogen receptor family in the rainbow trout: discovery of the novel ERalpha2 and both ERbeta isoforms. *Gene* 392, 164–173. doi: 10.1016/j.gene.2006.12.030
247. Navas, J. M., Anglade, I., Bailhache, T., Pakdel, F., Breton, B., Jego, P., et al. (1995). Do gonadotrophin-releasing hormone neurons express estrogen receptors in the rainbow trout? A double immunohistochemical study. *J. Comp. Neurol.* 363, 461–474. doi: 10.1002/cne.903630309
248. Nico, B., Frigeri, A., Nicchia, G. P., Quondamatteo, F., Herken, R., Errede, M., et al. (2001). Role of aquaporin-4 water channel in the development and integrity of the blood-brain barrier. *J. Cell Sci.* 114, 1297–1307.
249. Noctor, S. C., Flint, A. C., Weissman, T. A., Dammerman, R. S., and Kriegstein, A. R. (2001). Neurons derived from radial glial cells establish radial units in neocortex. *Nature* 409, 714–720. doi: 10.1038/350 55553
250. Okada, M., Makino, A., Nakajima, M., Okuyama, S., Furukawa, S., and Furukawa, Y. (2010). Estrogen stimulates proliferation and differentiation of neural stem/progenitor cells through different signal transduction pathways. *Int. J. Mol. Sci.* 11, 4114–4123. doi: 10.3390/ijms11104114
251. Olsson, P. E., Berg, A. H., von Hofsten, J., Grahn, B., Hellqvist, A., Larsson, A., et al. (2005). Molecular cloning and characterization of a nuclear androgen receptor activated by 11-ketotestosterone. *Reprod. Biol. Endocrinol.* 3:37. doi: 10.1186/1477-7827-3-37
252. Ormerod, B. K., and Galea, L. A. (2001). Reproductive status influences cell proliferation and cell survival in the dentate gyrus of adult female meadow voles: a possible regulatory role for estradiol. *Neuroscience* 102, 369–379. doi: 10.1016/S0306-4522(00)00474-7
253. Ormerod, B. K., and Galea, L. A. (2003). Reproductive status influences the survival of new cells in the dentate gyrus of adult male meadow voles. *Neurosci. Lett.* 346, 25–28. doi: 10.1016/S0304-3940(03)00546-9
254. Ortiz-Muñoz, G., Couret, D., Lapergue, B., Bruckert, E., Meseguer, E., Amarenco, P., et al. (2016). Dysfunctional HDL in acute stroke. *Atherosclerosis* 253, 75–80. doi: 10.1016/j.atherosclerosis.2016.08.035
255. Pakdel, F., Le Gac, F., Le Goff, P., and Valotaire, Y. (1990). Full-length sequence and *in vitro* expression of rainbow trout estrogen receptor cDN. *Mol. Cell. Endocrinol.* 71, 195–204. doi: 10.1016/0303-7207(90)90025-4
256. Pang, Y., and Thomas, P. (2009). Involvement of estradiol-17beta and its membrane receptor, G protein coupled receptor 30 (GPR30) in regulation of oocyte maturation in zebrafish, *Danio rario*. *Gen. Comp. Endocrinol.* 161, 58–61. doi: 10.1016/j.ygcen.2008.10.003
257. Pang, Y., Dong, J., and Thomas, P. (2008). Estrogen signaling characteristics of Atlantic croaker G protein-coupled receptor 30 (GPR30) and evidence

it is involved in maintenance of oocyte meiotic arrest. *Endocrinology* 149, 3410–3426. doi: 10.1210/en.2007-1663

258. Pang, Y., Dong, J., and Thomas, P. (2013). Characterization, neurosteroid binding and brain distribution of human membrane progesterone receptors delta and {epsilon} (mPRdelta and mPR{epsilon}) and mPRdelta involvement in neurosteroid inhibition of apoptosis. *Endocrinology* 154, 283–295. doi: 10.1210/en.2012-1772
259. Panzica, G. C., Castagna, C., Viglietti-Panzica, C., Russo, C., Tlemcani, O., and Balthazart, J. (1998). Organizational effects of estrogens on brain vasotocin and sexual behavior in quail. *J. Neurobiol.* 37, 684–699. doi: 10.1002/(SICI)1097-4695(199812)37:4<684::AID-NEU15>3.0.CO;2-U
260. Pardridge, W. M., and Mietus, L. J. (1979). Transport of steroid hormones through the rat blood-brain barrier. Primary role of albumin-bound hormone. *J. Clin. Investig.* 64, 145–154. doi: 10.1172/JCI109433
261. Parimisetty, A., Dorsemans, A. C., Awada, R., Ravanan, P., Diotel, N., and Lefebvre d'Hellencourt, C. (2016). Secret talk between adipose tissue and central nervous system via secreted factors-an emerging frontier in the neurodegenerative research. *J. Neuroinflammation* 13, 67. doi: 10.1186/s12974-016- 0530-x
262. Pasmanik, M., and Callard, G. V. (1985). Aromatase and 5 alpha-reductase in the teleost brain, spinal cord, and pituitary gland. *Gen. Comp. Endocrinol.* 60, 244–251. doi: 10.1016/0016-6480(85)90320-X
263. Pasmanik, M., and Callard, G. V. (1988). Changes in brain aromatase and 5 alpha-reductase activities correlate significantly with seasonal reproductive cycles in goldfish (*Carassius auratus*). *Endocrinology* 122, 1349–1356. doi: 10.1210/endo-122-4-1349
264. Pawlisch, B. A., and Remage-Healey, L. (2015). Neuroestrogen signaling in the songbird auditory cortex propagates into a sensorimotor network via an 'interface' nucleus. *Neuroscience* 284, 522–535. doi: 10.1016/j.neuroscience.2014.10.023
265. Pellegrini, E., Coumailleau, P., Kah, O., and Diotel, N. (2015). "Aromatase and estrogens: involvement in constitutive and regenerative neurogenesis in adult zebrafish," in*Estrogen Effects on Traumatic Brain Injury - Mechanisms of Neuroprotection and Repair,* ed A. Duncan Kelli (Amsterdam: Academic Press Elsevier), 51–71.
266. Pellegrini, E., Menuet, A., Lethimonier, C., Adrio, F., Gueguen, M. M., Tascon, C., et al. (2005). Relationships between aromatase and estrogen receptors in the brain of teleost fish. *Gen. Comp. Endocrinol.* 142, 60–66. doi: 10.1016/j.ygcen.2004.12.003
267. Pellegrini, E., Mouriec, K., Anglade, I., Menuet, A., Le Page, Y., Gueguen, M. M., et al. (2007). Identification of aromatase-positive radial glial cells as progenitorcells in the ventricular layer of the forebrain in zebrafish. *J. Comp. Neurol.* 501, 150–167. doi: 10.1002/cne.21222
268. Pellegrini, E., Vaillant, C., Diotel, N., Benquet, P., Brion, F., and Kah, O. (2013). "Expression, regulation and potential functions of aromatase in radial glial cells of the fish brain," in *Brain Aromatase, Estrogens, and Behavior*, eds Balthazart,
269. J. Ball, and F.Gregory (Oxford; New York, NY: University Press), 2013. Pelletier, G. (2010). Steroidogenic enzymes in the brain: morphological aspects. *Prog. Brain Res.* 181, 193–207. doi: 10.1016/S0079-6123(08)81011-4
270. Perkins, A., and Roselli, C. E. (2007). The ram as a model for behavioral neuroendocrinology. *Horm. Behav.* 52, 70–77. doi: 10.1016/j.yhbeh.2007.03.016
271. Petersen, S. L., Intlekofer, K. A., Moura-Conlon, P. J., Brewer, D. N., Del Pino Sans, J., and Lopez, J. A. (2013). Novel progesterone receptors: neural localization and possible functions. *Front. Neurosci.* 7:164. doi: 10.3389/fnins.2013.00164
272. Peterson, R. S., Lee, D. W., Fernando, G., and Schlinger, B. A. (2004). Radial glia express aromatase in the injured zebra finch brain. *J. Comp. Neurol.* 475, 261–269. doi: 10.1002/cne.20157
273. Peterson, R. S., Saldanha, C. J., and Schlinger, B. A. (2001). Rapid upregulation of aromatase mRNA and protein following neural injury in the zebra finch (*Taeniopygia guttata*). *J. Neuroendocrinol.* 13, 317–323. doi: 10.1046/j.1365-2826.2001.00647.x
274. Peterson, R. S., Yarram, L., Schlinger, B. A., and Saldanha, C. J. (2005). Aromatase is pre-synaptic and sexually dimorphic in the adult zebra finch brain. *Proc. Biol. Sci.* 272, 2089–2096. doi: 10.1098/rspb.2005.3181
275. Petralia, S. M., and Frye, C. A. (2005). In the ventral tegmental area picrotoxin blocks FGIN 1-27-induced increases in sexual behavior of rats and hamsters. *Psychopharmacology* 178, 174–182. doi: 10.1007/s00213-004-2001-9
276. Petrone, A. B., Rudy, C. C., Barr, T. L., Simpkins, J. W., and Reed, M. N. (2015). "Neuroprotective effects of estrogen following neural injury," in *Estrogen Effects on Traumatic Brain Injury - Mechanisms of Neuroprotection and Repair,*ed A. Duncan Kelli (Amsterdam: Academic Press Elsevier), 91–111.
277. Phan, A., Gabor, C. S., Favaro, K. J., Kaschack, S., Armstrong, J. N., MacLusky,
278. N. J., et al. (2012). Low doses of 17beta-estradiol rapidly improve learning and increase hippocampal dendritic spines. *Neuropsychopharmacology* 37, 2299–2309. doi: 10.1038/npp.2012.82
279. Pouso, P., Quintana, L., Bolatto, C., and Silva, A. C. (2010). Brain androgen receptor expression correlates with seasonal changes in the behavior of a weakly electric fish, *Brachyhypopomus gauderio*. *Horm. Behav.* 58, 729–736. doi: 10.1016/j.yhbeh.2010.07.005
280. Putnam, C. D., Brann, D. W., and Mahesh, V. B. (1991). Acute activation of the adrenocorticotropin-adrenal axis: effect on gonadotropin and prolactin secretion in the female rat. *Endocrinology* 128, 2558–2566. doi: 10.1210/endo-128-5-2558
281. Quan, G., Xie, C., Dietschy, J. M., and Turley, S. D. (2003). Ontogenesis and regulation of cholesterol metabolism in the central nervous system of the mouse. *Brain Res. Dev. Brain Res.* 146, 87–98. doi: 10.1016/j.devbrainres.2003.09.015
282. Ravi, V., and Venkatesh, B. (2008). Rapidly evolving fish genomes and teleost diversity. *Curr. Opin. Genet. Dev.* 18, 544–550. doi: 10.1016/j.gde.2008.11.001
283. Roncali, L., Nico, B., Ribatti, D., Bertossi, M., and Mancini, L. (1986). Microscopical and ultrastructural investigations on the development of the blood-brain barrier in the chick embryo optic tectum. *Acta Neuropathol.* 70, 193–201. doi: 10.1007/BF00686072
284. Roof, R. L., and Hall, E. D. (2000). Gender differences in acute CNS trauma and stroke: neuroprotective effects of estrogen and progesterone. *J. Neurotrauma* 17, 367–388. doi: 10.1089/neu.2000.17.367
285. Roselli, C. E., Cross, E., Poonyagariyagorn, H. K., and Stadelman, H. L. (2003). Role of aromatization in anticipatory and consummatory aspects of sexual behavior in male rats. *Horm. Behav.* 44, 146–151. doi: 10.1016/S0018-506X(03)00123-5
286. Roselli, C. F. (2007). Brain aromatase: roles in reproduction and neuroprotection. *J. Steroid Biochem. Mol. Biol.* 106, 143–150. doi: 10.1016/j.jsbmb.2007.05.014 Rosner, W. (2015). Free estradiol and sex hormone-binding globulin. *Steroids* 99, 113–116. doi: 10.1016/j.steroids.2014.08.005
287. Rossetti, M. F., Cambiasso, M. J., Holschbach, M. A., and Cabrera, R. (2016). Oestrogens and progestagens: synthesis and action in the brain. *J. Neuroendocrinol.* 28. doi: 10.1111/jne.12402
288. Rothenaigner, I., Krecsmarik, M., Hayes, J. A., Bahn, B., Lepier, A., Fortin, G., et al. (2011). Clonal analysis by distinct viral vectors identifies bona fide neural stem cells in the adult zebrafish telencephalon and characterizes their division properties and fate. *Development* 138, 1459–1469. doi: 10.1242/dev.058156
289. Roy, S. R., Wang, J., Rana, M. R., Nakashima, M., and Tokumoto, T. (2017). Characterization of membrane progestin receptor alpha (mPRalpha) of the medaka and role in the induction of oocyte maturation. *Biomed. Res.* 38, 79–87. doi: 10.2220/biomedres.38.79
290. Sabo-Attwood, T., Kroll, K. J., and Denslow, N. D. (2004). Differential expression of largemouth bass (*Micropterus salmoides*) estrogen receptor isotypes alpha, beta, and gamma by estradiol. *Mol. Cell. Endocrinol.* 218, 107–118. doi: 10.1016/j.mce.2003.12.007
291. Sager, T., Kashon, M., and Krajnak, K. (2017). Estrogen and environmental enrichment differentially affect neurogenesis, dendritic spine immunolabeling and synaptogenesis in the hippocampus of young and reproductively senescent female rats. *Neuroendocrinology*. doi: 10.1159/000479699
292. Sakamoto, H., Ukena, K., and Tsutsui, K. (2001a). Activity and localization of 3beta-hydroxysteroid dehydrogenase/ Delta5-Delta4-isomerase in the zebrafish central nervous system. *J. Comp. Neurol.* 439, 291–305. doi: 10.1002/cne.1351
293. Sakamoto, H., Ukena, K., and Tsutsui, K. (2001b). Effects of progesterone synthesized *de novo* in the developing Purkinje cell on its dendritic growth and synaptogenesis. *J. Neurosci.* 21, 6221–6232.
294. Sakamoto, H., Ukena, K., and Tsutsui, K. (2002). Dendritic spine formation in response to progesterone synthesized de novo in the developing Purkinje cell in rats. *Neurosci. Lett.* 322, 111–115. doi: 10.1016/S0304-3940(02)00077-0
295. Salbert, G., Bonnec, G., Le Goff, P., Boujard, D., Valotaire, Y., and Jego, P. (1991). Localization of the estradiol receptor mRNA in the forebrain of the rainbow trout. *Mol. Cell. Endocrinol.* 76, 173–180. doi: 10.1016/0303-7207(91)90271-S
296. Saldanha, C. J., Remage-Healey, L., and Schlinger, B. A. (2011). Synaptocrine

signaling: steroid synthesis and action at the synapse. *Endocr. Rev.* 32, 532–549. doi:10.1210/er.2011-0004

297. Sar, M., Lubahn, D. B., French, F. S., and Wilson, E. M. (1990). Immunohistochemical localization of the androgen receptor in rat and human tissues. *Endocrinology* 127, 3180–3186. doi: 10.1210/endo-127-6-3180

298. Sasano, H., Takashashi, K., Satoh, F., Nagura, H., and Harada, N. (1998). Aromatase in the human central nervous system. *Clin. Endocrinol.* 48, 325–329. doi:10.1046/j.1365-2265.1998.00390.x

299. Schlinger, B. A. (1997). The activity and expression of aromatase in songbirds. *Brain Res. Bull.* 44, 359–364. doi: 10.1016/S0361-9230(97)00215-3

300. Schlinger, B. A., and Remage-Healey, L. (2012). Neurosteroidogenesis: insights from studies of songbirds. *J. Neuroendocrinol.* 24, 16–21. doi: 10.1111/j.1365-2826.2011.02150.x

301. Schlinger, B. A., Pradhan, D. S., and Soma, K. K. (2008). 3beta-HSD activates DHEA in the songbird brain. *Neurochem. Int.* 52, 611–620. doi: 10.1016/j.neuint.2007.05.003

302. Schlinger, B. A., Soma, K. K., and London, S. E. (2001). Neurosteroids and brain sexual differentiation. *Trends Neurosci.* 24, 429–431. doi: 10.1016/S0166-2236(00)01855-5

303. Schmidt, K. L., Pradhan, D. S., Shah, A. H., Charlier, T. D., Chin, E. H., and Soma, K. K. (2008). Neurosteroids, immunosteroids, and the Balkanization of endocrinology. *Gen. Comp. Endocrinol.* 157, 266–274. doi: 10.1016/j.ygcen.2008.03.025

304. Schumacher, M., Guennoun, R., Stein, D. G., and De Nicola, A. F. (2007). Progesterone: therapeutic opportunities for neuroprotection and myelin repair. *Pharmacol. Ther.* 116, 77–106. doi: 10.1016/j.pharmthera.2007.06.001

305. Scordalakes, E. M., Imwalle, D. B., and Rissman, E. F. (2002). Oestrogen's masculine side: mediation of mating in male mice. *Reproduction* 124, 331–338. doi: 10.1530/rep.0.1240331

306. Sellers, K. J., Erli, F., Raval, P., Watson, I. A., Chen, D., and Srivastava, D. P. (2015). Rapid modulation of synaptogenesis and spinogenesis by 17beta-estradiol in primary cortical neurons. *Front. Cell. Neurosci.* 9:137. doi: 10.3389/fncel.2015.00137

307. Seredynski, A. L., Balthazart, J., Ball, G. F., and Cornil, C. A. (2015). Estrogen receptor beta activation rapidly modulates male sexual motivation through the transactivation of metabotropic glutamate receptor 1a. *J. Neurosci.* 35, 13110–13123. doi: 10.1523/JNEUROSCI.2056-15.2015

308. Seredynski, A. L., Balthazart, J., Christophe, V. J., Ball, G. F., and Cornil, C. A. (2013). Neuroestrogens rapidly regulate sexual motivation but not performance. *J. Neurosci.* 33, 164–174. doi: 10.1523/JNEUROSCI.2557-12.2013

309. Shah, A. H., Chin, E. H., Schmidt, K. L., and Soma, K. K. (2011). DHEA and estradiol levels in brain, gonads, adrenal glands, and plasma of developing male and female European starlings. *J. Comp. Physiol. A Neuroethol. Sens. Neural Behav. Physiol.* 197, 949–958. doi: 10.1007/s00359-011-0655-4

310. Shahrokhi, N., Haddad, M. K., Joukar, S., Shabani, M., Keshavarzi, Z., and Shahozehi, B. (2012). Neuroprotective antioxidant effect of sex steroid hormones in traumatic brain injury. *Pak. J. Pharm. Sci.* 25, 219–225.

311. Shi, Y., Liu, X., Zhu, P., Li, J., Sham, K. W., Cheng, S. H., et al. (2013). G-protein-coupled estrogen receptor 1 is involved in brain development during zebrafish (*Danio rerio*) embryogenesis. *Biochem. Biophys. Res. Commun.* 435, 21–27. doi: 10.1016/j.bbrc.2013.03.130

312. Shughrue, P. J., Lane, M. V., and Merchenthaler, I. (1997). Comparative distribution of estrogen receptor-alpha and -beta mRNA in the rat central nervous system. *J. Comp. Neurol.* 388, 507–525. doi: 10.1002/(SICI)1096- 9861(19971201)388:4<507::AID-CNE1>3.0.CO;2-6

313. Si, D., Li, J., Liu, J., Wang, X., Wei, Z., Tian, Q., et al. (2014). Progesterone protects blood-brain barrier function and improves neurological outcome following traumatic brain injury in rats. *Exp. Ther. Med.* 8, 1010–1014. doi: 10.3892/etm.2014.1840

314. Sinchak, K., Mills, R. H., Tao, L., LaPolt, P., Lu, J. K., and Micevych, P. (2003). Estrogen induces *de novo* progesterone synthesis in astrocytes. *Dev. Neurosci.* 25, 343–348. doi: 10.1159/000073511

315. Slewa-Younan, S., Green, A. M., Baguley, I. J., Gurka, J. A., and Marosszeky, J. E. (2004). Sex differences in injury severity and outcome measures after traumatic brain injury. *Arch. Phys. Med. Rehabil.* 85, 376–379. doi: 10.1016/j.apmr.2003.05.007

316. Socorro, S., Power, D. M., Olsson, P. E., and Canario, A. V. (2000). Two estrogen receptors expressed in the teleost fish, *Sparus aurata*: cDNA cloning, characterization and tissue distribution. *J. Endocrinol.* 166, 293–306. doi: 10.1677/joe.0.1660293

317. Södersten, P. (2013). "A historical and personal perspective on the aromatization revolution," in *Brain Aromatase, Estrogens, and Behavior*, eds J. Balthazart and G. F. Ball (New York, NY; Oxford UP), 281–314.

318. Sohrabji, F. (2015). "Cerebrovascular stroke: sex differences and the impact of Estrogens," in *Estrogen Effects on Traumatic Brain Injury - Mechanisms of Neuroprotection and Repair*, ed A. Duncan Kelli (Amsterdam: Academic Press Elsevier), 125–141.

319. Soma, K. K., Alday, N. A., Hau, M., and Schlinger, B. A. (2004). Dehydroepiandrosterone metabolism by 3beta-hydroxysteroid dehydrogenase/Delta5-Delta4 isomerase in adult zebra finch brain: sex difference and rapid effect of stress. *Endocrinology* 145, 1668–1677. doi: 10.1210/en.2003-0883

320. Soma, K. K., Sinchak, K., Lakhter, A., Schlinger, B. A., and Micevych, P. E. (2005). Neurosteroids and female reproduction: estrogen increases 3beta-HSD mRNA and activity in rat hypothalamus. *Endocrinology* 146, 4386–4390. doi: 10.1210/en.2005-0569

321. Sperry, T. S., and Thomas, P. (1999a). Characterization of two nuclear androgen receptors in Atlantic croaker: comparison of their biochemical properties and binding specificities. *Endocrinology* 140, 1602–1611. doi: 10.1210/endo.140.4.6631

322. Sperry, T. S., and Thomas, P. (1999b). Identification of two nuclear androgen receptors in kelp bass (*Paralabrax clathratus*) and their binding affinities for xenobiotics: comparison with Atlantic croaker (*Micropogonias undulatus*) androgen receptors. *Biol. Reprod.* 61, 1152–1161. doi: 10.1095/biolreprod61.4.1152

323. Spritzer, M. D., and Galea, L. A. (2007). Testosterone and dihydrotestosterone, but not estradiol, enhance survival of new hippocampal neurons in adult male rats. *Dev. Neurobiol.* 67, 1321–1333. doi: 10.1002/dneu.20457

324. Stephens, S. B., Tolson, K. P., Rouse, M. L. Jr., Poling, M. C., Hashimoto-Partyka, M. K., Mellon, P. L., et al. (2015). Absent progesterone signaling in kisspeptin neurons disrupts the LH surge and impairs fertility in female mice. *Endocrinology* 156, 3091–3097. doi: 10.1210/en.2015-1300

325. Sterling, R. J., Gasc, J. M., Sharp, P. J., Renoir, J. M., Tuohimaa, P., and Baulieu, E. E. (1987). The distribution of nuclear progesterone receptor in the hypothalamus and forebrain of the domestic hen. *Cell Tissue Res.* 248, 201–205. doi: 10.1007/BF01239981

326. Stewart, P. A., and Wiley, M. J. (1981). Structural and histochemical features of the avian blood-brain barrier. *J. Comp. Neurol.* 202, 157–167. doi: 10.1002/cne.902020203

327. Stone, D. J., Rozovsky, I., Morgan, T. E., Anderson, C. P., Hajian, H., and Finch, C. E. (1997). Astrocytes and microglia respond to estrogen with increased apoE mRNA *in vivo* and *in vitro*. *Exp. Neurol.* 143, 313–318. doi: 10.1006/exnr.1996.6360

328. Strobl-Mazzulla, P. H., Lethimonier, C., Gueguen, M. M., Karube, M., Fernandino, J. I., Yoshizaki, G., et al. (2008). Brain aromatase (Cyp19A2) and estrogen receptors, in larvae and adult pejerrey fish *Odontesthes bonariensis*: neuroanatomical and functional relations. *Gen. Comp. Endocrinol.* 158, 191–201. doi: 10.1016/j.ygcen.2008.07.006

329. Strobl-Mazzulla, P. H., Moncaut, N. P., López, G. C., Miranda, L. A., Canario, A. V., and Somoza, G. M. (2005). Brain aromatase from pejerrey fish (*Odontesthes bonariensis*): cDNA cloning, tissue expression, and immunohistochemical localization. *Gen. Comp. Endocrinol.* 143, 21–32. doi: 10.1016/j.ygcen.2005.02.026

330. Strobl-Mazzulla, P. H., Nuñez, A., Pellegrini, E., Gueguen, M. M., Kah, O., and Somoza, G. M. (2010). Progenitor radial cells and neurogenesis in pejerrey fish forebrain. *Brain Behav. Evol.* 76, 20–31. doi: 10.1159/000316022

331. Strömstedt, M., and Waterman, M. R. (1995). Messenger RNAs encoding steroidogenic enzymes are expressed in rodent brain. *Brain Res. Mol. Brain Res.* 34, 75–88. doi: 10.1016/0169-328X(95)00140-N

332. Sugiyama, D., Kusuhara, H., Shitara, Y., Abe, T., Meier, P. J., Sekine, T., et al. (2001). Characterization of the efflux transport of 17beta-estradiol-D-17beta- glucuronide from the brain across the blood-brain barrier. *J. Pharmacol. Exp. Ther.* 298, 316–322.

333. Sugiyama, N., Andersson, S., Lathe, R., Fan, X., Alonso-Magdalena, P., Schwend, T., et al. (2009). Spatiotemporal dynamics of the expression of estrogen receptors in the postnatal mouse brain. *Mol. Psychiatry* 14, 223–232. doi: 10.1038/mp.2008.118

334. Suzuki, S., Gerhold, L. M., Böttner, M., Rau, S. W., Dela Cruz, C., Yang, E., et al. (2007). Estradiol enhances neurogenesis following ischemic stroke through estrogen receptors alpha and beta. *J. Comp. Neurol.* 500, 1064–1075. doi: 10.1002/cne.21240
335. Takeo, J., and Yamashita, S. (1999). Two distinct isoforms of cDNA encoding rainbow trout androgen receptors. *J. Biol. Chem.* 274, 5674–5680.
336. Takeo, J., and Yamashita, S. (2000). Rainbow trout androgen receptor-alpha fails to distinguish between any of the natural androgens tested in transactivation assay, not just 11-ketotestosterone and testosterone. *Gen. Comp. Endocrinol.* 117, 200–206. doi: 10.1006/gcen.1999.7398
337. Tan, N. S., Lam, T. J., and Ding, J. L. (1995). The hormone-binding domain of *Oreochromis aureus* estrogen receptor gene: homology comparison with other steroid binding receptors. *DNA Seq.* 5, 371–379.
338. Tanapat, P., Hastings, N. B., and Gould, E. (2005). Ovarian steroids influence cell proliferation in the dentate gyrus of the adult female rat in a dose- and time-dependent manner. *J. Comp. Neurol.* 481, 252–265. doi: 10.1002/cne.20385
339. Tanapat, P., Hastings, N. B., Reeves, A. J., and Gould, E. (1999). Estrogen stimulates a transient increase in the number of new neurons in the dentate gyrus of the adult female rat. *J. Neurosci.* 19, 5792–5801.
340. Tang, H., Liu, Y., Li, J., Yin, Y., Li, G., Chen, Y., et al. (2016). Gene knockout of nuclear progesterone receptor provides insights into the regulation of ovulation by LH signaling in zebrafish. *Sci. Rep.* 6:28545. doi: 10.1038/srep28545
341. Taziaux, M., Keller, M., Bakker, J., and Balthazart, J. (2007). Sexual behavior activity tracks rapid changes in brain estrogen concentrations. *J. Neurosci.* 27, 6563–6572. doi: 10.1523/JNEUROSCI.1797-07.2007
342. Tchoudakova, A., Pathak, S., and Callard, G. V. (1999). Molecular cloning of an estrogen receptor beta subtype from the goldfish, *Carassius auratus*. *Gen. Comp. Endocrinol.* 113, 388–400. doi: 10.1006/gcen.1998.7217
343. Thomas, P. (2008). Characteristics of membrane progestin receptor alpha (mPRalpha) and progesterone membrane receptor component 1 (PGMRC1) and their roles in mediating rapid progestin actions. *Front. Neuroendocrinol.* 29, 292–312. doi: 10.1016/j.yfrne.2008.01.001
344. Thompson, R. R., George, K., Dempsey, J., and Walton, J. C. (2004). Visual sex discrimination in goldfish: seasonal, sexual, and androgenic influences. *Horm. Behav.* 46, 646–654. doi: 10.1016/j.yhbeh.2004.06.008
345. Thornton, J. W. (2001). Evolution of vertebrate steroid receptors from an ancestral estrogen receptor by ligand exploitation and serial genome expansions. *Proc. Natl. Acad. Sci. U.S.A.* 98, 5671–5676. doi: 10.1073/pnas.091 553298
346. Tikkanen, M. J., Vihma, V., Jauhiainen, M., Höckerstedt, A., Helisten, H., and Kaamanen, M. (2002). Lipoprotein-associated estrogens. *Cardiovasc. Res.* 56, 184–188. doi: 10.1016/S0008-6363(02)00535-7
347. Timmers, R. J., and Lambert, J. G. (1987). Measurement of aromatase activity in the brain of the African catfish, *Clarias gariepinus*–a comparison of two assay methods. *Comp. Biochem. Physiol. B Comp. Biochem.* 88, 453–456. doi: 10.1016/0305-0491(87)90325-7
348. Tokumoto, M., Nagahama, Y., Thomas, P., and Tokumoto, T. (2006). Cloning and identification of a membrane progestin receptor in goldfish ovaries and evidence it is an intermediary in oocyte meiotic maturation. *Gen. Comp. Endocrinol.* 145, 101–108. doi: 10.1016/j.ygcen.2005.07.002
349. Tokumoto, T., Tokumoto, M., Oshima, T., Shimizuguchi, K., Fukuda, T., Sugita, E., et al. (2012). Characterization of multiple membrane progestin receptor (mPR) subtypes from the goldfish ovary and their roles in the induction of oocyte maturation. *Gen. Comp. Endocrinol.* 177, 168–176. doi: 10.1016/j.ygcen.2012.03.005
350. Tomy, S., Wu, G. C., Huang, H. R., Dufour, S., and Chang, C. F. (2007). Developmental expression of key steroidogenic enzymes in the brain of protandrous black porgy fish, *Acanthopagrus schlegeli*. *J. Neuroendocrinol.* 19, 643–655. doi: 10.1111/j.1365-2826.2007.01572.x
351. Tong, S. K., Mouriec, K., Kuo, M. W., Pellegrini, E., Gueguen, M. M., Brion, F., et al. (2009). A cyp19a1b-gfp (aromatase B) transgenic zebrafish line that expresses GFP in radial glial cells. *Genesis* 47, 67–73. doi: 10.1002/dvg. 20459
352. Toran-Allerand, C. D. (2005). Estrogen and the brain: beyond ER-alpha, ER-beta, and 17beta-estradiol. *Ann. N. Y. Acad. Sci.* 1052, 136–144. doi: 10.1196/annals.1347.009
353. Toran-Allerand, C. D., Guan, X., MacLusky, N. J., Horvath, T. L., Diano, S., Singh, M., et al. (2002). ER-X: a novel, plasma membrane-associated, putative estrogen receptor that is regulated during development and after ischemic brain injury. *J. Neurosci.* 22, 8391–8401.
354. Tramontin, A. D., Wingfield, J. C., and Brenowitz, E. A. (2003). Androgens and estrogens induce seasonal-like growth of song nuclei in the adult songbird brain. *J. Neurobiol.* 57, 130–140. doi: 10.1002/neu.10263
355. Tran-Dinh, A., Diallo, D., Delbosc, S., Varela-Perez, L. M., Dang, Q. B., Lapergue, B., et al. (2013). HDL and endothelial protection. *Br. J. Pharmacol.* 169, 493–511. doi: 10.1111/bph.12174
356. Tsutsui, K. (2008). Progesterone biosynthesis and action in the developing neuron.
357. Endocrinology 149, 2757–2761. doi: 10.1210/en.2007-1592
358. Tsutsui, K. (2011). Neurosteroid biosynthesis and function in the brain of domestic birds. *Front. Endocrinol.* 2:37. doi: 10.3389/fendo.2011.00037
359. Tsutsui, K., and Ukena, K. (1999). Neurosteroids in the cerebellar Purkinje neuron and their actions (review). *Int. J. Mol. Med.* 4, 49–56. doi: 10.3892/ijmm.4.1.49 Tsutsui, K., and Yamazaki, T. (1995). Avian neurosteroids. I. Pregnenolone biosynthesis in the quail brain. *Brain Res.* 678, 1–9. doi: 10.1016/0006-8993(95)00116-8
360. Tsutsui, K., Haraguchi, S., Inoue, K., Miyabara, H., Suzuki, S., Ogura, Y., et al. (2009). Identification, biosynthesis, and function of 7alpha-hydroxypregnenolone, a new key neurosteroid controlling locomotor activity, in nonmammalian vertebrates. *Ann. N. Y. Acad. Sci.* 1163, 308–315. doi: 10.1111/j.1749-6632.2009.04426.x
361. Tsutsui, K., Matsunaga, M., Miyabara, H., and Ukena, K. (2006). Neurosteroid biosynthesis in the quail brain: a review. *J. Exp. Zool. A Comp. Exp. Biol.* 305, 733–742. doi: 10.1002/jez.a.302
362. Tsutsui, K., Ukena, K., Takase, M., Kohchi, C., and Lea, R. W. (1999). Neurosteroid biosynthesis in vertebrate brains. *Comp. Biochem. Physiol. C Pharmacol. Toxicol. Endocrinol.* 124, 121–129. doi: 10.1016/S0742-8413(99)00065-1
363. Ukena, K., Honda, Y., Inai, Y., Kohchi, C., Lea, R. W., and Tsutsui, K. (1999). Expression and activity of 3beta-hydroxysteroid dehydrogenase/Delta5-Delta4-isomerase in different regions of the avian brain. *Brain Res.* 818, 536–542. doi: 10.1016/S0006-8993(98)01296-7
364. Vance, J. E., and Hayashi, H. (2010). Formation and function of apolipoprotein E-containing lipoproteins in the nervous system. *Biochim. Biophys. Acta* 1801, 806–818. doi: 10.1016/j.bbalip.2010.02.007
365. Vitali, C., Wellington, C. L., and Calabresi, L. (2014). HDL and cholesterol handling in the brain. *Cardiovasc. Res.* 103, 405–413. doi: 10.1093/cvr/cvu148
366. Wakai, S., and Hirokawa, N. (1978). Development of the blood-brain barrier to horseradish peroxidase in the chick embryo. *Cell Tissue Res.* 195, 195–203. doi: 10.1007/BF00236719
367. Wang, C., Liu, D., Chen, W., Ge, W., Hong, W., Zhu, Y., et al. (2016). Progestin increases the expression of gonadotropins in pituitaries of male zebrafish. *J. Endocrinol.* 230, 143–156. doi: 10.1530/JOE-16-0073
368. Wang, L., Andersson, S., Warner, M., and Gustafsson, J. A. (2003). Estrogen receptor (ER)beta knockout mice reveal a role for ERbeta in migration of cortical neurons in the developing brain. *Proc. Natl. Acad. Sci. U.S.A.* 100, 703–708. doi: 10.1073/pnas.242735799
369. Waters, E. M., Thompson, L. I., Patel, P., Gonzales, A. D., Ye, H. Z., Filardo, E. J., et al. (2015). G-protein-coupled estrogen receptor 1 is anatomically positioned to modulate synaptic plasticity in the mouse hippocampus. *J. Neurosci.* 35, 2384–2397. doi: 10.1523/JNEUROSCI.1298-14.2015
370. Watson, J. T., and Adkins-Regan, E. (1989a). Testosterone implanted in the preoptic area of male Japanese quail must be aromatized to activate copulation. *Horm. Behav.* 23, 432–447. doi: 10.1016/0018-506X(89)90055-X
371. Watson, J. T., and Adkins-Regan, E. (1989b). Activation of sexual behavior by implantation of testosterone propionate and estradiol benzoate into the preoptic area of the male Japanese quail (*Coturnix japonica*). *Horm. Behav.* 23, 251–268. doi: 10.1016/0018-506X(89)90065-2
372. Weger, M., Diotel, N., Weger, B. D., Beil, T., Zaucker, A., Eachus, H. L., et al. (accepted). Expression profiling of the steroidogenic enzymes of glucocorticoid biosynthesis and the fdx1 co-factors in zebrafish. *J. Neuroendocrinol.*
373. Weidenfeld, J., Siegel, R. A., and Chowers, I. (1980). *In vitro* conversion of pregnenolone to progesterone by discrete brain areas of the male rat. *J. Steroid Biochem.* 13, 961–963. doi: 10.1016/0022-4731(80)90171-5
374. Weissman, T., Noctor, S. C., Clinton, B. K., Honig, L. S., and Kriegstein, A. R. (2003). Neurogenic radial glial cells in reptile, rodent and human: from mitosis to migration. *Cereb. Cortex* 13, 550–559. doi: 10.1093/cercor/13.6.550
375. Witt, K. A., and Sandoval, K. E. (2014). Steroids and the blood-brain barrier: therapeutic implications. *Adv. Pharmacol.* 71, 361–390. doi: 10.1016/bs.apha.2014.06.018
376. Xia, Z., Patiño, R., Gale, W. L., Maule, A. G., and Densmore, L. D. (1999).

Cloning, *in vitro* expression, and novel phylogenetic classification of a channel catfish estrogen receptor. *Gen. Comp. Endocrinol.* 113, 360–368. doi: 10.1006/gcen.1999.7196

377. Xiao, H., Deng, M., Yang, B., Hu, Z., and Tang, J. (2017). Pre-treatment of 17beta-estradiol Attenuates cerebral-ischemia-induced blood-brain barrier disruption in aged rats: involvement of antioxidant signaling. *Neuroendocrinology.* doi: 10.1159/000455866
378. Xing, L., Esau, C., and Trudeau, V. L. (2015). Direct regulation of aromatase B expression by 17beta-estradiol and dopamine D1 receptor agonist in adult radial glial cells. *Front. Neurosci.* 9:504. doi: 10.3389/fnins.2015.00310
379. Xing, L., Goswami, M., and Trudeau, V. L. (2014). Radial glial cell: critical functions and new perspective as a steroid synthetic cell. *Gen. Comp. Endocrinol.* 203, 181–185. doi: 10.1016/j.ygcen.2014.03.010
380. Xing, L., Martyniuk, C. J., Esau, C., Da Fonte, D. F., and Trudeau, V. L. (2016). Proteomic profiling reveals dopaminergic regulation of progenitor cell functions of goldfish radial glial cells *in vitro*. *J. Proteomics* 144, 123–132. doi: 10.1016/j.jprot.2016.05.003
381. Yague, J. G., Muñoz, A., de Monasterio-Schrader, P., Defelipe, J. Garcia-Segura, L. M., and Azcoitia, I. (2006). Aromatase expression in the human temporal cortex. *Neuroscience* 138, 389–401. doi: 10.1016/j.neuroscience.2005.11.054
382. Yu, L., Romero, D. G., Gomez-Sanchez, C. E., and Gomez-Sanchez, E. P. (2002). Steroidogenic enzyme gene expression in the human brain. *Mol. Cell. Endocrinol.* 190, 9–17. doi: 10.1016/S0303-7207(02)00041-2
383. Zempo, B., Kanda, S., Okubo, K., Akazome, Y., and Oka, Y. (2013). Anatomical distribution of sex steroid hormone receptors in the brain of female medaka. *J. Comp. Neurol.* 521, 1760–1780. doi: 10.1002/cne.23255
384. Zhang, J., and Liu, Q. (2015). Cholesterol metabolism and homeostasis in the brain. *Protein Cell* 6, 254–264. doi: 10.1007/s13238-014-0131-3
385. Zhang, P., Xie, M. Q., Ding, Y. Q., Liao, M., Qi, S. S., Chen, S. X., et al. (2015). Allopregnanolone enhances the neurogenesis of midbrain dopaminergic neurons in APPswe/PSEN1 mice. *Neuroscience* 290, 214–226. doi: 10.1016/j.neuroscience.2015.01.019
386. Zhang, W., Cheng, J., Vagnerova, K., Ivashkova, Y., Young, J., Cornea, A., et al. (2014). Effects of androgens on early post-ischemic neurogenesis in mice. *Transl. Stroke Res.* 5, 301–311. doi: 10.1007/s12975-013-0298-6
387. Zhang, Y., Wang, H., Qin, F., Liu, S., Wu, T., Li, M., et al. (2012). Molecular characterization of estrogen receptor genes in loach *Paramisgurnus dabryanus* and their expression upon 17alpha-ethinylestradiol exposure in juveniles. *Gen. Comp. Endocrinol.* 178, 194–205. doi: 10.1016/j.ygcen.2012. 06.004
388. Zhang, Z., Yang, R., Zhou, R., Li, L., Sokabe, M., and Chen, L. (2010). Progesterone promotes the survival of newborn neurons in the dentate gyrus of adult male mice. *Hippocampus* 20, 402–412. doi: 10.1002/hipo.20642
389. Zhao, Y., Wang, J., Liu, C., Jiang, C., Zhao, C., and Zhu, Z. (2011). Progesterone influences postischemic synaptogenesis in the CA1 region of the hippocampus in rats. *Synapse* 65, 880–891. doi: 10.1002/syn.20915
390. Zhu, Y., Bond, J., and Thomas, P. (2003). Identification, classification, and partial characterization of genes in humans and other vertebrates homologous to a fish membrane progestin receptor. *Proc. Natl. Acad. Sci. U.S.A.* 100, 2237–2242. doi: 10.1073/pnas.0436133100
391. Zhu, Y., Liu, D., Shaner, Z. C., Chen, S., Hong, W., and Stellwag, E. J. (2015). Nuclear progestin receptor (pgr) knockouts in zebrafish demonstrate role for pgr in ovulation but not in rapid non-genomic steroid mediated meiosis resumption. *Front. Endocrinol.* 6:37. doi: 10.3389/fendo.2015. 00037
392. Zuloaga, D. G., Yahn, S. L., Pang, Y., Quihuis, A. M., Oyola, M. G., Reyna, A., et al. (2012). Distribution and estrogen regulation of membrane progesterone receptor-beta in the female rat brain. *Endocrinology* 153, 4432–4443. doi: 10.1210/en.2012-1469
393. Zwain, I. H., and Yen, S. S. (1999). Neurosteroidogenesis in astrocytes, oligodendrocytes, and neurons of cerebral cortex of rat brain. *Endocrinology* 140, 3843–3852. doi: 10.1210/endo.140.8.6907

3

Src Kinase Dependent Rapid Non-Genomic Modulation of Hippocampal Spinogenesis Induced by Androgen and Estrogen

Mika Soma[1], *Jonghyuk Kim*[1], *Asami Kato*[1] *and Suguru Kawato*[1,2,3*]

[1] *Department of Cognitive Neuroscience, Faculty of Pharma-Science, Teikyo University, Itabashi, Japan,* [2] *Department of Urology, Graduate School of Medicine, Juntendo University, Hongo, Japan,* [3] *Department of Biophysics and Life Sciences, Graduate School of Arts and Sciences, The University of Tokyo, Meguro, Japan*

Correspondence:
Suguru Kawato
kawato@bio.c.u-tokyo.ac.jp

Dendritic spine is a small membranous protrusion from a neuron's dendrite that typically receives input from an axon terminal at the synapse. Memories are stored in synapses which consist of spines and presynapses. Rapid modulations of dendritic spines induced by hippocampal sex steroids, including dihydrotestosterone (DHT), testosterone (T), and estradiol (E2), are essential for synaptic plasticity. Molecular mechanisms underlying the rapid non-genomic modulation through synaptic receptors of androgen (AR) and estrogen (ER) as well as its downstream kinase signaling, however, have not been well understood. We investigated the possible involvement of Src tyrosine kinase in rapid changes of dendritic spines in response to androgen and estrogen, including DHT, T, and E2, using hippocampal slices from adult male rats. We found that the treatments with DHT (10 nM), T (10 nM), and E2 (1 nM) increased the total density of spines by ~1.22 to 1.26-fold within 2 h using super resolution confocal imaging of Lucifer Yellow-injected CA1 pyramidal neurons. We examined also morphological changes of spines in order to clarify differences between three sex steroids. From spine head diameter analysis, DHT increased middle- and large-head spines, whereas T increased small- and middle-head spines, and E2 increased small-head spines. Upon application of Src tyrosine kinase inhibitor, the spine increases induced through DHT, T, and E2 treatments were completely blocked. These results imply that Src kinase is essentially involved in sex steroid-induced non-genomic modulation of the spine density and morphology. These results also suggest that rapid effects of exogenously applied androgen and estrogen can occur in steroid-depleted conditions, including "acute" hippocampal slices and the hippocampus of gonadectomized animals.

Keywords: androgen, estrogen, Src kinase, spine, hippocampus, non-genomic, synapse

INTRODUCTION

Accumulating evidence over the past two decades supports the conclusion that some sex steroid responses in the brain involve rapid non-genomic mechanisms (Mukai et al., 2010) in addition to slow/genomic actions (Gould et al., 1990; Woolley et al., 1990; Woolley and McEwen, 1992; MacLusky et al., 2005). In rat and mouse hippocampus, androgen, and estrogen, including testosterone (T), dihydrotestosterone (DHT), and estradiol (E2), induced rapid modulation of dendritic spines, which occurred between 30 and 120 min after the application (MacLusky et al., 2005; Murakami et al., 2006; Mukai et al., 2007). Sex steroid-induced rapid effects were also observed in electrophysiological investigations, such as the long-term potentiation (LTP) (Foy et al., 1999; Bi et al., 2000; Grassi et al., 2011; Ooishi et al., 2012b; Hasegawa et al., 2015). E2-induced rapid synaptic modulation occurred not only *in vitro* but also *in vivo* conditions in the hippocampus (MacLusky et al., 2005) (Luine and Frankfurt, 2012; Luine, 2014). The rapid signaling of E2 may depend on multiple kinases, including mitogen-activated protein kinase (MAPK) and phosphoinositide 3-kinase (PI3K) in the hippocampus (Bi et al., 2000, 2001; Znamensky et al., 2003; Mannella and Brinton, 2006; Mukai et al., 2010; Luine, 2014; Tuscher et al., 2016). The contribution of many other essential serine/threonine kinases have also been studied. These important kinases are LIM domain kinase (LIMK), protein kinase A (PKA), and protein kinase C (PKC) all of which are essential for regulation of the synaptic plasticity (Frick, 2015; Hasegawa et al., 2015; Tuscher et al., 2016).

On the other hand, androgen (T and DHT)-induced rapid effects on synaptic modulation in the hippocampus or other brain regions have not been extensively investigated (Foradori et al., 2008; Hajszan et al., 2008), while rapid effects of androgen were extensively studied in prostate cancer cells and gonadal cells (Migliaccio et al., 2000; Cheng et al., 2007). We tried to examine molecular mechanisms of rapid effects in the hippocampus, and showed that DHT and T induced rapid increase of CA1 dendritic spines via non-genomic signaling, including activation of several serine/threonine kinases (including MAPK, LIMK, PKA, PKC; Hatanaka et al., 2015). Also in CA3 region, T, and DHT rapidly increased thorns in stratum lucidum via MAPK and PKC, but not via PKA (Hatanaka et al., 2009).

Rapid synaptic action may require new arrangement of sex steroid receptor systems. In the hippocampus, androgen receptor (AR), and estrogen receptor (ER), classic nuclear steroid receptors, appear to be primarily located in the glutamatergic neurons (Simerly et al., 1990; Clancy et al., 1992; Brown et al., 1995; Kerr et al., 1995; Mukai et al., 2007). AR and ER are located not only in the cytoplasm and the nuclei but also within dendritic spines (Tabori et al., 2005; Mukai et al., 2007; Hatanaka et al., 2015). Therefore, classic receptors AR and ER, localized in the synaptic membrane, could act as membrane receptors, triggering rapid effects of sex steroids as indicated from many recent investigations (Milner et al., 2005; Mukai et al., 2007, 2010; Pedram et al., 2007; Hojo et al., 2008; Hasegawa et al., 2015; Levin and Hammes, 2016). Synaptic membrane localization of these receptors might be accomplished via palmitoylation of receptors (Pedram et al., 2007; Levin and Hammes, 2016)

Since adult hippocampus locally synthesizes androgen and estrogen (Hojo et al., 2004), their levels in the hippocampus are key factors for action through synaptic AR and ER. Mass-spectrometric analysis revealed that the levels of androgen and estrogen in freshly isolated male hippocampus are higher than those in plasma (Hojo et al., 2009). The levels of male hippocampal sex steroids were ~17 nM for T, ~7 nM for DHT, and ~8 nM for E2 (Hojo et al., 2009), which levels are much higher than that of circulating T (~15 nM), DHT (~0.6 nM), and E2 (~0.01 nM). Importantly, after preparation of "acute" hippocampal slices, sex steroid levels were considerably decreased to below 0.5 nM due to recovery incubation in artificial cerebrospinal fluid (ACSF) (Hojo et al., 2009, 2011; Ooishi et al., 2012a,b; Hatanaka et al., 2015). Therefore, exogenous application of sex steroids may help to elevate steroid levels back to the *in vivo* situation.

We here investigated the possible involvement of Src tyrosine kinase in rapid spine modulation of DHT, T, and E2, with considering similarity and difference in signal pathways between DHT, T, and E2 in male rats. Although Src kinase was known to be activated by androgen and E2 in prostate and breast cancer cells (Migliaccio et al., 1996, 2000), its role in hippocampal synaptic plasticity has not been well-documented.

MATERIALS AND METHODS

Animals

Young adult male Wistar rats (12 week old, 320–360 g) were purchased from Tokyo Experimental Animals Supply (Japan). All animals were maintained under a 12 h light/12 h dark cycle and free access to food and water. The experimental procedure of this research was approved by the Committee for Animal Research of Teikyo University.

Chemicals

DHT, T and PP2 were purchased from Sigma-Aldrich (USA). Estradiol was from Wako Pure Chemicals (Japan). Lucifer Yellow was obtained from Molecular Probes (USA).

Slice Preparation

Adult male rats were deeply anesthetized by isoflurane and decapitated. Immediately after decapitation, the brain was removed from the skull and placed in ice-cold oxygenated (95% O_2, 5% CO_2) artificial cerebrospinal fluid (ACSF) containing (in mM): 124 NaCl, 5 KCl, 1.25 NaH_2PO_4, 2 $MgSO_4$, 2 $CaCl_2$, 22 $NaHCO_3$, and 10 D-glucose (all from Wako); pH was set at 7.4. The hippocampus was then dissected and 400 μm thick transverse slices to the long axis, from the middle third of the hippocampus, were prepared with a vibratome (Dosaka, Japan). These slices were "fresh" slices without ACSF incubation. Slices were then incubated in oxygenated ACSF for 2 h (slice recovery processes) in order to obtain widely used "acute slices."

Imaging and Analysis of Dendritic Spine Density and Morphology

Drug Treatments and Current Injection of Lucifer Yellow

The "acute" slices (used worldwide) were incubated for 2 h with 10 nM DHT, 10 nM T, or 1 nM E2, together with 4-amino-5-(4-chlorophenyl)-7-(dimethylethyl)pyrazolo[3,4-d]pyrimidine (PP2), a Src kinase inhibitor. Slices were then fixed with 4% paraformaldehyde in PBS at 4°C overnight. Neurons within slices were visualized by an injection of Lucifer Yellow (Molecular Probes, USA) under Nikon E600FN microscope (Japan) equipped with a C2400-79H infrared camera (Hamamatsu

Photonics, Japan) and with a 40× water immersion lens (Nikon, Japan).

Current injection was performed with glass electrode filled with 4% Lucifer Yellow for 2 min, using Axopatch 200B (Axon Instruments, USA). Approximately two neurons within a depth of 100–200 μm from the surface of a slice were injected with Lucifer Yellow (Duan et al., 2002).

Confocal Laser Microscopic Imaging and Analysis

The imaging was performed from sequential z-series scans with super-resolution confocal microscope (Zeiss LSM880; Carl Zeiss, Germany) using Airy Scan Mode, at high zoom (× 3.0) with a 63 × oil immersion lens, NA 1.4. For Lucifer Yellow, the excitation and emission wavelengths were 458 and 515 nm, respectively. For analysis of spines, three-dimensional image was reconstructed from ~30 sequential z-series sections of every 0.45 μm. The applied zoom factor (×3.0) yielded 23 pixels per 1 μm. The confocal lateral resolution was ~0.14 μm. The z-axis resolution was ~0.40 μm. Our resolution limits were regarded to be sufficient to allow the determination of the head diameter of spines in addition to the density of spines. Confocal images were deconvoluted with the measured point spread function using Processing Mode of LSM880.

The density of spines as well as the head diameter were analyzed with Spiso-3D (automated software calculating mathematically geometrical parameters of spines) developed by Bioinformatics Project of Kawato's group (Mukai et al., 2011). Spiso-3D has an equivalent capacity with Neurolucida (MicroBrightField, USA), furthermore, Spiso-3D considerably reduces human errors and experimenter labor. The single apical dendrite was analyzed separately. The spine density was calculated from the number of spines along secondary dendrites having a total length of 40–60 μm. These dendrites were present within the stratum radiatum, between 100 and 200 μm from the soma. Spine shapes were classified into three categories as follows. (1) A small-head spine, whose head diameter is smaller than 0.4 μm. (2) A middle-head spine, which has 0.4–0.5 μm spine head. (3) A large-head spine, whose head diameter is larger than 0.5 μm. These three categories were useful to distinguish different responses upon kinase inhibitor application. Small-, middle-, and large-head spines probably have different number of α-amino-3-hydroxy-5-methyl-4-isoxazolepropionic acid (AMPA) receptors, and therefore these three types of spines might have different efficiency in memory storage. The number of AMPA receptors (including GluR1 subunits) in the spine increases as the size of postsynapse increases, whereas the number of N-methyl-D-aspartate (NMDA) receptors (including NR2B subunits) might be relatively constant (Shinohara et al., 2008). Because the majority of spines (>93–95%) had a distinct head, and stubby spines and filopodia did not contribute much to overall changes, we analyzed spines having a distinct head.

Statistical Analysis

Drug-treated dendrite images were used for spine analysis, and typical images were shown in **Figures 1–4**. Each dendrite has ~50 μm in length including ~50 spines. For statistical analysis, we employed two-way ANOVA, followed by Tukey-Kramer multiple comparison's test. For each steroid application analysis, we used ~50 dendrites with 2,300–2,700 spines obtained from 3 rats, 12 slices, 30 neurons. For control dendrite analysis without steroid application, we used 80 dendrites with ~4,000 spines from 6 rats, 24 slices, 50 neurons.

RESULTS

We investigated the involvement of Src protein kinase in the modulation effects of DHT, T, and E2 on spinogenesis. Dendritic spine imaging was performed for Lucifer Yellow-injected glutamatergic neurons in acute hippocampal slices of male rats. We analyzed secondary branches of the apical dendrites located 100–200 μm distant from the pyramidal cell body around the middle of the stratum radiatum of CA1 region.

Analysis of Spine Head Diameter as Well as the Total Spine Density

The morphological changes in spine head diameter induced after 2 h treatments of drugs were analyzed. Since observing the total spine density cannot describe well the complicated different kinase effects, the changes in spine head diameter distribution were also analyzed. Because the majority of spines (>93–95%) had distinct heads and necks, and stubby spines and filopodia did not contribute much to overall changes (<5–7%), we analyzed spines having distinct heads. We classified these spines with clear heads into three categories based on their head diameter, e.g., 0.2–0.4 μm as small-head spines, 0.4–0.5 μm as middle-head spines, and larger than 0.5 μm as large-head spines.

Statistical analyses based on classification of the spines into three categories were performed. In control slices (without sex steroids supplementation), the spine density was 0.52 spines/μm for small-head spines, 0.30 spines/μm for middle-head spines, and 0.20 spines/μm for large-head spines (**Figure 1**). In order to investigate intracellular signaling pathways of kinases involved in the sex steroid-induced spinogenesis, here, we analyzed the contribution of Src protein kinase by blocking Src kinase with a selective inhibitor, PP2.

DHT Effects and Src Kinase Blocking

The treatments with DHT and PP2 induced significant changes in the total spine density ($F = 20.46$, $p < 0.0001$, two-way ANOVA). After 2 h treatment with 10 nM DHT, the total spine density was significantly increased to 1.26 spines/μm from the control density of 1.04 spines/μm ($p < 0.0001$ for control vs. DHT, Tukey–Kramer multiple comparison's test) (see **Figure 1**). This increase in the total spine density was suppressed by blocking of Src kinase through co-incubation of 10 nM DHT and 10 μM PP2 ($p < 0.0001$ for DHT vs. PP2+ DHT, Tukey–Kramer multiple comparison's test).

From spine head diameter analysis, after 2 h treatments with DHT, the density of middle- and large-head spines significantly increased ($p = 0.0304$ for middle-head and $p < 0.0001$ for large-head, for control vs. DHT, Tukey–Kramer), while the density of small-head spines was not significantly altered. Blocking Src kinase by PP2 abolished the DHT effects on the dendritic spine densities, by decreasing the density of the middle-head spines

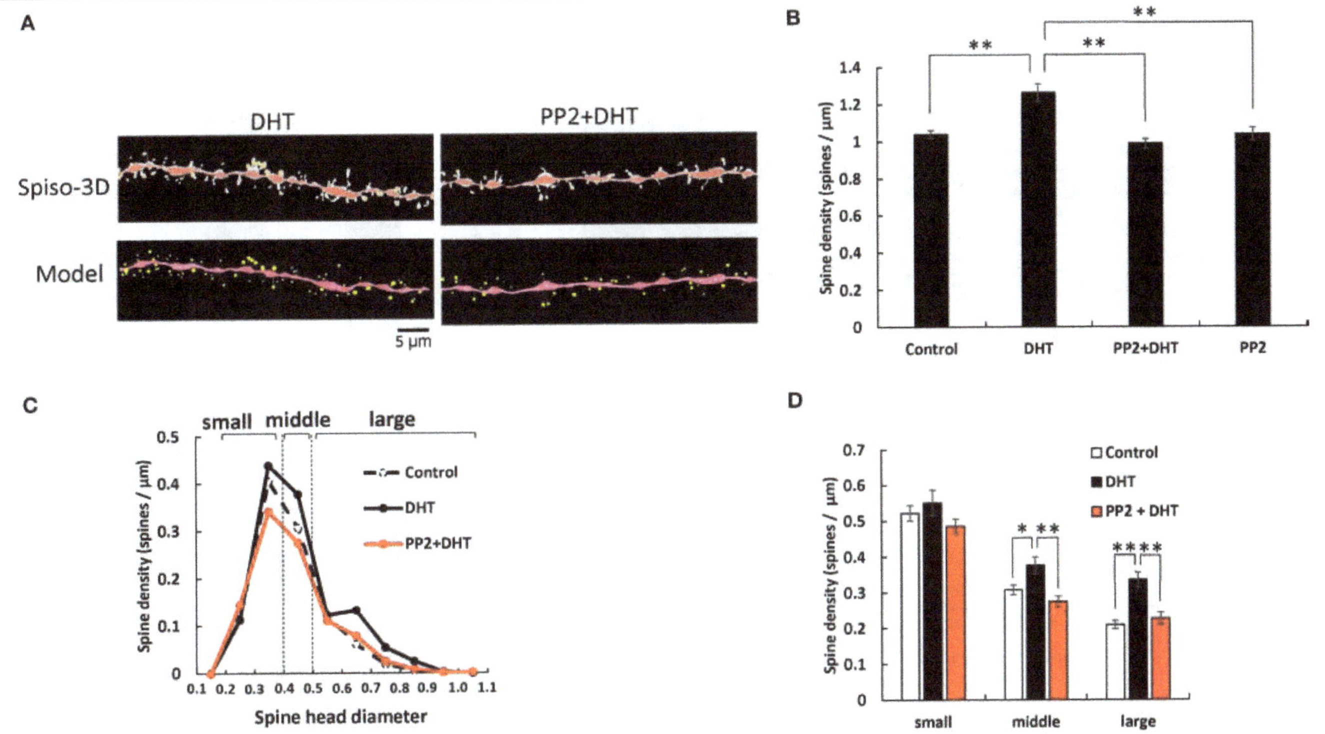

FIGURE 1 | Effects of Src kinase blocker (PP2) on DHT-induced spine increase and change in morphology in hippocampal slices. **(A)** Spines were analyzed along the secondary dendrites of pyramidal neurons in the stratum radiatum of CA1 neurons. Dendrite after DHT-treatment for 2 h (DHT) and dendrite after DHT plus PP2 treatment for 2 h (PP2+DHT). (Spiso) shows the image of dendrite and spines analyzed with Spiso-3D software. Maximal intensity projections onto XY plane is shown. Traced dendrite is shown in red color and spines are indicated in yellow color. (Model) shows 3 dimensional model illustration of (Spiso) image. Bar, 5 μm. **(B)** Effect of treatments by DHT or PP2 on the total spine density in CA1 neurons. Vertical axis is the average number of spines per 1 μm of dendrite. A 2 h treatment in ACSF without drugs (Control), with 10 nM DHT (DHT), with 10 nM DHT and 10 μM PP2 (PP2 + DHT), and with PP2 only (PP2). **(C)** Histogram of spine head diameters after a 2 h treatment in ACSF without drugs (Control, black dashed line), with 10 nM DHT (black line), with 10 nM DHT and 10 μM PP2 (red line). Spines were classified into three categories depending on their head diameter, e.g., 0.2–0.4 μm as small-head spines, 0.4–0.5 μm as middle-head spines, and larger than 0.5 μm as large-head spines. Vertical axis is the number of spines per 1 μm of dendrite. **(D)** Density of three subtypes of spines. Abbreviations are same as in **(B)**. Vertical axis is the number of spines per 1 μm of dendrite. From left to right, small-head spines (small), middle-head spines (middle), and large-head spines (large) type. ACSF without drugs (Control, open column), DHT (black column), PP2 + DHT (red column). Vertical axis is the number of spines per 1 μm of dendrite. Results are represented as mean ± SEM. Statistical significance yielded $^{*}P < 0.05$, $^{**}P < 0.01$ vs. DHT sample. For DHT, PP2+DHT, and PP2 only treatments, we investigated, 50 dendrites with 2,300–2,700 spines from 3 rats, 12 slices, and 30 neurons. For control, we used 80 dendrites with ~4,000 spines from 6 rats, 24 slices and 50 neurons.

and large-head spines ($p = 0.0016$ for middle and $p = 0.0004$ for large-head, for DHT vs. PP2+ DHT, Tukey–Kramer), while significant changes in the small-head spines did not occur (**Figures 1B–D**).

Note that, only PP2 did not significantly affect the total spine density, implying that the observed inhibitory effects are not due to simple non-specific effects by blockers (**Figure 1B**).

T Effects and Src Kinase Blocking

T and PP2 treatments induced significant changes in the total spine density ($F = 25.68$, $p < 0.0001$, two-way ANOVA). The total spine density was significantly increased to 1.31 spines/μm through 2 h incubation with 10 nM T ($p < 0.0001$ for control vs. T, Tukey–Kramer) (see **Figure 2**). This increase in the total spine density was suppressed by blocking Src kinase through co-incubation of 10 nM T and 10 μM PP2 ($p < 0.0001$ for T vs. PP2+T, Tukey–Kramer) (**Figure 2B**).

From spine head diameter analysis, upon treatments with T, the density of small- and middle-head spines significantly increased ($p = 0.0004$ for small-head and $p = 0.0005$ for middle-head, Tukey–Kramer), while the density of large-head spines was not significantly altered. Inhibition of Src kinase abolished the effect of T on the spine density, by decreasing the density of small-and middle-head spines ($p = 0.0248$ for small-head and $p < 0.0001$ for middle-head, Tukey–Kramer), while there were no significant changes in large-head spines (**Figures 2B–D**).

E2 Effects and Src Kinase Blocking

E2 and PP2 treatments induced significant changes in the total spine density ($F = 19.71$, $p < 0.0001$, two-way ANOVA). After 2 h treatments with 1 nM E2, the total spine density was significantly increased to 1.29 spines/μm ($p < 0.0001$ for control vs. E2, Tukey–Kramer) (**Figure 3**). This increase in the total spine density was suppressed by blocking of Src kinase through

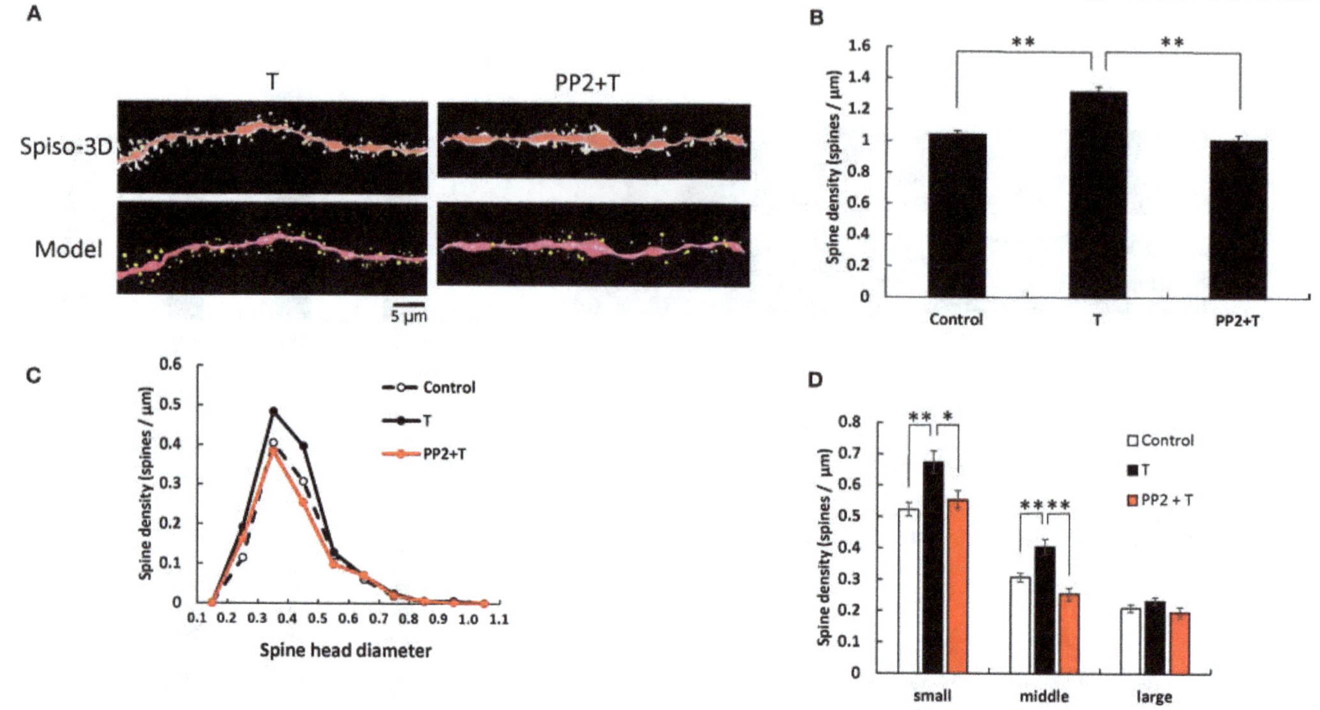

FIGURE 2 | Effects of Src kinase blocker on T-induced spine increase and change in morphology in hippocampal slices. **(A)** Spines were analyzed along the secondary dendrites of pyramidal neurons in the stratum radiatum of CA1 neurons as in **Figure 1**. Dendrite after T-treatment for 2 h (T) and dendrite after T plus PP2 treatment for 2 h (PP2+T). (Spiso) shows the image of dendrite and spines analyzed with Spiso-3D software. Maximal intensity projections onto XY plane is shown. Traced dendrite is shown in red color and spines are indicated in yellow color. (Model) shows 3 dimensional model illustration of (Spiso) image. Bar, 5 μm. **(B)** Effect of treatments by T or PP2 on the total spine density in CA1 neurons. Vertical axis is the average number of spines per 1 μm of dendrite. A 2 h treatment in ACSF without drugs (Control), with 10 nM T (T), with 10 nM T and 10 μM PP2 (PP2 + T). **(C)** Histogram of spine head diameters after a 2 h treatment in ACSF without drugs (Control, black dashed line), with 10 nM T (black line), with 10 nM T and 10 μM PP2 (PP2 + T, red line). **(D)** Density of three subtypes of spines. Abbreviations are same as in **(B)**. From left to right, small-head spines (small), middle-head spines (middle), and large-head spines (large) type. ACSF without drugs (Control, open column), T (black column), PP2 + T (red column). Results are represented as mean ± SEM. Statistical significance yielded $^{*}P < 0.05$, $^{**}P < 0.01$ vs. T sample. For T and PP2 + T treatments, we investigated 50 dendrites with 2300–2700 spines from 3 rats, 12 slices, 30 neurons. For control, we used 80 dendrites with ~4,000 spines from 6 rats, 24 slices, and 50 neurons.

co-incubation of 1 nM E2 and 10 μM PP2 ($p < 0.0001$ for E2 vs. PP2+ E2, Tukey–Kramer) (**Figure 3A**).

From spine head diameter analysis, treatments with E2 significantly increased the density of small-head spines ($p = 0.0079$, Tukey–Kramer), while the density of middle- and large-head spines was not significantly altered. Blocking Src kinase by PP2 suppressed the effects of E2, by decreasing the density of small-head spines ($p = 0.0075$, Tukey–Kramer), while significant change was not observed in middle- and large-head spines (**Figures 3B–D**).

Improvement of Image Analysis With Super Resolution Confocal Microscopy

Airy scan mode of LSM880 super resolution confocal microscopy is equipped with 32 channel area detectors with honeycomb arrangement in the back of confocal pinhole. With these detectors we can directly measure the main part of the point spread function with which we perform deconvolution of confocal images. Therefore, the resultant final spine images were much clearer particularly for neck images with super resolution confocal microscopic imaging (**Figure 4A**) than those with conventional confocal microscopic imaging (**Figure 4B**) which uses blind deconvolution method with AutoDeblur software (AutoQuant, USA). Particularly necks of spines were clearly observed in Airy Scan mode, while sometimes spine heads spatially isolated from dendrites, without visible necks which connect spine heads to the dendritic shafts, were observed with conventional confocal microscopic imaging (**Figure 4B**). Identification of necks is critical in classification of spine types between stubby type (without neck) and spines with necks (thin and mushroom types).

We quantitatively compared control dendritic spines (without steroid supplementation) obtained from super resolution confocal microscopic analysis (LSM880) with those obtained from conventional confocal microscopic analysis (with Zeiss PASCAL confocal microscopy) (Hasegawa et al., 2015). We observed no significant difference in spine densities within experimental error concerning not only the total spine density but also the head diameter distribution, between these two confocal microscopic analyses. (**Figures 4C–E**). However, the ratio of large-head spine population and middle-head

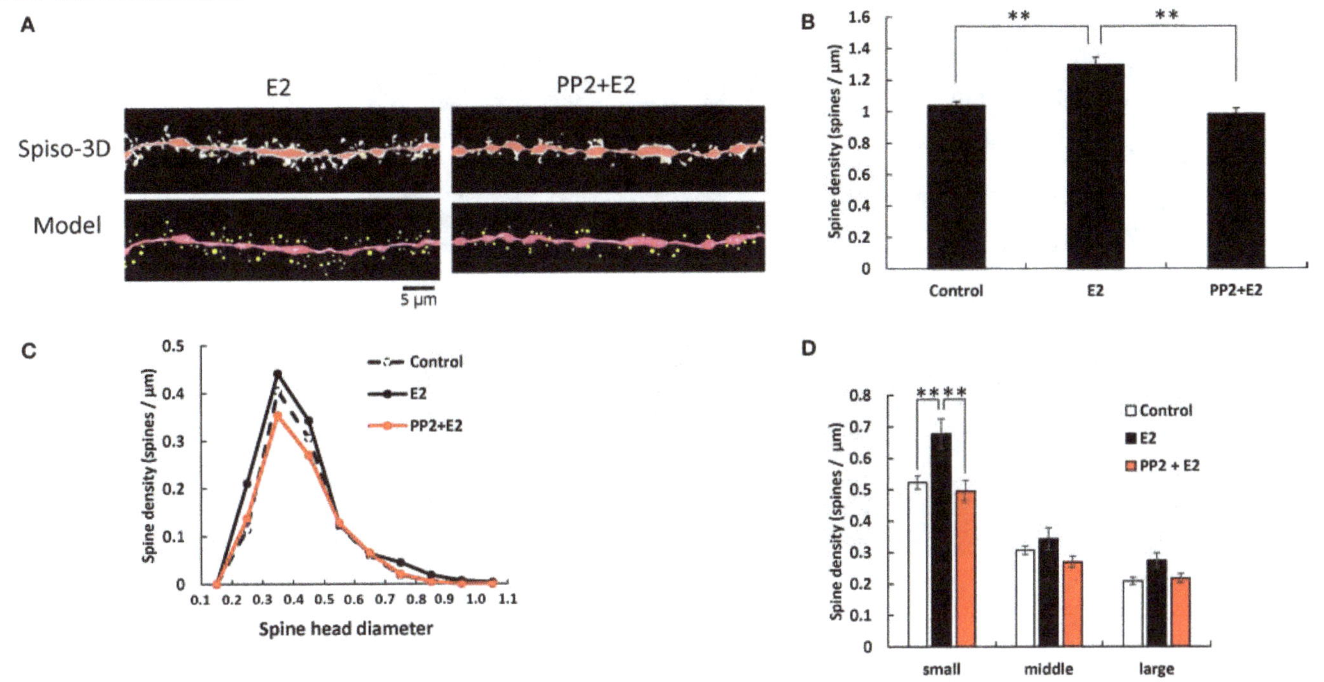

FIGURE 3 | Effects of Src kinase blocker on E2-induced spine increase and change in morphology. **(A)** Spines were analyzed along the secondary dendrites of pyramidal neurons in the stratum radiatum of CA1 neurons as in **Figure 1**. Dendrite after E2-treatment for 2 h (E2) and dendrite after E2 plus PP2 treatment for 2 h (PP2+E2). (Spiso) shows the image of dendrite and spines analyzed with Spiso-3D software. Maximal intensity projections onto XY plane is shown. Traced dendrite is shown in red color and spines are indicated in yellow color. (Model) shows 3 dimensional model illustration of (Spiso) image. Bar, 5 μm. **(B)** Effect of treatments by E2 and PP2 on the total spine density. Vertical axis is the average number of spines per 1 μm of dendrite. A 2 h treatment in ACSF without drugs (Control), with 1 nM E2 (E2), and with 1 nM E2 and 10 μM PP2 (PP2 + E2). **(C)** Histogram of spine head diameters. A 2 h treatment in ACSF without drugs (Control, dashed line), with E2 (black line), with E2 + PP2 (red line). **(D)** Density of three subtypes of spines. From left to right, small-head spines (small), middle-head spines (middle), and large-head spines (large) type. In each group, control (open column), E2 (black column), and PP2+E2 (red column). Results are represented as mean ± SEM. Statistical significance was defined as $^*p < 0.05$, $^{**}p < 0.01$ vs. E2 sample. For E2 and PP2+E2 treatments, we investigated 50 dendrites with 2300–2700 spines from 3 rats, 12 slices, and 30 neurons. For control, we used 80 dendrites with ~4,000 spines from 6 rats, 24 slices, and 50 neurons.

spine population was little bit higher in super resolution than conventional confocal analysis.

DISCUSSION

We consider and discuss about Src kinase dependent signaling mechanisms in non-genomic modulation of sex steroid-induced dendritic spinogenesis.

Src Kinase-Mediated Signaling With Sex Steroids Treatments in Peripheral Tissues

Involvement of Src kinase (nonreceptor tyrosine kinase) in non-genomic rapid signaling upon androgen and estrogen stimulation has been extensively investigated in non-neuronal cells, including prostate cancer cells (e.g., LNCaP cells) (Migliaccio et al., 2000), breast cancer cells (e.g., MCF-7 cells) (Migliaccio et al., 1996), epithelial cells (Castoria et al., 2004), and Sertoli cells (Cheng et al., 2007).

Both T and E2 induced complex formation of AR, ERβ and Src kinase in LNCaP (Migliaccio et al., 2000). E2-induced complex formation of ERα with Src kinase was observed in MCF-7 cells (Migliaccio et al., 2000). Src kinase phosphorylated Erk MAPK in MCF-7 cells (Migliaccio et al., 1996). Upon T stimulation in Sertoli cells, association of AR with Src kinase occurred, leading to activation of Erk MAPK (Cheng et al., 2007).

Taken together, upon stimulation of T or E2, AR or ER may form complex with Src kinase, leading to activation of MAPK in prostate cancer cells, breast cancer cells, or other gonadal tissues (Foradori et al., 2008). Androgen-induced Ca influx may be a trigger of these events in these cells (Rusanescu et al., 1995; Foradori et al., 2008). Src kinase activation is induced by dephosphorylation of tyrosine residue, and this might occur within complexes of AR, ER, and Src kinase, via AR binding to SH3 domain or via ER binding to SH2 domain (Migliaccio et al., 2000). Note that Src kinase is anchored to the membrane via myristoylation (**Figure 5**; Kim et al., 2017).

Src Kinase-Mediated Signaling With Sex Steroid Treatments in Neurons

We observed association of Src kinase, Erk MAPK, and ERα with post synaptic density (PSD), using Western blotting of PSD fractions prepared from male rat hippocampi, implying the spine membrane binding of Src kinase, MAPK, and ER (Mukai et al., 2007). Therefore, from the current results in combination

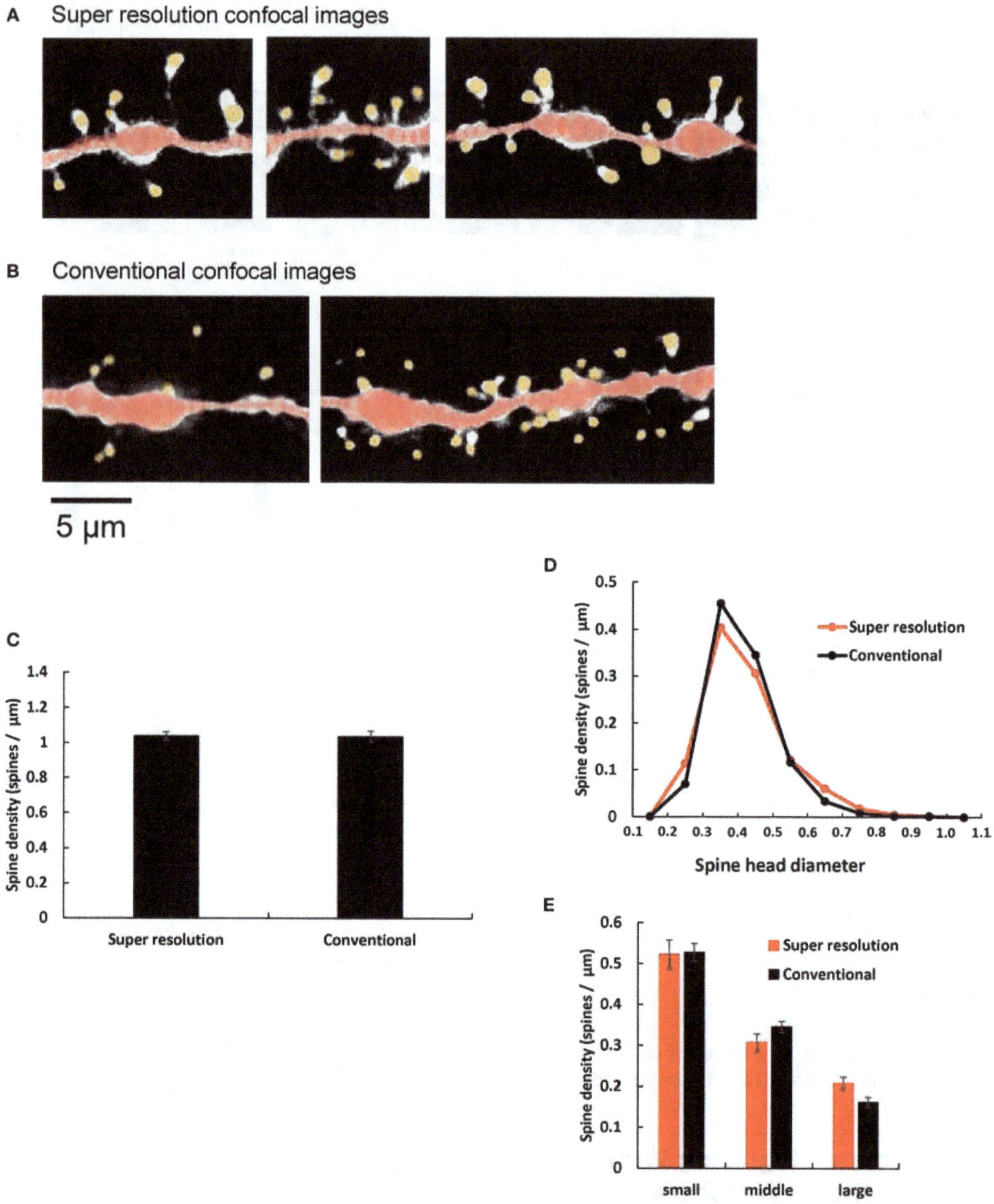

FIGURE 4 | Comparison of spine images obtained by super resolution confocal microscopy and conventional confocal microscopy. **(A,B)** Typical dendrites with spines of CA1 neurons are shown after analysis with Spiso-3D software. Maximal intensity projections onto XY plane are shown. Traced dendrites are shown in red color and spines are indicated in yellow color. Images are obtained with **(A)** Super resolution confocal microscopy and **(B)** Conventional confocal microscopy. Bar, 5 μm. **(C)** Comparison of the total spine density of control dendrites (without steroid supplementation) obtained with super resolution confocal microscopy (Super resolution) and Conventional confocal microscopy (Conventional). Vertical axis is the average number of spines per 1 μm of dendrite. **(D)** Histogram of spine head diameters of control. Super resolution (red line), and Conventional (black line). **(E)** Density of three subtypes of spines of control dendrites. From left to right, small-head spines (small), middle-head spines (middle), and large-head spines (large). In each group, Super resolution (red column), and Conventional (black column). Abbreviations are same as in **(C)**. Results are represented as mean ± SEM. No statistical significance was observed. For Super resolution, we investigated 80 dendrites with ~4,000 spines, 6 rats, 24 slices, and 50 neurons. For Conventional, we used 40 dendrites with ~2,000 spines from 4 rats, 10 slices, and 21 neurons.

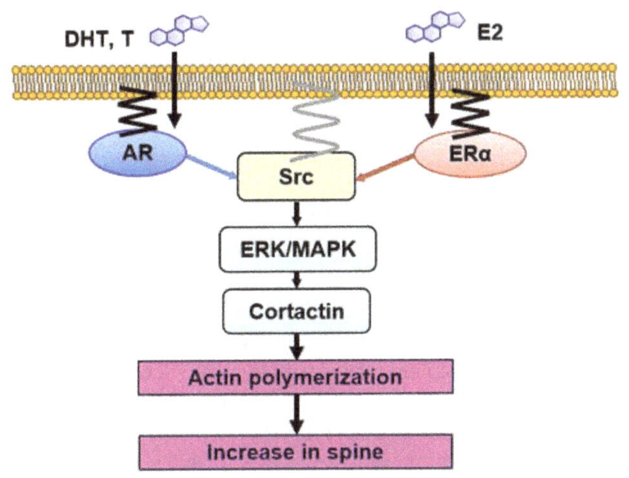

FIGURE 5 | Model illustration of Src kinase-mediated signaling in non-genomic effects of sex steroids on spinogenesis. DHT, T and E2 bind to synaptic receptors (AR and ER) within spines. Then, Src kinase may form complex with AR and ER, resulting in activation of Src kinase. Erk MAPK is then activated, leading to phosphorylation of cortactin, resulting in actin polymerization and new spine formation. AR and ER are anchored to the membrane via palmitoylation. Src kinase is localized to the membrane via myristoylation.

with the results from endocrine tissues (see section Src Kinase-Mediated Signaling With Sex Steroids Treatments in Peripheral Tissues), we can speculate that Src kinase-mediated signaling, triggered by sex steroids in hippocampal spines, may occur as follows: upon T, DHT, and E2 binding to their synaptic receptors (AR and ERα), these receptors activate Src kinase via conformational change of Src, leading to phosphorylation of Erk MAPK (**Figure 5**).

Until recently, however, inadequate amounts of investigations had been accumulated for Src kinase signaling upon androgen and estrogen stimulation in central nervous systems. In one of a few reports, Src tyrosine kinase involvement was suggested from PP2-induced suppression of E2-enhanced LTP in acute hippocampal slices (Bi et al., 2000). Chronic DHT-treatment for 24 h elevated Ca concentrations in the endoplasmic reticulum of primary hippocampal neurons, but this might not directly contribute to non-genomic actions (Foradori et al., 2007).

On the other hand, downstream signaling of Src kinase, from MAPK to spine increase, has been extensively studied in neurons (see section MAPK-Mediated Signaling, Downstream of Src Kinase in Spinogenesis).

MAPK-Mediated Signaling, Downstream of Src Kinase in Spinogenesis

Erk MAPK (serine/threonine kinase) was involved in the rapid non-genomic effects on CA1 hippocampal spinogenesis through DHT, T, and E2 treatments (Hasegawa et al., 2015; Hatanaka et al., 2015). These results were obtained by using MAPK inhibitors, U0126 and PD98059. E2-induced rapid CA1 spinogenesis via Erk MAPK was found in the male and female hippocampus (Mukai et al., 2007; Phan et al., 2011; Luine and Frankfurt, 2012). *In vivo* E2 infusion induced CA1 spinogenesis as well as phosphorylation of Erk MAPK in female ovariectomized (OVX) mouse hippocampus (Frick et al., 2015; Tuscher et al., 2016). T and DHT individually phosphorylated Erk MAPK within 1 h, leading to neuroprotection in primary cultured hippocampal neurons (Nguyen et al., 2005).

Since both steroid receptors (AR and ER), Src kinase and MAPK are present in dendritic spines, an efficient coupling between these proteins could occur in spines, resulting in activation of Src kinase, followed by activation of Erk MAPK (**Figure 5**) (Milner et al., 2005; Tabori et al., 2005; Mukai et al., 2007; Hojo et al., 2008; Hatanaka et al., 2015).

In spinogenesis, the target of Erk MAPK may be cortactin. Erk MAPK phosphorylates cortactin which is associated with actin (MacQueen et al., 2003). Cortactin interacts with both F-actin and actin-related protein (Arp) 2/3 complex as well as scaffold protein Shank (Weed et al., 1998; Campbell et al., 1999), leading to promotion of actin fiber remodeling within spines. Therefore, it is possible that DHT, T, and E2 might modulate spines via cortactin-actin pathway. Cortactin has multiple phosphorylation sites, such as Ser^{113}, Ser^{405}, and Ser^{418}, which are putative phosphorylation sites of MAPK (Campbell et al., 1999). Phosphorylation of cortactin triggered by DHT, T, and E2 may promote assembly of actin cytoskeleton, which either leads to increasing spines or modulating the spine morphology (Hering and Sheng, 2003). The involvement of cortactin in androgen-induced modulation of spines is suggested from the results that AR inhibitor induced actin depolymerization via tyrosine phosphorylation of cortactin (Anahara et al., 2006).

Localization of AR and ER in Spines

The involvement of classic AR in androgen-induced rapid action was indicated from suppressing effects of hydroxyflutamide, a specific inhibitor of AR, on androgen-induced spinogenesis in acute slices of male rat hippocampus (Hatanaka et al., 2015). The AR immunostaining was localized in CA1 neurons with optical microscopic analysis, and synaptic localization of AR was indicated with immuno-electron microscopic analysis (Tabori et al., 2005). Western blot analysis showed the AR expression in PSD fractions as well as in nuclear and cytoplasmic fractions, which implies that AR localized in the PSD can participate in the T- and DHT-induced spine increase (Hatanaka et al., 2015). These results suggest that AR localized in spines could mediate androgen-induced rapid spine increase through activation of Src kinase and MAPK.

The involvement of classic ER in rapid E2 action was indicated from suppressing effects of ICI182,780 (ICI), a specific antagonist of both ER, on E2-induced spinogenesis in male hippocampal slices (Mukai et al., 2007; Hasegawa et al., 2015). Involvement of ERα or ERβ in rapid spinogenesis was also examined by using estrogen receptor agonists. ERα agonist, (propyl-pyrazole-trinyl) tris-phenol (PPT), unlike ERβ agonist such as (4-hydroxyphenyl)-propionitrile (DPN), acutely increased the density of spines in hippocampal CA1 neurons in male rat slices (Hasegawa et al., 2015) and OVX female mice (Phan et al., 2011). These results support the exclusive involvement of ERα in rapid signaling. ERαKO mice and ERβKO mice studies further confirmed the involvement of ERα, but not ERβ, in the rapid E2 signaling (Murakami et al., 2015).

Expression of ERα in neurons of CA1 in rat and mouse hippocampus was demonstrated by immunostaining with purified antibody RC-19 (Mukai et al., 2007). ERα was located in spines in addition to nuclei/cytoplasm, as revealed by the immunogold electron-microscopic analyses (Mukai et al., 2007). Spine membrane localization of AR and ER may be accomplished via palmitoylation of receptors (**Figure 5**), as judged from recent studies, including the finding that some populations of ERα and ERβ were plasma membrane-bound in cultured breast cancer cells MCF-7 (Pedram et al., 2006), and they were anchored via palmitoylation (Pedram et al., 2007).

Difference Between DHT, T, and E2 in Rapid Effects on Spine Density and Morphology in CA1

Although treatments with DHT, T, and E2 increased the total spine density to almost the same level, three subclass analysis showed clear differences between DHT, T, and E2 in modulation of the spine morphology of hippocampal CA1 neurons (**Figures 1–3**). DHT treatments considerably increased the density of large-head spines. On the other hand, all the small- and middle-head spines were increased with T treatments, whereas E2 increased only small-head spines. Since large-head spines have significantly more AMPA receptors than small-head spines (Shinohara et al., 2008), DHT might increase synapses with higher memory storage capacity than T and E2.

The T-effect is not dependent on the conversion from T to E2, and neither from T to DHT. This is concluded from the fact that T-effect was not blocked by inhibition of P450arom (E2 synthetase) and 5α-reductase (DHT synthetase) (Hatanaka et al., 2015). Moreover, the effect of T was blocked by AR antagonist. T-effect must be therefore directly mediated by AR, and not mediated by E2.

Difference in Sex Steroid Levels Between Acute Hippocampal Slices and *in Vivo* Hippocampus

Sex steroid levels in the hippocampus play a key role for rapid action through synaptic AR and ER as modulators of synaptic plasticity. The average concentrations of male rat hippocampal DHT, T, and E2 *in vivo* were determined to be ~7, 17, and 8 nM, respectively, in freshly isolated hippocampi, with mass-spectrometric analysis (Hojo et al., 2008, 2009) (Okamoto et al., 2012). These hippocampal sex steroid levels are significantly higher than plasma sex steroid levels, due to hippocampal synthesis of sex steroids, in addition to penetration of T (~15 nM in plasma) to the hippocampus via blood circulation (Hojo et al., 2009). Interestingly, E2 level in the male hippocampus (~8 nM) is higher than that in female (0.6–4.3 nM), due to conversion of high level T into E2 within the hippocampus by P450arom (Kato et al., 2013). Importantly in "acute" slices (used for current analysis of synaptic plasticity), the levels of DHT, T, and E2 decreased to below 0.5 nM due to the slice recovery incubation for 2 h with ACSF after fresh slice preparations (Hojo et al., 2009, 2011; Ooishi et al., 2012a,b). In the current study, the exogenous application of 10 nM DHT, 10 nM T, and 1 nM E2 individually was used to rapidly elevate the hippocampal sex steroid levels from the steroid-depleted levels in "acute" slice (<0.5 nM), to nearly the endogenous levels of male rat (Ooishi et al., 2012a), resulting in rapid action of sex steroids.

Toward *in Vivo* Analysis of Sex Steroid Effects on Spine Modulation

The currently obtained knowledge encourages analysis of *in vivo* mechanisms of rapid sex steroid actions on spines. Recent *in vivo* investigations implied that E2 treatments with s.c. injection rapidly (within 30–40 min) increased the spine density in CA1 hippocampal neurons of OVX female mice (Phan et al., 2011, 2012; Jacome et al., 2016; Tuscher et al., 2016). These *in vivo* investigations can be interpreted that E2 supplementation recovered the spine density, because OVX surgery once decreased spine density as well as declined hippocampal E2 level due to depletion of circulating E2 (Kato et al., 2013). Such approaches in combination with kinase inhibitors may be useful to analyze *in vivo* molecular mechanisms of rapid synaptic modulation by E2 in female rodents. Concerning male rodents, approaches with castration followed by rapid androgen supplementation could be promising to analyze mechanisms of rapid modulation effects of androgen on spines, because castration decreases hippocampal T and DHT as well as the spine density.

AUTHOR CONTRIBUTIONS

SK: conceived and designed the study; MS, JK, and AK: conducted the experiments and analysis of the data; SK: wrote the manuscript. All authors provided feedback on the manuscript.

ACKNOWLEDGMENTS

We thank Mr. J. Murakami, Mr. W. Tokuyama for spine data analysis. Profs. K. Inoue, J. Kurihara, and A. Kittaka (Teikyo University) are acknowledged for helpful discussions.

REFERENCES

1. Anahara, R., Toyama, Y., Maekawa, M., Yoshida, M., Kai, M., et al. (2006). Anti-estrogen ICI 182.780 and anti-androgen flutamide induce tyrosine phosphorylation of cortactin in the ectoplasmic specialization between the Sertoli cell and spermatids in the mouse testis. *Biochem. Biophys. Res. Commun.* 346, 276–280. doi: 10.1016/j.bbrc.2006. 05.125
2. Bi, R., Broutman, G., Foy, M. R., Thompson, R. F., and Baudry, M. (2000). The tyrosine kinase and mitogen-activated protein kinase pathways mediate multiple effects of estrogen in hippocampus. *Proc. Natl. Acad. Sci. U.S.A.* 97, 3602–3607. doi: 10.1073/pnas.97.7.3602
3. Bi, R., Foy, M. R., Vouimba, R. M., Thompson, R. F., and Baudry, M. (2001). Cyclic changes in estradiol regulate synaptic plasticity through the MAP kinase pathway. *Proc. Natl. Acad. Sci. U.S.A.* 98, 13391–13395. doi: 10.1073/pnas.241507698
4. Brown, T. J., Sharma, M., Heisler, L. E., Karsan, N., Walters, M. J., and MacLusky, N. J. (1995). *In vitro* labeling of gonadal steroid hormone

receptors in brain tissue sections. *Steroids* 60, 726–737. doi: 10.1016/0039-128X(95)00107-2

5. Campbell, D. H., Sutherland, R. L., and Daly, R. J. (1999). Signaling pathways and structural domains required for phosphorylation of EMS1/cortactin. *Cancer Res.* 59, 5376–5385.
6. Castoria, G., Lombardi, M., Barone, M. V., Bilancio, A., Di Domenico, M., et al. (2004). Rapid signalling pathway activation by androgens in epithelial and stromal cells. *Steroids* 69, 517–522. doi: 10.1016/j.steroids.2004.05.001
7. Cheng, J., Watkins, S. C., and Walker, W. H. (2007). Testosterone activates mitogen-activated protein kinase via Src kinase and the epidermal growth factor receptor in sertoli cells. *Endocrinology* 148, 2066–2074. doi:10.1210/en.2006-1465
8. Clancy, A. N., Bonsall, R. W., and Michael, R. P. (1992). Immunohistochemical labeling of androgen receptors in the brain of rat and monkey. *Life Sci.* 50, 409–417. doi: 10.1016/0024-3205(92)90375-Y
9. Duan, H., Wearne, S. L., Morrison, J. H., and Hof, P. R. (2002). Quantitative analysis of the dendritic morphology of corticocortical projection neurons in the macaque monkey association cortex. *Neuroscience* 114, 349–359. doi:10.1016/S0306-4522(02)00305-6
10. Foradori, C. D., Weiser, M. J., and Handa, R. J. (2008). Non- genomic actions of androgens. *Front. Neuroendocrinol.* 29, 169–181. doi:10.1016/j.yfrne.2007.10.005
11. Foradori, C. D., Werner, S. B., Sandau, U. S., Clapp, T. R., and Handa, R. J. (2007). Activation of the androgen receptor alters the intracellular calcium response to glutamate in primary hippocampal neurons and modulates sarco/endoplasmic reticulum calcium ATPase 2 transcription. *Neuroscience* 149, 155–164. doi: 10.1016/j.neuroscience.2007.06.054
12. Foy, M. R., Xu, J., Xie, X., Brinton, R. D., Thompson, R. F., and Berger, T. W. (1999). 17beta-estradiol enhances NMDA receptor-mediated EPSPs and long-term potentiation. *J. Neurophysiol.* 81, 925–929. doi: 10.1152/jn.1999.81.2.925
13. Frick, K. M. (2015). Molecular mechanisms underlying the memory-enhancing effects of estradiol. *Horm. Behav.* 74, 4–18. doi: 10.1016/j.yhbeh.2015.05.001
14. Frick, K. M., Kim, J., Tuscher, J. J., and Fortress, A. M. (2015). Sex steroid hormones matter for learning and memory: estrogenic regulation of hippocampal function in male and female rodents. *Learn. Mem.* 22, 472–493. doi:10.1101/lm.037267.114
15. Gould, E., Woolley, C. S., Frankfurt, M., and McEwen, B. S. (1990). Gonadal steroids regulate dendritic spine density in hippocampal pyramidal cells in adulthood. *J. Neurosci.* 10, 1286–1291. doi: 10.1523/JNEUROSCI. 10-04-01286.1990
16. Grassi, S., Tozzi, A., Costa, C., Tantucci, M., Colcelli, E., et al. (2011). Neural 17beta-estradiol facilitates long-term potentiation in the hippocampal CA1 region. *Neuroscience* 192, 67–73. doi: 10.1016/j.neuroscience.2011.06.078
17. Hajszan, T., MacLusky, N. J., and Leranth, C. (2008). Role of androgens and the androgen receptor in remodeling of spine synapses in limbic brain areas. *Horm. Behav.* 53, 638–646. doi: 10.1016/j.yhbeh.2007.12.007
18. Hasegawa, Y., Hojo, Y., Kojima, H., Ikeda, M., Hotta, K., et al. (2015). Estradiol rapidly modulates synaptic plasticity of hippocampal neurons: involvement of kinase networks. *Brain Res.* 1621, 147–161. doi: 10.1016/j.brainres.2014.12.056
19. Hatanaka, Y., Hojo, Y., Mukai, H., Murakami, G., Komatsuzaki, Y., et al. (2015). Rapid increase of spines by dihydrotestosterone and testosterone in hippocampal neurons: dependence on synaptic androgen receptor and kinase networks. *Brain Res.* 1621, 121–132. doi: 10.1016/j.brainres.2014.12.011
20. Hatanaka, Y., Mukai, H., Mitsuhashi, K., Hojo, Y., Murakami, G., et al. (2009). Androgen rapidly increases dendritic thorns of CA3 neurons in male rat hippocampus. *Biochem. Biophys. Res. Commun.* 381, 728–732. doi: 10.1016/j.bbrc.2009.02.130
21. Hering, H., and Sheng, M. (2003). Activity-dependent redistribution and essential role of cortactin in dendritic spine morphogenesis. *J. Neurosci.* 23, 11759–11769. doi: 10.1523/JNEUROSCI.23-37-11759.2003
22. Hojo, Y., Hattori, T. A., Enami, T., Furukawa, A., Suzuki, K., et al. (2004). Adult male rat hippocampus synthesizes estradiol from pregnenolone by cytochromes P45017alpha and P450 aromatase localized in neurons. *Proc. Natl. Acad. Sci. U.S.A.* 101, 865–870. doi: 10.1073/pnas.2630225100
23. Hojo, Y., Higo, S., Ishii, H., Ooishi, Y., Mukai, H., et al. (2009). Comparison between hippocampus-synthesized and circulation-derived sex steroids in the hippocampus. *Endocrinology* 150, 5106–5112. doi: 10.1210/en.2009-0305
24. Hojo, Y., Higo, S., Kawato, S., Hatanaka, Y., Ooishi, Y., et al. (2011). Hippocampal synthesis of sex steroids and corticosteroids: essential for modulation of synaptic plasticity. *Front. Endocrinol.* 2:43. doi: 10.3389/fendo.2011.00043
25. Hojo, Y., Murakami, G., Mukai, H., Higo, S., Hatanaka, Y., et al. (2008). Estrogen synthesis in the brain–role in synaptic plasticity and memory. *Mol. Cell Endocrinol.* 290, 31–43. doi: 10.1016/j.mce.2008.04.017
26. Jacome, L. F., Barateli, K., Buitrago, D., Lema, F., Frankfurt, M., and Luine, V. N. (2016). Gonadal hormones rapidly enhance spatial memory and increase hippocampal spine density in male rats. *Endocrinology* 157, 1357–1362. doi:10.1210/en.2015-1959
27. Kato, A., Hojo, Y., Higo, S., Komatsuzaki, Y., Murakami, G., et al. (2013). Female hippocampal estrogens have a significant correlation with cyclic fluctuation of hippocampal spines. *Front. Neural. Circuits* 7:149. doi: 10.3389/fncir.2013.00149
28. Kerr, J. E., Allore, R. J., Beck, S. G., and Handa, R. J. (1995). Distribution and hormonal regulation of androgen receptor (AR) and AR messenger ribonucleic acid in the rat hippocampus. *Endocrinology* 136, 3213–3221. doi:10.1210/endo.136.8.7628354
29. Kim, S., Alsaidan, O. A., Goodwin, O., Li, Q., Sulejmani, E., Han, Z., et al. (2017). Blocking myristoylation of src inhibits its kinase activity and suppresses prostate cancer progression. *Cancer Res.* 77, 6950–6962. doi: 10.1158/0008-5472.CAN-17-0981
30. Levin, E. R., and Hammes, S. R. (2016). Nuclear receptors outside the nucleus: extranuclear signalling by steroid receptors. *Nat. Rev. Mol. Cell Biol.* 17, 783–797. doi: 10.1038/nrm.2016.122
31. Luine, V. N. (2014). Estradiol and cognitive function: past, present and future. *Horm. Behav.* 66, 602–618. doi: 10.1016/j.yhbeh.2014.08.011
32. Luine, V. N., and Frankfurt, M. (2012). Estrogens facilitate memory processing through membrane mediated mechanisms and alterations in spine density. *Front. Neuroendocrinol.* 33, 388–402. doi: 10.1016/j.yfrne.2012.07.004
33. MacLusky, N. J., Luine, V. N., Hajszan, T., and Leranth, C. (2005). The 17alpha and 17beta isomers of estradiol both induce rapid spine synapse formation in the CA1 hippocampal subfield of ovariectomized female rats. *Endocrinology* 146, 287–293. doi: 10.1210/en.2004-0730
34. MacQueen, G. M., Campbell, S., McEwen, B. S., Macdonald, K., Amano, S., et al. (2003). Course of illness, hippocampal function, and hippocampal volume in major depression. *Proc. Natl. Acad. Sci. U.S.A.* 100, 1387–1392. doi:10.1073/pnas.0337481100
35. Mannella, P., and Brinton, R. D. (2006). Estrogen receptor protein interaction with phosphatidylinositol 3-kinase leads to activation of phosphorylated Akt and extracellular signal-regulated kinase 1/2 in the same population of cortical neurons: a unified mechanism of estrogen action. *J. Neurosci.* 26, 9439–9447. doi: 10.1523/JNEUROSCI.1443-06.2006
36. Migliaccio, A., Castoria, G., Di Domenico, M., de Falco, A., Bilancio, A., et al. (2000). Steroid-induced androgen receptor-oestradiol receptor beta-Src complex triggers prostate cancer cell proliferation. *EMBO J.* 19, 5406–5417. doi:10.1093/emboj/19.20.5406
37. Migliaccio, A., Di Domenico, M., Castoria, G., de Falco, A., Bontempo, P., et al. (1996). Tyrosine kinase/p21ras/MAP-kinase pathway activation by estradiol- receptor complex in MCF-7 cells. *EMBO J.* 15, 1292–1300.
38. Milner, T. A., Ayoola, K., Drake, C. T., Herrick, S. P., Tabori, N. E., et al. (2005). Ultrastructural localization of estrogen receptor beta immunoreactivity in the rat hippocampal formation. *J. Comp. Neurol.* 491, 81–95. doi: 10.1002/cne.20724
39. Mukai, H., Hatanaka, Y., Mitsuhashi, K., Hojo, Y., Komatsuzaki, Y., et al. (2011). Automated analysis of spines from confocal laser microscopy images: application to the discrimination of androgen and estrogen effects on spinogenesis. *Cereb Cortex.* 21, 2704–2711. doi: 10.1093/cercor/ bhr059
40. Mukai, H., Kimoto, T., Hojo, Y., Kawato, S., Murakami, G., et al. (2010). Modulation of synaptic plasticity by brain estrogen in the hippocampus. *Biochim. Biophys. Acta* 1800, 1030–1044. doi: 10.1016/j.bbagen.2009.11.002
41. Mukai, H., Tsurugizawa, T., Murakami, G., Kominami, S., Ishii, H., et al. (2007). Rapid modulation of long-term depression and spinogenesis via synaptic estrogen receptors in hippocampal principal neurons. *J. Neurochem.* 100, 950–967. doi: 10.1111/j.1471-4159.2006.04264.x
42. Murakami, G., Hojo, Y., Ogiue-Ikeda, M., Mukai, H., Chambon, P., et al. (2015). Estrogen receptor KO mice study on rapid modulation of spines and long-term depression in the hippocampus. *Brain Res.* 1621, 133–146. doi:10.1016/j.brainres.2014.12.002
43. Murakami, G., Tsurugizawa, T., Hatanaka, Y., Komatsuzaki, Y., Tanabe, N., et al. (2006). Comparison between basal and apical dendritic spines in estrogen-induced rapid spinogenesis of CA1 principal neurons in the

adult hippocampus. *Biochem. Biophys. Res. Commun.* 351, 553–558. doi: 10.1016/j.bbrc.2006.10.066

44. Nguyen, T. V., Yao, M., and Pike, C. J. (2005). Androgens activate mitogen-activated protein kinase signaling: role in neuroprotection. *J. Neurochem.* 94, 1639–1651. doi: 10.1111/j.1471-4159.2005.03318.x
45. Okamoto, M., Hojo, Y., Inoue, K., Matsui, T., Kawato, S., et al. (2012). Mild exercise increases dihydrotestosterone in hippocampus providing evidence for androgenic mediation of neurogenesis. *Proc. Natl. Acad. Sci. U.S.A.* 109, 13100–13105. doi: 10.1073/pnas.1210023109
46. Ooishi, Y., Kawato, S., Hojo, Y., Hatanaka, Y., Higo, S., et al. (2012a). Modulation of synaptic plasticity in the hippocampus by hippocampus-derived estrogen and androgen. *J Steroid Biochem Mol. Biol.* 131, 37–51. doi: 10.1016/j.jsbmb.2011.10.004
47. Ooishi, Y., Mukai, H., Hojo, Y., Murakami, G., Hasegawa, Y., et al. (2012b). Estradiol rapidly rescues synaptic transmission from corticosterone-induced suppression via synaptic/extranuclear steroid receptors in the hippocampus. *Cereb Cortex* 22, 926–936. doi: 10.1093/cercor/bhr164
48. Pedram, A., Razandi, M., and Levin, E. R. (2006). Nature of functional estrogen receptors at the plasma membrane. *Mol. Endocrinol.* 20, 1996–2009. doi: 10.1210/me.2005-0525
49. Pedram, A., Razandi, M., Sainson, R. C., Kim, J. K., Hughes, C. C., and Levin, E. R. (2007). A conserved mechanism for steroid receptor translocation to the plasma membrane. *J. Biol. Chem.* 282:22278. doi: 10.1074/jbc.M611877200
50. Phan, A., Gabor, C. S., Favaro, K. J., Kaschack, S., Armstrong, J. N., et al. (2012). Low doses of 17beta-estradiol rapidly improve learning and increase hippocampal dendritic spines. *Neuropsychopharmacology* 37, 2299–2309. doi: 10.1038/npp.2012.82
51. Phan, A., Lancaster, K. E., Armstrong, J. N., MacLusky, N. J., and Choleris, E. (2011). Rapid effects of estrogen receptor alpha and beta selective agonists on learning and dendritic spines in female mice. *Endocrinology* 152, 1492–1502. doi: 10.1210/en.2010-1273
52. Rusanescu, G., Qi, H., Thomas, S. M., Brugge, J. S., and Halegoua, S. (1995). Calcium influx induces neurite growth through a Src-Ras signaling cassette. *Neuron* 15, 1415–1425. doi: 10.1016/0896-6273(95)90019-5
53. Shinohara, Y., Hirase, H., Watanabe, M., Itakura, M., Takahashi, M., and Shigemoto, R. (2008). Left-right asymmetry of the hippocampal synapses with differential subunit allocation of glutamate receptors. *Proc. Natl. Acad. Sci. U.S.A.* 105, 19498–19503. doi: 10.1073/pnas.0807461105
54. Simerly, R. B., Chang, C., Muramatsu, M., and Swanson, L. W. (1990). Distribution of androgen and estrogen receptor mRNA-containing cells in the rat brain: an *in situ* hybridization study. *J. Comp. Neurol.* 294, 76–95. doi: 10.1002/cne.902940107
55. Tabori, N. E., Stewart, L. S., Znamensky, V., Romeo, R. D., Alves, S. E., et al. (2005). Ultrastructural evidence that androgen receptors are located at extranuclear sites in the rat hippocampal formation. *Neuroscience* 130, 151–163. doi: 10.1016/j.neuroscience.2004.08.048
56. Tuscher, J. J., Luine, V., Frankfurt, M., and Frick, K. M. (2016). Estradiol-Mediated spine changes in the dorsal hippocampus and medial prefrontal cortex of ovariectomized female mice depend on ERK and mTOR activation in the dorsal hippocampus. *J. Neurosci.* 36, 1483–1489. doi: 10.1523/JNEUROSCI.3135-15.2016
57. Weed, S. A., Du, Y., and Parsons, J. T. (1998). Translocation of cortactin to the cell periphery is mediated by the small GTPase Rac1. *J. Cell Sci.* 111 (Pt 16), 2433–2443.
58. Woolley, C. S., Gould, E., and McEwen, B. S. (1990). Exposure to excess glucocorticoids alters dendritic morphology of adult hippocampal pyramidal neurons. *Brain Res.* 531, 225–231. doi: 10.1016/0006-8993(90) 90778-A
59. Woolley, C. S., and McEwen, B. S. (1992). Estradiol mediates fluctuation in hippocampal synapse density during the estrous cycle in the adult rat. *J. Neurosci.* 12, 2549–2554.
60. Znamensky, V., Akama, K. T., McEwen, B. S., and Milner, T. A. (2003). Estrogen levels regulate the subcellular distribution of phosphorylated Akt in hippocampal CA1 dendrites. *J. Neurosci.* 23, 2340–2347. doi: 10.1523/JNEUROSCI.23-06-02340.2003

4

Temporal Expression Patterns of Genes Related to Sex Steroid Action in Sexually Dimorphic Nuclei During Puberty

*Moeko Kanaya[†], Masahiro Morishita and Shinji Tsukahara**

Division of Life Science, Graduate School of Science and Engineering, Saitama University, Saitama, Japan

Correspondence:
Shinji Tsukahara
stsuka@mail.saitama-u.ac.jp

Sex steroids play a major role in sexually dimorphic brain development during not only the perinatal period but also the pubertal period. We previously showed that, in male mice, the estrogen receptor-α (*Esr1*) and aromatase (*Cyp19a1*) genes are essential to the sexually dimorphic formation of the anteroventral periventricular nucleus (AVPV) and the principal nucleus of the bed nucleus of the stria terminalis (BNSTp), but the estrogen receptor-β (*Esr2*) gene is not necessary. We also showed that the androgen receptor (*Ar*) gene is essential to the sexually dimorphic formation of the BNSTp. These genes are expressed in the AVPV and BNSTp of perinatal mice. However, it remains unknown whether these genes are expressed in the AVPV and BNSTp during puberty, and whether the expression, if any, differs by sex, age, and brain region. Here, we dissected the AVPV and BNSTp from Nissl-stained brain sections of male and female mice on postnatal day (PD) 20 (prepuberty), PD30 (puberty onset in females), PD40 (puberty onset in males), and PD60 (young adult) using a laser microdissection system. We then examined the mRNA levels of *Esr1*, *Esr2*, *Cyp19a1*, and *Ar* in these brain regions. In the AVPV, *Esr1* mRNA levels were greater in females than males during PD20–60. *Esr2* and *Ar* mRNA expressions did not differ between sexes. *Ar* mRNA levels were higher at PD30 than PD20. *Cyp19a1* mRNA was not detected in the AVPV at PD20–60. In the BNSTp, *Esr1* and *Esr2* mRNA levels were higher in females than in males during PD20–60, although the mRNA levels of *Cyp19a1* and *Ar* did not differ between sexes. Additionally, we revealed that orchiectomy at PD20 induced a failure of normal formation of the male BNSTp and testosterone replacement in the prepubertal period rescued the effect of orchiectomy at PD20. Taken together, it is suggested that pubertal testosterone transported to the AVPV is not converted to estradiol there and does not act *via* ESR1 and ESR2. By contrast, the formation of the male BNSTp may be affected by testicular testosterone during puberty *via* AR and/or *via* ESR1 after conversion to estradiol by CYP19A1.

Keywords: aromatase, puberty, sex steroids, sexual differentiation, sexually dimorphic nucleus, sex steroid receptor, anteroventral periventricular nucleus, principal nucleus of the bed nucleus of the stria terminalis

INTRODUCTION

Sexually dimorphic nuclei underlie sex- and gender-specific functions in the brain. The anteroventral periventricular nucleus (AVPV) of the hypothalamus in rodents is a sexually dimorphic nucleus that is larger in size and contains more neurons in females than in males (1–4). Specifically, the female AVPV contains a larger number of neurons expressing tyrosine hydroxylase (TH) (3) and kisspeptin (5, 6). TH neurons in the AVPV promote parental behavior in female mice (7). Although TH neurons in the AVPV do not promote parental behavior in male mice, they suppress inter-male aggression (7). Kisspeptin neurons in the female AVPV appear to participate in the estradiol-induced surge of luteinizing hormone (8, 9). The principal nucleus of the bed nucleus of the stria terminalis (BNSTp) is a sexually dimorphic nucleus in the forebrain that is larger and contains a greater number of neurons in male rodents (10–13). Males have a greater number of vasopressin neurons in the BNSTp, which are involved in anxiety, aggressive behavior, and stress responses (14), and which project to the lateral septum (15–17). These differences in vasopressin neurons may underlie behavioral sex differences, particularly as male rodents exhibit more anxiety-related behavior than females (18, 19).

In male rodents, sexually dimorphic nuclei are formed by the influence of testicular testosterone during the perinatal period (20, 21). Like the AVPV in male rats, the AVPV in female rats treated with testosterone postnatally is smaller and contains fewer TH neurons and kisspeptin neurons in adulthood (6, 22). We previously showed that the volume and number of neurons in the AVPV are increased in male mice with deletion of the estrogen receptor-α (*Esr1*) and aromatase (*Cyp19a1*) genes, but are not affected by deletion of the estrogen receptor-β (*Esr2*) or androgen receptor (*Ar*) gene (23). These previous findings suggest that *Esr1* and *Cyp19a1* are essential to the formation of the male AVPV, but *Esr2* and *Ar* are not necessary. In support of this notion, *Esr1* and *Cyp19a1* mRNAs are expressed in the AVPV in perinatal mice (23). Postnatal treatment with estradiol, as well as testosterone, reduces the number of neurons in the AVPV in adult female rats (24). Thus, testicular testosterone in the perinatal period might be converted by CYP19A1 in the AVPV to estradiol, which signals through ESR1 to defeminize the morphology of the AVPV.

Perinatal testicular testosterone also affects the BNSTp, although the effects are opposite to those on the AVPV. The volume and number of neurons in the BNSTp in adult male rats are decreased by neonatal orchiectomy (12). Postnatal treatment with testosterone or estradiol increases the number of neurons in the BNSTp of adult female mice (25). The volume and number of neurons in the BNSTp in male mice are reduced to levels similar to those in females by deletion of *Esr1* or *Cyp19a1*, but not *Esr2* (26). *Esr1* and *Cyp19a1* are expressed in the BNSTp in perinatal mice (23). These findings suggest that the formation of the male BNSTp involves the action of estradiol (produced by the aromatization of testosterone) *via* ESR1 during the perinatal period. Additionally, the AR plays an important role in the formation of the male BNSTp, because the volume and number of neurons in the BNSTp are smaller in male *Ar* knockout (KO) mice, compared with wild-type males, similar to females (23). *Ar* is not expressed in the murine BNSTp prenatally, but begins expression early in the postnatal period (23, 27). The formation of the male BNSTp might require not only estradiol, formed from the aromatization of testosterone, acting *via* ESR1 in the perinatal period, but also testosterone acting *via* AR postnatally.

Accumulating evidence shows that testicular testosterone during the perinatal period is essential for the sexually dimorphic formation of brain structures. However, the formation of sexually dimorphic nuclei is affected by pubertal gonadal hormones as well (28, 29). In male mice, the BNSTp contains a comparatively greater number of calbindin neurons (30). This sex difference in calbindin neurons emerges before puberty, and increases further as calbindin neurons continue to increase in males and decrease in females during the pubertal and adolescent periods (31, 32). Testicular hormones during puberty also contribute to the formation of the male BNSTp, because the increase in calbindin neurons in the male BNSTp is perturbed by prepubertal orchiectomy, although the decrease in the female BNSTp is not altered by prepubertal ovariectomy (32). The sexually dimorphic formation of the AVPV might be influenced by pubertal ovarian hormones. Prepubertal ovariectomy decreases the volume and number of neurons in the AVPV in female rats (33). Thus, gonadal hormones during puberty play an important role in the sexually dimorphic formation of the AVPV and BNSTp; however, it remains unknown whether genes related to gonadal hormone actions are expressed in the sexually dimorphic nuclei during puberty.

In this study, we aimed to determine whether the AVPV and BNSTp of pubertal mice express genes involved in gonadal hormone actions, and whether the expression, if any, varies by sex, age, and brain-region. First, using tissue samples isolated precisely and accurately from the AVPV and BNSTp of peripubertal mice, we evaluated the mRNA expression patterns of *Esr1*, *Cyp19a1*, and *Ar*, which play an essential role in the sexually dimorphic formation of the AVPV and/or BNSTp (23, 26), as well as that of *Esr2*. As a result, the mRNA of *Cyp19a1* was expressed in the BNSTp, but not in the AVPV of peripubertal mice, suggesting that the BNSTp of male mice is affected by estradiol, which is converted from testicular testosterone by CYP19A1 locally there during puberty, but the AVPV is not. Next, to determine whether testicular testosterone during puberty contributes to the formation of the male BNSTp, we investigated the effects of prepubertal orchiectomy and testosterone replacement on the morphology of the BNSTp in adulthood with reference to calbindin expression.

MATERIALS AND METHODS

Animals

Adult male and female C57BL/6J mice for breeding were purchased from Sankyo Labo Service Corporation (Tokyo, Japan). Offspring derived from mating in our facility were housed with dams in the same cages until weaning on postnatal day (PD) 21 (PD0 = day of birth). All animals were bred and housed in a room with a controlled temperature (22°C) and a 12-h light/12-h dark cycle (lights on: 08:00–20:00). Standard diet and tap water were available *ad libitum*. All animal experimental procedures were approved by the Animal Care and Experimentation Committee of Saitama University and were conducted in accordance with the Guidelines for the Care and Use of Experimental Animals of Saitama University.

Gene Expression Analysis of the AVPV and BNSTp in Peripubertal Mice

Brain Tissue Collection

Male and female mice of different ages {PD20, prepuberty; PD30, puberty onset in females; PD40, puberty onset in males; and PD60, young adult [see review by Piekarski et al. (34)]} were deeply anesthetized by intraperitoneal injection of sodium pentobarbital (64.8 mg/kg body weight) and decapitated. Fresh brains were quickly frozen in hexane chilled to −80°C and stored at −80°C until further processing. There are several studies showing that the levels of *Esr1* mRNA and protein in the preoptic area (35, 36) and the number of ESR1- and AR-immunoreactive cells in the BNSTp (37, 38) are affected by circulating estradiol. Therefore, we compared the mRNA levels of *Esr1*, *Esr2*, *Cyp19a1*, and *Ar* in the AVPV and BNSTp of diestrous and proestrous female mice. When collecting brains from females on PD40 or PD60, vaginal smears were performed starting on the day of vaginal opening, and animals in the diestrous or proestrous phase were sacrificed between 12:00 hours and 14:00 hours on PD40 or PD60. As a result, unexpectedly, diestrous and proestrous female mice did not differ with regard to the mRNA levels of *Esr1*, *Esr2*, and *Ar* in the AVPV and BNSTp (data not shown). *Cyp19a1* mRNA was not detected in the AVPV on PD40 and PD60. *Cyp19a1* mRNA in the BNSTp did not differ between diestrous and proestrous females on PD40 and PD60 (data not shown). In this study, diestrous and proestrous female mice of the same age were therefore combined into a single group. The numbers of animals used for this study were as follows: PD20 male, $n = 6$; PD20 female, $n = 4$; PD30 male, $n = 4$; PD30 female, $n = 5$; PD40 male, $n = 4$; PD40 female, $n = 6$; PD60 male, $n = 4$; PD60 female, $n = 8$.

Isolation of the AVPV and BNSTp

The AVPV and BNSTp were dissected using a laser microdissection (LMD) system (Leica LMD 7000; Leica Microsystems, Wetzlar, Germany) in accordance with the procedure reported previously, with slight modification (23). Briefly, frozen brains were coronally cut at a thickness of 30 μm on a cryostat. Brain sections containing the AVPV and BNSTp were obtained in the coronal plane 0.38–0.02 mm rostral to the bregma and 0.10–0.34 mm caudal to the bregma, respectively, according to the mouse brain atlas (39). Brain sections containing the AVPV or BNSTp were mounted on PEN membrane slides (Leica Microsystems), fixed with ice-cold 5% acetic acid in ethanol for 3 min, stained with ice-cold 0.2% cresyl fast violet for 1 min, rinsed in 100% ethanol for 1 min, and dried with cool air. The AVPV and BNSTp were then dissected out from cresyl fast violet-stained brain sections by the LMD system and collected in a tube containing 70 μL RNA extraction buffer and 5 μL carrier RNA working solution (4 ng/μL) from the RNeasy Micro Kit (Qiagen, Valencia, CA, USA). To confirm whether the AVPV and BNSTp were precisely collected, we measured the volume of the nuclei. If the AVPV and BNSTp were correctly isolated, a sex difference in the volume of the nuclei could be found. The areas of the dissected tissue fragments were recorded by the LMD system. We calculated the volume of the acquired tissues by multiplying total of the areas of the dissected tissue fragments by the thickness of brain sections (30 μm) for each sample.

Quantification of mRNA Levels

Total RNA was extracted and purified using the RNeasy Micro Kit (Qiagen) according to the manufacturer's protocol. First-strand cDNA was synthesized using the TaKaRa Prime Script RT reagent kit (TaKaRa Bio, Otsu, Japan). For each sample, total RNA (approximately 160 ng) was reverse-transcribed to first-strand cDNA in a final volume of 15 μL Prime Script buffer containing Prime Script RT Enzyme Mix I (0.75 μL) and random hexamers (75 pmol). Standard samples for *Esr1*, *Cyp19a1*, *Ar*, and glyceraldehyde-3-phosphate dehydrogenase (*Gapdh*), a housekeeping gene, were prepared by mixing an equal amount of each cDNA sample and serially diluting in EASY Dilution solution (TaKaRa Bio). To prepare standard samples for *Esr2*, cDNA obtained from the hypothalamus of adult mice was serially diluted.

Quantitative polymerase chain reaction (qPCR) was performed using a Light Cycler ST300 (Roche Diagnostics, Mannheim, Germany). A 2-μL aliquot of standard or unknown sample was amplified in a 20-μL reaction mixture containing 200 nM of each gene-specific primer [*Gapdh* forward primer: CACTGCCACC CAGAAGA, *Gapdh* reverse primer: TCCACGACGGACACATT; other genes were designed according to our previous study (23)] and 10 μL of 2× SYBR Premix Ex Taq (TaKaRa Bio). The thermocycling parameters for qPCR were 30 s at 95°C, followed by 40 cycles of 95°C for 5 s and 60°C for 20 s. After qPCR, melting curve analysis was performed to assess the specificity of the PCR products. This analysis showed that the melting curves for the PCR products all had a single peak (data not shown).

qPCR analysis for *Gapdh* mRNA in the AVPV and BNSTp revealed that *Gapdh* mRNA levels in these nuclei did not differ significantly by sex or age (data not shown). Therefore, the amount of *Esr1*, *Esr2*, *Cyp19a1*, and *Ar* mRNAs was normalized by dividing by the amount of *Gapdh* mRNA for each sample.

Morphological Analysis of the BNSTp in Male Mice

Prepubertal Orchiectomy and Testosterone Replacement

At PD20, male mice were orchiectomized and subcutaneously implanted with a Silastic tube [1.02 mm inner diameter, 2.16 mm outer diameter, 10.9 mm in total length (effective length: 6.9 mm); Dow Corning Corporation, Midland, MI, USA] containing testosterone (Sigma-Aldrich, St. Louis, MO, USA; $n = 5$) or cholesterol (Wako Pure Chemical Industries, Osaka, Japan; $n = 5$). The testosterone implantation was designed to produce the levels of serum testosterone in young male mice (Tsukahara, unpublished data). Surgery was performed under isoflurane inhalational anesthesia (concentration, 1.5% in air; flow rate, 1 L/min). Additionally, we prepared gonadally intact males ($n = 5$).

Tissue Preparation

At 10 weeks of ages, all animals were deeply anesthetized by intraperitoneal injection of sodium pentobarbital (64.8 mg/kg body weight) and transcardially perfused with 0.05 M ice-cold phosphate-buffered saline (PBS; pH, 7.4) followed by ice-cold 4% paraformaldehyde in 0.05 M phosphate buffer (pH, 7.4). Brains were postfixed with the same fixative at 4°C overnight and then immersed in 30% sucrose in 0.05 M phosphate buffer at 4°C for 2 days. Fixed brains were quickly frozen, coronally sectioned at a thickness of 30 μm using a cryostat, and collected at 60-μm intervals.

Immunohistochemistry for Calbindin

Brain sections were rinsed in 0.05 M PBS containing 1% Triton X-100 (PBST) and placed in 0.6% H_2O_2 in PBST for 30 min at room temperature. The sections were then placed in 5% normal goat serum in PBST for 1 h at room temperature and were reacted with a mouse monoclonal anti-calbindin antibody (1:15,000; C9848; Sigma-Aldrich; RRID: AB_476894) in 5% normal goat serum-containing PBST at 4°C over two nights. After rinsing in PBST, the sections were reacted with peroxidase-labeled polymer conjugated to goat anti-mouse immunoglobulin (K4001, Dako, Carpinteria, CA, USA) for 1 h at room temperature. Calbindin immunoreactivity was visualized with a chromogenic substrate, 3,3′-diaminobenzidine (liquid DAB plus substrate chromogen system, Dako). Immunostained sections were mounted on gelatin-coated glass slides, air dried, dehydrated in ascending ethanol, cleared with xylene, and cover-slipped with a mounting medium.

Morphometric Analysis

The volumes of the BNSTp and the number of calbindin-immunopositive (calbindin-ir) cells in the BNSTp were measured using a light microscope equipped with a charge-coupled device camera (CX9000; MBF Bioscience, Williston, VT, USA) and a computer running Stereo Investigator software (MBF Bioscience). The outlines of the BNSTp on the left of the midline were traced to measure the volume. Calbindin-ir cells in the BNSTp were then counted using the optical fractionator method. Detailed parameters of the stereological analyses are as follows: section thickness, 30 μm; section interval, 60 μm; sampling grid size, 150 μm × 150 μm; counting frame size, 50 μm × 50 μm; dissector height, 13–16 μm; and guard zone height, 1.5 μm.

Statistical Analysis

Two-way analysis of variance (ANOVA) was used to assess the effects of sex and age and the interaction between main factors on AVPV and BNSTp volume and the mRNA levels of target genes. The test of simple main effects was conducted when the interaction between main factors was significant in the two-way ANOVA. If there was a significant effect of age, but no significant interaction between sex and age, Bonferroni *post hoc* test was used to compare the mRNA levels of target genes between the different age groups. Differences in BNSTp volume and the number of calbindin-ir cells in the BNSTp among intact males, males subjected to prepubertal orchiectomy and cholesterol-implantation, and males subjected to prepubertal orchiectomy and testosterone implantation were analyzed with one-way ANOVA followed by Bonferroni *post hoc* test where appropriate. IBM SPSS Statistics v20.0 (IBM, Armonk, NY, USA) was used for data analyses. $P < 0.05$ was considered statistically significant. A *post hoc* power analysis was carried out after data has been collected to determine the power in this study using G*Power 3 (40), a free power analysis program.

RESULTS

AVPV and BNSTp Volume on PD20–60

Tissues from the AVPV were collected from cresyl fast violet-stained brain sections using the LMD system for accuracy and precision (**Figure 1A**). Two-way ANOVA indicated that the volume of the AVPV was significantly larger in females than in males [$F_{1,32} = 13.86$, $p < 0.005$, power $(1 - \beta) = 0.98$; **Figure 1B** inset], and that it increased significantly with age from PD20 to PD60 [$F_{3,32} = 4.70$, $p < 0.01$, power $(1 - \beta) = 0.93$; **Figure 1B**], although there was no significant interaction between sex and age [power $(1 - \beta) = 0.10$]. AVPV tissue volumes in PD30 mice were significantly greater ($p < 0.05$) than PD20 mice and did not differ from those in PD40 and PD60 mice.

Tissues from the BNSTp were isolated from cresyl fast violet-stained brain sections using the LMD system (**Figure 2A**). BNSTp volume was significantly greater in PD20–60 males than in

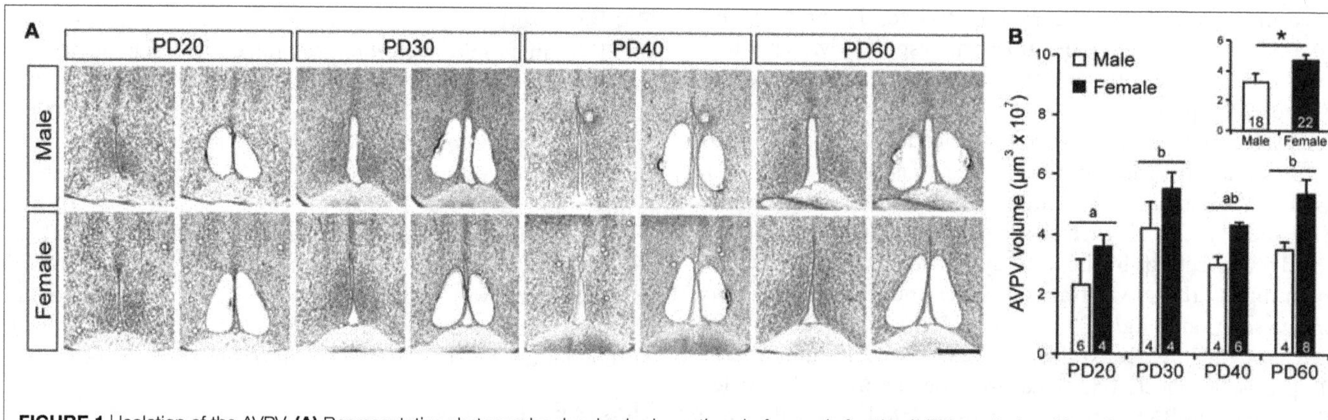

FIGURE 1 | Isolation of the AVPV. **(A)** Representative photographs showing brain sections before and after the AVPV was isolated in male and female mice on PD20–60. Scale bar indicates 400 μm. **(B)** The volume of AVPV tissues isolated from the brain of male and female mice on PD20, PD30, PD40, and PD60. The inset graph in panel **(B)** indicates the average volume of the AVPV in all ages. The numbers in the columns indicate the numbers of animals. Values are the mean ± SEM. Differences in values that are significantly ($p < 0.05$) different from each other are indicated with letters. *$p < 0.05$.

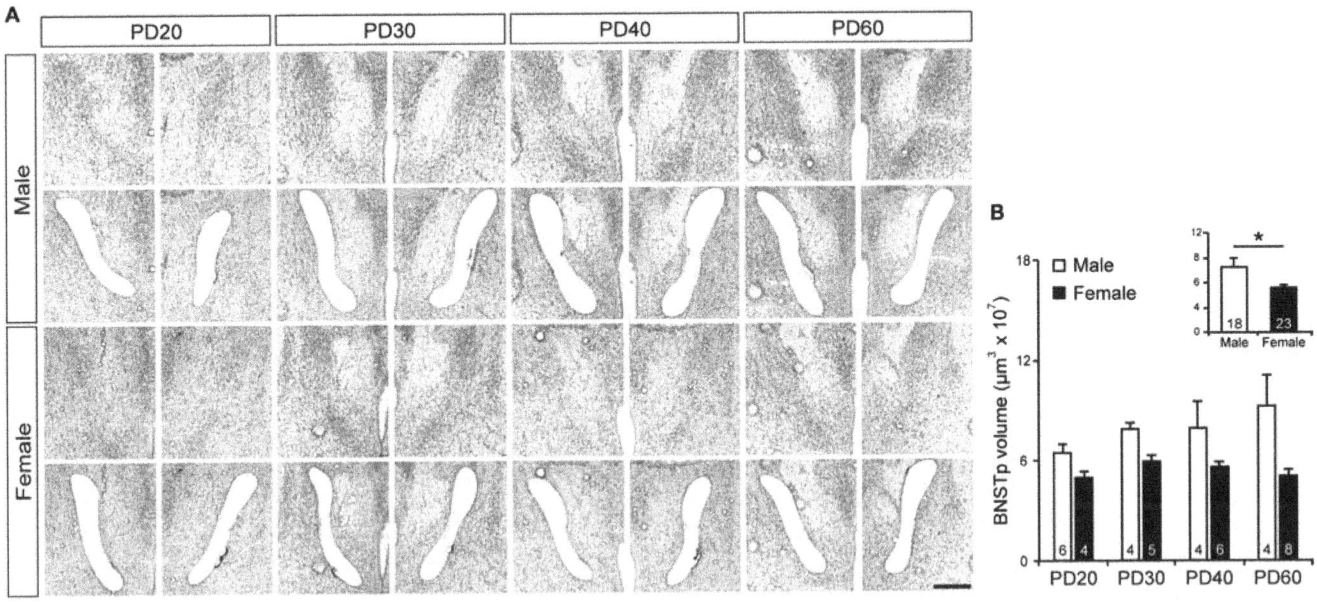

FIGURE 2 | Isolation of the BNSTp. **(A)** Representative photographs showing brain sections before and after the BNSTp was isolated in male and female mice on PD20–60. Scale bar indicates 400 μm. **(B)** The volume of BNSTp tissues isolated from the brain of male and female mice on PD20, PD30, PD40, and PD60. The inset graph in panel **(B)** indicates the average volume of the BNSTp in all ages. The numbers in the columns indicate the numbers of animals. Values are the mean ± SEM. $^{*}p < 0.05$.

PD20–60 females [$F_{1,33} = 16.33, p < 0.0001$, power $(1 - \beta) = 0.99$; **Figure 2B** inset]. The main effect of age and the interaction between sex and age on BNSTp volume were not significant [power $(1 - \beta) = 0.68$ and 0.58, respectively; **Figure 2B**].

Expression of *Esr1*, *Esr2*, *Cyp19a1*, and *Ar* mRNA in the AVPV on PD20–60

Although the effect of age and interaction between sex and age on *Esr1* mRNA levels were not significant [power $(1 - \beta) = 0.68$ and 0.63, respectively], *Esr1* mRNA levels in the AVPV at PD20–60 were significantly higher in females than in males [$F_{1,32} = 35.75$, $p < 0.0001$, power $(1 - \beta) = 1.00$; **Figure 3A** inset]. *Esr2* mRNA levels in the AVPV were not significantly affected by sex, age, and their interaction [power $(1 - \beta) = 0.56$, 0.25 and 0.20, respectively; **Figure 3B**]. *Ar* mRNA levels in the AVPV was affected significantly by age [$F_{3,32} = 3.03, p < 0.05$, power $(1 - \beta) = 0.76$], but not by sex [power $(1 - \beta) = 0.53$] and the interaction between sex and age [power $(1 - \beta) = 0.34$]. *Ar* mRNA levels in the AVPV of PD30 mice were significantly higher ($p < 0.05$) than those of PD20 mice and comparable with those of PD40 and PD60 mice (**Figure 3C**). *Cyp19a1* mRNA in the AVPV on PD20–60 was at an undetectable level in most animals in either sex. *Cyp19a1* mRNA was detectable in one female each on PD20, PD30, and PD40, in two males at PD30, and in two males and two females at PD60, but at the limit of detection by qPCR (data not shown).

Expression of *Esr1*, *Esr2*, *Cyp19a1*, and *Ar* mRNA in the BNSTp on PD20–60

There was a significant effect of sex [$F_{1,33} = 51.56, p < 0.0001$, power $(1 - \beta) = 1.00$] on *Esr1* mRNA levels in the BNSTp during PD20–60 (**Figure 4A** inset). However, the *Esr1* mRNA levels were not significantly affected by age [power $(1 - \beta) = 0.12$] and by interaction between sex and age [power $(1 - \beta) = 0.51$]. *Esr2* mRNA levels in the BNSTp were significantly higher in females than in males at PD20–60 [$F_{1,33} = 4.35$, $p < 0.05$, power $(1 - \beta) = 0.62$; **Figure 4B** inset], although they did not significantly change with age [power $(1 - \beta) = 0.07$] and were not affected by the interaction between sex and age [power $(1 - \beta) = 0.08$] (**Figure 4B**). Unlike the AVPV, the BNSTp expressed *Cyp19a1* mRNA at PD20–60 (**Figure 4C**). *Cyp19a1* mRNA levels in the BNSTp did not significantly change with sex and age [power $(1 - \beta) = 0.22$ and 0.24, respectively]. The interaction of sex and age was also not significant on the *Cyp19a1* mRNA levels [power $(1 - \beta) = 0.22$]. *Ar* mRNA levels in the BNSTp during PD20–60 were not significantly impacted by sex, age, and their interaction [power $(1 - \beta) = 0.24$, 0.73 and 0.40, respectively] (**Figure 4D**).

Effects of Prepubertal Orchiectomy and Testosterone Replacement on the BNSTp in Male Mice

One-way ANOVA revealed that BNSTp volume [$F_{2,12} = 7.07$, $p < 0.01$, power $(1 - \beta) = 0.92$] and the number of calbindin-ir cells in the BNSTp [$F_{2,12} = 6.98, p < 0.05$, power $(1 - \beta) = 0.92$] of adult male mice were significantly different among the experimental groups. BNSTp volume in males that were orchiectomized and implanted with cholesterol at PD20 was significantly smaller ($p < 0.05$) than that in gonadally intact males (**Figures 5A,B**). However, BNSTp volume in males that were orchiectomized and implanted with testosterone at PD20 was similar to that in

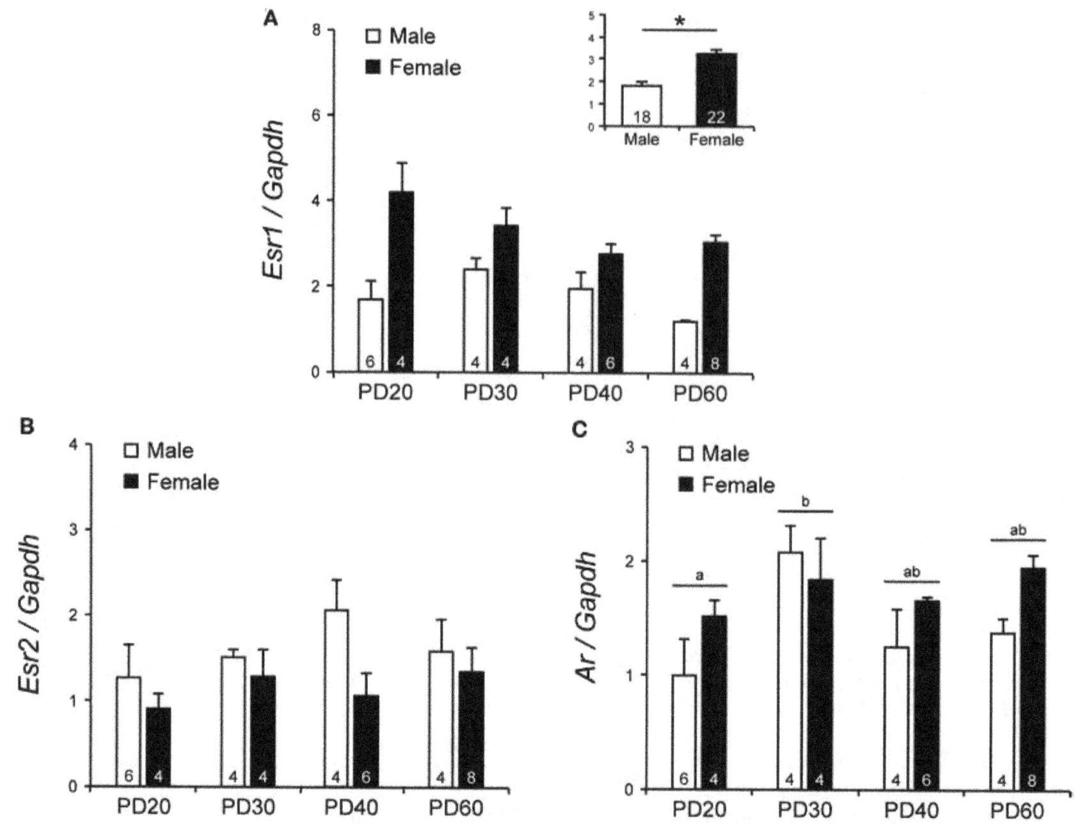

FIGURE 3 | The mRNA levels of *Esr1*, *Esr2*, and *Ar* in the AVPV of peripubertal mice. The mRNA levels of *Esr1* **(A)**, *Esr2* **(B)**, and *Ar* **(C)** in male and female mice on PD20, PD30, PD40, and PD60. The inset graph in panel **(A)** indicates the average mRNA level of *Esr1* in all ages. The numbers in the columns indicate the numbers of animals. Values are the mean ± SEM. Differences in values that are significantly (p < 0.05) different from each other are indicated with letters. *p < 0.05.

gonadally intact males and was significantly greater ($p < 0.05$) than that in the orchidectomzied and cholesterol-implanted males (**Figures 5A,B**). Likewise, the number of calbindin-ir cells in the BNSTp was significantly smaller ($p < 0.05$) in the orchiectomized and cholesterol-implanted males than in gonadally intact males (**Figure 5C**). The cell number in the orchiectomized and testosterone-implanted males was significantly larger ($p < 0.05$) than that in the orchiectomized and cholesterol-implanted males and was similar to that in gonadally intact males.

DISCUSSION

Here, we examined the mRNA levels of *Esr1*, *Esr2*, *Cyp19a1*, and *Ar* in the AVPV and BNSTp of peripubertal mice. To the best of our knowledge, this is the first study to examine these mRNA expressions to investigate the role of gonadal hormones during puberty in the formation of sexually dimorphic structures in the AVPV and BNSTp. We revealed that these genes are expressed in a sex-, age-, and region-specific manner. Especially, *Cyp19a1* mRNA was expressed in the BNSTp but not in the AVPV on PD20–60. This suggests that the AVPV and BNSTp respond differentially to testicular testosterone, which might contribute to the sexually dimorphic development of these brain structures.

Role of Sex Steroids in the Development of the AVPV

We previously showed that the volume and neuron number in the AVPV of male mice lacking *Esr1* and *Cyp19a1* are larger than those of wild-type males and similar to those of females, although the volume and neuron number in the AVPV of male mice lacking *Esr2* are comparable to those of wild-type males (23). We further showed that the AVPV expresses *Esr1* and *Cyp19a1* in the perinatal period (23). Additionally, it has been reported that administration of testosterone to postnatal female rats reduces AVPV volume and the number of TH and kisspeptin neurons in this structure in adulthood (6, 22). In this study, we found that the AVPV expressed *Esr1* and *Esr2*, but not *Cyp19a1* during PD20–60. This finding suggests that testicular testosterone in the peripubertal period is not converted to estradiol locally in the AVPV and does not affect the AVPV of male mice *via* ESR1 and ESR2, although it is not ruled out that estradiol produced elsewhere can affect the AVPV. Taken together, it is suggested that the morphology of the male AVPV might be organized by estradiol, which is synthesized from testicular testosterone by CYP19A1 (aromatase) expressed locally in the AVPV, which signals *via* ESR1 in the perinatal, but not pubertal period. Here, we found that *Ar* mRNA was expressed in the AVPV during puberty. However, AR-mediated testosterone signaling might

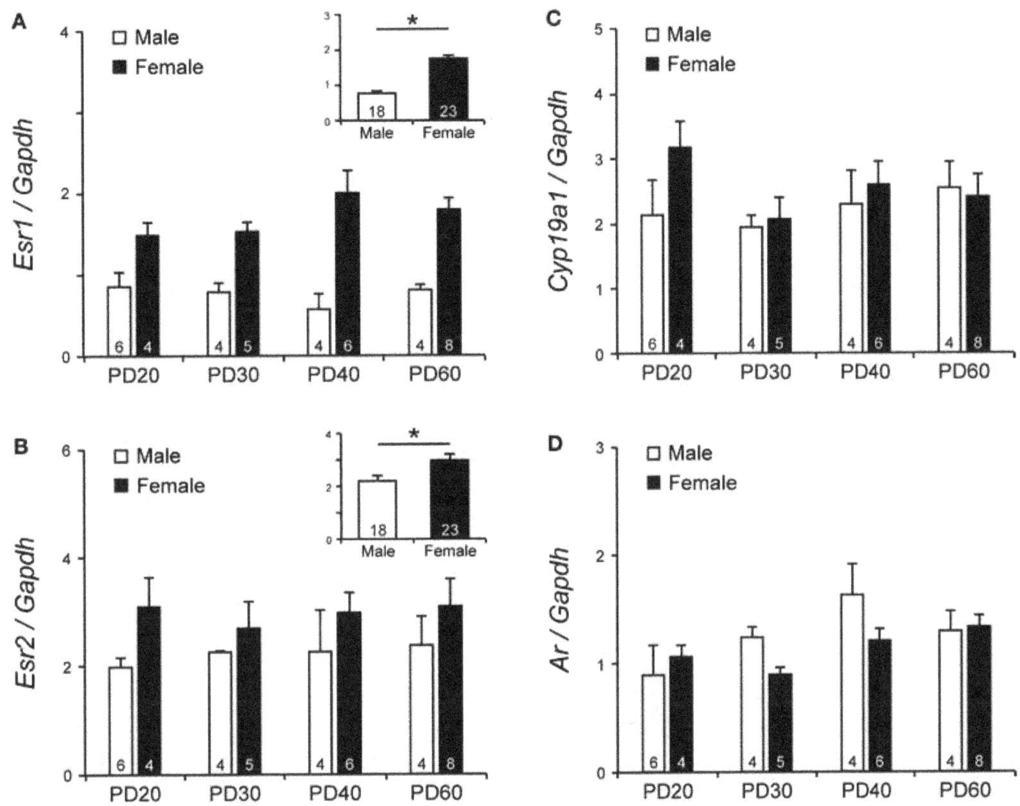

FIGURE 4 | The mRNA levels of *Esr1*, *Esr2*, *Cyp19a1*, and *Ar* in the BNSTp of peripubertal mice. The mRNA levels of *Esr1* **(A)**, *Esr2* **(B)**, *Cyp19a1* **(C)**, and *Ar* **(D)** in male and female mice on PD20, PD30, PD40 and PD60. The inset graphs in panels **(A,B)** indicate the average mRNA level of *Esr1* and *Esr2* in all ages, respectively. The numbers in the columns indicate the numbers of animals. Values are the mean ± SEM. $^*p < 0.05$.

not be necessary for the organization of the AVPV in male mice, because the volume and neuron number in the AVPV of *Ar* KO male mice is comparable to those of wild-type male mice (23). Additionally, the AVPV in male rats appears to be not affected by prepubertal orchiectomy (33), suggesting that testicular hormones during puberty contribute minimally to the organization of the AVPV in male mice.

Esr1 and *Esr2* were expressed in the female AVPV from PD20 to PD60. Given that ovaries begin to produce estradiol on PD7 (41), ovarian estradiol could act on the AVPV through ESR1 and ESR2 during the peripubertal period. We found here that AVPV volume increased from PD20 to PD30, and remained high on PD60, and that it was greater in female mice compared with male mice. During puberty in rats, newborn cells are incorporated into the AVPV, more so in females than in males, and this incorporation of new cells is suppressed by ovariectomy on PD20 (33). Thus, ovarian estradiol, signaling through ESR1 and/or ESR2 during puberty, might promote the generation of AVPV cells, which could contribute to the sexually dimorphic development of the AVPV.

Role of Sex Steroids in the Development of the BNSTp

We previously reported that the masculinization of the BNSTp is disrupted in male mice lacking *Esr1*, *Cyp19a1*, or *Ar*, but not *Esr2* (23). We further found that the BNSTp expresses mRNAs of *Esr1* and *Cyp19a1* in the perinatal period and *Ar* mRNA in the postnatal period (23). Neonatal orchiectomy decreases the volume and number of neurons in the BNSTp of adult male rats (12), and early postnatal treatment with testosterone or estradiol increases the number of neurons in the BNSTp of adult female mice (25). These findings suggest that testosterone, acting through AR, during the postnatal period, and aromatized testosterone (estradiol), acting through ESR1, during the perinatal period help to masculinize the morphology of the BNSTp. In addition, it is thought that pubertal gonadal hormones affect the formation of the BNSTp. The BNSTp in prepubertal male mice has a greater volume and contains a larger number of calbindin neurons than the BNSTp of female mice of the same age (31, 32), and these sex differences become more pronounced over time, with a gradual increase in these parameters in males and a gradual decrease in females during puberty (31, 32). The increase in the volume and calbindin neuron number of the male BNSTp is suppressed by orchiectomy on PD20 (32). In this study, we confirmed that orchiectomy at PD20 reduced BNSTp volume and calbindin-ir cell number of the BNSTp in adult male mice. Moreover, we revealed that a compensatory treatment with testosterone could rescue the effects of orchiectomy at PD20 on the BNSTp in male mice. These findings suggest that testicular testosterone during puberty plays an important role in the formation of the male

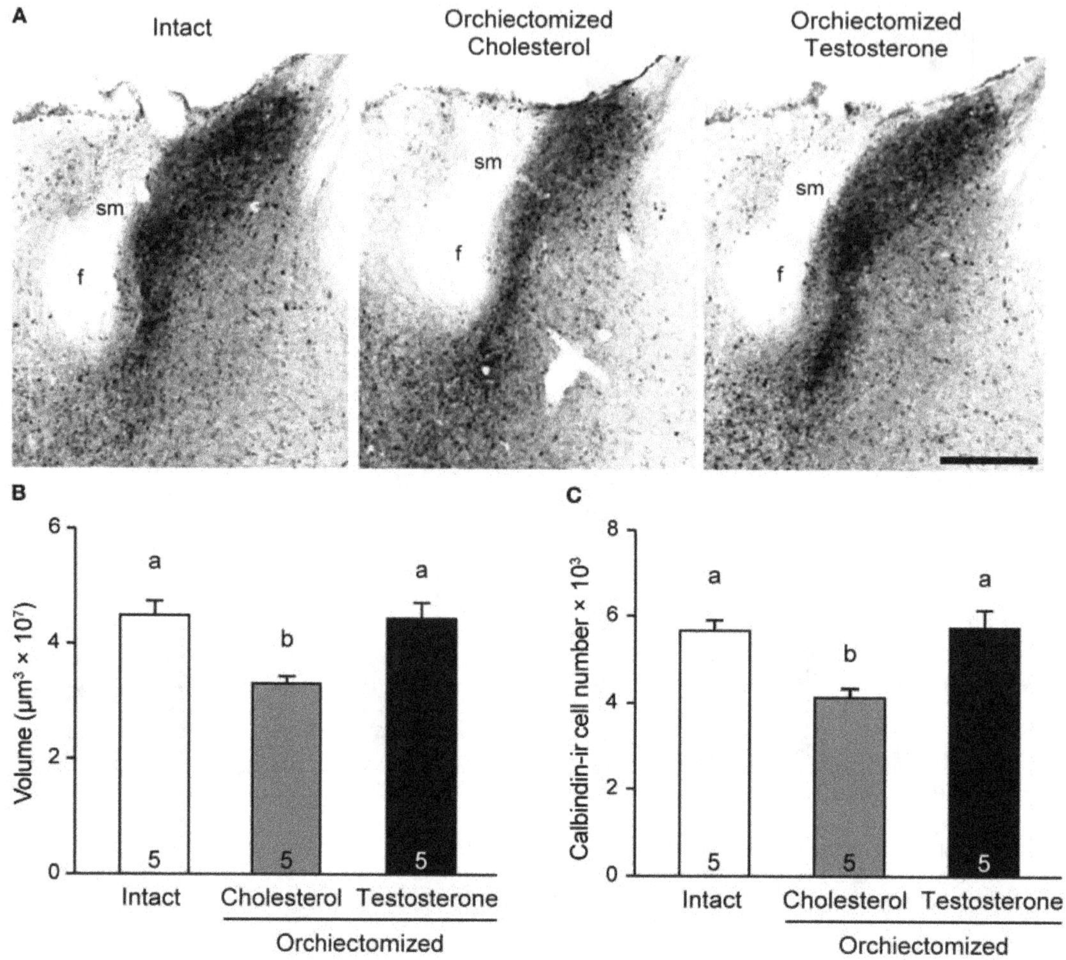

FIGURE 5 | Effects of peripubertal testicular testosterone on the BNSTp in male mice. **(A)** Representative photomicrographs of brain sections from a gonadally intact adult male mouse, an adult male mouse subjected to orchiectomy and cholesterol implantation at PD20, and an adult male mouse subjected to orchiectomy and testosterone implantation at PD20. Scale bar indicates 300 μm. f, fornix; sm, stria medullaris of the thalamus. **(B)** The volume of the BNSTp in adult male mice. **(C)** The number of the calbindin-ir cells in the BNSTp of adult male mice. The numbers in the columns indicate the numbers of animals. Differences in values that are significantly ($p < 0.05$) different from each other are indicated with letters.

BNSTp. It was reported that the volume of the BNSTp in adult male rats is reduced by orchiectomy in adulthood (42), whereas orchiectomy in adulthood has no effect on BNSTp volume in guinea pigs (43). Therefore, the results of our current study do not exclude the notion that the formation of the male BNSTp requires testicular testosterone in the postpubertal period as well as the pubertal period. Considering that the BNSTp from PD20 to PD60 expressed the mRNAs of *Esr1*, *Cyp19a1*, and *Ar*, we can deduce that the masculinization of the BNSTp is affected both by testicular testosterone acting *via* AR and by estradiol, which is synthesized locally in the BNSTp by CYP19A1 from testicular testosterone and acts *via* ESR1, during the pubertal period. Thus, unlike the defeminization of the AVPV, the masuclinization of the BNSTp is likely established by testicular testosterone and estradiol not only in the perinatal period, but also in the pubertal period. In comparison, the volume and number of calbindin neurons in the BNSTp are lower in adult females than in PD20 females, and ovariectomy on PD20 does not affect the reduction in BNSTp volume or neuron number during puberty (32). Unlike the formation of the male BNSTp, the formation of the female BNSTp may be independent of ovarian hormones during puberty, despite the mRNA expression of *Esr1* and *Esr2* in this brain structure.

On PD4, the mRNA levels of *Esr1* and *Cyp19a1* in the BNSTp of *Ar* KO male mice are higher than those in wild-type male mice (23). This suggests that testosterone acting *via* AR suppresses the mRNA expression of *Esr1* and *Cyp19a1* in the male BNSTp, thereby reducing estradiol signaling in the early postnatal period. In male mice, the testosterone concentration in blood is gradually increased before puberty and it is higher levels during puberty (PD35 and PD40) (44). Therefore, if the inhibitory action of testosterone on *Esr1* and *Cyp19a1* mRNA expressions persists until puberty, the action of a large amount of testosterone *via* AR and lower ESR1 expression in the male BNSTp during puberty might stimulate male-specific development of this structure, as more testosterone would be available to bind the AR (as a lower amount would be converted to estradiol, which would also have fewer receptors to signal through). Nonetheless, it was reported that *Cyp19a1* mRNA and aromatase activity in the bed nucleus of the stria terminalis (BST) including the BNSTp of adult male rats are enhanced by testosterone actions *via* AR (45, 46). If this mechanism is functional during puberty as well as adult period, pubertal testosterone may facilitate estrogen production, followed by enhancement of estrogen signaling *via* ESR. Indeed, a marked less ESR1 in the male BNSTp than in the female BNSTp on PD20–60 may be due to a downregulation of ESR1 by a large amount of aromatized testosterone. Taken together, further experiments are required to determine the relevance between testosterone action *via* AR and estradiol action *via* ESR1 in the BNSTp during puberty in the sexually dimorphic formation of the BNSTp.

Microscopic Isolation of Target Tissues

In this study, we isolated the AVPV and BNSTp from the brain using the LMD system. The LMD system enables precise and accurate isolation of target regions in sample tissues. This allowed us to detect sex-, age-, and region-dependent differences in the mRNA expression of genes related to sex steroid signaling. In the AVPV, we found that *Esr1* mRNA levels were greater in females at PD20–60. However, in one study, the expression of ESR1 protein in the AVPV on PD25 did not differ between the sexes (47). There might be a sex difference in the posttranscriptional stability of *Esr1* mRNA and/or the posttranslational stability of ESR1 protein. In the BNSTp, one study reported that greater *Esr1* mRNA expression in female mice is not observed at PD20, but appears by PD60 (48). Another study reported that the murine BNSTp on PD25 contains a greater number of ESR1-immunoreactive cells in females compared with males (47). In this study, although we did not find a significant difference in *Esr1* mRNA levels between sexes at each age, we observed higher mRNA levels of *Esr1* in female mice at PD20–60. Our current study showed no sex difference in *Cyp19a1* mRNA expression in the BNSTp. Another study showed that *Cyp19a1* mRNA expression in the BST is greater

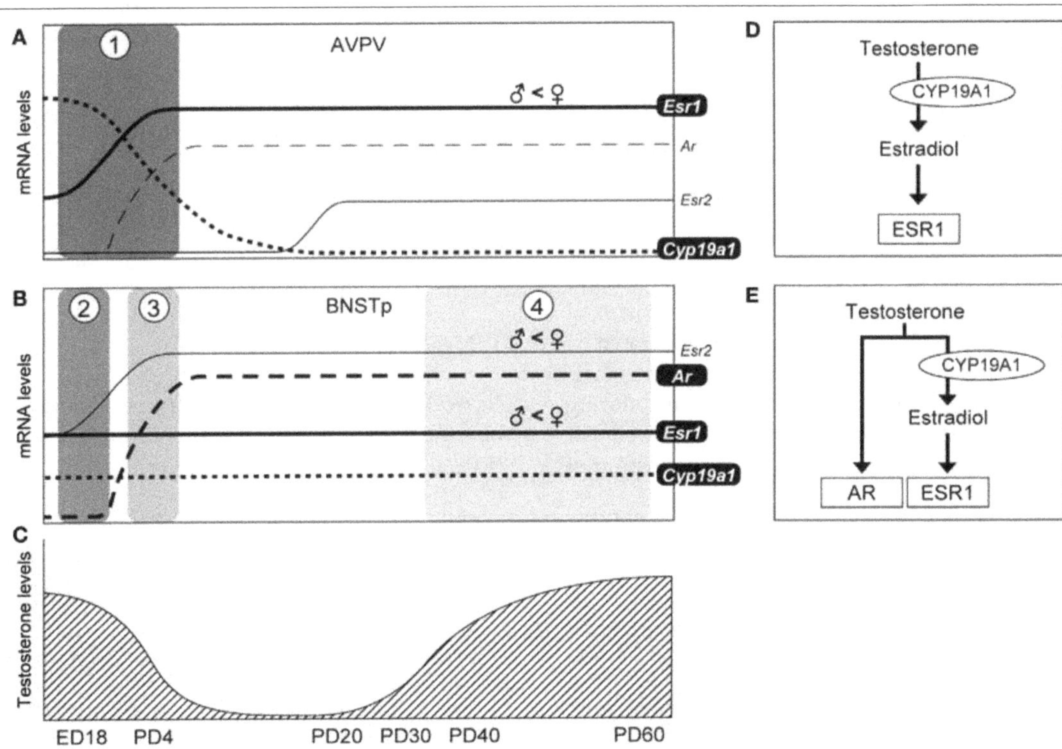

FIGURE 6 | Schematic illustration of the temporal expression patterns of genes in the AVPV and BNSTp and possible testicular testosterone actions on the formation of the AVPV and BNSTp in male mice. In the AVPV [*panel* **(A)**], based upon our previous (23) and current studies, *Esr1* mRNA expression (*solid line*) increases from embryonic day 18 (ED18) to PD4 and continues in the pubertal period. *Cyp19a1* mRNA level (*dotted line*) decreases from ED18 to PD4 and is not expressed by PD20. *Esr1* and *Cyp19a1* are essential to the formation of the male AVPV, but *Esr2* and *Ar* are not necessary (23). Testicular testosterone production reaches a peak level at ED18 and decreases after birth (50), and again is increased from PD35 (44) [*panel* **(C)**]. The temporal patterns of *Esr1*, *Cyp19a1*, and testicular testosterone may indicate that the male AVPV is organized by estradiol (formed by the aromatization of testosterone) signaling through ESR1 during the perinatal period [*boxed phase 1 in panel* **(A)** and *panel* **(D)**]. In the BNSTp [*panel* **(B)**], based upon our previous (23) and current studies, *Esr1* mRNA (*solid line*) is expressed during the perinatal period, and is also expressed during the pubertal period. *Cyp19a1* mRNA level (*dotted line*) is stably expressed in the perinatal and pubertal periods. *Ar* mRNA (*broken line*) is not expressed in the late fetal period (ED18), but expressed in the postnatal (PD4) and pubertal periods. *Esr1*, *Cyp19a1*, and *AR* are requisite for the sexual differentiation of the male BNSTp (23, 26). The patterns of *Esr1*, *Cyp19a1*, *Ar*, and testicular testosterone levels may indicate that the male BNSTp is formed by the action of estradiol (formed by the aromatization of testicular testosterone) *via* ESR1 in the fetal period [*boxed phase 2 in panel* **(B)** and *panel* **(D)**], and both the action of estradiol *via* ESR1 and testicular testosterone *via* AR in the postnatal [*boxed phase 3 in panel* **(B)** and *panel* **(E)**] and pubertal [*boxed phase 4 in panel* **(B)** and *panel* **(E)**] periods.

in male mice than in female mice (49). This discordance may be due to a difference of target area. Target area in the previous study was the BST that includes some sub-nuclei (lateral division–dorsal, intermediate, posterior and ventral parts; and medial division–anterior, ventral parts, etc.). By contrast, our current study targeted only the BNSTp (the principal nucleus of the BST posterior division).

In this study, the volume of the AVPV and BNSTp was measured. We found that volume of the AVPV was larger in female mice than that in male mice through PD20 to PD60, although the sex difference was no found at each age. It was previously reported that the sexual dimorphism in AVPV volume in rats emerges between PD30 and PD40 (2). Considering species differences, it is plausible that we correctly isolated AVPV tissues enough to detect sex- and age-related alterations. Regarding the BNSTp, we found a male-biased difference in the volume on PD20–PD60. This sex difference may be resulted from an increase in the volume of the male BNSTp during puberty as reported previously (28, 31, 32). In this study, there was a tendency that the volume of the male BNSTp increased with age. Taken together, the results that sex differences and age-related alterations in the volume of the AVPV and BNSTp could be acquired in the LMD system may guarantee the accuracy of mRNA expression analysis in the current study.

In conclusion, pubertal testosterone is not converted to estradiol locally in the AVPV because of the absence of *Cyp19a1* mRNA. This suggests that estradiol synthesized in the AVPV itself is not able to act on the AVPV. Our previous study showed that *Esr1* and *Cyp19a1* are necessary genes for the defeminization of the AVPV, but *Esr2* and *Ar* are not, and that *Esr1* and *Cyp19a1* mRNAs are expressed in the AVPV in the perinatal period (23). Collectively, the male AVPV might be generated by estradiol (formed by the aromatization of testosterone) signaling through ESR1 during the perinatal period, but not during puberty (**Figure 6**). Additionally, our previous study showed that *Esr1*, *Cyp19a1*, and *Ar* are necessary for the masculinization of the BNSTp, but *Esr2* is not (23, 26). Furthermore, we previously reported that the BNSTp expresses *Esr1* and *Cyp19a1* mRNAs in the perinatal period and *Ar* mRNA in the postnatal period (23). In this study, we found that the BNSTp expresses *Esr1*, *Cyp19a1*, and *Ar* in the pubertal period. Additionally, the results of the histological analysis of the BNSTp suggest that testicular testosterone during puberty affects the formation of the BNSTp in male mice. The findings of our current study may indicate that the masculinization of the BNSTp is affected by testosterone, *via* AR, and by estradiol (formed by the aromatization of testosterone) *via* ESR1 during puberty. Thus, the sexually dimorphic development of the BNSTp in males might be accomplished by testicular testosterone in the postnatal and pubertal periods as well as by estradiol derived from testosterone in the perinatal and pubertal periods (**Figure 6**).

ETHICS STATEMENT

All animal experimental procedures were approved by the Animal Care and Experimentation Committee of Saitama University and were conducted in accordance with the Guidelines for the Care and Use of Experimental Animals of Saitama University.

AUTHOR CONTRIBUTIONS

MK performed the experiments, analyzed the data, and prepared the manuscript. MM performed the experiments and analyzed the data. ST designed the experiments, analyzed the data, and prepared the manuscript.

FUNDING

This work was supported by Grants-in-Aid for Scientific Research from the Japan Society for the Promotion of Science (No. 17K08567 to ST).

REFERENCES

1. Bleier R, Byne W, Siggelkow I. Cytoarchitectonic sexual dimorphisms of the medial preoptic and anterior hypothalamic areas in guinea pig, rat, hamster, and mouse. *J Comp Neurol* (1982) 212(2):118–30. doi:10.1002/cne.902120203
2. Davis EC, Shryne JE, Gorski RA. Structural sexual dimorphisms in the anteroventral periventricular nucleus of the rat hypothalamus are sensitive to gonadal steroids perinatally, but develop peripubertally. *Neuroendocrinology* (1996) 63(2):142–8. doi:10.1159/000126950
3. Simerly RB, Swanson LW, Gorski RA. The distribution of monoaminergic cells and fibers in a periventricular preoptic nucleus involved in the control of gonadotropin release: immunohistochemical evidence for a dopaminergic sexual dimorphism. *Brain Res* (1985) 330(1):55–64. doi:10.1016/0006-8993(85)90007-1
4. Sumida H, Nishizuka M, Kano Y, Arai Y. Sex differences in the anteroventral periventricular nucleus of the preoptic area and in the related effects of androgen in prenatal rats. *Neurosci Lett* (1993) 151(1):41–4. doi:10.1016/0304-3940(93)90040-R
5. Clarkson J, Herbison AE. Postnatal development of kisspeptin neurons in mouse hypothalamus; sexual dimorphism and projections to gonadotropin-releasing hormone neurons. *Endocrinology* (2006) 147(12):5817–25. doi:10.1210/en.2006-0787
6. Kauffman AS, Gottsch ML, Roa J, Byquist AC, Crown A, Clifton DK, et al. Sexual differentiation of Kiss1 gene expression in the brain of the rat. *Endocrinology* (2007) 148(4):1774–83. doi:10.1210/en.2006-1540
7. Scott N, Prigge M, Yizhar O, Kimchi T. A sexually dimorphic hypothalamic circuit controls maternal care and oxytocin secretion. *Nature* (2015) 525(7570):519–22. doi:10.1038/nature15378
8. Smith JT, Popa SM, Clifton DK, Hoffman GE, Steiner RA. Kiss1 neurons in the forebrain as central processors for generating the preovulatory luteinizing hormone surge. *J Neurosci* (2006) 26(25):6687–94. doi:10.1523/JNEUROSCI.1618-06.2006
9. Robertson JL, Clifton DK, de la Iglesia HO, Steiner RA, Kauffman AS. Circadian regulation of Kiss1 neurons: implications for timing the preovulatory gonadotropin-releasing hormone/luteinizing hormone surge. *Endocrinology* (2009) 150(8):3664–71. doi:10.1210/en.2009-0247
10. Forger NG, Rosen GJ, Waters EM, Jacob D, Simerly RB, de Vries GJ. Deletion of Bax eliminates sex differences in the mouse forebrain. *Proc Natl Acad Sci U S A* (2004) 101(37):13666–71. doi:10.1073/pnas.0404644101
11. del Abril A, Segovia S, Guillamon A. The bed nucleus of the stria terminalis in the rat: regional sex differences controlled by gonadal steroids early after birth. *Brain Res* (1987) 429(2):295–300. doi:10.1016/0165-3806(87)90110-6
12. Guillamon A, Segovia S, del Abril A. Early effects of gonadal steroids on the neuron number in the medial posterior region and the lateral division of the

bed nucleus of the stria terminalis in the rat. *Brain Res Dev Brain Res* (1988) 44(2):281–90. doi:10.1016/0165-3806(88)90226-X
13. Hines M, Allen LS, Gorski RA. Sex differences in subregions of the medial nucleus of the amygdala and the bed nucleus of the stria terminalis of the rat. *Brain Res* (1992) 579(2):321–6. doi:10.1016/0006-8993(92)90068-K
14. Caldwell HK, Lee HJ, Macbeth AH, Young WS III. Vasopressin: behavioral roles of an "original" neuropeptide. *Prog Neurobiol* (2008) 84(1):1–24. doi:10.1016/j.pneurobio.2007.10.007
15. Rood BD, Stott RT, You S, Smith CJ, Woodbury ME, De Vries GJ. Site of origin of and sex differences in the vasopressin innervation of the mouse (*Mus musculus*) brain. *J Comp Neurol* (2013) 521(10):2321–58. doi:10.1002/cne.23288
16. Rood BD, Murray EK, Laroche J, Yang MK, Blaustein JD, De Vries GJ. Absence of progestin receptors alters distribution of vasopressin fibers but not sexual differentiation of vasopressin system in mice. *Neuroscience* (2008) 154(3):911–21. doi:10.1016/j.neuroscience.2008.03.087
17. De Vries GJ, al-Shamma HA. Sex differences in hormonal responses of vasopressin pathways in the rat brain. *J Neurobiol* (1990) 21(5):686–93. doi:10.1002/neu.480210503
18. Bielsky IF, Hu SB, Ren X, Terwilliger EF, Young LJ. The V1a vasopressin receptor is necessary and sufficient for normal social recognition: a gene replacement study. *Neuron* (2005) 47(4):503–13. doi:10.1016/j.neuron.2005.06.031
19. Bielsky IF, Hu SB, Young LJ. Sexual dimorphism in the vasopressin system: lack of an altered behavioral phenotype in female V1a receptor knockout mice. *Behav Brain Res* (2005) 164(1):132–6. doi:10.1016/j.bbr.2005.06.005
20. Forger NG. Control of cell number in the sexually dimorphic brain and spinal cord. *J Neuroendocrinol* (2009) 21(4):393–9. doi:10.1111/j.1365-2826.2009.01825.x
21. Tsukahara S. Sex differences and the roles of sex steroids in apoptosis of sexually dimorphic nuclei of the preoptic area in postnatal rats. *J Neuroendocrinol* (2009) 21(4):370–6. doi:10.1111/j.1365-2826.2009.01855.x
22. Simerly RB. Hormonal control of the development and regulation of tyrosine hydroxylase expression within a sexually dimorphic population of dopaminergic cells in the hypothalamus. *Brain Res Mol Brain Res* (1989) 6(4):297–310. doi:10.1016/0169-328X(89)90075-2
23. Kanaya M, Tsuda MC, Sagoshi S, Nagata K, Morimoto C, Thu CK, et al. Regional difference in sex steroid action on formation of morphological sex differences in the anteroventral periventricular nucleus and principal nucleus of the bed nucleus of the stria terminalis. *PLoS One* (2014) 9(11):e112616. doi:10.1371/journal.pone.0112616
24. Patchev AV, Gotz F, Rohde W. Differential role of estrogen receptor isoforms in sex-specific brain organization. *FASEB J* (2004) 18(13):1568–70. doi:10.1096/fj.04-1959fje
25. Hisasue S, Seney ML, Immerman E, Forger NG. Control of cell number in the bed nucleus of the stria terminalis of mice: role of testosterone metabolites and estrogen receptor subtypes. *J Sex Med* (2010) 7(4 Pt 1):1401–9. doi:10.1111/j.1743-6109.2009.01669.x
26. Tsukahara S, Tsuda MC, Kurihara R, Kato Y, Kuroda Y, Nakata M, et al. Effects of aromatase or estrogen receptor gene deletion on masculinization of the principal nucleus of the bed nucleus of the stria terminalis of mice. *Neuroendocrinology* (2011) 94(2):137–47. doi:10.1159/000327541
27. Juntti SA, Tollkuhn J, Wu MV, Fraser EJ, Soderborg T, Tan S, et al. The androgen receptor governs the execution, but not programming, of male sexual and territorial behaviors. *Neuron* (2010) 66(2):260–72. doi:10.1016/j.neuron.2010.03.024
28. Schulz KM, Zehr JL, Salas-Ramirez KY, Sisk CL. Testosterone programs adult social behavior before and during, but not after, adolescence. *Endocrinology* (2009) 150(8):3690–8. doi:10.1210/en.2008-1708
29. Juraska JM, Sisk CL, DonCarlos LL. Sexual differentiation of the adolescent rodent brain: hormonal influences and developmental mechanisms. *Horm Behav* (2013) 64(2):203–10. doi:10.1016/j.yhbeh.2013.05.010
30. Gilmore RF, Varnum MM, Forger NG. Effects of blocking developmental cell death on sexually dimorphic calbindin cell groups in the preoptic area and bed nucleus of the stria terminalis. *Biol Sex Differ* (2012) 3:5. doi:10.1186/2042-6410-3-5
31. Wittmann W, McLennan IS. The bed nucleus of the stria terminalis has developmental and adult forms in mice, with the male bias in the developmental form being dependent on testicular AMH. *Horm Behav* (2013) 64(4):605–10. doi:10.1016/j.yhbeh.2013.08.017
32. Morishita M, Maejima S, Tsukahara S. Gonadal hormone-dependent sexual differentiation of a female-biased sexually dimorphic cell group in the principal nucleus of the bed nucleus of the stria terminalis in mice. *Endocrinology* (2017) 158(10):3512–25. doi:10.1210/en.2017-00240
33. Ahmed EI, Zehr JL, Schulz KM, Lorenz BH, DonCarlos LL, Sisk CL. Pubertal hormones modulate the addition of new cells to sexually dimorphic brain regions. *Nat Neurosci* (2008) 11(9):995–7. doi:10.1038/nn.2178
34. Piekarski DJ, Johnson CM, Boivin JR, Thomas AW, Lin WC, Delevich K, et al. Does puberty mark a transition in sensitive periods for plasticity in the associative neocortex? *Brain Res* (2017) 1654(Pt B):123–44. doi:10.1016/j.brainres.2016.08.042
35. Shughrue PJ, Bushnell CD, Dorsa DM. Estrogen receptor messenger ribonucleic acid in female rat brain during the estrous cycle: a comparison with ovariectomized females and intact males. *Endocrinology* (1992) 131(1):381–8. doi:10.1210/endo.131.1.1612018
36. Zhou Y, Shughrue PJ, Dorsa DM. Estrogen receptor protein is differentially regulated in the preoptic area of the brain and in the uterus during the rat estrous cycle. *Neuroendocrinology* (1995) 61(3):276–83. doi:10.1159/000126849
37. Leite C, Madeira MD, Sa SI. Effects of sex steroids and estrogen receptor agonists on the expression of estrogen receptor alpha in the principal division of the bed nucleus of the stria terminalis of female rats. *Brain Res* (2014) 1582:99–106. doi:10.1016/j.brainres.2014.07.041
38. Feng Y, Weijdegard B, Wang T, Egecioglu E, Fernandez-Rodriguez J, Huhtaniemi I, et al. Spatiotemporal expression of androgen receptors in the female rat brain during the oestrous cycle and the impact of exogenous androgen administration: a comparison with gonadally intact males. *Mol Cell Endocrinol* (2010) 321(2):161–74. doi:10.1016/j.mce.2010.02.029
39. Franklin KBJ, Paxinos G. *The Mouse Brain in Stereotaxic Coordinates*. 3rd ed. San Diego, CA: Academic Press (2008).
40. Faul F, Erdfelder E, Lang AG, Buchner A. G*Power 3: a flexible statistical power analysis program for the social, behavioral, and biomedical sciences. *Behav Res Methods* (2007) 39(2):175–91. doi:10.3758/BF03193146
41. Mannan MA, O'Shaughnessy PJ. Steroidogenesis during postnatal development in the mouse ovary. *J Endocrinol* (1991) 130(1):101–6. doi:10.1677/joe.0.1300101
42. Malsbury CW, McKay K. Neurotrophic effects of testosterone on the medial nucleus of the amygdala in adult male rats. *J Neuroendocrinol* (1994) 6(1):57–69. doi:10.1111/j.1365-2826.1994.tb00555.x
43. Hines M, Davis FC, Coquelin A, Goy RW, Gorski RA. Sexually dimorphic regions in the medial preoptic area and the bed nucleus of the stria terminalis of the guinea pig brain: a description and an investigation of their relationship to gonadal steroids in adulthood. *J Neurosci* (1985) 5(1):40–7. doi:10.1523/JNEUROSCI.05-01-00040.1985
44. Stephens SB, Chahal N, Munaganuru N, Parra RA, Kauffman AS. Estrogen stimulation of Kiss1 expression in the medial amygdala involves estrogen receptor-alpha but not estrogen receptor-beta. *Endocrinology* (2016) 157(10):4021–31. doi:10.1210/en.2016-1431
45. Roselli CE. Sex differences in androgen receptors and aromatase activity in microdissected regions of the rat brain. *Endocrinology* (1991) 128(3):1310–6. doi:10.1210/endo-128-3-1310
46. Roselli CE, Resko JA. Sex differences in androgen-regulated expression of cytochrome P450 aromatase in the rat brain. *J Steroid Biochem Mol Biol* (1997) 61(3–6):365–74. doi:10.1016/S0960-0760(97)80034-9
47. Brock O, De Mees C, Bakker J. Hypothalamic expression of oestrogen receptor alpha and androgen receptor is sex-, age- and region-dependent in mice. *J Neuroendocrinol* (2015) 27(4):264–76. doi:10.1111/jne.12258
48. Kelly DA, Varnum MM, Krentzel AA, Krug S, Forger NG. Differential control of sex differences in estrogen receptor alpha in the bed nucleus of the stria terminalis and anteroventral periventricular nucleus. *Endocrinology* (2013) 154(10):3836–46. doi:10.1210/en.2013-1239
49. Stanic D, Dubois S, Chua HK, Tonge B, Rinehart N, Horne MK, et al. Characterization of aromatase expression in the adult male and female mouse brain. I. Coexistence with oestrogen receptors alpha and beta, and androgen receptors. *PLoS One* (2014) 9(3):e90451. doi:10.1371/journal.pone.0090451

5

Neurosteroid Actions in Memory and Neurologic/ Neuropsychiatric Disorders

*Marcia H. Ratner, Vidhya Kumaresan and David H. Farb**

Laboratory of Molecular Neurobiology, Department of Pharmacology and Experimental Therapeutics, Boston University School of Medicine, Boston, MA, United States

Correspondence:
David H. Farb
dfarb@bu.edu

Memory dysfunction is a symptomatic feature of many neurologic and neuropsychiatric disorders; however, the basic underlying mechanisms of memory and altered states of circuitry function associated with disorders of memory remain a vast unexplored territory. The initial discovery of endogenous neurosteroids triggered a quest to elucidate their role as neuromodulators in normal and diseased brain function. In this review, based on the perspective of our own research, the advances leading to the discovery of positive and negative neurosteroid allosteric modulators of GABA type-A ($GABA_A$), NMDA, and non-NMDA type glutamate receptors are brought together in a historical and conceptual framework. We extend the analysis toward a state-of-the art view of how neurosteroid modulation of neural circuitry function may affect memory and memory deficits. By aggregating the results from multiple laboratories using both animal models for disease and human clinical research on neuropsychiatric and age-related neurodegenerative disorders, elements of a circuitry level view begins to emerge. Lastly, the effects of both endogenously active and exogenously administered neurosteroids on neural networks across the life span of women and men point to a possible underlying pharmacological connectome by which these neuromodulators might act to modulate memory across diverse altered states of mind.

Keywords: neurosteroid, memory, anxiety, depression, schizophrenia, allopregnanolone, pregnenolone sulfate, Alzheimer's disease

INTRODUCTION

A major question in neuroscience since the initial discovery that somatically released gut peptides could alter central nervous system (CNS) function relates to whether and how the body can influence or modulate brain function. The science of neuroendocrinology was advanced conceptually 50 years ago by the independent discoveries of Schally, Leeman and Reichlin, demonstrating that the gut peptides thyrotropin-releasing hormone (TRH) (1, 2) and substance P (3, 4) were synthesized, stored, and released in the hypothalamus as endogenous neuromodulators. The demonstration of local synthesis of neuropeptides within the CNS presented a non-canonical mechanism for gut peptides to act as chemical neurotransmitters at synapses, without transport via the systemic circulation and transport across the blood-brain barrier (BBB).

The BBB does not impair access of sex steroids to the CNS to the same extent as gut peptides. Lipophilic steroid hormones, such as progesterone, estradiol and testosterone cross the BBB and readily gain access to the CNS (5) where they can serve as agonists of steroid hormone receptors that in turn act at genomic response elements. In the early 1980s, several lines of evidence from Etienne, Baulieu, and Robel (6–9) challenged the central dogma that neuroactive steroids were exclusively synthesized peripherally, demonstrating for the first time that steroids could be synthesized from cholesterol within the CNS.

Such steroids were called *neurosteroids* and an intensive search began to identify which steroids belonged to this group and to define their function. An early clue came from the research of Selye (10) showing that steroids could have anesthetic effects. Four decades later, in 1983, radiolabeling studies by Sapolsky, McEwen, and Rainbow revealed uptake of corticosterone in the stratum oriens and apical dendrite regions of the hippocampus, suggesting that GABAergic interneurons in these regions might possess corticosterone receptors (11). Corticosterone treatment had been shown to affect GABA uptake in the hippocampus, possibly suggesting a mechanism for hormonal modulation of memory. In a seemingly unrelated study, while investigating the pharmacological mechanism of action of the synthetic steroid anesthetic alphaxalone, Harrison and Simmonds (12) demonstrated that alphaxalone and barbiturates shared a common mechanism of action via augmenting $GABA_AR$ action. Subsequent research by multiple investigators demonstrated that several reduced metabolites of progesterone and deoxycorticosterone act as positive allosteric modulators of $GABA_ARs$ (13–17), much like benzodiazepines (18, 19). Other research (20, 21) also suggested that neurosteroids might be capable of modulating inhibitory GABAergic neurotransmission.

As new ideas emerged from clinical studies by Andrew Herzog in the mid 1980s concerning the possible role of estrogen and progesterone in catamenial epilepsy (22), we hypothesized that progesterone might act as a positive allosteric modulator of the $GABA_AR$. This led to the early work of Fong-sen Wu and Terrell Gibbs in my lab (23) showing that progesterone did in fact modulate $GABA_A$ and glycine receptors. Unexpectedly, we also found that pregnenolone sulfate (PregS), a novel negatively charged steroid derived from the sulfation of pregnenolone (PREG), potentiated N-methyl-D-aspartate receptor (NMDAR) function (24) (**Figure 1** and **Table 1**).

Over the ensuing 25 years, endogenous neurosteroids have been implicated in learning and memory function, hippocampal information processes, and synaptic plasticity (28, 29, 48, 59–63). Neurosteroids have also been implicated in the etiology and treatment of learning and memory disturbances associated with certain neuropsychiatric disorders, including schizophrenia, depression, and anxiety (50, 64–66) (**Table 2**).

Memory dysfunction is frequently comorbid with age-related neurodegenerative diseases, such as Alzheimer's disease (AD) (84). From a therapeutic standpoint, the lack of an effective treatment for memory disorders extends beyond neurodegeneration to a wide range of neuropsychiatric disorders, such as depression and schizoprhenia.

Memory dysfunction seriously impacts performance of routine tasks necessary for a productive and healthy life, including the ability to maintain gainful employment and compliance with treatment plans (85). This review summarizes the field from the perspective of our own research, which has spanned the past three decades, and attempts to bring together state-of-the-art findings related to the role of neurosteroids in memory dysfunction, as seen in patients with schizophrenia, depression, and anxiety disorders. We believe that a greater understanding of how steroids modulate neural network activity will help lay the foundation for a unifying theory of neurosteroid action in the brain centered on a systems level "pharmacological connectome."

SYNTHESIS, STRUCTURE, TRANSPORT AND CELLULAR TARGETS OF NEUROSTEROIDS

Synthesis and Translocation

Neurosteroid synthesis involves translocation of cholesterol across the mitochondrial membrane by transport proteins, such as the steroidogenic acute regulatory protein (StAR protein), the translocator protein (TSPO), voltage-dependent anion channel (VDAC) protein and the adenine nucleotide transporter (ANT) protein (86–89). The conversion of cholesterol to PREG is catalyzed by the enzyme cytochrome P450 side chain cleavage (P450 scc) located on chromosome 15 in humans (90). Other enzymes that play a role in the biosynthesis of neurosteroids include 5α-reductase and 3α-hydroxysteroid dehydrogenase (91–93). These two enzymes are involved in the biosynthesis of allopregnanolone (ALLO) and tetrahydrodeoxycorticosterone (THDOC); the identification of neurons that express these enzymes in the rodent cerebral cortex, hippocampus, olfactory bulb, amygdala, and thalamus suggests that ALLO and THDOC can be synthesized locally from precursors within the CNS (94).

The sulfation and desulfation of neurosteroids further alters both the pharmacokinetic and pharmacodynamic properties of these endogenous neuromodulators (95). In humans, sulfation of PREG to PregS is catalyzed by SULT2B1a, whereas SULT2B1b

---

Abbreviations: ACTH, adrenocorticotropic hormone; AD, Alzheimer's disease; ALLO, allopregnanolone; AMPA, α-amino-3-hydroxy-5-methyl-4-isoxazolepropionic acid; ANT, adenine nucleotide transporter protein; BBB, blood-brain barrier; BNST, bed nucleus of the stria terminalis; CB1, cannabinoid receptor 1; CICR, Ca^{2+}-induced Ca^{2+} release; CNS, central nervous system; DA, dopamine; DAT, dopamine transporter; DAT KO, dopamine transporter knockout; DHEA, dehydroepiandrosterone; DHEAS, dehydroepiandrosterone sulfate; GABA, gamma-aminobutyric acid; GAD, generalized anxiety disorder; GLIC, Gloeobacter ligand-gated ion channels; GnRH, gonadotrophin-releasing hormone; HPA axis, hypothalamic-pituitary-adrenal axis; HRSA, Hamilton Rating Scale for Anxiety; IL-6, interleukin-6; L-Type VGCC, L-type voltage-gated Ca^{2+} channel; LTD, long-term depression; LTP, long-term potentiation; MCI, mild cognitive impairment; NMDA, N-methyl-D-aspartate; OATPs, organic anion transporting peptides; ORAI1, Ca^{2+} release-activated Ca^{2+} channel protein 1; PAHS, pregnanolone hemisuccinate; pCREB, phosphorylated CREB; PET, positron emission tomography; PCOS, polycystic ovary syndrome; PREG, pregnenolone; PregS, pregnenolone sulfate; PTSD, post-traumatic stress disorder; PV, parvalbumin; PXR, pregnane xenobiotic receptor; P450 scc, cytochrome P450 side chain cleavage; sEPSC, spontaneous excitatory post-synaptic currents; 5-HT, serotonin; SSRIs, selective serotonin reuptake inhibitors; StAR protein, steroidogenic acute regulatory protein; STIM1, stromal interaction molecule 1; THDOC, tetrahydrodeoxycorticosterone; TRH, thyrotropin-releasing hormone; TRP channels, transient receptor potential channels; TSPO, translocator protein; VDAC, voltage-dependent anion channel.

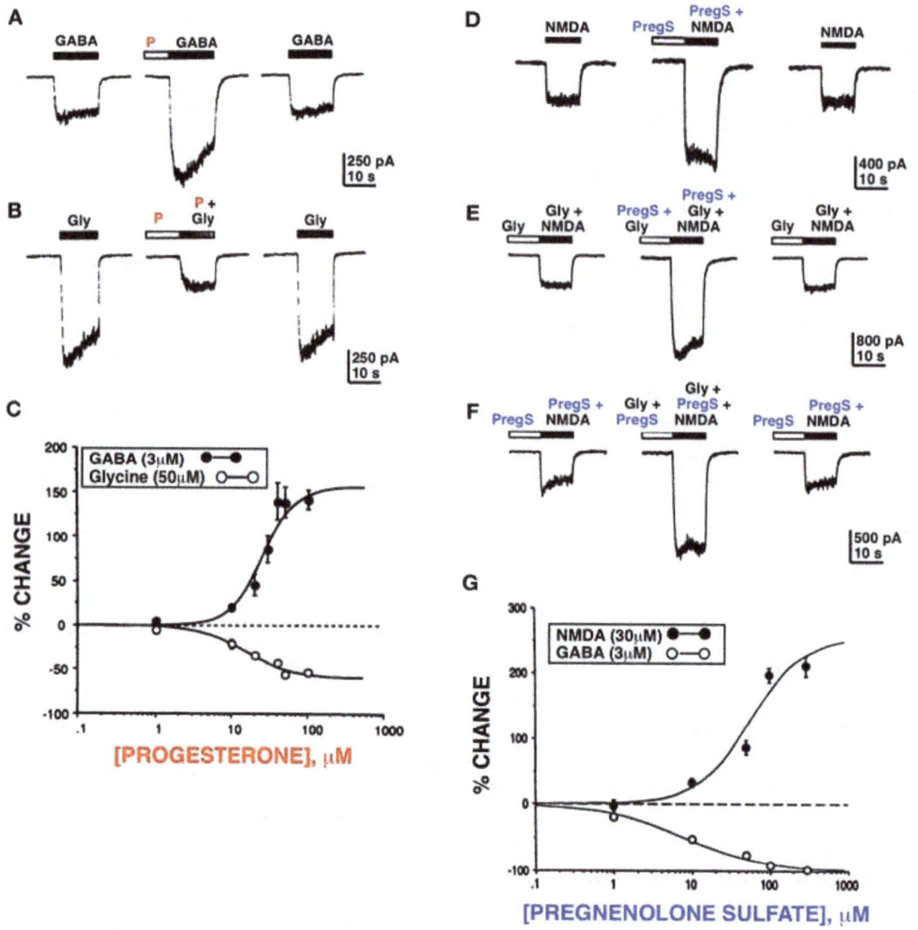

FIGURE 1 | Progesterone and PregS differentially modulate whole cell currents induced by GABA, glycine and NMDA. Progesterone (P) (100 μM) potentiates the GABA response **(A)** and inhibits the glycine **(B)** response. **(C)** Dose response curves for progesterone modulation of GABA and glycine currents; enhancement of the GABA response by progesterone occurs over the same concentration range as inhibition of the glycine response. **(D)** PregS (100 μM) potentiates the NMDA response (normal media [Gly]). **(E)** PregS and glycine potentiate NMDA response by different mechanisms. **(F)** In the presence of the maximal concentration (10 μM) of glycine, PregS (100 μM) enhances (179 ± 17.1%; $n = 4$) the response induced by 30 μM of NMDA; **(F)** In the presence of near maximal concentration of PregS (100 μM), glycine (10 μM) reversibly potentiates (210 ± 36.5%; $n = 4$) the NMDA response. **(G)** Dose response curves for PregS modulation of NMDA and GABA currents. Enhancement of the NMDA response by PregS occurs over the same concentration range as inhibition of the GABA response (*Horizontal bar above each trace represents period of drug application*) [Modified from Wu et al. (23, 24) with Permission].

preferentially catalyzes the sulfation of 3beta-hydroxysteroids. Non-human primate studies suggest that age-dependent changes in the expression of these enzymes could play a role in age-related changes in cognitive function (96, 97).

Neurosteroids and their sulfated conjugates can be characterized based on their core backbone structures as pregnanes, pregnenes, androstanes, progesterones, and deoxycorticosterones. Neurosteroids in these respective subcategories include: pregnanolone and pregnanolone sulfate; PREG and PregS; dehydroepiandrosterone (DHEA) and dehydroepiandrosterone sulfate (DHEAS); progesterone and ALLO; and, deoxycorticosterone and THDOC (98). While delineating the neurological function of sulfated neurosteroids remains a frontier in neuroendocrinology, some fundamental progress has been made these past few decades.

Physiological Actions

The physiologic effects of neurosteroids are mediated through direct interactions with neurotransmitter receptors and transporters, and indirectly via promotion of second-messenger signaling cascades (47, 48, 99–103). Their rapid non-genomic effects are exerted via the allosteric modulation of inhibitory and excitatory receptors located in the surface membrane. In some cases, neurosteroids exert genomic effects, at least in part, by activation of intracellular steroid receptors (104). The degree to which neurosteroids produce genomic and non-genomic effects depends on the extent to which they are metabolized (e.g., PREG to progesterone), and the extent to which the parent molecule and its neuroactive metabolites modulate extra- and intracellular receptors (104).

The modulation of GABAergic neurotransmission by neurosteroids is mediated by interactions with allosteric sites

TABLE 1 | Historical discoveries in pregnene series neurosteroids.

References	System and methodology	Key findings and novel outcomes
Majewska and Schwartz (21); Majewska, (25)	Measurement of inhibition of GABA-mediated uptake of labeled chloride in rat brain synaptosome preparations	Demonstration of a possible receptor target for PregS as an inhibitor of $GABA_A$ receptors
Wu et al. (24); Farb et al. (26)	Whole cell patch clamp of NMDARs currents in cultured chick spinal cord neurons	PregS and related sulfated neurosteroids of the pregnene series potentiate NMDARs acting as functional neuromodulators in glutamatergic synaptic transmission
Irwin et al. (27)	Micro-spectrofluorimetric measurement of intracellular calcium in primary neuronal cultures of rat hippocampus	Neurosteroids, such as PregS modulate excitation-inhibition balance in the CNS
Flood et al. (28–30); Plescia et al. (31); Plescia et al. (32); Abdel-Hafiz, (33)	Behavioral assays in rodent models	Pregnene group neurosteroid-mediated enhancement of cognitive function. Subsequent studies provide further demonstration that PREG and its metabolite, PregS, enhances memory.
Park-Chung et al. (34)	Whole cell patch clamp in cultured chick spinal cord neurons	Elucidation of subunit-specific effects of PregS and demonstration that pregnene neurosteroids modulate excitatory ionotropic GluRs.
Park-Chung et al. (35, 36)	Whole cell recordings in cultured chick spinal cord neurons. Structure-activity studies using recordings from recombinant NMDAR expressed in *Xenopus* oocytes	Identification of PregS binding site. First demonstration that steroids function by binding to an extracellular site on NMDAR.
Yaghoubi et al. (37); Malayev et al. (38); Cameron et al. (39)	Voltage clamp recordings of recombinant NMDAR in *Xenopus* oocytes. Bacterial cultures. Intrinsic fluorescence spectroscopy.	PregS positively modulates GluN2A- and GluN2B-containing NMDARs. PregS inhibits GluN2C- and GluN2D-containing NMDARs and AMPA/kainate receptors.
Partridge and Valenzuela, (40); Sliwinski et al. (41); Sabeti et al. (42)	Measurement of long-term potentiation using hippocampal slice electrophysiology	PregS modulates synaptic strength critical for learning and memory. nM PregS: modulates LTP via NMDARs; modulates presynaptic release of glutamate; voltage-gated Ca^{2+} channel induced LTP potentiation.
Jang et al. (43); Horak et al. (44); Kostakis et al. (45)	Electrophysiology; molecular modeling; recombinant chimeric NMDARs, with altered residues by means of site directed mutagenesis expressed in *Xenopus* oocytes.	PregS exhibits a rich modulatory repertoire enabled by the structural diversity of NMDARs. The extracellular steroid-modulatory site (SMD1) contains the J/K helices and contiguous TMD4. Extracellular loop between TMD3 and 4 mediates both excitatory and inhibitory effects.
Petrovic et al. (46)	Voltage-clamp studies in HEK293 cells expressing NR1/NR2B NMDARs and cultured rat hippocampal neurons.	PregS influences NMDAR-dependent responses via a phosphorylation dependent mechanism.
Kostakis et al. (47); Smith et al. (48)	Whole cell recordings of recombinant receptors expressed in oocytes and $[Ca^{2+}]$i imaging using and primary neuronal cultures of embryonic cortical neurons	First demonstration that physiologically relevant concentrations of PregS modulate synaptic plasticity *in vitro.* Picomolar concentrations are sufficient to increase intracellular Ca^{2+}. Increased intracellular Ca^{2+} increases surface GluN1-NMDARs and CREB activation. PregS mediated modulation of NMDARs results in delayed onset potentiation occurs via a non-canonical G-protein and Ca^{2+} dependent manner. This potentiation is absent when the J/K helices and TMD4 of GluN2B are replaced with that of GluN2D further establishing the subunit-dependent action of PregS and importantly the extracellular binding site of PregS.
Smith et al. (48); Adamusová et al. (49)	$[Ca^{2+}]$i imaging studies using primary rat hippocampal neuronal cultures and HEK293 cells	Picomolar to femtomolar concentrations of PregS increases intracellular $Ca2^{+}$
Marx et al. (50–52); Ritsner et al. (53)	Human subjects for clinical effects	Adjunctive treatment with PREG in schizophrenia and schizoaffective disorders shown to reduce negative symptoms and improve positive symptoms of verbal memory and attention. Post-treatment elevation of ALLO and PregS correlate with enhancement of cognitive function. Metabolism of PREG to PregS likely ameliorating NMDAR hypofunction implicated in schizophrenia.
Wilding et al. (54)	Whole cell recordings and molecular modeling using recombinant chimeric GluN and GluK2 receptor constructs in HEK 293 cells	Confirmation of binding sites and relationship to specific receptor domains elucidated. Confirmed extracellularly directed binding site for PregS. Requirement of TMD likely for pore formation.
Paul et al. (55); Linsenbardt et al. (56)	Investigations of synthetic PregS analogs and oxysterols as therapeutics using *in vitro* and *ex vivo* electrophysiological methods	The major brain-derived cholesterol metabolite, 24(S)-hydroxy cholesterol modulates NMDARs by binding to an intracellular site. This intracellular oxysterol binding site is distinct from the extracellular site that bind PregS.
Vyklicky et al. (57)	Electrophysiological investigations of *de novo* missense mutations of the hGluN2B expressed in HEK cells.	Missense mutations of the hGluN2B subunit located in membrane domains lead to multiple defects that manifest by the NMDAR loss of function that can be rectified by steroids.
Chisari et al. (58)	Hippocampal slice electrophysiology, *in vitro* electrophysiological recordings from cultured hippocampal neurons and *Xenopus* oocytes. expressing recombinant NMDARs.	Analogs of PregS and oxysterols, such as KK169 shown to exhibit properties of PregS.

TABLE 2 | Neurosteroids in human neurologic and neuropsychiatric disorders.

Disorder	Neurosteroid(s)	Clinical response	Memory
ALZHEIMER'S DISEASE			
Temporal cortex: Naylor et al. (67)	Increased DHEA and PREG decrease ALLO levels	ALLO levels inversely correlate with Braak and Braak neuropathological stage	NR
Striatum and cerebellum: Hypothalamus: Weill-Engerer et al. (60)	Low PregS and DHEAS Low DHEAS	Negative correlation between cortical β-amyloid and PregS in striatum and cerebellum Negative correlation between levels of pTau and DHEAS	NR
DHEAS: Carlson et al. (68)	Increases in plasma	AD risk not linked with DHEAS	Increased memory performance
Cortisol: Csernansky et al. (69)	Increases in plasma	More rapid disease progression	Increased memory performance
Cortisol: Carlson et al. (68)	Decreases in plasma	No relationship to AD risk	Increased Delayed Route Recall
DHEA in women: Rasmuson et al. (70)	Increases in serum	Associated with AD risk	NR
DHEA and DHEAS in men: Aldred and Mecocci (71)	Decreases in plasma	Associated with AD risk	NR
Cortisol in men: Rasmuson et al. (70)	Increases in serum	Associated with AD risk	NR
aMCI in men: Cherrier et al. (72)	Testosterone treatment	Reduced depression	Improved verbal memory
MOOD DISORDERS			
GAD in elderly: Mantella et al. (73)	Increased saliva cortisol	Positive correlation between symptoms and saliva cortisol	NR
Generalized social phobia in men: Heydari and Le Mellédo (74)	Decreased plasma PregS	PregS levels lower in generalized social phobia subjects	NR
PTSD in women: Rasmusson et al. (75)	Decreased CSF ALLO	ALLO/DHEA correlates negatively with PTSD and Profile of Mood States depression dejection scores	NR
PTSD in men: Rasmusson et al. (76)	ALLO and pregnanolone CSF	Negative correlation between ALLO + pregnanolone and symptoms severity	NR
Acute stress: Droogleever Fortuyn et al. (77)	Increased plasma ALLO	Peripheral benzodiazepine receptor density increased in blood platelets	NR
Acute psychosocial stress in elderly: Wolf et al. (78)	DHEA at 50 mg/kg/day for 2 weeks	DHEAS lower than in young adults. DHEA replacement increases DHEAS	Enhanced attention; Impaired declarative memory and recall, but not spatial memory.
Dysphoria: Premenstrual Girdler et al. (79)	Increased plasma ALLO/progesterone	Greater levels of premenstrual anxiety	NR
Post-partum depression: Kanes et al. (80, 81)	ALLO	Reduction in hamilton depression rating scale scores.	NR
SCHIZOPHRENIA			
Marx et al. (50)	Adjunctive PREG	Improves negative symptoms and ameliorates cognitive deficits	NR
Marx et al. (51)	Treatment with PREG for 8 weeks	Increases serum PREG and its metabolites ALLO and PregS	Increased serum PREG aligns with BACS score
CATAMENIAL EPILEPSY			
Herzog (22) Herzog and Frye (82)	Progesterone ALLO	Associated with progesterone No association between serum ALLO and seizure frequencies in women treated with progesterone stratified by catamenial vs. non-catamenial epilepsy Serum ALLO correlated with seizure reduction in progesterone-treated women who reported a 3-fold or greater perimenstrual increase in average daily seizure frequency	NR
Partial intractable epilepsy: Valencia-Sanchez et al. (83)	Adjunctive progesterone	No effect on catamenial or non-catamenial seizures	NR

NR, not reported.

on $GABA_AR$s (105–109), and neurosteroids appear to play a role in regulating the expression of specific $GABA_AR$ subunits (63). Classical uncharged neurosteroids modulate inhibitory GABA receptors and neurotransmission. Neurosteroids that are known to be relatively potent positive modulators of GABAergic neurotransmission include ALLO, pregnanolone, and TDHOC.

PregS is a relatively potent positive allosteric modulator of NMDAR-mediated synaptic transmission, while pregnanolone sulfate is a relatively potent negative allosteric modulator of NMDAR-mediated glutamatergic neurotransmission (24, 35, 110).

PregS is the most widely studied neurosteroid that potentiates NMDARs (111, 112). 17-hydroxy-PREG is metabolized to DHEA by cytochrome P450 17α-hydroxylase/17,20-lyase. The sulfated form of DHEA, like the sulfated form of PREG (i.e., PregS), is also an NMDAR potentiator. Electrophysiology studies of recombinant NMDARs expressed in *Xenopus* oocytes have established that the effects of PregS are dependent on NMDAR subunit composition. PregS potentiates GluN2A- and GluN2B-NMDARs, whereas it negatively modulates GluN2C- and GluN2D-NMDARs (38). Long known to be critical for learning and memory, transient activation of NMDARs is required for induction of long-term potentiation (LTP) or strengthening of synaptic transmission, as well as long-term depression (LTD) or weakening of synaptic transmission (113). Activation of NMDARs is crucial for many forms of activity-dependent plasticity responsible for learning and memory in the hippocampus and other brain nuclei (114–118).

PregS also acts as a negative allosteric modulator of GABA, glycine, kainate, and α-amino-3-hydroxy-5-methyl-4-isoxazolepropionic acid (AMPA) receptors (34). The synthetic analog of PregS, PREG hemisuccinate, and other related PREG derivatives bearing a negative charge, potentiate the NMDA response (119). This observation suggests that positive modulation of NMDARs is not mediated by the sulfate group *per se*. Additional studies using other synthetic analogs of PregS revealed that a negatively charged moiety at the C3 position is, however, essential for positive modulation of NMDARs (35). PregS may also influence NMDAR-dependent responses via a phosphorylation-dependent mechanism (46). Low nanomolar concentrations of PregS induce a delayed onset increase of the neuronal response to NMDA and trafficking of NMDAR to the cell surface through an intracellular Ca^{2+} ($[Ca^{2+}]i$)-dependent and non-canonical mechanism involving G-proteins (47) (**Figure 2**). Moreover, low picomolar PregS concentrations appear to be sufficient to increase $[Ca^{2+}]i$ and CREB phosphorylation (48).

Effects of PregS on NMDARs are diverse (15). NMDARs possess at least two distinct modulatory sites (38). PregS increases the frequency and duration of NMDA-mediated channel opening while it inhibits AMPA and $GABA_AR$s (24, 110). PregS effects are dependent on the subunit composition of NMDARs (45, 120). PregS potentiates recombinant NMDARs with GluN1-1a/GluN2B through a steroid modulating domain in GluN2B that also modulates tonic proton inhibition and is pH independent. PregS-mediated potentiation of GluN-2C-NMDARs is similarly pH-dependent. On the other hand, PregS-mediated potentiation of GluN2A and 2D-NMDARs is enhanced at reduced pH. The presence of GluN1-1b subunit with an N-terminal exon-5 splicing insert modulates the extent of proton-dependent PregS potentiation (43, 45). The differential pH sensitivity of the NMDAR isoforms to modulation by PregS is likely to be critical in view of the importance of proton sensors in CNS health and disease (45). PregS acts at a site distinct from the PregS site and inhibits NMDARs irrespective of subunit composition (35, 38, 46).

PregS increases spontaneous excitatory post-synaptic currents (sEPSC) frequency but not amplitude. This demonstrates PregS-mediated presynaptic regulation of spontaneous glutamate release and points to a potential significant impact of PregS on hippocampal function. Presynaptic transient receptor potential channel (TRP channel) receptor activation by PregS modulates glutamate release and increases sEPSC in acutely isolated hilar neurons of the dentate gyrus, an increase that is blocked by TRP channel antagonists (121). Dong et al. (122) had previously demonstrated presynaptic effects of PregS. Lee et al. (121) identified a role for PregS in eliciting presynaptic plasticity by altering intracellular Ca^{2+} via Ca^{2+}-induced Ca^{2+} release (CICR). Moreover, PregS modulates CICR, which is a key mediator of neuronal plasticity. PregS may affect CICR indirectly by activation of NMDARs or L-type voltage-gated Ca^{2+} channels (L-Type VGCCs) and not by direct activation of the Ca^{2+} release-activated Ca^{2+} channel protein 1 (ORAI1) or stromal interaction molecule 1 (STIM1).

DHEA, which is structurally similar to PREG, is the most abundantly expressed neurosteroid in the human body. This neurosteroid is synthesized in the brain, and higher concentrations are found in the brain than in plasma (123). DHEA and DHEAS are neuroprotective, acting via NMDA and AMPA receptors (124, 125). DHEA also appears to play a role in neuronal cell differentiation and programmed cell death via interactions with neurotrophic tyrosine kinase receptors (126, 127). DHEAS, which is structurally similar to PregS except for substitution of carbonyl oxygen for the acetyl group at C17 on the steroid D ring, potentiates NMDA-mediated Ca^{2+} currents and inhibits $GABA_AR$-mediated chloride currents (124, 128–131). Neurosteroids are neuroprotective and reduce neuroinflammation (124, 125, 132, 133).

The Modulatory Recognition Sites

There is a paucity of information on the direct binding of neurosteroids to receptors and of the mechanisms underpinning neuromodulation (39, 134). The ability of neurosteroids to bind to and activate specific categories and subtypes of neuronal receptors is influenced by: (1) conjugation of the parent molecule with a sulfate group; (2) geometry (planar vs. bent); and (3) charge (38, 119). The complexity of neurosteroid-mediated effects, for instance gating of $GABA_AR$ (109, 135–139) and subunit-specific modulation of glycine and NMDARs (140), suggest the likelihood of multiple binding sites that contribute to potentiating and inhibitory effects (39). The effects of neurosteroids on $GABA_AR$s also appears to involve modulation

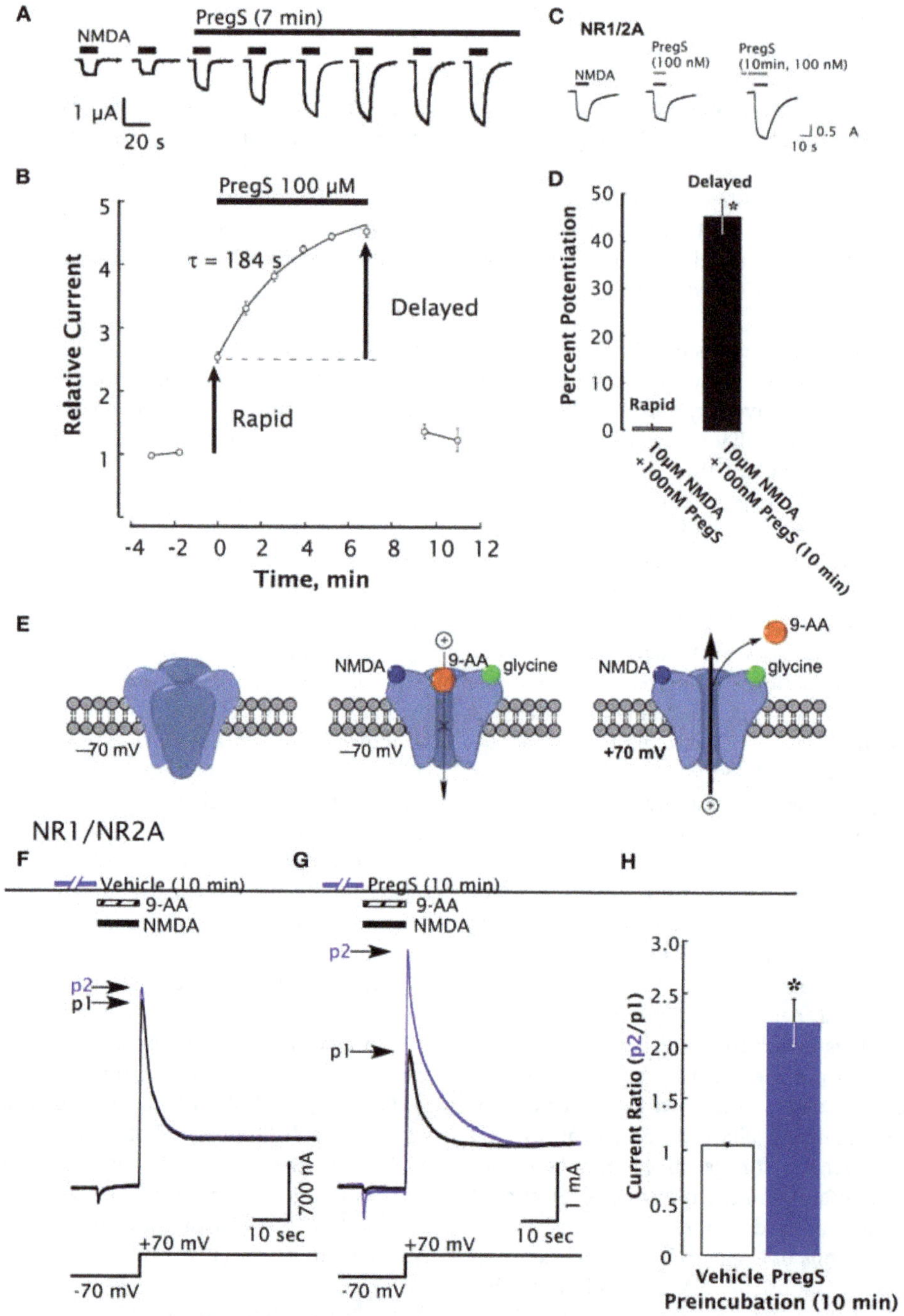

FIGURE 2 | Delayed-onset potentiation of NMDARs is induced by PregS. Two-electrode whole-cell voltage clamp recording from *Xenopus oocytes* expressing NR1/2A subunits following application of PregS (100 μM) and NMDA (300 μM). **(A)** Potentiation of the NMDA response by PregS. Black bars indicate successive applications of NMDA. **(B)** Peak NMDA-induced currents determined as in **(A)** are normalized to the average response before application of PregS beginning at $t = 0$. Smooth curve reflects an exponential fit ($t = 184$ s). Error bars indicate S.E.M. ($n = 3$). Arrows indicate rapid and delayed components of potentiation. **(D)** In oocytes expressing NR1/2A receptors, delayed potentiation but not rapid potentiation is induced by 100 nM PregS. **(D)** Averaged values of normalized peak current responses for rapid and delayed increase. When added simultaneously with NMDA, PregS produces a negligible potentiation of the NMDA response (1 ± 2%), whereas after 10 min pre-incubation with 100 nM PregS, the response to NMDA was enhanced by 45 ± 3%. Error bars represent S.E.M ($n = 8$–10). *Indicates a significant difference between rapid and delayed potentiation ($P < 0.0005$). **(E)** Cartoon shows NMDA and 9-aminoacridine (9-AA) (100 μM) co-applied to *Xenopus oocytes* expressing NR1/2A receptors results in a transient inward current as NMDA-activated channels are blocked by 9-AA (a voltage-dependent open-channel blocker). As the holding potential is switched from −70 to +70 mV, an outward tail current reflecting 9-AA unblock of NMDAR channels ensues (black traces). Cells were then exposed to vehicle (Ba-Ringer) **(F)** or PregS **(G)** for 10 min, and the 9-AA block and unblock sequences were repeated (blue traces). Peak tail currents after baseline subtraction are expressed relative to the control current (black trace) from the same cell (p2/p1). **(H)** The peak current ratio p2/p1 for PregS-treated oocytes (blue bar; $n = 8$) is significantly higher than for vehicle-treated oocytes (white bar; $n = 6$). *Relative current $P < 0.00001$, unpaired 2-tail *t*-test [From Kostakis et al. (47) with Permission].

of δ subunit-containing receptors which play a role in tonic inhibition (141–145).

The receptor transmembrane domain plays a role in neurosteroid-mediated modulation of NMDARs (43) (**Figure 3**) and $GABA_A$Rs (109, 146, 147). Residues in the α1-subunit M1 and/or M2 membrane domains of the $GABA_A$Rs are critical for neurosteroid action (109) (**Figure 4**) Recent studies using Gloeobacter ligand-gated ion channels (GLIC), a prototypic pentameric ligand-gated ion channel that is a homolog to the nicotinic acetylcholine receptor, have identified putative intersubunit and intrasubunit neurosteroid binding sites for ALLO within the transmembrane domain (134) (**Figure 5**). Using this innovative approach, Cheng et al. (134) found that substitutions at the 12 and 15 positions on the neurosteroid backbone altered modulation of GLIC channel activity, demonstrating the functional role of both sites. The interaction of neurosteroids with $GABA_A$R is stereoselective, suggesting that the binding sites for these compounds are of a specific dimension and shape (12, 34, 148).

The results suggest that interactions between the extracellular domain and transmembrane domains play an essential role in the positive and negative modulatory actions of neurosteroids (149). Another important factor determining neurosteroid-dependent modulation of cell function is localization of the neurosteroid. Recent studies have started investigating this aspect using both endogenous neurosteroids and their synthetic

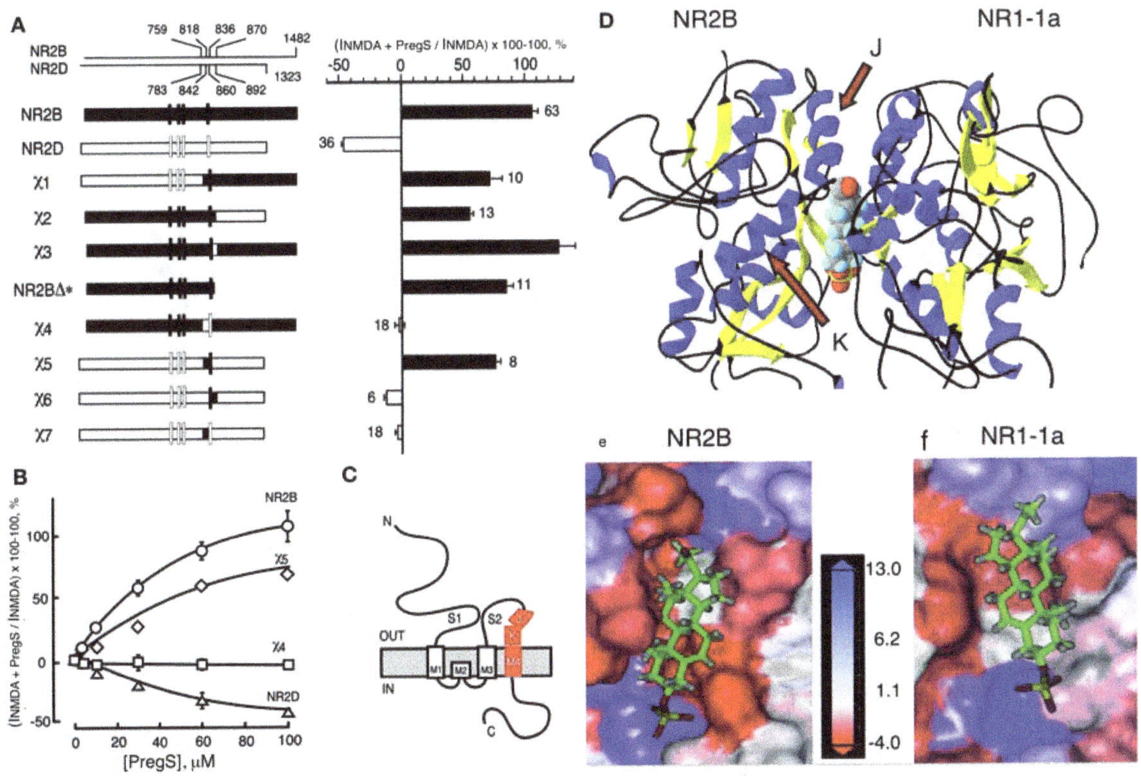

FIGURE 3 | Steroid modulatory domain of NMDARs. **(A)** (Left) Schematic representation of wildtype NR2B, NR2D, and the NR2B, NR2D chimeras. The contribution of NR2B and NR2D to chimeras is depicted in black and white, respectively. The scales at the top indicate the residue numbers in the wildtype subunits at junctions. Vertical bars represent the four hydrophobic membrane domains. (Right) Percent increase in the NMDA glycine response (elicited by 300 μM NMDA and 50 μM glycine in oocytes expressing NR1-1a and NR2 subunits) in the presence of 100 μM PS is indicated. Error bars are SEMs. Numbers adjacent to the error bars indicate the number of oocytes used in the study. **(B)** Concentration–response curves of PregS modulation for receptors containing NR2B (○), NR2D (Δ), χ4 (), and χ5 (◇), were determined in the presence of saturating concentrations of NMDA (300 μM) and glycine (50 μM). The EC50 (NMDA) for NR1-1a χ4 and NR1-1a_NR2B are both 22 ± 1 μM, and EC50 (glycine) is 0.30 ± 0.02 and 0.10 ± 0.02 μM, respectively. **(C)** The topological representation of the NR2B subunit and the location of the identified segment are depicted in red. Membrane domains are denoted as M1–M4. The amino terminus (N) is located on the extracellular side and the carboxyl terminus **(C)** on the intracellular side of the plasma membrane. **(D)** Molecular modeling of potential binding pocket for PregS. The dimer comprising the S1/S2 domains of NR2B and NR1-1a is depicted in a 3D ribbon structure with helices colored in blue and sheets colored in yellow with PregS docked at the interface between the two subunits. Our finding that both J and K helices (see arrows) and M4 of the NR2B subunit are required to confer PS potentiation indicates that M4 is also critical in coupling allosteric modulation from extracellular binding regions to the gating mechanism. **(E)** Detailed view of the potential binding pocket for PregS on NR2B. **(F)** Detailed view of the potential binding pocket for PregS on NR1-1a. NR1-1a or NR2B have been removed from the models to show the hydrophobic pocket on NR2B **(E)** or NR1-1a **(F)**, respectively. The receptor surface is colored according to a hydrophobicity scale with hydrophobic residues in red and charged residues in blue. PregS is depicted in a stick configuration and colored by the atom type with hydrogen in white, carbon in green, oxygen in red, and sulfur in yellow. Our finding that both J and K helices (see arrows) and M4 of the NR2B subunit are required to confer PS potentiation indicates that M4 is also critical in coupling allosteric modulation from extracellular binding regions to the gating mechanism [From Jang et al. (43) with Permission].

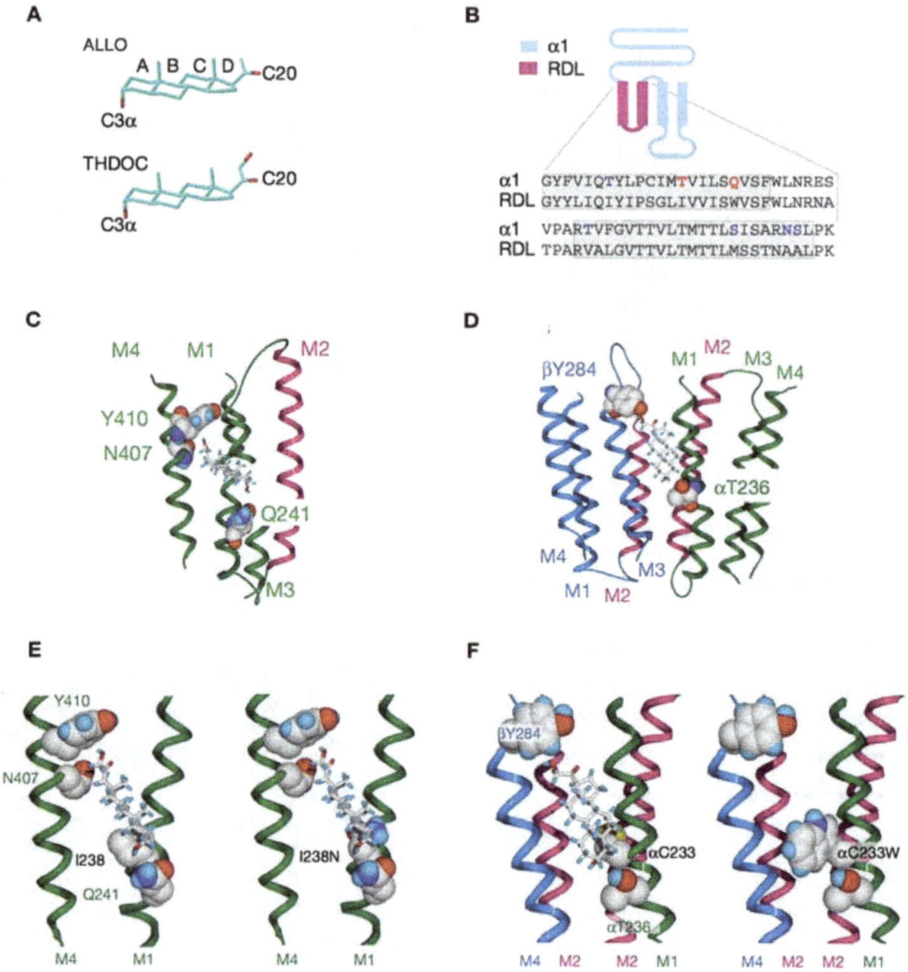

FIGURE 4 | Activation of GABA$_A$Rs by neurosteroids, such as ALLO and THDOC depends on occupancy of both the activation and potentiation sites on the transmembrane domain. **(A)** Regulation of GABA$_A$R, is dependent on the C3a hydroxyl group on the A-ring and the C20 ketone on the D-ring shown here in structures of ALLO and THDOC. **(B)** *Neurosteroid activity is determined by α-subunit M1 domain residues.* Replacement of membrane domains M1 through to the end of M2 in the murine α1 and β2 subunits with the corresponding sequence from the RDL subunit, forming the chimeras αR and βR, respectively, was the first modification used to established their GABA$_A$R pharmacology. Potentiation and direct activation of GABA$_A$Rs by THDOC and ALLO was abolished in chimeric receptors incorporating αR; receptors containing βR were indistinguishable from the wild type. Polar residues in α1 (blue) are in bold, with Thr 236 and Gln 241 (red) highlighted. The transmembrane domains are boxed. **(C)** *Neurosteroid potentiation requires α-subunit M1 and M4 membrane domains.* Ribbon structure of α subunit viewed from the lipid bilayer showing αGln 241, αAsn 407, and αTyr 410 docking with a THDOC molecule. The channel lining the M2 membrane domain is shown in purple (a section of M3 domain is omitted for clarity). **(D)** *Neurosteroid activation binding site spans the β/α-subunit interface.* View of transmembrane region (extracellular and cytoplasmic domains removed) with a bound THDOC molecule. Replacing αThr 236 with non-hydrogen-bonding isoleucine or valine reduces the agonist potency of ALLO and THDOC. **(E)** *Neurosteroid potentiation requires α-subunit M1 and M4 membrane domains.* Homology model of THDOC bound to the potentiation site between M1 and M4 membrane domains of the [David: should the following show alpha or beta symbol?] α subunit (M3 membrane domain removed from figure for clarity). Ile 238 is predicted to lie close to the A-ring of THDOC (left). Introduction of a similar-sized but polar side chain at residue 238, such as replacement with asparagine repels the steroid (right). **(F)** Replacement of Cys 233 (left) with tryptophan (right) increases the steric hindrance for THDOC binding to βTyr 284 and αThr 236 [From Figures 1, 3, 4 of Hosie et al. (109)].

analogs. Neurosteroids that can permeate cell membranes can be localized within different intracellular compartments. This compartmentalization is likely to be of importance to the therapeutic function of the neurosteroid (150).

Other known molecular targets of neurosteroids include various TRP channels (151, 152), serotonin receptors and L-Type VGCCs (42). Subtypes of the TRP channels expressed in mammals include TRPC (canonical), TRPV (vallinoid), TRPM (melastatin), and TRPA (ankyrin) channels. PregS modulates Ca^{2+} influx via TRPM3 channels in pancreatic beta cells (151). In addition, TRPM3 is also activated by related substances PREG, DHEA and DHEA sulfate in these studies. Although previous studies by Chen and Wu (153) suggest that PregS activates TRPV1, also known as the capsaicin receptor, other members of the TRPV and TRPM subfamily tested by Wagner and colleagues were not activated by PregS.

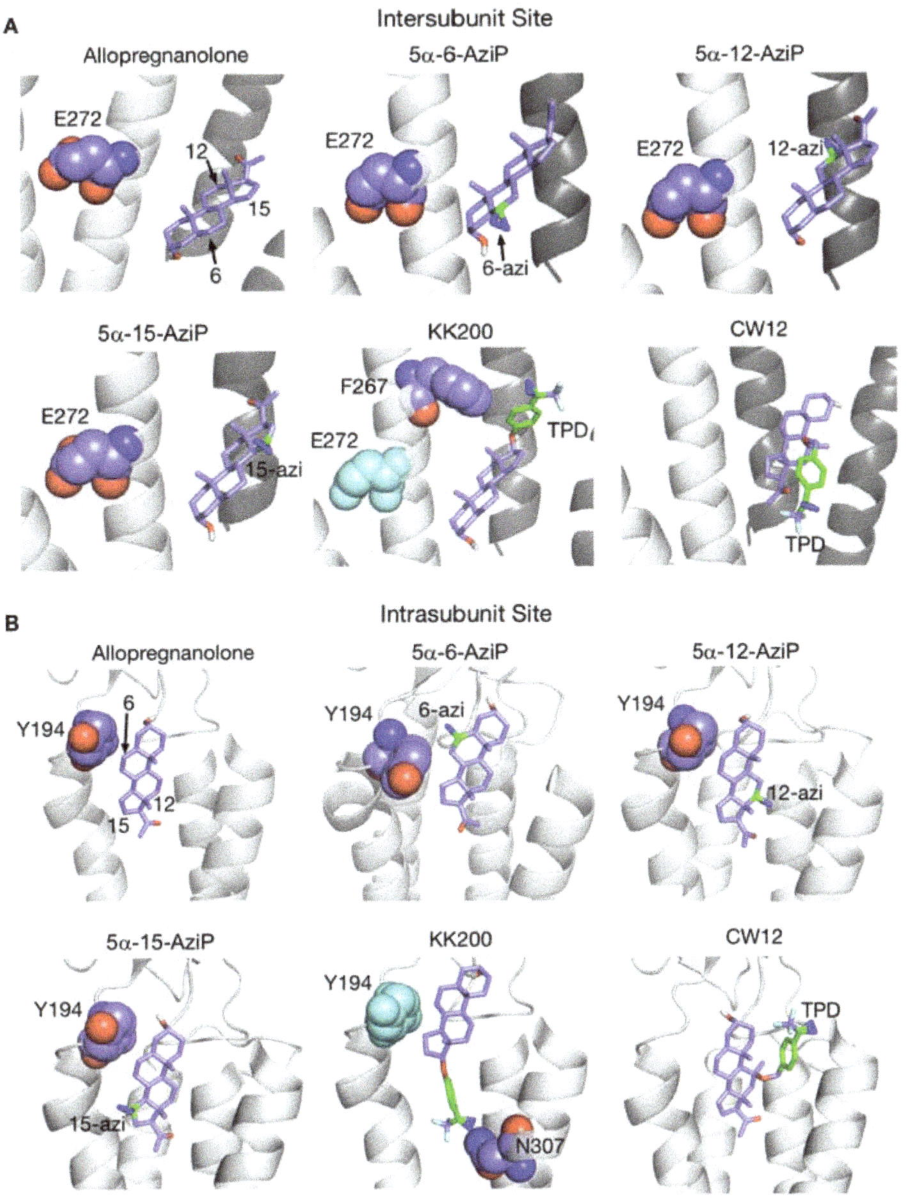

FIGURE 5 | Docking positions of ALLO and photolabeling reagents in the intersubunit and intrasubunit sites. **(A)** Intersubunit docking sites; the photolabeled residues for Glu-272 (5α-6-AziP, 5α-12-AziP, 5α-15-AziP) and Phe-267 (KK200), are shown as purple spheres. **(B)** The intrasubunit docking sites; the photolabeled residues, Tyr-194 (5α-6-AziP) and Asn-307 (KK200), are shown as purple spheres [From Cheng et al. (134), with Permission].

TRPM3 channels are expressed at glutamatergic synapses in neonatal Purkinje cells (154). The effect of PregS on AMPA receptor-mediated miniature excitatory post-synaptic current (mEPSC) frequency is blocked by lanthanide^{3+}, a non-selective TRP channel blocker (155), providing support for TRPM3 as a target for PregS modulation of glutamate release. Valenzuela et al. (156) demonstrated that PregS activates silent synapses by promoting Ca^{2+} influx in a TRP channel-dependent manner, increasing presynaptic glutamate release, and insertion of AMPARs into the post-synaptic membrane (**Figure 6**). Based on these results, Valenzuela et al. developed a working model to explain the actions of PregS at glutamatergic synapses (**Figure 7**). This model is consistent with the recent discovery of delayed onset potentiation of the NMDA response reported by Kostakis et al. (47). We subsequently demonstrated that the phenomenon of delayed onset potentiation of the NMDAR response induced by PregS occurs at physiologically relevant picomolar concentrations and is coupled to a downstream signal transduction pathway associated with learning and memory function (**Figures 8, 9**).

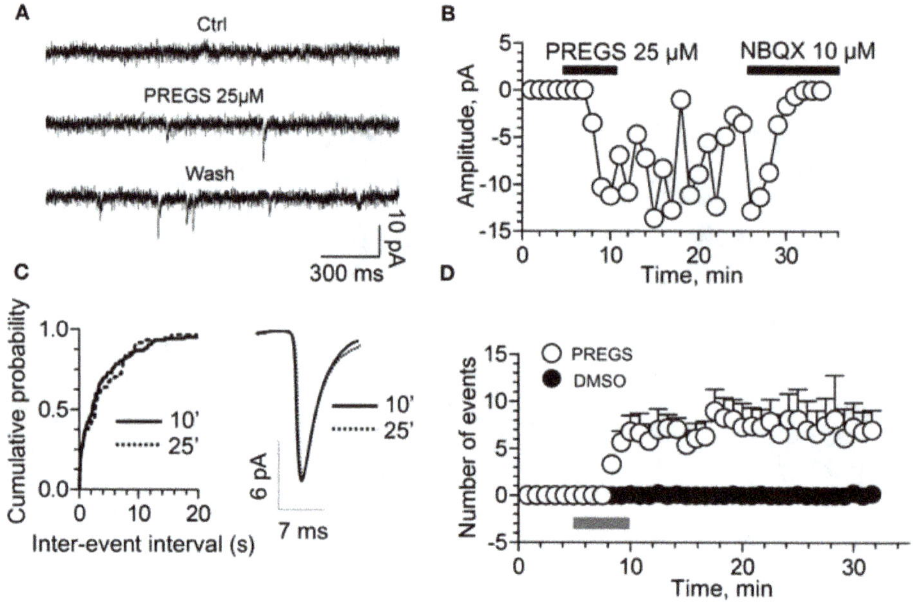

FIGURE 6 | PregS activates silent synapses. **(A)** Sample traces of whole-cell patch-clamp recording from CA1 pyramidal neurons in hippocampal slices from a P3 rat reveal mEPSCs after 25 μM PregS exposure. This effect, which is absent under control conditions, is not reversed by washout. **(B)** Depiction of the time course for the recordings shown in figure **(A)**. Note that NBQX blocks this effect, indicating it is mediated by AMPA receptors. **(C)** Cumulative probability plot. The distribution of the mEPSC inter-event intervals at 10 vs. 25 min is not influenced by PregS exposure. Average mEPSC traces illustrating the lack of an effect of PregS on mEPSC amplitude at these time points. **(D)** Summary figure showing effects of vehicle (DMSO) and PregS (application represented by the gray bar) on the number of events as a function of time ($n = 8$–12) [From Valenzuela et al. (156) with Permission].

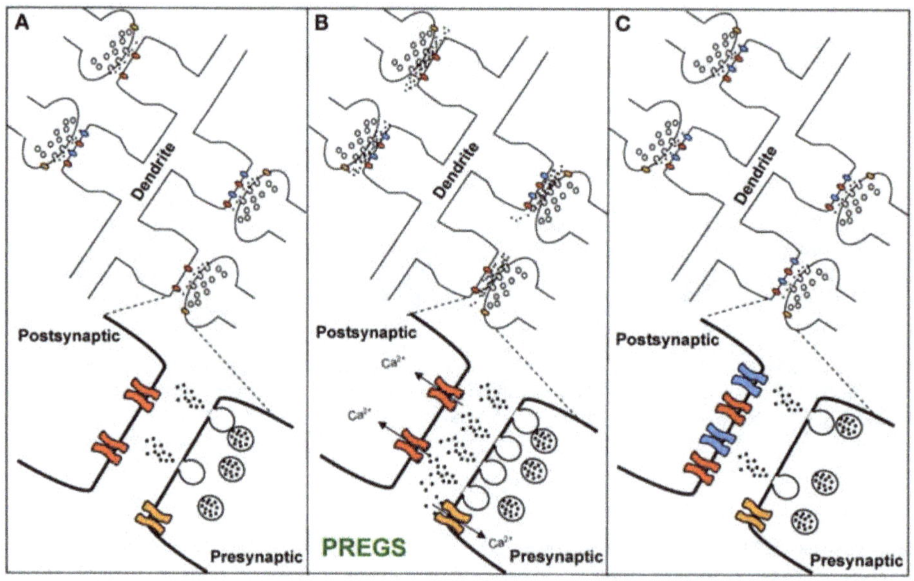

FIGURE 7 | Working model for the action of PregS and related neurosteroids at glutamatergic synapses in immature CA1 hippocampal pyramidal cells. **(A)** Under control conditions, neonatal CA1 hippocampal pyramidal neurons could have a mixture of glutamatergic synapses containing both post-synaptic AMPARs (blue) and NMDARs (red) (active synapses) or only post-synaptic NMDARs (silent synapses at rest). A "*silent synapse*" is enlarged. Presynaptic NMDARs are shown in orange. **(B)** PregS increases Ca^{2+} influx through presynaptic NMDARs, leading to an increase in the probability of glutamate release and activation of post-synaptic NMDARs. Pre- and post-synaptic NMDARs at these synapses are proposed to contain NR2D subunits, making them less sensitive to Mg^{2+} block. **(C)** Glutamate release probability returns to baseline levels after PregS washout. The post-synaptic increase in $[Ca^{2+}]$ shown in panel B elicits delayed insertion of AMPARs only in "*silent synapses*" [From Valenzuela et al. (156) with Permission].

Modulation of TRP channels has been proposed as a therapeutic target for age-related neurologic disorders, such as AD (157). TRPA1 channels regulate astrocyte resting Ca^{2+} and inhibitory synapse efficacy (158). The TRPA1 channel has also been implicated in astrocytic hyperactivity and synaptic dysfunction mediated by Aβ in mouse models of AD (159). Recognized differences in TRPA1 channels across species have been cited as confounding the translational value of results from preclinical rodent models (160). For example, human TRPA1 activity is suppressed by caffeine but mouse TRPA1 channels are activated (161). More work is needed to fully elucidate the role of neurosteroids as functional modulators of the different subtypes of TRPs expressed in the brain.

Transport of Negatively Charged Steroids Across Cell Membranes

Sulfated steroids, namely PregS and DHEAS, are unique in that they are highly negatively charged and thus do not pass across cell membranes without specific transporters. It therefore seems unlikely, although not impossible, that PregS or DHEAS could rapidly associate with a receptor present within the cell without a specific membrane transporter. Our results show that PregS acts extracellularly (35) and that PREG is inactive as a modulator (36–38, 162). For these reasons, PregS more closely resembles the characteristics of classical neurotransmitters, such as acetylcholine, in which the parent molecule bears a full positive charge and is active only at an extracellularly directed recognition site while the immediate breakdown products (choline + acetic acid) are inactive. However, with respect to the neuronal membrane, PregS exhibits full effect even when applied extracellularly to cultured cortical and hippocampal neurons (27, 48) internally dialyzed with the same concentration of PregS via the whole cell patch clamp recording configuration (47).

The recognition site for steroids, such as estrogen (ER), progesterone and its metabolite ALLO is now relatively well-described. For instance, membrane-bound ER receptors, such as ERα localize at the cell surface where they regulate cell signaling mediated by ER produced in the CNS; this function is in addition to their well-recognized classical intracellular localizations where these receptors function to modulate transcription (163–166).

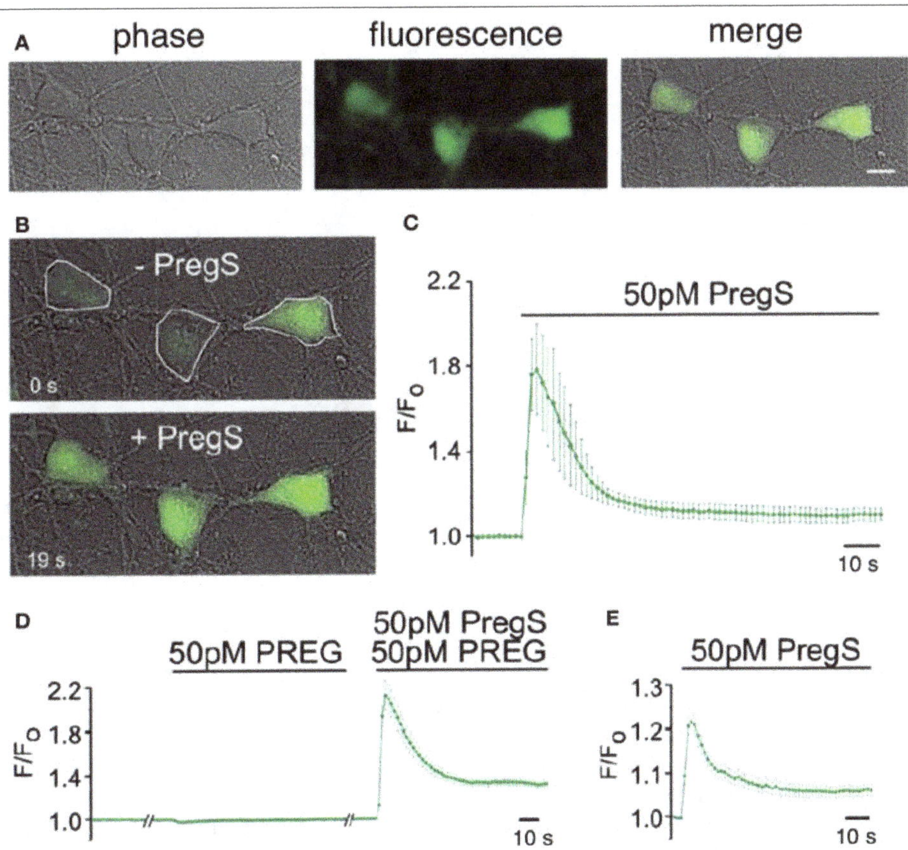

FIGURE 8 | Picomolar concentrations of PregS increase $[Ca^{2+}]_i$ in primary cultured cortical neurons. **(A)** Phase-contrast (left), fluorescence (middle), and merged (right) image of a field of cortical neurons. **(B)** Before (top, 0 s) and after (bottom, 19 s) application of 50 pM PregS. Regions of interest defined morphologically as neuronal cell bodies are outlined in white. **(C)** Mean 6 S.E.M. fluorescence intensity normalized to average initial intensity of the same cell (F/Fo) for 3 neurons in **(B)**. **(D)** Baseline Ca^{2+} fluorescence is shown in the (left) trace. PREG (50 pM) does not increase $[Ca^{2+}]$l (middle trace), whereas a subsequent application of 50 pM PregS in the presence of 50 pM PREG increases $[Ca^{2+}]$i. (right trace) (mean 6 S.E.M., 30 neurons). **(E)** 50 pM PregS increases $[Ca^{2+}]$i in primary cultured hippocampal neurons. Scale bar for **(A,B)**: 10 mm. [From Smith et al. (48) with Permission].

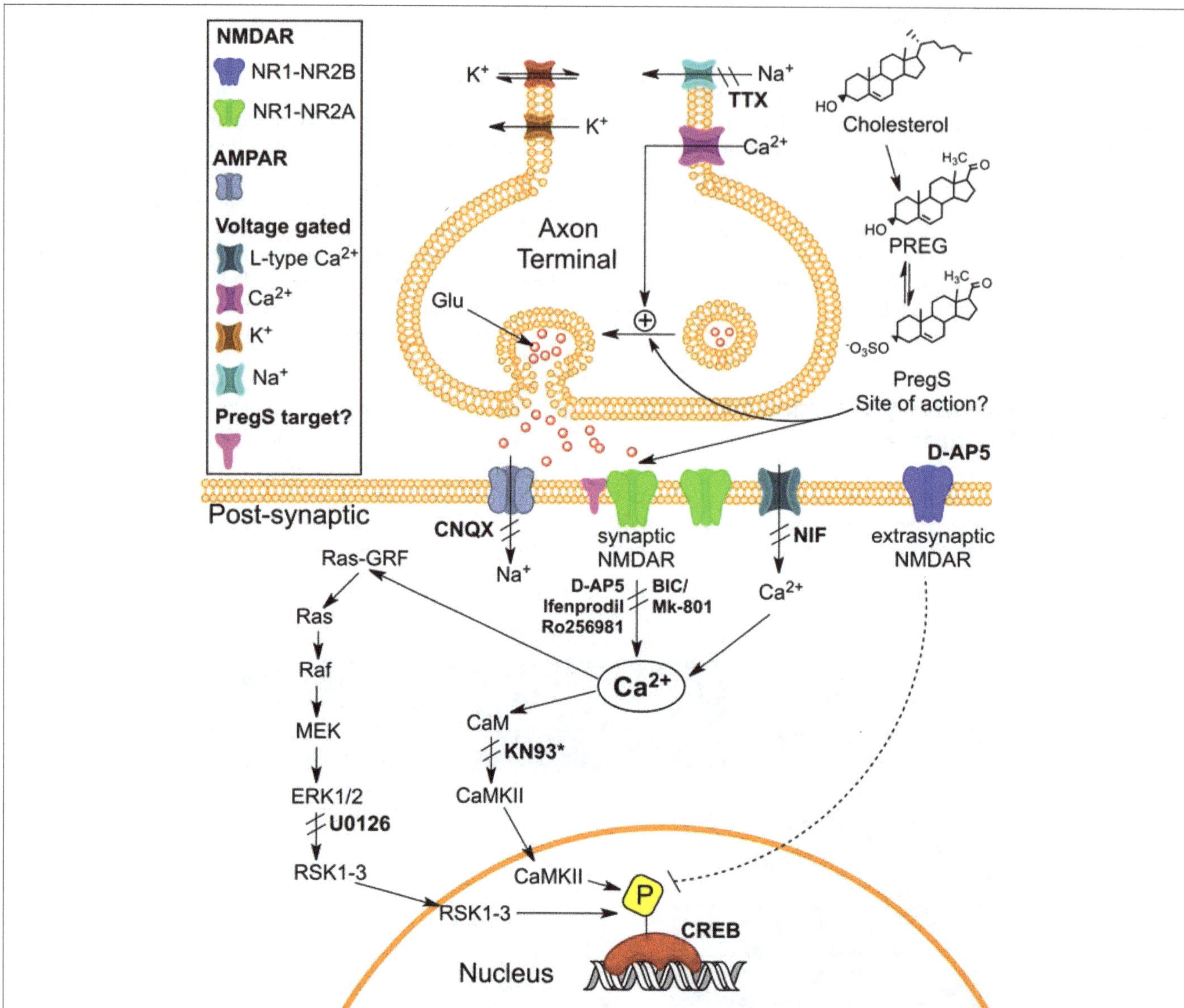

FIGURE 9 | Schematic illustrating pathways that may underlie pM PregS-induced $[Ca^{2+}]i$ and pCREB increases. Diagram illustrates 50 pM PregS-stimulated increase in $[Ca^{2+}]i$ via voltage-gated Na+ channels, NMDARs, and $Ca^{2+}L$ and 50 pM PregS-induced pCREB increases via synaptic NMDAR and ERK activation. Inhibitors used in the study are in bold. *KN93 did not inhibit PregS-induced pCREB increases. [From Smith et al. (48) with Permission].

Interestingly, activation of these membrane receptors leads to rapid, non-genomic effects and regulates neuronal plasticity in the CNS (166–171).

An extracellular site of activation for PregS on endogenous NMDARs in primary rat hippocampal and chick spinal cord neurons in culture, as well as receptors expressed in *Xenopus* oocytes, was demonstrated by Farb et al. (26). Extracellular application of PregS activates NMDARs, whereas intracellular dialysis with PregS fails to elicit a neuronal response or to inhibit PregS applied extracellularly (35). An extracellularly directed PregS -binding domain and obligatory transmembrane domain TM4 participate in the positive allosteric modulation of NMDAR activation by neurotransmitter co-agonists glutamate and glycine [(43, 44) and reviewed by (62, 172)].

These findings were recently confirmed and extended by Wilding et al. (54), who generated chimeric receptors by replacing specific domains of the NMDAR with homologous domains from kainate receptors expressed in non-neuronal HEK293 cells to elucidate the contribution of specific domains to pore formation and allosteric modulation of the NMDARs. By contrast, potentiation by the dihydroxysterol does not require the ligand-binding domain but instead requires a membrane proximal portion of the carboxy terminal domain of the

NMDAR, consistent with an intracellularly directed site for receptor activation. Recently, Chisari et al. (58) have described the characterization of compound analogs of PregS, such as KK169. Like PregS, KK169 has the ability to potentiate NMDAR function, and possesses several characteristics that are consistent with an action for PregS and related sulfated steroids at a cell surface-oriented activation domain (35, 43). Interestingly, KK169 does not inhibit oxysterol potentiation of the NMDAR, consistent with its action at an extracellularly directed binding site (similar to that for PregS). However, some sequestration of KK169 was observed in cultured hippocampal neurons, revealing a possible mechanism for membrane transport and accumulation.

These considerations also relate to question of whether PregS might be able to cross the BBB, with the clear expectation that a specific transmembrane transporter would be needed. In fact, such a transporter has been observed in non-fenestrated intracerebral capillaries (173–177) and could well be present in glia and/or neurons, providing a possible pathway toward sequestration.

NEUROSTEROIDS AND MEMORY FUNCTION

PREG was initially thought of only as a precursor for other steroids and not as an active modulator. Fluorescence spectroscopy studies of the binding of PREG and the related sulfated neurosteroid 3α-hydroxy-5β-pregnan-20-one sulfate, which differentially modulate NMDA and AMPA receptors, suggest that the differential effects of these sulfated neurosteroids on current flow may be related to their binding at the SIS2 and amino terminal domains of these receptors (39). Cannabinoid receptor 1 (CB1) has been identified as a molecular target for PREG (178). Tetrahydrocannabinol or THC, the active ingredient in cannabis, induces PREG synthesis in a CB1 receptor-dependent manner. PREG then acts as an allosteric negative modulator of CB1 receptor in an autocrine-paracrine loop in the brain acting to ameliorate cannabis intoxication. CB1 receptor activation is well-known to modulate learning and memory function by depressing neurotransmitter release. Interestingly, two cannabinoid receptor-mediated signaling cascades have been identified: one is PREG sensitive and targets the vesicular protein Munc-18-1, thereby depressing transmitter release; the other is PREG-insensitive and involves the lateral perforant path of the hippocampus (179). When given as an adjunctive treatment to patients diagnosed with schizophrenia, PREG both improves negative symptoms and ameliorates cognitive deficits (50).

Although controversy still remains with respect to the ability of systemically administered sulfated neurosteroids to cross the BBB, acute treatment with PregS, which is well-recognized for its actions as a positive allosteric modulator of NMDARs, has been associated with an improvement in learning and memory function (21, 24, 31, 34, 35, 162, 180–185). The influx of the sulfated compounds is dependent upon transporters, such as organic anion transporting peptides (OATPs) situated in the BBB and choroid plexus (173, 177, 186) (**Figure 10**).

The role of these transporters in the efflux of negatively charged sulfate steroids across the BBB from the CNS into the systemic circulation is fairly well-established; however, the specific mechanisms associated with brain influx have not been fully elucidated, despite the finding that systemic administration of sulfated steroids produces effects on cognition including improved learning and memory function (31, 173, 176). It had been suggested, based on studies looking at the expression of 17α-Hydroxylase/C17-20-lyase and hydroxysteroid sulfotransferase, that sulfated steroids, such as DHEAS are unlikely to be synthesized *de novo* within the human hippocampus (186). This work has led to the suggestion that sulfated neurosteroids must be transported from the periphery into the CNS, but this hypothesis has not been validated (186). Using *in situ* rat brain perfusion, Qaiser et al. (176) found that PregS enters the brain more rapidly than DHEAS and that both sulfated steroids undergo extensive desulfation mediated by sulfatase located in the capillary fraction of the BBB. While more work is clearly needed to parse out these complex relationships (95), systemic administration of conjugated neurosteroids can nevertheless result in increased CNS levels of the unsulfated neurosteroids (176).

Whether or not the cognitive enhancing effects are due to PregS or PREG remains to be determined. However, the cognitive enhancing effects of PregS in healthy subjects are unlikely to be due to the PREG metabolite ALLO since acute administration of this and other GABAergic modulating neurosteroids to healthy subjects inhibits learning and memory function in a manner similar to benzodiazepines (187–191). On the contrary, ALLO may play a role in the effects of PREG seen in patients with schizophrenia and other neuropsychiatric and neurologic disorders in which neural network activity is dysregulated (51).

Unlike synthetic pharmaceuticals, the literature reporting on the role of neurosteroids in learning and memory function includes some studies looking at the role of endogenous levels and other studies looking at the effects of systemically administered neurosteroids. Because of this, there are several important factors that must be considered when interpreting the results of these studies, including: (1) metabolism of the parent neurosteroid molecule and active metabolites may have a different mechanisms of action; (2) dosing schedules can be acute or chronic; and (3) pharmacokinetic and pharmacodynamic interactions between the neurosteroids and endogenous levels of circulating steroid hormones can fluctuate over time.

Performance on tests of memory function also depends on when neurosteroids are administered in relationship to training or testing. For example, administration of neurosteroids before training can influence both acquisition and consolidation of new information, whereas administration after training is expected to influence consolidation and recall but not acquisition. The type of memory function being assessed (e.g., working memory vs. long-term memory) may also be

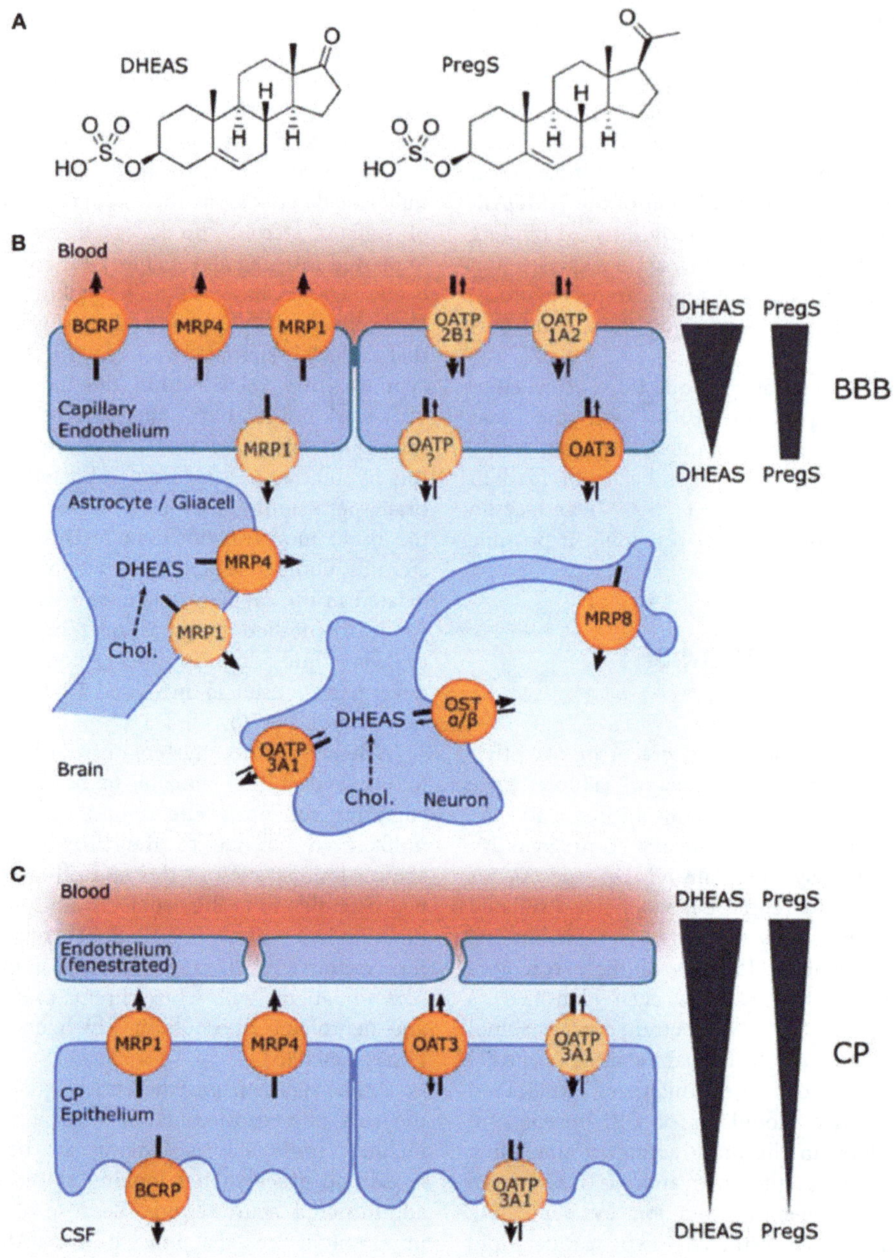

FIGURE 10 | Schematic illustration of ABC and SLC transporters putatively involved in DHEAS and PregS transport and their proposed localization. **(A)** Structures of DHEAS and PregS. **(B,C)** The ATP-binding cassette (ABC) and solute carrier (SLC)-type membrane proteins facilitate transport of neurosteroids at the BBB and in the choroid plexus (CP) The ABC transporters BCRP (ABCG2), MRP1, MRP4, and MRP8 (ABCC1, ABCC4, and ABCC11) facilitate efflux of conjugated steroids. The solute carriers OAT3 (SLC22A3), OATP1A2 (SLCO1A2), OATP2B1 (SLCO2B1), and OSTa/ß (SLC51A/B) are implicated in secretion of sulfated steroids from neurons and glial cells and in their transport across the BBB as well as blood–CSF barrier in the CP. Arrows indicate the directions of substrate transport. Proteins for which there is little or controversial evidence for expression and localization in the basal or apical membrane are indicated in light orange and by a dashed line. The DHEAS and PregS concentration gradients across the BBB and in the CP are depicted on the right [From Grube et al. (177) with Permission].

more or less sensitive to the effects of neurosteroids. Finally, the age and cognitive status of the study subjects must be considered. Each of these factors is explored in greater detail below.

Mechanism of Action and Metabolism of Parent Molecule to Active Metabolites

Neurosteroids are metabolized to other neurosteroids that can also influence neurologic function. For example, PREG is a lipophilic precursor of ALLO, which is also a metabolite of progesterone. Administration of a loading dose of PREG is associated with an increase in serum ALLO levels (192). Although PREG is preferentially metabolized to ALLO, it is also metabolized to progesterone and DHEA (51, 52, 104). The extent to which a neurosteroid, such as PREG is metabolized to progesterone and vice versa determines whether the dose administered will modulate extra- or intracellular receptors to produce non-genomic vs. genomic effects (104).

Administration of 5α-reductase inhibitors, such as finasteride appears to prevent the metabolism of progesterone to ALLO and may thereby influence the neuromodulatory effects of endogenous as well as exogenous sources of these neurosteroids (193–195). Studies looking at the direct infusion of PregS into the nucleus basalis show that this neurosteroid improves spatial memory function in rats and increases acetylcholine release in the basolateral amygdala and frontoparietal cortex (196). Despite these promnestic effect, the metabolism of sulfated neurosteroids, such as PregS by sulfatases, coupled with limited transport across the BBB, has impeded the development of this compound as a novel therapeutic. This limitation can be overcome by using synthetic analogs (132).

Acute vs. Chronic Dosing Schedules

Acute administration of ALLO improves memory function in one mouse model of AD (197), but other studies using rodent models suggest that chronic exposure to ALLO may actually cause memory deficits and exacerbate disease-related functional impairments (198–200). The observation that ALLO transiently increases CREB phosphorylation and increases indicators of neurogenesis in wildtype rats (201) suggests that the acute and chronic effects may not be the same. The translational relevance of these observations to human subjects is unclear since, although men show an age-related decrease in serum ALLO, a similar age-dependent reduction in circulating levels of this neurosteroid is not seen in women (202). On the contrary, women show changes in circulating levels of ALLO that correlate with transient changes in circulating levels of steroid hormones (202). Interestingly, acute systemic administration of ALLO appears to interfere with episodic memory function in healthy women without impairing semantic or working memory function (203), suggesting that brain regions involved in these distinct memory processes, such as the frontal lobes and hippocampus are differentially modulated by this neurosteroid.

Studies looking at brain region-specific effects of neurosteroids on memory function have served to further elucidate the role these neuromodulators play in the acquisition, consolidation and retrieval of information. Systemic administration of the $GABA_AR$ positive modulator ALLO to mice interferes with acquisition and consolidation on a hippocampal-dependent novel object recognition task (204, 205). ALLO impairs memory acquisition/encoding in rodent models when it is injected into the nucleus basalis magnocellularis *before* an acquisition trial, implicating inhibition of cholinergic neurotransmission in the effects of ALLO on memory acquisition (181). Intrahippocampal administration of ALLO into the CA1 subregion *after* the acquisition phase of a passive avoidance paradigm has no measurable effect on retention (206).

Age-Dependent Effects of Neurosteroids

Neuroactive steroid hormones levels change during development, with aging and across the estrous cycle (207, 208). Age-dependent effects of neurosteroids on memory function are seen in rodents and humans. For example, neonatal exposure of female rats to estradiol has been associated with reduced brain levels of ALLO and improved learning and memory function in adulthood (209). It has been suggested, based largely on work in animal models, that enduring changes in $GABA_ARs$ expression induced by developmental exposure to steroid hormones, such as progesterone and its metabolites play a role in hippocampal neuronal excitability and in the etiology of sex-dependent neuropsychiatric disorders and memory deficits later in life (209–211). Administration of the 5α-reductase inhibitor, finasteride to pregnant rat dams late in gestation impairs cognitive and neuroendocrine function in their juvenile offspring (210). Treatment of neonatal female rats with estradiol increases the expression of extrasynaptic α4/δ subunit-containing $GABA_ARs$ and improves performance in the Morris water maze during adulthood (209).

In humans, serum levels of ALLO are normally stable during the first 2 years of life (212). Obese children have been reported to have elevated circulating levels of ALLO, but how this influences their learning and memory function later in life has not been elucidated (213). In post-menopausal women, the effects of ALLO on mood appears to be dose dependent and to follow an inverted U-shaped cure (214). The major contributor to endogenous levels of ALLO is the corpus luteum of the ovary and, not too surprisingly, serum levels of ALLO increase during puberty and with polycystic ovary syndrome (PCOS) (202, 212, 215–218). Functional imaging studies indicate that activity within the right superior and inferior parietal lobes is increased during performance of working memory tasks in untreated women with PCOS. The observed increase in neuronal activity is attenuated by antiandrogen therapy (219).

During the menstrual cycle in humans, ALLO and progesterone levels rise together, with the highest concentrations reached in the luteal phase (202, 220–223). Encoding of emotional memories appears to be better in the luteal phase than in follicular phase (207). It has been suggested that cyclical fluctuations in circulating steroid hormone levels can influence encoding and recall of emotional stimuli, and therefore may play a role in the expression of post-traumatic stress disorder (PTSD) symptomology (224, 225).

In rodents, the onset of puberty is associated with an increase in the expression α4β8 $GABA_ARs$ on dendrites of CA1 hippocampal pyramidal cells (226–228). There is also evidence to suggest that synaptic pruning is influenced by neurosteroids during puberty. Optimal spine density may depend in part on expression and modulation of α4β8 $GABA_ARs$ during puberty, which in turn appears necessary for optimal learning and memory function in adulthood (229). The estrus cycle influences memory function in female rodents (230). Spatial learning and memory deficits observed on the morning of proestrus phase in rodent are associated with an increased expression of α4β δ $GABA_A$Rs on CA1 pyramidal cell dendrites (230). There is a reversible decrease in the expression of δ-$GABA_A$Rs in parvalbumin containing interneurons in the CA3 hippocampal subregion during pregnancy in rodents, and this change is associated with increased levels of ALLO (231). Reduced expression of δ-$GABA_A$Rs and increased ALLO may serve to counterbalance each other during pregnancy so that tonic inhibition is maintained. It has been suggested that dysregulation of this delicate balance alters cortical activity in the γ frequency range and that measuring drug-induced changes in cortical γ activity could serve as a non-invasive objective biomarker for predicting the efficacy of pharmacological interventions (231). A non-invasive objective biomarker of this type could prove to be very useful in open label studies.

Timing of Neurosteroid Administration in Relationship to Effect on Memory Function

Learning and memory function can be broken down into three phases: (1) acquisition; (encoding); (2) consolidation; and (3) retrieval (recall). As a result, in addition to their unique and sometimes complex mechanisms of action, the timing of neurosteroid administration can also influence performance on specific tests sensitive to the different aspects of learning and memory function. For example, post-acquisition administration of PregS is associated with improved retention in rodents on a passive avoidance paradigm, indicating that this positive modulator of glutamatergic neurotransmission facilitates consolidation (206). Systemic administration of PregS enhances acquisition (31), while direct infusion of this neurosteroid into the lateral septum 30 min before training appears to interfere with acquisition (185). This seeming discrepancy between the two studies can likely be explained by the complexity of the septo-hippocampal interaction and Pregs-induced increase in excitation and/or decreased excitation within the septum (232).

Specific Type of Memory Function Being Assessed

But what about the specific type of memory function being assessed with a specific task; how might this affect interpretation of behavioral response to neurosteroids? Different types of memories require activation of different brain regions. Regional changes in activation are also associated with specific neuropsychiatric and neurologic disorders. Problems with attention, concentration, and motivation can interfere with encoding of new information and, thus, with performance on tests of memory function (233). While the hippocampus is involved in most aspects of learning and memory function, certain types of memory appear to depend less on activation of this brain region than on other regions (234).

The role of neurosteroids in semantic memory function can only be effectively studied in humans who have the inherent ability to verbally express what they know about the world (235). Humans are also capable of using non-episodic strategies on tests looking at the temporal aspects of an episodic memory (236). This distinction can be very important when parsing out the effects of neurosteroid on episodic vs. semantic memory function. For example, systemic administration of ALLO impairs episodic memory but not working or semantic memory function in healthy adult women (203). The effects of neurosteroids on semantic memory function in schizophrenia has not been elucidated; however, PREG is metabolized to ALLO and PregS, both of which appear to improve working memory function in this patient population (51, 52, 65, 237, 238). Whether this effect on performance is mediated by PREG, ALLO, or PregS alone or via a combination of all three neurosteroids has not been determined.

The effects of neurosteroids on learning and memory for fear-inducing stimuli appears to be different in males and females, who show different brain levels of ALLO at baseline as well. Augmenting levels of ALLO in the bed nucleus of the stria terminalis (BNST) of males, who have lower levels of ALLO at baseline, promotes contextual freezing. By contrast, reducing intra-BNST levels of ALLO in females, who have higher brain ALLO levels at baseline, enhances the expression of contextual freezing (239). In addition to differences in responding due to sex-related baseline levels of neurosteroids, different aspects of memory function depend on recruitment of different brain regions, as well as on activation of different subregions within the hippocampus (e.g., dorsal vs. ventral hippocampus) (240).

Learning and memory of coordinated motor activities involves activation of the cerebellum where neurosteroids are synthesized *de novo* by Purkinje cells (241–243). It has recently been suggested that 17β-estradiol may also play a role in cerebellar motor memory formation in male rats (244). Animal studies also suggest that the glutamate-nitric oxide-cyclic GMP pathway is impaired in the cerebellum and cortex of subjects with hyperammonemia due to hepatic failure. Ammonia-induced disruption of this pathway has been implicated in impaired performance on certain types of procedural tasks that depend in part on optimization of motor performance. Restoring the pathway and cyclic GMP levels in the brain restores learning ability. The role of neurosteroids in cerebellar function and the acquisition of motor skills has not been fully elucidated. Elevated levels of GABAergic neurosteroids have been associated with hepatic failure, and it has been suggested that PregS may be of clinical benefit in the treatment of deficits in motor coordination and memory disturbances associated with hyperammonia seen in this patient population (245).

Where within the pharmacological connectome do neurosteroids act to modulate different types of learning and memory function *in vivo*? Not too surprisingly, direct infusion of agonists and antagonists into the brain regions implicated in these different types of memory can either augment or inhibit learning and memory function. For example, the effects of the neurosteroid ALLO on acquisition and extinction of memories associated with exposure to powerful emotion-evoking or fear-inducing stimuli are state independent when it is injected into the amygdala and hippocampus, but state-dependent when injected into the BNST (246). Due to the high concentration of $GABA_A$ receptors in the basolateral amygdala, infusion of

GABAergic neurosteroids, such as ALLO into this brain region interferes with the acquisition and expression of the contextual and auditory cue-induced freezing responses in male rats (246).

Age and Cognitive Status of Subjects at Time of Testing

Neurosteroids are implicated in age- and disease state-dependent impairments in learning and memory function (247–249). Because aging subjects can be comorbid for neuropsychiatric disorders, such as depression and age-related neurodegenerative diseases that both affect memory function (250), understanding the role of neurosteroids in age-related changes in memory function can shed light on potential therapeutic targets suitable for this unique patient population.

Low brain levels of ALLO have been associated with memory impairments in aged rats as well as in human subjects diagnosed with AD (67, 248). In addition, post-mortem studies of human subjects with AD reveal increased brain levels of DHEA and PREG (67). Autopsy studies in humans indicate that brain testosterone levels are lower in patients with AD in comparison to normal men (251) and free testosterone has been implicated as a risk factor for probable AD based on clinical diagnostic criteria (252). However, although low testosterone has been implicated in cognitive deficits in healthy men, testosterone replacement therapy does not appear to significantly improve memory function in cognitively impaired older men with low testosterone (253). It is important to point out that although *in vivo* biomarkers are expected to enhance the pathophysiological specificity of the diagnosis of AD dementia in future studies, most published studies to date looking at the role of neurosteroids on memory function have used core clinical criteria for the diagnosis of possible/probable AD type dementia. Interpretation of such results is hampered in human studies as inclusion of subjects who will ultimately not meet the definitive diagnostic criteria for AD at autopsy is a possible confounding factor.

Decreased plasma levels of DHEA and DHEAS have also been reported in humans with AD (71). It has been suggested that patients meeting clinical criteria for probable AD who have higher baseline levels of DHEAS may perform better on memory tasks than those with lower levels, while by contrast patients with lower circulating levels of cortisol may perform better than those with higher plasma cortisol (68). Men with probable AD based on clinical features of the disease show diurnal changes in cortisol levels characterized by a significant increases at 03 h 00 not seen in healthy elderly men. This increase in cortisol levels occurs despite a slight decrease in levels of adrenocorticotropic hormone (70). Increased levels of DHEA, adrenocorticotropic hormone (ACTH), and interleukin-6 (IL-6) are seen in the morning in women diagnosed with clinical symptoms consistent with AD (70). Cortisol levels are important to the different sleep stages.

Although sleep disturbances are implicated in AD, it is not entirely clear how the aforementioned diurnal changes in cortisol influence sleep and memory consolidation. Sleep plays a role in memory consolidation, and neurosteroids, such as PregS and ALLO can modulate activity within brain regions, such as the pedunculopontine tegmentum nucleus implicated in regulation of sleep (248, 254, 255). Neurosteroids, such as PregS have been implicated in disturbances of sleep and cognitive dysfunction in AD rodent models (247, 256). It has been suggested that the promnestic effects of PregS are mediated by an increase in paradoxical (a.k.a., rapid eye movement; REM) sleep (257, 258), but whether or not the effects of PregS on memory function in subjects with neuropsychiatric disorders and age-related neurodegenerative disease are mediated by enhancement of REM and/or non-REM sleep has not been fully elucidated (259, 260).

Positron emission tomography (PET) imaging studies using the high-affinity sigma-1 (σ-1) receptor selective PET tracer [18F]1-(3-Fluoropropyl)-4-[4-cyanophenoxy) methyl]piperidine ([18F]FPS) as a radioligand suggest that neurosteroids including DHEA bind to σ-1 receptors *in vivo* (261). Sigma-1 receptors modulate NMDA-mediated responses (262, 263). Agonists of the σ-1 receptor, which acts as a molecular chaperone on mitochondria-associated endoplasmic reticulum membranes, appear to provide neuroprotection in rodent models of AD (264).

PET scans using the radiotracer [carbonyl-(11)C]WAY-100635 indicate that progesterone and DHEAS modulate serotonin 1A (5-HT1A) receptor binding *in vivo* (265, 266). While there is evidence of disrupted serotonergic neurotransmission in AD (267), the role of neurosteroids, such as DHEAS in the progression of this age-related neurodegenerative disease has not been fully elucidated.

Hyperactivity of entorhinal cortical and hippocampal circuits are also thought to underlie neurodegenerative disorders, such as AD and mild cognitive impairment (MCI) (268–272). Early synaptic dysfunction or "synaptopathy" at the level of inhibitory interneurons within the entorhinal cortex and CA3 hippocampal subregion leads to hyperactivity of pyramidal cells, which appears to play a role in the progression of AD neuropathology (e.g., tauopathy) (271, 272). This hyperactivity may be due in part to reduced responsiveness of pyramidal neurons to GABAergic inhibitory inputs (272). Other studies implicate a loss of GABAergic interneurons in aging rat models of MCI, suggesting that multiple mechanisms may play a role and/or may interact to contribute to hyperactivity (273, 274). Studies using human tissue from patients with late stage AD reveal hippocampal subregion- and strata specific changes in receptor subunit expression that could potentially influence memory function (275). For example, $\alpha 5$ subunit expression, which is implicated in learning and memory function, is increased in the pyramidal layer and oriens of the CA1 subregion. In addition, expression of the $\alpha 1$ subunit, which is implicated in sedation, is increased in all strata of the CA3 subregion and in the granule cell layer and hilus of the dentate gyrus. An increase in $\alpha 2$ subunit expression, which has been implicated in anxiety, is seen in the oriens and radiatum in the CA3 subregion. Expression of $\alpha 2$ is increased in the oriens of the CA1 subregion, but is decreased in the pyramidal layer. There is a decrease in $\beta 3$ subunit expression in the granular and molecular layers of the dentate gyrus, while expression of $\alpha 3$ and $\beta 1$ subunits remain unchanged.

ALLO may be useful in attenuating the hyperactivity implicated in early stage AD (201, 276). In mouse models, ALLO appears to increase neurogenesis, reduce amyloid deposition and improve performance on learning and memory tests, suggesting that it may serve as a regenerative therapeutic (197, 277–279). A clinical trial for ALLO is ongoing. Other investigations indicate that chronic treatment with riluzole, which includes a reduction in glutamatergic neurotransmission among its mechanisms of action, attenuates the spread of tauopathy in rodent models (280). Is it possible that neurosteroids, such as pregnanolone sulfate and its synthetic analog pregnanolone hemisuccinate, which negatively modulate glutamatergic neurotransmission, may also have potential therapeutic applications in AD and age-related MCI.

Upregulation of TSPO expression has been implicated in neuropsychiatric disorders and neurodegenerative disease (281–283). Oxidative stress is associated with induction of neurosteroid biosynthesis in the human brain (284), and TSPO ligands (*N,N*-dialkyl-2-phenylindol-3-ylglyoxylamides) that also show anxiolytic activity promote a reduction in oxidative stress and pro-inflammatory enzymes in glial cells via promotion of neurosteroid synthesis (133). The role of this pathway in the progression of neurodegenerative diseases associated with memory impairments, such as AD has not been fully elucidated. However, increasing oxidative stress by treating oligodendrocytes with beta-amyloid is associated with an increase in the synthesis of DHEA (284), which provides some neuroprotection in a rodent model of AD (285).

Radioligands are being used to measure TSPO expression *in vivo*. PET scans using 11C-PBR28 as a radiolabeled tracer indicate that binding to TSPO is greater in patients with early-onset AD than in those with late-onset disease. Binding to TSPO is also inversely correlated with gray matter volume and performance on measures of cognitive function in all patients with AD. Early-onset patients have greater 11C-PBR28 binding than late-onset patients. Additionally, an increase in TSPO binding is not seen in patients with age-related MCI, even though these patients show increased amyloid pathology as assessed by Pittsburgh Compound B PET scans and hippocampal atrophy as assessed by volumetric analysis of MRI scans (282). The largest differences in TSPO binding in these groups are seen in the temporal and parietal cortices.

These findings collectively point to a potential therapeutic use for neurosteroids in age-related neurodegenerative diseases. The unique modulatory properties of neurosteroids make these particularly well-suited for targeting comorbid anxiety and depression as well as memory deficits in these patient populations.

THE ROLE OF NEUROSTEROIDS IN MEMORY DEFICITS ASSOCIATED WITH STRESS AND ANXIETY DISORDERS

Three large scale major neural networks—the default mode network, central executive network, and salience network—contribute to cognitive processing within the human brain and function together to facilitate adaptive responses of the CNS (286). The *default mode network* plays a role in episodic memory function and self-related cognitive activities including autobiographical memories. Key functional nodes within the *default mode network,* which includes the hippocampus, amygdala, and medial prefrontal cortex, have been implicated in AD and epilepsy (287, 288). The frontal parietal connections of the *central executive network* control attention, working memory, and executive function.

Connections within the central executive network have been implicated in schizophrenia (289). Responses to emotional changes and reward stimuli are dependent on intact function of the *salience network*, within which the anterior insula, anterior cingulate cortex and amygdala, ventral tegmental area, and thalamus function together to segregate the most relevant and rewarding among internal and extra-personal stimuli in order to guide behavior. Stronger connectivity within the salience network has been associated with increased anxiety (290, 291). Pathological activation of the salience and default networks can interfere with the process of switching between these two networks, which would have a differential impact on mood and memory functionality. Neurosteroids can therefore differentially modulate these three major neural networks central to memory processing.

Neurosteroids play a role in anxiety and in the learning and memory deficits associated with certain anxiety disorders. Treatment of subjects under acute psychosocial stress with DHEA (50 mg/day) both improves attention but also impairs declarative memory function (78), suggesting that the benefits in one cognitive domain may be offset by deficits in another at this dose. Neurosteroid modulation of GABAergic neurotransmission in the central amygdala has been implicated in anxiety (131) and the effects of ALLO on anxiety appear to be mediated in part via modulation of activity within the amygdala, which in turn influences neural activity in brain regions involved in learning and memory function (64, 192, 292) (**Figures 11, 12**). Although the role of 5α-reductase inhibition in the memory deficits associated with anxiety disorders has not been fully elucidated, it has nevertheless been suggested that serum and brain levels of ALLO are increased by 5α-reductase inhibition.

The BNST, which is also referred to as the extended amygdala, receives input from the hippocampus and shares reciprocal projections with the paraventricular nucleus of the thalamus (246, 293–296). This brain regions play a role in adaptive responses of the hypothalamic-pituitary-adrenal axis (HPA axis) to fear-inducing stimuli (239, 246, 296). The effects of ALLO on acquisition and extinction of hippocampal-dependent memories associated with fear-inducing stimuli appear to be state-dependent following direct injections of this neurosteroid into the BNST. Direct injections of ALLO into the BNST during conditioning or testing suppressed contextual fear, but this effect was not seen when the neurosteroid was injected into the BNST during both procedures (246).

Selective serotonin reuptake inhibitors (SSRIs) increase brain levels of ALLO in humans and animals, suggesting that the anxiolytic effects of SSRIs may be related in part to their effect on CNS levels of this endogenous GABAergic modulator (93, 297–301). Patients with anxiety disorders often self-medicate with ethanol. Acute exposure to ethanol also increases brain levels of ALLO (302). By contrast, preclinical studies in a rat

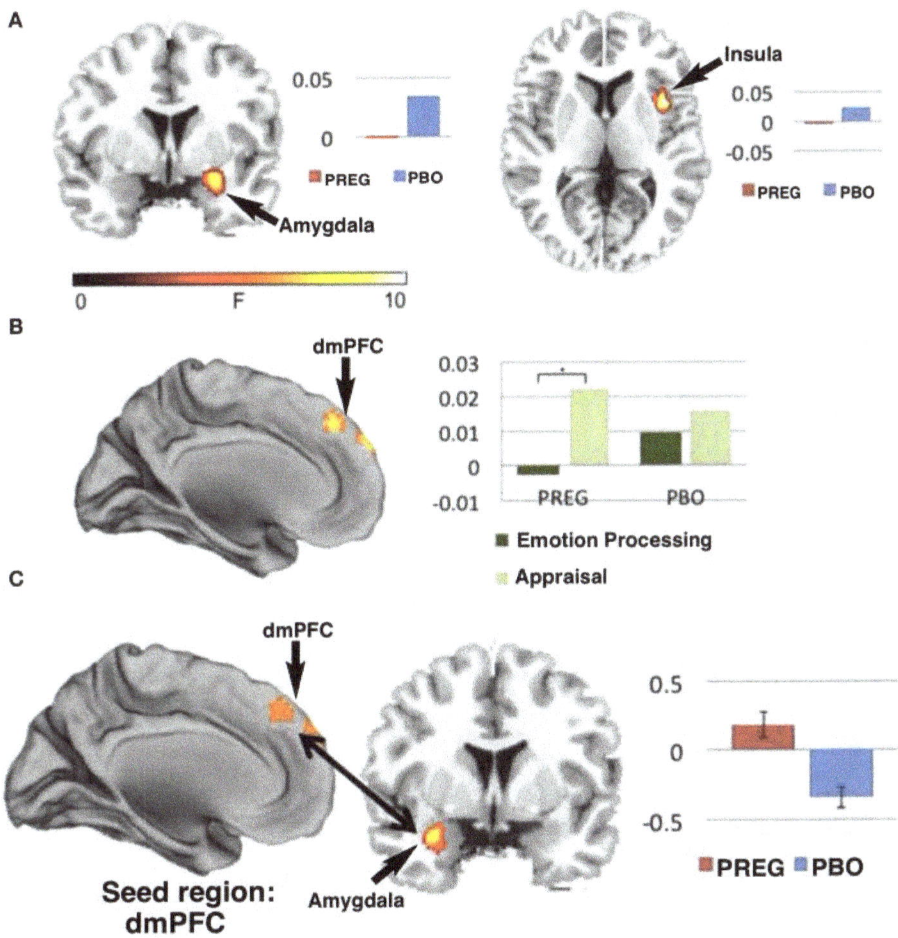

FIGURE 11 | Functional MRI studies show that treatment with PREG enhances activation of neural circuitry involved in emotional regulation as measured by a Shifted-Attention Emotion Appraisal (SEAT) paradigm. The SEAT task is designed to probe multiple aspects of emotional regulation in response to presentation of images depicting neutral, angry, or fearful expressions superimposed on pictures of indoor or outdoor scenes. Sixteen subjects were treated with PREG and 15 were treated with placebo (PBO). Subjects viewed the stimuli through MR-compatible goggles and responded using an MRI-compatible button box. Maps of cerebral activation in each condition indicated that: **(A)** There was a significant ($p < 0.05$) main effect of drug in the amygdala [Montreal Institute (MNI) coronal (y) plane coordinate = 2] and right insula [MNI axial (z) plane coordinate = −6] such that, treatment with PREG decreased activity in these two regions across all conditions and face types. **(B)** Treatment with PREG increased activation in dorsal medial prefrontal cortex (dmPFC) [MNI sagittal (x) plane coordinate = 0] during appraisal. **(C)** PREG treatment also significantly ($p < 0.001$) increased functional connectivity between the dmPFC and left amygdala during appraisal. Self-reported anxiety was inversely correlated ($r = -0.52$, $p = 0.046$) with functional connectivity between the dmPFC and amygdala in the PREG group. Percent signal change is displayed next to each figure [Modified from Sripada et al. (192) with Permission].

model suggest that chronic intermittent exposure to ethanol is associated with decreased ALLO levels in the hippocampus. Although protein levels were not reported, in this study, mRNA levels for 5alpha-reductase and 3alpha-HSD were noted to be reduced in the hippocampus of these rats, which also had impaired performance on a hippocampal-dependent memory test and increased sensitivity to the anxiolytic effects of alphaxalone (303). Could targeting neurosteroidogenesis (304) and/or steroid metabolism be a viable strategy for the treatment of patients presenting with comorbid anxiety and alcohol use disorders?

When compared with normal subjects and patients with major depression, elderly patients with generalized anxiety disorder (GAD) show more deficits on tests of short-term memory function (305). The severity of GAD has been found to positively correlate with cortisol levels in saliva of older adults (73). Elevated salivary cortisol in older adults is associated with impaired performance on tests of memory function (306). Treatment of older adults presenting with GAD and elevated baseline cortisol with SSRIs is associated with a reduction in salivary cortisol that correlates with reductions in anxiety (307). SSRIs increase levels of ALLO (299). and ALLO restores hippocampal-dependent learning and memory function in a rodent model of AD (308). AD is associated with non-cognitive behavioral and psychological symptoms, which can include paranoia and anxiety; therefore, ALLO may be well-suited for targeting these as well as the cognitive deficits associated with this form of dementia (309).

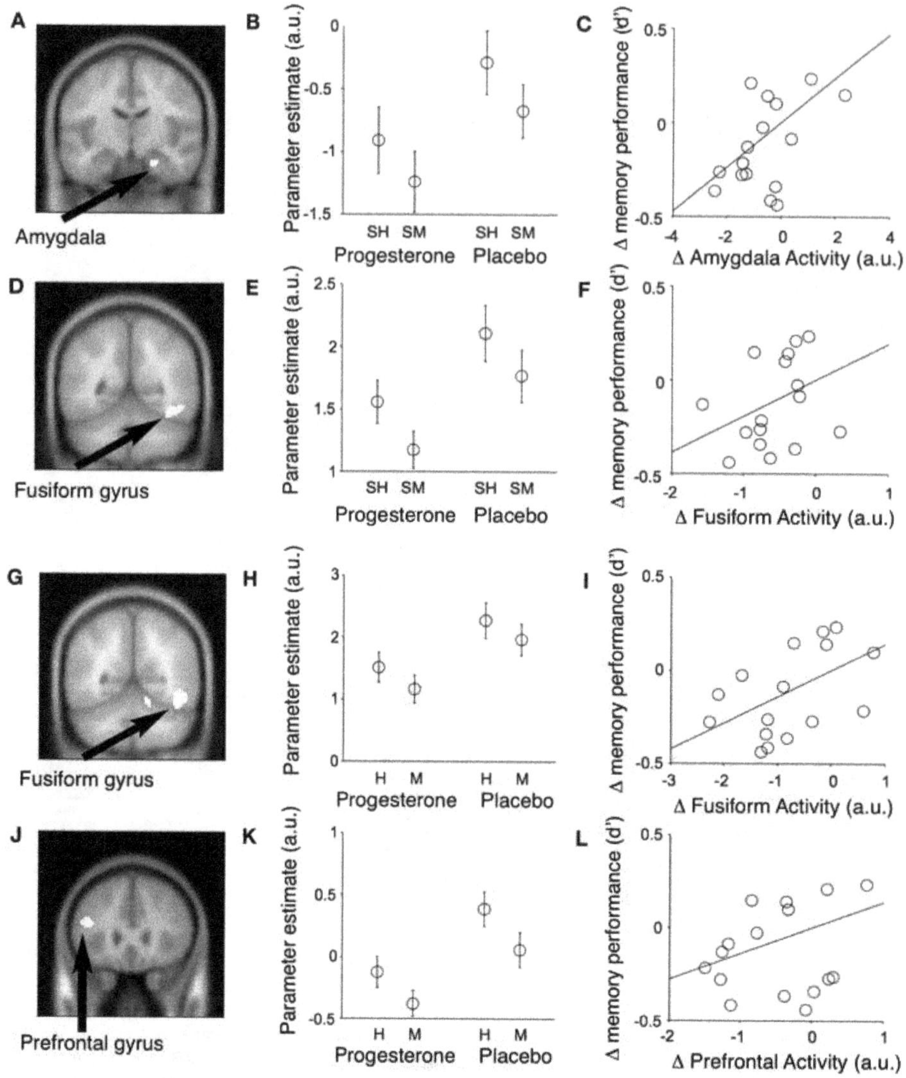

FIGURE 12 | Event-related fMRI studies in female subjects showing effects of progesterone on brain regions involved in the encoding and retrieval of memories of faces. Results of conjunction analyses for the relationships between neural activity in different brain regions and memory performance across subjects. **(A)** During encoding of memories for faces, progesterone administration was associated with reduced activity in the right amygdala (MNI coronal (y) plane coordinate = −12; $p < 0.001$, uncorrected) and fusiform gyrus [MNI coronal (y) plane coordinate = −52] which predicted a decrease in memory performance across subjects. **(B)** Parameter estimates for mean activity within each significant conjunction cluster (SH = subsequent hits; SM = subsequent misses; a.u. = arbitrary units; mean ± SEM). **(C)** The progesterone-induced decrease in amygdalar activity predicted the decrease in memory performance across subjects [recognition memory accuracy = d′]. **(D–F)** Identical figures for the significant conjunction of main effects in the right fusiform gyrus and memory performance. Progesterone reduces activity in the fusiform and inferior frontal gyri and impairs performance during retrieval of memories for faces. **(G)** Significant conjunction of main effect of memory (i.e., hits > misses) and main effect of drug [i.e., placebo (faces > null events) > progesterone (faces > null events)] in the right fusiform gyrus [MNI coronal (y) plane coordinate = −56; $p < 0.001$, uncorrected]. **(H)** Parameter estimates of the conjunction cluster (arbitrary units; mean ± SEM). **(I)** Progesterone-induced reduction in fusiform gyrus activity predicted the decrease in memory performance across subjects [recognition memory accuracy (d′)]. **(J–L)** Identical figures for the significant conjunction of main effects in the left inferior frontal gyrus [MNI coronal (y) plane coordinate = 26]. H, Hits; M, misses; a.u., arbitrary units. H, Hits; M, misses; a.u., arbitrary units [Modified from van Wingen et al. (64) with Permission].

Cortisol seems to enhance treatment outcomes in a small group (males and females) treated with exposure-based group therapy (310). In addition, high endogenous estradiol vs. low estradiol correlates with better treatment outcomes in exposure therapy (311) in female patients with spider phobias. Investigations of neural network activity using intracranial electroencephalography in human subjects indicate that β-frequency coherence (13–30 Hz) between the amygdala and hippocampus encodes variations in mood (312). Stress may mediate changes in mood and cognition in early adolescence and may play a role in the expression of psychopathologies in adulthood. During stress, corticotropin-releasing hormone promotes an increase in adrenocorticotropic hormone release. This promotes an increase in the concentration of cholesterol at the inner mitochondria membrane of the adrenal cortical cell via activation of the steroidogenic acute regulatory protein. Cholesterol is then converted to PREG and its steroid metabolites, including PregS, cortisol, corticosterone, DHEA, and ALLO (77, 87, 313, 314).

DHEA and DHEAS appear to counteract the negative effects of increased cortisol on working memory function in women and men, respectively (315, 316). A dose-dependent inverted U-shaped response to DHEAS is observed on tests of learning and memory function in male mice (30). By contrast, DHEA is effective in a wider range of doses, suggesting it would be a better choice as a therapeutic (30). Although a positive correlation between DHEAS and cognitive function has been observed in women and men, more research is needed to determine if the effects of DHEA and DHEAS on learning and memory function in humans are sex, dose, and disease state dependent (30, 317, 318).

The response to stress appears to be influenced in part by circulating steroid hormones. Stress increases associative learning and dendritic spine density in the hippocampus of male rats, but impairs associative learning and reduces spine density in females (319). The potential effects of neurosteroids on development of anxiety disorders can be observed during puberty, which is not only associated with increase in levels of reproductive hormones but also with the onset of many psychiatric disorders, including GAD, social anxiety, and panic attacks (320–326). Anxiety symptoms have been found to increase from middle to late adolescence (323), with a particularly high prevalence of all anxiety disorders reported among adolescent girls (324, 327, 328). Of particular interest in this setting are the neurosteroids ALLO (in human and rat) and pregnanolone (in human only), metabolites of the reproductive hormone progesterone that are also produced in the brain in response to stress (79, 329).

Animal studies suggest that developmental exposure to ALLO influences subsequent responsivity to anxiolytics in adulthood (206, 330–332). Acute stress is associated with an increase in plasma ALLO levels that correlates with an increase in expression of the TSPO, also known as the peripheral benzodiazepine receptor. Because the TSPO plays a role in steroidogenesis, it has been considered as a therapeutic target for treatment of anxiety disorders (77, 333). It is interesting to note, that ALLO levels have been found to be decreased relative to controls in the CSF of women with chronic stress disorders, such as PTSD (75). A subsequent study from this group observed a negative correlation between CSF levels of total GABAergic neurosteroids levels (ALLO plus pregnanolone) and PTSD symptoms in men (76). This study also found an association between PTSD and reduced 5α-reductase mediated biosynthesis of ALLO in men, which is in contrast to the block at 3α-HSD previously observed in women with PTSD. Other studies have found that administration of sodium lactate and cholecystokinin tetrapeptide to persons diagnosed with panic disorder decreases plasma concentrations of both pregnanolone and ALLO, and increases the concentration of the functional antagonistic isomer 3β,5α-tetrahydroprogesterone (334). These findings suggest that both acute stress and chronic stress give rise to unique effects on ALLO levels in men and women. Although studies in post-menopausal women did not reveal any benefit on tests of short-term memory function, it has nevertheless been suggested that replenishing this neurosteroid may have beneficial effects on memory function in certain populations with age-related memory deficits (335, 336).

Restoration of altered endogenous neurosteroid levels via modulation of steroidogenesis mediated by pregnane xenobiotic receptors (PXR) and the endocannabinoid system has been suggested as an alternative to direct administration of neurosteroids (89, 178, 337). Because PREG is a precursor for all steroid hormones, it seems plausible that promotion of cortisol synthesis during stress may attenuate synthesis of other steroid hormones, but this suggestion has not been substantiated.

These findings suggest that changes in endogenous brain levels of neurosteroids associated with age, sex, stress, and administration of SSRIs may play a key role in the onset and clinical response to pharmacologic interventions in certain anxiety disorders. Supporting this hypothesis are findings related to the effects of ALLO on gonadotrophin-releasing hormone (GnRH), the primary chemical messenger implicated in the onset of puberty and sexual maturation (338). Central precocious puberty is associated with ALLO, which has been found to suppress the release of hypothalamic GnRH via allosteric modulation of $GABA_A$Rs (339, 340). Although inhibition of GnRH release is increased by ALLO administration before puberty and in adulthood, it is paradoxically reduced during puberty (212).

The reduction in GnRH release during puberty is also associated with increased excitability of pyramidal cells in hippocampal region CA1. This effect appears to be due in part to inhibition of α4-containing $GABA_A$Rs, which are expressed at higher levels than normal in the CA1 region of the hippocampus during puberty. $GABA_A$Rs of the α4β2δ subtype, which have a δ subunit instead of a γ subunit, play a role in tonic inhibition in areas, such as the dentate gyrus and cortex (341). $GABA_A$R-mediated conductance is normally inhibitory; however, the reversal potential of $GABA_A$R-mediated post-synaptic current in dentate gyrus granule cells is "positive" to the resting membrane potential, making membrane hyperpolarization of $GABA_A$Rs unlikely in this region. Inhibition of shunting appears to play a role in overcoming this process, such that non-hyperpolarizing inhibitory conductance reduces the depolarizing effect of post-synaptic potentials by decreasing proximal membrane resistance (342). In the dentate gyrus and cortex, the GABAergic current is inward (i.e., chloride flux is outward) (342, 343), and thus inhibition in these areas is enhanced by ALLO. However, in the CA1 hippocampal subregion the current is normally outward (344), and thus increased expression of α4β2δ GABA receptors paradoxically results in ALLO attenuating rather than enhancing inhibition. The reduction in currents generated by ALLO at α4β2δ $GABA_A$R is dependent upon the presence of arginine 353 in the intracellular loop of α4, where it may serve as a chloride modulatory site (345). This polarity-dependent decrease in inhibition mediated by ALLO may have important implications for how we approach the memory deficits associated with anxiety disorders, which may prove to be amenable to therapeutic strategies targeting the expression and/or activity of $GABA_A$Rs of the α4β2δ subtype (346).

THE ROLE OF NEUROSTEROIDS IN MEMORY DEFICITS ASSOCIATED WITH DEPRESSION

Changes in neurosteroid levels have been implicated in onset of depression and in the actions of medications used to treat depression. Animal studies using a synthetic analog of ALLO suggest that fluctuations in neurosteroids levels may also influence motivation to learn via modulation of dopaminergic pathways (347). The effects of ALLO on mood in women appear to follow an inverted U-shaped curve (214). SSRI treatment has been associated with increased brain levels of ALLO, suggesting that the memory enhancing effects of SSRIs in this patient population may be related in part to the actions of this neurosteroid (93, 297, 348, 349). Preclinical animal studies suggest that modulation of GABAergic neurotransmission by DHEA may also have therapeutic potential in the treatment of memory deficits associated with depression (350).

It is not entirely clear how ALLO, which is a positive allosteric modulator of GABAergic neurotransmission, acts to improve memory function in this patient population, but it has been suggested that stress-induced changes in GABA receptor expression levels are likely to play a role in the etiology of depression. This hypothesis is supported by preclinical studies showing that early life traumatic stress is associated with chronic anxiety, spatial memory deficits and reduced expression of $GABA_A$R subunits in the adult rat brains (351).

It has been suggested that PREG and its metabolites may be efficacious in the treatment of depressive disorders. Treatment of depression poses several challenges and this is especially true in the treatment of depression in bipolar disorder (BPD). In a study conducted by Brown et al. (352), 80 adults with BPD and depressive mood state were treated with PREG or placebo as add-on therapy for 12 weeks. Outcome measures included the 17-item Hamilton Scale for Depression, Hamilton Rating Scale for Anxiety (HRSA) and Young Mania Rating Scale. Assessment of serum neurosteroid levels at baseline and treatment completion (week 12) revealed large baseline-to exit changes in neurosteroids in the PREG treatment group. In the PREG group, unlike the placebo group, HRSA changes negatively correlated with ALLO and PREG levels, indicative of reduced anxiety. The results of this small study should be interpreted with caution because subjects were taking a wide variety of medications including lithium, antidepressants (unspecified), sedative hypnotics/anxiolytics (unspecified), antipsychotics (unspecified), and stimulants (unspecified) and they were not stratified based on the drugs they were taking for their depression.

THE ROLE OF NEUROSTEROIDS IN MEMORY DEFICITS ASSOCIATED WITH SCHIZOPHRENIA

The cognitive deficits associated with schizophrenia are caused by multiple factors, and elucidating a single causative part of the cognitive component would provide some hope for understanding memory and a basis for therapeutic discovery. Neural circuitry-based studies highlight cortical disinhibition as a critical factor in schizophrenia affecting GABAergic interneurons (parvalbumin, SOM/NPY/CCK/expressing interneurons). GAD67 deficiencies together with changes in $GABA_A$R expression, in particular the α2 subunit, are known (353–356). Hypofunction of NMDARs, particularly in inhibitory parvalbumin (PV) interneurons (357), may initiate the disease process, leading to decreased inhibition of pyramidal neurons. NMDAR hypofunction in inhibitory interneurons is implicated in the observed GABAergic deficits (358–364). Whatever the specific path for initiating dynamical imbalance or dysregulation of the circuitry, the resultant hyperactivity of downstream pyramidal neurons ultimately leads to dysregulated neural network activity, excitotoxicity, and eventually frank neuronal loss. Note that hypofunction of NMDARs expressed in pyramidal neurons themselves is also likely (365). Disruptions of neural network activity during sleep, including reduced sleep spindle activity, has been associated with impaired sleep dependent memory consolidation in schizophrenia (260).

Synchronous activity of PV interneurons generates gamma oscillations which are observed during performance of cognitive tasks. Cognitive deficits are thought to arise from a disturbance of these high frequency oscillations in the gamma range due to reduced excitatory drive to cortical PV interneurons (366, 367) with resultant network hypersynchrony (368, 369). Manipulations of various receptors such as α5 type $GABA_A$Rs and sodium channels have been shown to enhance cognition (356). The glutamate hypothesis of schizophrenia underscores the importance of NMDARs in neuropsychiatric disorders. NMDARs are critical for the generation of gamma oscillations, and dysfunctional NMDARs result in psychosis and deficits in specific cognitive domains. Genetically engineered mice lacking NMDARs show deficits in habituation, working memory and associative learning (370).

Enhancing NMDAR function is therefore vital for enhancing cognition in healthy individuals and those with neuropsychiatric disorders (111). However, attempts to enhance NMDAR neurotransmission thus far have not been successful (371). A recent meta-analysis of currently available NMDAR positive allosteric modulators reveals that these are ineffective in alleviating cognitive impairments (371). Maintaining a critical balance in NMDAR activation is optimal for avoiding the negative consequences of NMDAR stimulation a, making PregS, DHEAS and their analogs highly suitable candidates. Subunit selective modulation, combined with its ability to potentiate receptor function without overstimulation, renders

PregS a likely and highly suitable positive modulator of NMDARs (111, 371).

PREG and ALLO have been investigated as potential therapeutics for treating memory deficits associated with schizophrenia (50, 65, 238). Acute administration of either clozapine or olanzapine increases brain and plasma levels of PREG, which is a precursor of ALLO and PregS (372). Adrenalectomy prevents clozapine-induced increase in hippocampal PREG. By contrast, significant increases in PREG levels in rat hippocampus are not observed following acute administration of aripiprazole, quetiapine, or ziprasidone administration. This suggests that the effects of second-generation antipsychotics on memory function may be due in part to increased brain levels of PREG and/or PregS (28, 48, 51, 62, 373).

We have previously demonstrated that low picomolar concentrations of PregS are sufficient to increase $[Ca^{2+}]i$ and CREB phosphorylation (48). There is some evidence that sulfotransferase 4A1 haplotype 1 (SULT4A1-1)-positive subjects show a better response to olanzapine than do SULT4A1-1 negative subjects. However, the exact role this sulfotransferase isozyme plays in the formation of PregS from PREG and the amelioration of learning and memory deficits in humans with schizophrenia treated with second-generation antipsychotics has not yet been established (374). ALLO-mediated modulation of GABAergic neurotransmission has also been implicated in the antipsychotic effects of clozapine and olanzapine in rodent models (375–377).

Multiple clinical and preclinical studies have examined the effects of neurosteroids, PREG, PregS and DHEA on memory and other cognitive attributes. Cognitive deficits are a core feature of schizophrenia (378). Recent clinical trials in patients with schizophrenia suggest that treatment with PREG as add-on therapy alleviates cognitive deficits (50). In patients receiving PREG, plasma levels of its immediate metabolite, PregS (positive modulator of NMDARs) and ALLO (positive modulator of $GABA_ARs$) are elevated, suggesting a possible role for PregS in improvement of learning and memory function (50). Earlier studies (28) had also described the cognition enhancing effects of PregS (29).

Neurosteroids, Dopamine Knockout Mouse Model and Schizophrenia

Dopamine (DA) is a neuromodulator and a key player in several neural disorders in which cognitive deficits are characteristic, such as schizophrenia, attention deficit hyperactivity disorder, and depression (379–381). The dopamine transporter (DAT) mediates re-uptake of extracellular DA, thus terminating DA receptor activation. DAT, a member of the Na^+/Cl^--dependent family of neurotransmitter transporters (382) is therefore a major therapeutic target for schizophrenia and other disorders (383–385). Several transgenic models have been generated with changes in DAT expression or function or mutations in the DAT gene (386). These models have proven to be crucial in elucidating neurotransmitter and neuromodulator function (or mechanistic underpinnings) of neuropsychiatric disorders (381, 387).

Wong et al. (373) have used a DAT knockout (DAT KO) mouse model exhibiting symptoms characteristic of schizophrenia to investigate the effects of PregS treatment on learning and memory function. Systemic administration of PregS, which is able to cross the BBB, alleviates positive and negative symptoms as well as cognitive deficits in the DAT KO mouse. Long-term systemic treatment with PregS rescues impaired episodic memory and poor discriminative abilities in the DAT KO mice without adverse effects. Consistent with observed reductions in cognitive deficits, long-term PregS

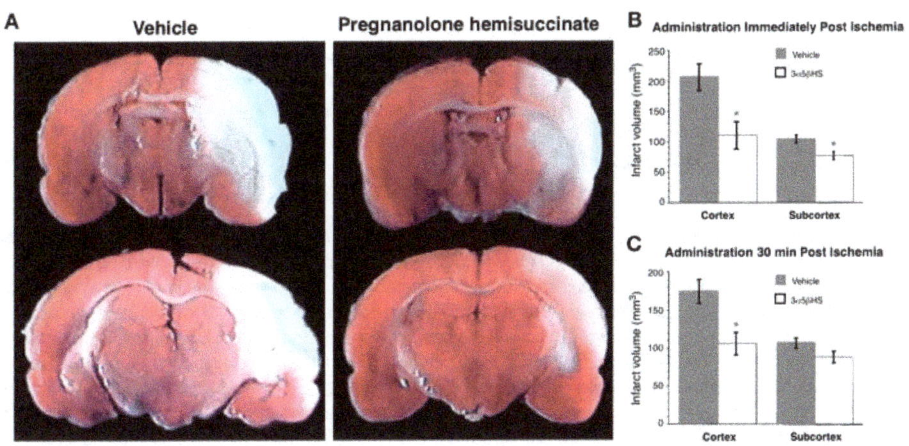

FIGURE 13 | Pregnanolone hemisuccinate (3α5βHS) is neuroprotective in an *in vivo* model of stroke. Rats were infused with either vehicle or 3α5βHS (6.9 mg/kg/h; 6.9 mg/kg loading dose), beginning immediately or 30 min after initiation of medial cerebral artery occlusion. Infusion of 3α5βHS was continued for an additional 22 h, at which time the rats were euthanized and their brains harvested and stained with 2,3,5-triphenyl tetrazolium Cl. **(A)** Representative coronal sections from animals receiving vehicle or 3α5βHS infusions immediately after initiation of ischemia. Infarct area appears pale. **(B)** Administration of 3α5βHS immediately after the onset of ischemia significantly reduced the volume of the cortical infarct from 206 ± 22 to 110 ± 21 mm^3 ($P < 0.005$) and subcortical infarct was reduced from 103 ± 6 to 76 ± 6 mm^3 ($^*P < 0.005$) (vehicle, $n = 9$; 3α5βHS, $n = 10$). **(C)** When 3α5βHS was administered 30 min after the onset of ischemia the volume of cortical infarct was reduced from 173 ± 15 to 106 ± 15 mm^3 ($^*P < 0.005$; $n = 13$), with no reduction apparent in the subcortical region [From Weaver et al. (132) with Permission].

treatment increases expression of the obligatory NMDAR subunit GluN1 in the hippocampus. Earlier, our laboratory characterized some of the mechanisms involved in increased expression of NMDAR subunits and demonstrated that PregS increases surface GluN1 in oocytes expressing recombinant NMDAR subunits in a non-canonical GPCR- and Ca^{2+}-dependent manner (47) (**Figure 2**).

SYNTHETIC NEUROSTEROIDS AS POTENTIAL COGNITIVE ENHANCERS

The findings reviewed herein suggest that the memory deficits seen in patients with schizophrenia, depression and anxiety disorders are influenced by changes in endogenous neurosteroid levels. Because not all systemically administered endogenously occurring neurosteroids readily cross the BBB and because these compounds can be metabolized to hormonally active steroids with different mechanisms of action, the therapeutic potential of these compounds is limited. For this reason, synthetic analogs of neurosteroids, which are more resistant to metabolism and better able to cross the BBB, are under investigation for use as anxiolytics, antidepressants, cognitive enhancers, anesthetics, and anticonvulsants (132, 388, 389). For example, synthetic neuroactive steroids bearing a hemisuccinate group are more resistant to hydrolysis than the corresponding sulfate esters and are partly unionized at physiological pH, allowing increased passage across the BBB. One such synthetic

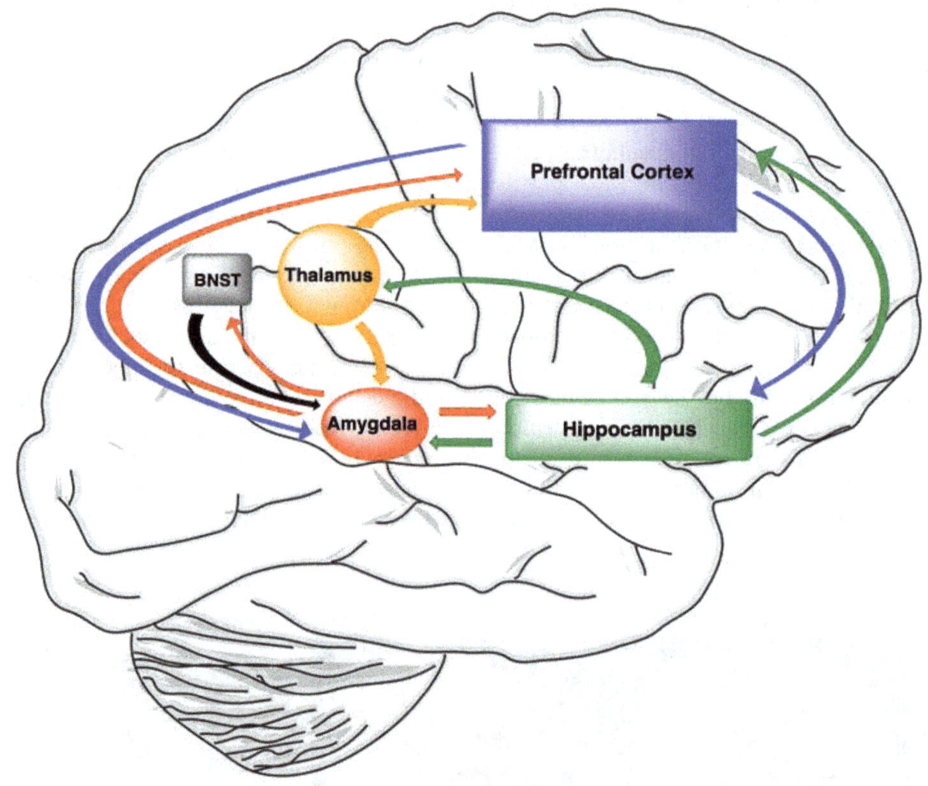

FIGURE 14 | Pharmacologic connectivity pathways implicated in neurosteroidal modulation of memory function. Neural networks that project to and/or share reciprocal connections with the hippocampus are modulated by neurosteroids as well as neurotransmitters. As a result, learning and memory deficits are associated with many of neurologic and neuropsychiatric disorders in which neurosteroids are implicated. The amygdala (shown in red), which is implicated in anxiety disorders, shares reciprocal connections with the hippocampus (shown in green). Progesterone, which is metabolized to ALLO, modulates emotional memory function by influencing amygdalar activity (64). The effects of neurosteroids on learning and memory for fear-inducing stimuli appears to be different in males and females which show different brain levels of ALLO at baseline as well (395). Neuroactive steroids, such as ALLO that enhance inhibitory neurotransmission can provide symptomatic relief from anxiety by reducing intra-network connectivity in the salience network and the amygdala (75, 192, 290, 291). ALLO induces an increase in functional connectivity between the amygdala and prefrontal cortex (shown in blue), which is involved in processing of complex social and non-social stimuli. However, the increased inhibition associated higher levels of ALLO can also interfere with episodic memory function which depends on intact functional connectivity between the hippocampus and the pre-cuneus (not shown) (203). Interestingly, both PREG, which is metabolized to ALLO, and PregS, which is a positive modulator of NMDARs, improve working memory function in patients with schizophrenia in which cortical disinhibition due to hypofunction of excitatory NMDARs on PV interneurons in the prefrontal cortex has been implicated (51, 52, 65, 237, 238). Parahippocampal and hippocampal structures including, the trisynaptic circuit receives sensory and emotional inputs from sensory modalities via the thalamus (shown in orange) and the amygdala, respectively (396–398). The impact of powerful emotion-evoking stimuli are state independent when ALLO is injected into the amygdala and hippocampus, but state-dependent when it is injected into the BNST (shown in gray) (246). The response of the hippocampal trisynaptic circuit to neurosteroids also depends on disease state-dependent changes in neurosteroid biosynthesis and receptor expression (399–401), as well as age-related changes in steroid hormone levels which converge to influence the responsivity of this circuit to endogenous and exogenous sources of neurosteroids and their synthetic analogs (229, 401–403).

neuroactive steroid, pregnanolone hemisuccinate, produces sedation and neuroprotection in mice and rats (132). Weaver et al. (132) demonstrated that pregnanolone hemisuccinate (PAHS) inhibits NMDA-induced currents and cell death in primary cultures of hippocampal neurons. Additionally, administration of a non-sedating dose of PAHS to rats following focal cerebral ischemia reduces cortical and subcortical infarct size (**Figure 13**).

Ganaxolone (3-hydroxy-3-methyl-5-pregnane-20-one), an orally bioavailable synthetic analog of ALLO, is a positive allosteric modulator of $GABA_AR$ with promising basic and early-stage clinical outcomes as a potential novel treatment for PTSD (388, 390–392). Based on the mechanism of action of ganaxolone and work in preclinical animal models suggesting improved spatial memory function in an animal model of Angelman Syndrome (393), future investigation looking at the clinical value of this agent in anxiety disorders appears warranted. Another synthetic analog of ALLO, 3β-ethenyl-3α-hydroxy-5α-pregnan-20-one (Co 3-0593), has been found to have anxiolytic effects comparable to benzodiazepines after both subcutaneous and oral administration in rodents. An absence of tolerance to this synthetic neuroactive steroid is suggested by the observation that its effects were maintained with chronic administration (394).

Current research into the function of PregS is impeded by the lack of selective/specific antagonists and by a lack of knowledge of validated binding site(s). These drawbacks are further exacerbated by the susceptibility of the essential 3-hydroxysulfate to hydrolysis by sulfatases. To overcome these limitations, we and others are using PregS analogs to decipher mechanistic aspects of PregS-mediated effects on learning and memory function. We recently reported that low nanomolar concentration of PregS induce a delayed-onset increase of the neuronal response to NMDA and trafficking of NMDAR to the cell surface through an intracellular ($[Ca^{2+}]i$)-dependent mechanism (47) (**Figure 2**). Moreover, we have demonstrated that low picomolar PregS increases $[Ca^{2+}]i$ and CREB phosphorylation and the frequency of spontaneous excitatory post-synaptic currents (48) (**Figures 8, 9**). More work is needed to determine if the synthetic analog of PregS, PREG hemisuccinate, has the potential to overcome the limitations associated with systemic administration of PregS.

CONCLUSIONS

The effects of neurosteroids in memory function in neuropsychiatric and neurologic disorders reflect their modulatory interactions exerted via selective binding at the amino and transmembrane domains of specific subunits comprising GABA and glutamate receptors, among others. Age- and disease state-dependent changes in endogenous levels of neurosteroids appear to play a role in the emergence of the unique functional imbalances implicated in specific neuropsychiatric disorders and the associated memory deficits, which are mediated in part by changes in neural network activity within specific brain regions implicated in the encoding, consolidation, and retrieval of memories. It may be helpful to think of these findings in terms of a *pharmacological connectome* that reflects the interactions of neurosteroids with various neural networks involved with the encoding and recall of memories. We believe that a neural circuitry framework will help to guide future investigations into the potential role of neurosteroids and their synthetic analogs as neurotherapeutics for memory dysfunction (**Figure 14**).

AUTHOR CONTRIBUTIONS

All authors listed have made a substantial, direct and intellectual contribution to the work, and approved it for publication.

FUNDING

NIH/NIA Grant Number: AG056947.

REFERENCES

1. Schally AV, Redding TW, Bowers CY, Barrett JF. Isolation and properties of porcine thyrotropin-releasing hormone. *J Biol Chem.* (1969) 244:4077–88.
2. Mitnick M, Reichlin S. Thyrotropin-releasing hormone: biosynthesis by rat hypothalamic fragments *in vitro*. *Science.* (1971) 172:1241–3. doi: 10.1126/science.172.3989.124
3. Leeman SE, Hammerschlag R. Stimulation of salivary secretion by a factor extracted from hypothalamic tissue. *Endocrinology.* (1967) 81:803–10. doi: 10.1210/endo-81-4-803
4. Chang MM, Leeman SE. Isolation of a sialogogic peptide from bovine hypothalamic tissue and its characterization as substance P. *J Biol Chem.* (1970) 245:4784–90.
5. Pardridge WM, Mietus LJ. Transport of steroid hormones through the rat blood-brain barrier. Primary role of albumin-bound hormone. *J Clin Invest.* (1979) 64:145–54. doi: 10.1172/JCI109433
6. Corpéchot C, Robel P, Axelson M, Sjövall J, Baulieu EE. Characterization and measurement of dehydroepiandrosterone sulfate in rat brain. *Proc Natl Acad Sci USA.* (1981) 78:4704–7.
7. Corpéchot C, Synguelakis M, Talha S, Axelson M, Sjövall J, Vihko R, et al. Pregnenolone and its sulfate ester in the rat brain. *Brain Res.* (1983) 270:119–25. doi: 10.1016/0006-8993(83)90797-7
8. Robel P, Bourreau E, Corpéchot C, Dang DC, Halberg F, Clarke C, et al. Neuro-steroids: 3 beta-hydroxy-delta 5-derivatives in rat and monkey brain. *J Steroid Biochem.* (1987) 27:649–55.
9. Morfin R, Young J, Corpéchot C, Egestad B, Sjövall J, Baulieu EE. Neurosteroids: pregnenolone in human sciatic nerves. *Proc Natl Acad Sci USA.* (1992) 89:6790–3. doi: 10.1073/pnas.89.15.6790
10. Selye H. Anaesthetic effects of steroid hormones. *Proc Soc Exp Biol Med.* (1941) 46:116–21.
11. Sapolsky RM, McEwen BS, Rainbow TC. Quantitative autoradiography of [3H]corticosterone receptors in rat brain. *Brain Res.* (1983) 271:331–4.
12. Harrison NL, Simmonds MA. Modulation of the GABA receptor complex by a steroid anaesthetic. *Brain Res.* (1984) 323:287–92. doi: 10.1016/0006-8993(84)90299-3
13. Harrison NL, Vicini S, Barker JL. A steroid anesthetic prolongs inhibitory postsynaptic currents in cultured rat hippocampal neurons. *J Neurosci.* (1987) 7:604–9. doi: 10.1523/JNEUROSCI.07-02-00604.1987

14. Barker JL, Harrison NL, Lange GD, Owen DG. Potentiation of gamma-aminobutyric-acid-activated chloride conductance by a steroid anaesthetic in cultured rat spinal neurones. *J Physiol.* (1987) 386:485–501.
15. Callachan H, Cottrell GA, Hather NY, Lambert JJ, Nooney JM, Peters JA. Modulation of the GABAA receptor by progesterone metabolites. *Proc R Soc Lond B Biol Sci.* (1987) 231:359–69. doi: 10.1098/rspb.1987.0049
16. Gee KW, Chang WC, Brinton RE, McEwen BS. GABA-dependent modulation of the Cl- ionophore by steroids in rat brain. *Eur J Pharmacol.* (1987) 136:419–23. doi: 10.1016/0014-2999(87)90317-7
17. Peters JA, Kirkness EF, Callachan H, Lambert JJ, Turner AJ. Modulation of the GABAA receptor by depressant barbiturates and pregnane steroids. *Br J Pharmacol.* (1988) 94:1257–69.
18. Choi DW, Farb DH, Fischbach GD. Chlordiazepoxide selectively augments GABA action in spinal cord cell cultures. *Nature.* (1977) 269:342–4.
19. Macdonald RL, Barker JL. Different actions of anticonvulsant and anesthetic barbiturates revealed by use of cultured mammalian neurons. *Science.* (1978) 200:775–7.
20. Majewska MD, Harrison NL, Schwartz RD, Barker JL, Paul SM. Steroid hormone metabolites are barbiturate-like modulators of the GABA receptor. *Science.* (1986) 232:1004–7. doi: 10.1126/science.2422758
21. Majewska MD, Schwartz RD. Pregnenolone-sulfate: an endogenous antagonist of the gamma-aminobutyric acid receptor complex in brain? *Brain Res.* (1987) 404:355–60. doi: 10.1016/0006-8993(87)91394-1
22. Herzog AG. Intermittent progesterone therapy and frequency of complex partial seizures in women with menstrual disorders. *Neurology.* (1986) 36:1607–10.
23. Wu FS, Gibbs TT, Farb DH. Inverse modulation of gamma-aminobutyric acid- and glycine-induced currents by progesterone. *Mol Pharmacol.* (1990) 37:597–602.
24. Wu FS, Gibbs TT, Farb DH. Pregnenolone sulfate: a positive allosteric modulator at the N-methyl-D-aspartate receptor. *Mol Pharmacol.* (1991) 40:333–6.
25. Majewska MD. Interaction of ethanol with the GABAA receptor in the rat brain: possible involvement of endogenous steroids. *Alcohol.* (1988) 5:269–73. doi: 10.1016/0741-8329(88)90064-X
26. Farb DH, Gibbs TT, Wu FS, Gyenes M, Friedman L, Russek SJ. Steroid modulation of amino acid neurotransmitter receptors. *Adv Biochem Psychopharmacol.* (1992) 47:119–31.
27. Irwin RP, Maragakis NJ, Rogawski MA, Purdy RH, Farb DH, Paul SM. Pregnenolone sulfate augments NMDA receptor mediated increases in intracellular Ca^{2+} in cultured rat hippocampal neurons. *Neurosci Lett.* (1992) 141:30–4. doi: 10.1016/0304-3940(92)90327-4
28. Flood JF, Morley JE, Roberts E. Memory-enhancing effects in male mice of pregnenolone and steroids metabolically derived from it. *Proc Natl Acad Sci USA.* (1992) 89:1567–71. doi: 10.1073/pnas.89.5.1567
29. Flood JF, Morley JE, Roberts E. Pregnenolone sulfate enhances post-training memory processes when injected in very low doses into limbic system structures: the amygdala is by far the most sensitive. *Proc Natl Acad Sci USA.* (1995) 92:10806–10. doi: 10.1073/pnas.92.23.10806
30. Flood JF, Smith GE, Roberts E. Dehydroepiandrosterone and its sulfate enhance memory retention in mice. *Brain Res.* (1988) 447:269–78. doi: 10.1016/0006-8993(88)91129-8
31. Plescia F, Marino RA, Cannizzaro E, Brancato A, Cannizzaro C. The role of pregnenolone sulphate in spatial orientation-acquisition and retention: an interplay between cognitive potentiation and mood regulation. *Behav Processes.* (2013) 99:130–7. doi: 10.1016/j.beproc.2013.07.001
32. Plescia F, Sardo P, Rizzo V, Cacace S, Marino RA, Brancato A, et al. Pregnenolone sulphate enhances spatial orientation and object discrimination in adult male rats: evidence from a behavioural and electrophysiological study. *Behav Brain Res.* (2014) 258:193–201. doi: 10.1016/j.bbr.2013.10.026
33. Abdel-Hafiz L, Chao OY, Huston JP, Nikolaus S, Spieler RE, de Souza Silva MA, et al. Promnestic effects of intranasally applied pregnenolone in rats. *Neurobiol Learn Mem.* (2016) 133:185–95. doi: 10.1016/j.nlm.2016.07.012
34. Park-Chung M, Wu FS, Farb DH. 3 alpha-Hydroxy-5 beta-pregnan-20-one sulfate: a negative modulator of the NMDA-induced current in cultured neurons. *Mol Pharmacol.* (1994) 46:146–50.
35. Park-Chung M, Wu FS, Purdy RH, Malayev AA, Gibbs TT, Farb DH. Distinct sites for inverse modulation of N-methyl-D-aspartate receptors by sulfated steroids. *Mol Pharmacol.* (1997) 52:1113–23. doi: 10.1124/mol.52.6.1113
36. Park-Chung M, Malayev A, Purdy RH, Gibbs TT, Farb DH. Sulfated and unsulfated steroids modulate gamma-aminobutyric acidA receptor function through distinct sites. *Brain Res.* (1999) 830:72–87.
37. Yaghoubi N, Malayev A, Russek SJ, Gibbs TT, Farb DH. Neurosteroid modulation of recombinant ionotropic glutamate receptors. *Brain Res.* (1998) 803:153–60. doi: 10.1016/S0006-8993(98)00644-1
38. Malayev A, Gibbs TT, Farb DH. Inhibition of the NMDA response by pregnenolone sulphate reveals subtype selective modulation of NMDA receptors by sulphated steroids. *Br J Pharmacol.* (2002) 135:901–9. doi: 10.1038/sj.bjp.0704543
39. Cameron K, Bartle E, Roark R, Fanelli D, Pham M, Pollard B, et al. Neurosteroid binding to the amino terminal and glutamate binding domains of ionotropic glutamate receptors. *Steroids.* (2012) 77:774–9. doi: 10.1016/j.steroids.2012.03.011
40. Partridge LD, Valenzuela CF. Neurosteroid-induced enhancement of glutamate transmission in rat hippocampal slices. *Neurosci Lett.* (2001) 301:103–6. doi: 10.1016/S0304-3940(01)01613-5
41. Sliwinski A, Monnet FP, Schumacher M, Morin-Surun MP. Pregnenolone sulfate enhances long-term potentiation in CA1 in rat hippocampus slices through the modulation of N-methyl-D-aspartate receptors. *J Neurosci Res.* (2004) 78:691–701. doi: 10.1002/jnr.20332
42. Sabeti J, Nelson TE, Purdy RH, Gruol DL. Steroid pregnenolone sulfate enhances NMDA-receptor-independent long-term potentiation at hippocampal CA1 synapses: role for L-type calcium channels and sigma-receptors. *Hippocampus.* (2007) 17:349–69. doi: 10.1002/hipo.20273
43. Jang MK, Mierke DF, Russek SJ, Farb DH. A steroid modulatory domain on NR2B controls N-methyl-D-aspartate receptor proton sensitivity. *Proc Natl Acad Sci USA.* (2004) 101:8198–203. doi: 10.1073/pnas.0401838101
44. Horak M, Vlcek K, Chodounska H, Vyklicky L Jr. Subtype-dependence of N-methyl-D-aspartate receptor modulation by pregnenolone sulfate. *Neuroscience.* (2006) 137:93–102. doi: 10.1016/j.neuroscience.2005.08.058
45. Kostakis E, Jang MK, Russek SJ, Gibbs TT, Farb DH. A steroid modulatory domain in NR2A collaborates with NR1 exon-5 to control NMDAR modulation by pregnenolone sulfate and protons. *J Neurochem.* (2011) 119:486–96. doi: 10.1111/j.1471-4159.2011.07442.x
46. Petrovic M, Sedlacek M, Cais O, Horak M, Chodounska H, Vyklicky L Jr. Pregnenolone sulfate modulation of N-methyl-D-aspartate receptors is phosphorylation dependent. *Neuroscience.* (2009) 160:616–28. doi: 10.1016/j.neuroscience.2009.02.052
47. Kostakis E, Smith C, Jang MK, Martin SC, Richards KG, Russek SJ, et al. The neuroactive steroid pregnenolone sulfate stimulates trafficking of functional N-methyl D-aspartate receptors to the cell surface via a noncanonical, G protein, and Ca^{2+}-dependent mechanism. *Mol Pharmacol.* (2013) 84:261–74. doi: 10.1124/mol.113.085696
48. Smith CC, Martin SC, Sugunan K, Russek SJ, Gibbs TT, Farb DH. A role for picomolar concentrations of pregnenolone sulfate in synaptic activity-dependent Ca^{2+} signaling and CREB activation. *Mol Pharmacol.* (2014) 86:390–8. doi: 10.1124/mol.114.094128
49. Adamusová E, Cais O, Vyklický V, Kudová E, Chodounská H, Horák M, et al. Pregnenolone sulfate activates NMDA receptor channels. *Physiol Res.* (2013) 62:731–6.
50. Marx CE, Lee J, Subramaniam M, Rapisarda A, Bautista DC, Chan E, et al. Proof-of-concept randomized controlled trial of pregnenolone in schizophrenia. *Psychopharmacology (Berl).* (2014) 231:3647–62. doi: 10.1007/s00213-014-3673-4
51. Marx CE, Keefe RS, Buchanan RW, Hamer RM, Kilts JD, Bradford DW, et al. Proof-of-concept trial with the neurosteroid pregnenolone targeting cognitive and negative symptoms in schizophrenia. *Neuropsychopharmacology.* (2009) 34:1885–903. doi: 10.1038/npp.2009.26
52. Marx CE, Bradford DW, Hamer RM, Naylor JC, Allen TB, Lieberman JA, et al. Pregnenolone as a novel therapeutic candidate in schizophrenia:

emerging preclinical and clinical evidence. *Neuroscience.* (2011) 191:78–90. doi: 10.1016/j.neuroscience.2011.06.076

53. Ritsner MS, Bawakny H, Kreinin A. Pregnenolone treatment reduces severity of negative symptoms in recent-onset schizophrenia: an 8-week, double-blind, randomized add-on two-center trial. *Psychiatry Clin Neurosci.* (2014) 68:432–40. doi: 10.1111/pcn.12150
54. Wilding TJ, Lopez MN, Huettner JE. Chimeric glutamate receptor subunits reveal the transmembrane domain is sufficient for NMDA receptor pore properties but some positive allosteric modulators require additional domains. *J Neurosci.* (2016) 36:8815–25. doi: 10.1523/JNEUROSCI.0345-16.2016
55. Paul SM, Doherty JJ, Robichaud AJ, Belfort GM, Chow BY, Hammond RS, et al. The major brain cholesterol metabolite 24(S)-hydroxycholesterol is a potent allosteric modulator of N-methyl-D-aspartate receptors. *J Neurosci.* (2013) 33:17290–300. doi: 10.1523/JNEUROSCI.2619-13.2013
56. Linsenbardt AJ, Taylor A, Emnett CM, Doherty JJ, Krishnan K, Covey DF, et al. Different oxysterols have opposing actions at N-methyl-D-aspartate receptors. *Neuropharmacology.* (2014) 85:232–42. doi: 10.1016/j.neuropharm.2014.05.027
57. Vyklicky V, Krausova B, Cerny J, Ladislav M, Smejkalova T, Kysilov B, et al. Surface expression, function, and pharmacology of disease-associated mutations in the membrane domain of the human GluN2B Subunit. *Front Mol Neurosci.* (2018) 11:110. doi: 10.3389/fnmol.2018.00110
58. Chisari M, Wilding TJ, Brunwasser S, Krishnan K, Qian M, Benz A, et al. Visualizing pregnenolone sulfate-like modulators of NMDA receptor function reveals intracellular and plasma-membrane localization. *Neuropharmacology.* (2018) 144:91–103. doi: 10.1016/j.neuropharm.2018.10.015
59. Vallée M, Mayo W, Darnaudéry M, Corpéchot C, Young J, Koehl M, et al. Neurosteroids: deficient cognitive performance in aged rats depends on low pregnenolone sulfate levels in the hippocampus. *Proc Natl Acad Sci USA.* (1997) 94:14865–70. doi: 10.1073/pnas.94.26.14865
60. Weill-Engerer S, David JP, Sazdovitch V, Liere P, Eychenne B, Pianos A, et al. Neurosteroid quantification in human brain regions: comparison between Alzheimer's and nondemented patients. *J Clin Endocrinol Metab.* (2002) 87:5138–43. doi: 10.1210/jc.2002-020878
61. Scullin CS, and Partridge LD. Modulation by pregnenolone sulfate of filtering properties in the hippocampal trisynaptic circuit. *Hippocampus.* (2012) 22:2184–98. doi: 10.1002/hipo.22038
62. Smith CC, Gibbs TT, Farb DH. Pregnenolone sulfate as a modulator of synaptic plasticity. *Psychopharmacology (Berl).* (2014) 231:3537–56. doi: 10.1007/s00213-014-3643-x
63. Reddy DS, Gangisetty O, Wu X. PR-independent neurosteroid regulation of α2-GABA-A receptors in the hippocampus subfields. *Brain Res.* (2017) 1659:142–7. doi: 10.1016/j.brainres.2017.01.030
64. van Wingen G, van Broekhoven F, Verkes RJ, Petersson KM, Bäckström T, Buitelaar J, et al. How progesterone impairs memory for biologically salient stimuli in healthy young women. *J Neurosci.* (2007) 27:11416–23. doi: 10.1523/JNEUROSCI.1715-07.2007
65. Kreinin A, Bawakny N, Ritsner MS. Adjunctive pregnenolone ameliorates the cognitive deficits in recent-onset schizophrenia: an 8-week, randomized, double-blind, placebo-controlled trial. *Clin Schizophr Relat Psychoses.* (2017) 10:201–10. doi: 10.3371/CSRP.KRBA.013114
66. Farb DH, Ratner MH. Targeting the modulation of neural circuitry for the treatment of anxiety disorders. *Pharmacol Rev.* (2014) 66:1002–32. doi: 10.1124/pr.114.009126
67. Naylor JC, Kilts JD, Hulette CM, Steffens DC, Blazer DG, Ervin JF, et al. Allopregnanolone levels are reduced in temporal cortex in patients with Alzheimer's disease compared to cognitively intact control subjects. *Biochim Biophys Acta.* (2010) 1801:951–9. doi: 10.1016/j.bbalip.2010.05.006
68. Carlson LE, Sherwin BB, Chertkow HM. Relationships between dehydroepiandrosterone sulfate (DHEAS) and cortisol (CRT) plasma levels and everyday memory in Alzheimer's disease patients compared to healthy controls. *Horm Behav.* (1999) 35:254–63. doi: 10.1006/hbeh.19 99.1518
69. Csernansky JG, Dong H, Fagan AM, Wang L, Xiong C, Holtzman DM, et al. Plasma cortisol and progression of dementia in subjects with Alzheimer-type dementia. *Am J Psychiatry.* (2006) 163:2164–9. doi: 10.1176/ajp.2006.163.12.2164
70. Rasmuson S, Näsman B, Olsson T. Increased serum levels of dehydroepiandrosterone (DHEA) and interleukin-6 (IL-6) in women with mild to moderate Alzheimer's disease. *Int Psychogeriatr.* (2011) 23:1386–92. doi: 10.1017/S1041610211000810
71. Aldred S, Mecocci P. Decreased dehydroepiandrosterone (DHEA) and dehydroepiandrosterone sulfate (DHEAS) concentrations in plasma of Alzheimer's disease (AD) patients. *Arch Gerontol Geriatr.* (2010) 51:e16–8. doi: 10.1016/j.archger.2009.07.001
72. Cherrier MM, Anderson K, Shofer J, Millard S, Matsumoto AM. Testosterone treatment of men with mild cognitive impairment and low testosterone levels. *Am J Alzheimers Dis Other Demen.* (2015) 30:421–30. doi: 10.1177/1533317514556874
73. Mantella RC, Butters MA, Amico JA, Mazumdar S, Rollman BL, Begley AE, et al. Salivary cortisol is associated with diagnosis and severity of late-life generalized anxiety disorder. *Psychoneuroendocrinology.* (2008) 33:773–81. doi: 10.1016/j.psyneuen.2008.03.002
74. Heydari B, Le Mellédo JM. Low pregnenolone sulphate plasma concentrations in patients with generalized social phobia. *Psychol Med.* (2002) 32:929–33. doi: 10.1017/S0033291702005238
75. Rasmusson AM, Pinna G, Paliwal P, Weisman D, Gottschalk C, Charney D, et al. Decreased cerebrospinal fluid allopregnanolone levels in women with posttraumatic stress disorder. *Biol Psychiatry.* (2006) 60:704–13. doi: 10.1016/j.biopsych.2006.03.026
76. Rasmusson AM, King MW, Valovski I, Gregor K, Scioli-Salter E, Pineles SL, et al. Relationships between cerebrospinal fluid GABAergic neurosteroid levels and symptom severity in men with PTSD. *Psychoneuroendocrinology.* (2018) 102:95–104. doi: 10.1016/j.psyneuen.2018.11.027
77. Droogleever Fortuyn HA, van Broekhoven F, Span PN, Bäckström T, Zitman FG, Verkes RJ. Effects of PhD examination stress on allopregnanolone and cortisol plasma levels and peripheral benzodiazepine receptor density. *Psychoneuroendocrinology.* (2004) 29:1341–4. doi: 10.1016/j.psyneuen.2004.02.003
78. Wolf OT, Kudielka BM, Hellhammer DH, Hellhammer J, Kirschbaum, C. Opposing effects of DHEA replacement in elderly subjects on declarative memory and attention after exposure to a laboratory stressor. *Psychoneuroendocrinology.* (1998) 23:617–29. doi: 10.1016/S0306-4530(98)00032-8
79. Girdler SS, Straneva PA, Light KC, Pedersen CA, Morrow AL. Allopregnanolone levels and reactivity to mental stress in premenstrual dysphoric disorder. *Biol Psychiatry.* (2001) 49:788–97. doi: 10.1016/S0006-3223(00)01044-1
80. Kanes SJ, Colquhoun H, Doherty J, Raines S, Hoffmann E, Rubinow DR, et al. Open-label, proof-of-concept study of brexanolone in the treatment of severe postpartum depression. *Hum Psychopharmacol.* (2017) 32:e2576. doi: 10.1002/hup.2576
81. Kanes S, Colquhoun H, Gunduz-Bruce H, Raines S, Arnold R, Schacterle A, et al. Brexanolone (SAGE-547 injection) in post-partum depression: a randomised controlled trial. *Lancet.* (2017) 390:480–9. doi: 10.1016/S0140-6736(17)31264-3
82. Herzog AG, Frye CA, Progesterone Trial Study Group. Allopregnanolone levels and seizure frequency in progesterone-treated women with epilepsy. *Neurology.* (2014) 83:345–8. doi: 10.1212/WNL.0000000000000623
83. Valencia-Sanchez C, Crepeau AZ, Hoerth MT, Butler KA, Almader-Douglas D, Wingerchuk DM, et al. Is adjunctive progesterone effective in reducing seizure frequency in patients with intractable catamenial epilepsy? A critically appraised topic. *Neurologist.* (2018) 23:108–12. doi: 10.1097/NRL.0000000000000167
84. Caraci F, Spampinato SF, Morgese MG, Tascedda F, Salluzzo MG, Giambirtone MC, et al. Neurobiological links between depression and AD: the role of TGF-β1 signaling as a new pharmacological target. *Pharmacol Res.* (2018) 130:374–84. doi: 10.1016/j.phrs.2018.02.007
85. McIntyre RS, Cha DS, Soczynska JK, Woldeyohannes HO, Gallaugher LA, Kudlow P, et al. Cognitive deficits and functional outcomes in major depressive disorder: determinants, substrates, and treatment interventions. *Depress Anxiety.* (2013) 30:515–27. doi: 10.1002/da.22063

86. Kallen CB, Billheimer JT, Summers SA, Stayrook SE, Lewis M, Strauss JF III. Steroidogenic acute regulatory protein (StAR) is a sterol transfer protein. *J Biol Chem.* (1998) 273:26285–8.
87. Liu J, Rone MB, Papadopoulos V. Protein-protein interactions mediate mitochondrial cholesterol transport and steroid biosynthesis. *J Biol Chem.* (2006) 281:38879–93. doi: 10.1074/jbc.M608820200
88. Bose M, Whittal RM, Miller WL, Bose HS. Steroidogenic activity of StAR requires contact with mitochondrial VDAC1 and phosphate carrier protein. *J Biol Chem.* (2008) 283:8837–45. doi: 10.1074/jbc.M709221200
89. Porcu P, Barron AM, Frye CA, Walf AA, Yang SY, He XY, et al. Neurosteroidogenesis today: novel targets for neuroactive steroid synthesis and action and their relevance for translational research. *J Neuroendocrinol.* (2016) 28:12351. doi: 10.1111/jne.12351
90. Chung BC, Matteson KJ, Voutilainen R, Mohandas TK, Miller WL. Human cholesterol side-chain cleavage enzyme, P450scc: cDNA cloning, assignment of the gene to chromosome 15, and expression in the placenta. *Proc Natl Acad Sci USA.* (1986) 83:8962–6. doi: 10.1073/pnas.83.23.8962
91. Penning TM, Pawlowski JE, Schlegel BP, Jez JM, Lin HK, Hoog SS, et al. Mammalian 3 alpha-hydroxysteroid dehydrogenases. *Steroids.* (1996) 61:508–23. doi: 10.1016/S0039-128X(96)00093-1
92. Penning TM, Jin Y, Heredia VV, Lewis M. Structure-function relationships in 3alpha-hydroxysteroid dehydrogenases: a comparison of the rat and human isoforms. *J Steroid Biochem Mol Biol.* (2003) 85:247–55. doi: 10.1016/S0960-0760(03)00236-X
93. Griffin LD, Mellon SH. Selective serotonin reuptake inhibitors directly alter activity of neurosteroidogenic enzymes. *Proc Natl Acad Sci USA.* (1999) 96:13512–7. doi: 10.1073/pnas.96.23.13512
94. Agís-Balboa RC, Pinna G, Zhubi A, Maloku E, Veldic M, Costa E, Guidotti A. Characterization of brain neurons that express enzymes mediating neurosteroid biosynthesis. *Proc Natl Acad Sci USA.* (2006) 103:14602–7. doi: 10.1073/pnas.0606544103
95. Mueller JW, Gilligan LC, Idkowiak J, Arlt W, Foster PA. The regulation of steroid action by sulfation and desulfation. *Endocr Rev.* (2015) 36:526–63. doi: 10.1210/er.2015-1036
96. Sorwell KG, Kohama SG, Urbanski HF. Perimenopausal regulation of steroidogenesis in the nonhuman primate. *Neurobiol Aging.* (2012) 33:1487.e1–13. doi: 10.1016/j.neurobiolaging.2011.05.004
97. Sorwell KG, Renner L, Weiss AR, Neuringer M, Kohama SG, Urbanski HF. Cognition in aged rhesus monkeys: effect of DHEA and correlation with steroidogenic gene expression. *Genes Brain Behav.* (2017) 16:361–8. doi: 10.1111/gbb.12351
98. Baulieu EE, Robel P, Schumacher M. Neurosteroids: beginning of the story. *Int Rev Neurobiol.* (2001) 46:1–32. doi: 10.1016/S0074-7742(01)46057-0
99. Chen L, Cai W, Chen L, Zhou R, Furuya K, Sokabe M. Modulatory metaplasticity induced by pregnenolone sulfate in the rat hippocampus: a leftward shift in LTP/LTD-frequency curve. *Hippocampus.* (2010) 20:499–512. doi: 10.1002/hipo.20649
100. Carrigan CN, Patel SA, Cox HD, Bolstad ES, Gerdes JM, Smith WE, et al. The development of benzo- and naphtho-fused quinoline-2,4-dicarboxylic acids as vesicular glutamate transporter (VGLUT) inhibitors reveals a possible role for neuroactive steroids. *Bioorg Med Chem Lett.* (2014) 24:850–4. doi: 10.1016/j.bmcl.2013.12.086
101. Shimizu H, Ishizuka Y, Yamazaki H, Shirao T. Allopregnanolone increases mature excitatory synapses along dendrites via protein kinase A signaling. *Neuroscience.* (2015) 305:139–45. doi: 10.1016/j.neuroscience.2015.07.079
102. Miller PS, Scott S, Masiulis S, De Colibus L, Pardon E, Steyaert J, Aricescu AR. Structural basis for GABAA receptor potentiation by neurosteroids. *Nat Struct Mol Biol.* (2017) 24:986–992. doi: 10.1038/nsmb.3484
103. Grosser G, Bennien J, Sánchez-Guijo A, Bakhaus K, Döring B, Hartmann M, et al. Transport of steroid 3-sulfates and steroid 17-sulfates by the sodium-dependent organic anion transporter SOAT (SLC10A6). *J Steroid Biochem Mol Biol.* (2018) 179:20–5. doi: 10.1016/j.jsbmb.2017.09.013
104. Rupprecht R, Berning B, Hauser CA, Holsboer F, Reul JM. Steroid receptor-mediated effects of neuroactive steroids: characterization of structure-activity relationship. *Eur J Pharmacol.* (1996) 303:227–34. doi: 10.1016/0014-2999(96)00036-2
105. Yang P, Jones BL, Henderson LP. Mechanisms of anabolic androgenic steroid modulation of alpha(1)beta(3)gamma(2L) GABA(A) receptors. *Neuropharmacology.* (2002) 43:619–33. doi: 10.1016/S0028-3908(02)00155-7
106. Lambert JJ, Peters JA, Sturgess NC, Hales TG. Steroid modulation of the GABAA receptor complex: electrophysiological studies. *Ciba Found Symp.* (1990) 153:56–71. doi: 10.1016/1044-5765(91)90020-O
107. Belelli D, Casula A, Ling A, Lambert JJ. The influence of subunit composition on the interaction of neurosteroids with GABA(A) receptors. *Neuropharmacology.* (2002) 43:651–61. doi: 10.1016/S0028-3908(02)00172-7
108. Harney SC, Frenguelli BG, Lambert JJ. Phosphorylation influences neurosteroid modulation of synaptic GABAA receptors in rat CA1 and dentate gyrus neurones. *Neuropharmacology.* (2003) 45:873–83. doi: 10.1016/S0028-3908(03)00251-X
109. Hosie AM, Wilkins ME, da Silva HM, Smart TG. Endogenous neurosteroids regulate GABAA receptors through two discrete transmembrane sites. *Nature.* (2006) 444:486–9. doi: 10.1038/nature05324
110. Bowlby MR. Pregnenolone sulfate potentiation of N-methyl-D-aspartate receptor channels in hippocampal neurons. *Mol Pharmacol.* (1993) 43:813–9.
111. Collingridge GL, Volianskis A, Bannister N, France G, Hanna L, Mercier M, et al. The NMDA receptor as a target for cognitive enhancement. *Neuropharmacology.* (2013) 64:13–26. doi: 10.1016/j.neuropharm.2012.06.051
112. Hackos DH, Hanson JE. Diverse modes of NMDA receptor positive allosteric modulation: mechanisms and consequences. *Neuropharmacology.* (2017) 112:34–45. doi: 10.1016/j.neuropharm.2016.07.037
113. Collingridge GL, Kehl SJ, McLennan H. Excitatory amino acids in synaptic transmission in the Schaffer collateral-commissural pathway of the rat hippocampus. *J Physiol.* (1983) 334:33–46. doi: 10.1113/jphysiol.1983.sp014478
114. Morris RG, Anderson E, Lynch GS, Baudry M. Selective impairment of learning and blockade of long-term potentiation by an N-methyl-D-aspartate receptor antagonist, AP5. *Nature.* (1986) 319:774–6. doi: 10.1038/319774a0
115. Bashir ZI, Alford S, Davies SN, Randall AD, Collingridge GL. Long-term potentiation of NMDA receptor-mediated synaptic transmission in the hippocampus. *Nature.* (1991) 349:156–8. doi: 10.1038/349156a0
116. Asztely F, Wigström H, Gustafsson B. The relative contribution of NMDA receptor channels in the expression of long-term potentiation in the hippocampal CA1 region. *Eur J Neurosci.* (1992) 4:681–90. doi: 10.1111/j.1460-9568.1992.tb00177.x
117. Cui LN, Inenaga K, Nagatomo T, Yamashita H. Sodium nitroprusside modulates NMDA response in the rat supraoptic neurons *in vitro*. *Brain Res Bull.* (1994) 35:253–60. doi: 10.1016/0361-9230(94)90131-7
118. Traynelis SF, Wollmuth LP, McBain CJ, Menniti FS, Vance KM, Ogden KK, et al. Glutamate receptor ion channels: structure, regulation, and function. *Pharmacol Rev.* (2010) 62:405–96. doi: 10.1124/pr.109.002451
119. Weaver CE, Land MB, Malayev AA, Purdy RH, Richards KG, Gibbs TT, Farb DH. Geometry and charge determine the pharmacological effects of steroids on the N-methyl-D-aspartate receptor. *J Pharmacol Exp Ther.* (2000) 293:747–54.
120. Korinek M, Kapras V, Vyklicky V, Adamusova E, Borovska J, Vales K, et al. Neurosteroid modulation of N-methyl-D-aspartate receptors: molecular mechanism and behavioral effects. *Steroids.* (2011) 76:1409–18. doi: 10.1016/j.steroids.2011.09.002
121. Lee KH, Cho JH, Choi IS, Park HM, Lee MG, Choi BJ, Jang IS. Pregnenolone sulfate enhances spontaneous glutamate release by inducing presynaptic Ca^{2+}-induced Ca^{2+} release. *Neuroscience.* (2010) 171:106–16. doi: 10.1016/j.neuroscience.2010.07.057
122. Dong Y, Fu YM, Sun JL, Zhu YH, Sun FY, Zheng P. Neurosteroid enhances glutamate release in rat prelimbic cortex via activation of alpha1-adrenergic and sigma1 receptors. *Cell Mol Life Sci.* (2005) 62:1003–14. doi: 10.1007/s00018-005-5004-8
123. Maninger N, Wolkowitz OM, Reus VI, Epel ES, Mellon SH. Neurobiological and neuropsychiatric effects of dehydroepiandrosterone (DHEA) and DHEA sulfate (DHEAS). *Front Neuroendocrinol.* (2009) 30:65–91. doi: 10.1016/j.yfrne.2008.11.002
124. Kimonides VG, Khatibi NH, Svendsen CN, Sofroniew MV, Herbert J. Dehydroepiandrosterone (DHEA) and DHEA-sulfate (DHEAS) protect

hippocampal neurons against excitatory amino acid-induced neurotoxicity. *Proc Natl Acad Sci USA.* (1998) 95:1852–7. doi: 10.1073/pnas.95.4.1852

125. Borowicz KK, Piskorska B, Banach M, Czuczwar SJ. Neuroprotective actions of neurosteroids. *Front Endocrinol (Lausanne).* (2011) 2:50. doi: 10.3389/fendo.2011.00050
126. Ulmann L, Rodeau JL, Danoux L, Contet-Audonneau JL, Pauly G, Schlichter R. Dehydroepiandrosterone and neurotrophins favor axonal growth in a sensory neuron-keratinocyte coculture model. *Neuroscience.* (2009) 159:514–25. doi: 10.1016/j.neuroscience.2009.01.018
127. Lazaridis I, Charalampopoulos I, Alexaki VI, Avlonitis N, Pediaditakis I, Efstathopoulos P, et al. Neurosteroid dehydroepiandrosterone interacts with nerve growth factor (NGF) receptors, preventing neuronal apoptosis. *PLoS Biol.* (2011) 9:e1001051. doi: 10.1371/journal.pbio.1001051
128. Shen W, Mennerick S, Zorumski EC, Covey DF, Zorumski CF. Pregnenolone sulfate and dehydroepiandrosterone sulfate inhibit GABA-gated chloride currents in Xenopus oocytes expressing picrotoxin-insensitive GABA(A) receptors. *Neuropharmacology.* (1999) 38:267–71. doi: 10.1016/S0028-3908(98)00172-5
129. Johansson T, Le Grevès P. The effect of dehydroepiandrosterone sulfate and allopregnanolone sulfate on the binding of [(3)H]ifenprodil to the N-methyl-d-aspartate receptor in rat frontal cortex membrane. *J Steroid Biochem Mol Biol.* (2005) 94:263–6. doi: 10.1016/j.jsbmb.2005.01.020
130. Twede V, Tartaglia AL, Covey DF, Bamber BA. The neurosteroids dehydroepiandrosterone sulfate and pregnenolone sulfate inhibit the UNC-49 GABA receptor through a common set of residues. *Mol Pharmacol.* (2007) 72:1322–9. doi: 10.1124/mol.107.034058
131. Wang C, Marx CE, Morrow AL, Wilson WA, Moore SD. Neurosteroid modulation of GABAergic neurotransmission in the central amygdala: a role for NMDA receptors. *Neurosci Lett.* (2007) 415:118–23. doi: 10.1016/j.neulet.2007.01.004
132. Weaver CE, Marek P, Park-Chung M, Tam SW, and Farb DH. Neuroprotective activity of a new class of steroidal inhibitors of the N-methyl-D-aspartate receptor. *Proc Natl Acad Sci USA.* (1997) 94:10450–4. doi: 10.1073/pnas.94.19.10450
133. Santoro A, Mattace Raso G, Taliani S, Da Pozzo E, Simorini F, Costa B, et al. TSPO-ligands prevent oxidative damage and inflammatory response in C6 glioma cells by neurosteroid synthesis. *Eur J Pharm Sci.* (2016) 88:124–31. doi: 10.1016/j.ejps.2016.04.006
134. Cheng WWL, Chen ZW, Bracamontes JR, Budelier MM, Krishnan K, Shin DJ, et al. Mapping two neurosteroid-modulatory sites in the prototypic pentameric ligand-gated ion channel GLIC. *J Biol Chem.* (2018) 293:3013–27. doi: 10.1074/jbc.RA117.000359
135. Majewska MD, Demirgören S, London ED. Binding of pregnenolone sulfate to rat brain membranes suggests multiple sites of steroid action at the GABAA receptor. *Eur J Pharmacol.* (1990) 189:307–15. doi: 10.1016/0922-4106(90)90124-G
136. Majewska MD, Demirgören S, Spivak CE, London ED. The neurosteroid dehydroepiandrosterone sulfate is an allosteric antagonist of the GABAA receptor. *Brain Res.* (1990) 526:143–6. doi: 10.1016/0006-8993(90) 90261-9
137. Akk G, Bracamontes JR, Covey DF, Evers A, Dao T, Steinbach JH. Neuroactive steroids have multiple actions to potentiate GABAA receptors. *J Physiol.* (2004) 558:59–74. doi: 10.1113/jphysiol.2004.066571
138. Akk G, Covey DF, Evers AS, Steinbach JH, Zorumski CF, Mennerick S. Mechanisms of neurosteroid interactions with GABA(A) receptors. *Pharmacol Ther.* (2007) 116:35–57. doi: 10.1016/j.pharmthera.2007.03.004
139. Akk G, Covey DF, Evers AS, Mennerick S, Zorumski CF, Steinbach JH. Kinetic and structural determinants for GABA-A receptor potentiation by neuroactive steroids. *Curr Neuropharmacol.* (2010) 8:18–25. doi: 10.2174/157015910790909458
140. Maksay G, Laube B, Betz H. Subunit-specific modulation of glycine receptors by neurosteroids. *Neuropharmacology.* (2001) 41:369–76. doi: 10.1016/S0028-3908(01)00071-5
141. Mihalek RM, Banerjee PK, Korpi ER, Quinlan JJ, Firestone LL, Mi ZP, et al. Attenuated sensitivity to neuroactive steroids in gamma-aminobutyrate type A receptor delta subunit knockout mice. *Proc Natl Acad Sci USA.* (1999) 96:12905–10. doi: 10.1073/pnas.96.22.12905
142. Mihalek RM, Bowers BJ, Wehner JM, Kralic JE, VanDoren MJ, Morrow AL, et al. GABA(A)-receptor delta subunit knockout mice have multiple defects in behavioral responses to ethanol. *Alcohol Clin Exp Res.* (2001) 25:1708–18. doi: 10.1111/j.1530-0277.2001.tb02179.x
143. Spigelman I, Li Z, Liang J, Cagetti E, Samzadeh S, Mihalek RM, et al. Reduced inhibition and sensitivity to neurosteroids in hippocampus of mice lacking the GABA(A) receptor delta subunit. *J Neurophysiol.* (2003) 90:903–10. doi: 10.1152/jn.01022.2002
144. Stell BM, Brickley SG, Tang CY, Farrant M, Mody I. Neuroactive steroids reduce neuronal excitability by selectively enhancing tonic inhibition mediated by delta subunit-containing GABAA receptors. *Proc Natl Acad Sci USA.* (2003) 100:14439–44. doi: 10.1073/pnas.2435457100
145. Whissell PD, Lecker I, Wang DS, Yu J, Orser BA. Altered expression of δGABAA receptors in health and disease. *Neuropharmacology.* (2015) 88:24–35. doi: 10.1016/j.neuropharm.2014.08.003
146. Rick CE, Ye Q, Finn SE, Harrison NL. Neurosteroids act on the GABAA receptor at sites on the N-terminal side of the middle of TM2. *Neuroreport.* (1998) 9:379–83. doi: 10.1097/00001756-199802160-00004
147. Hosie AM, Clarke L, da Silva H, Smart TG. Conserved site for neurosteroid modulation of $GABA_A$receptors. *Neuropharmacology.* (2009) 56:149–54. doi: 10.1016/j.neuropharm.2008.07.050
148. Covey DF, Nathan D, Kalkbrenner M, Nilsson KR, Hu Y, Zorumski CF, et al. Enantioselectivity of pregnanolone-induced gamma-aminobutyric acid(A) receptor modulation and anesthesia. *J Pharmacol Exp Ther.* (2000) 293:1009–16.
149. Ghosh B, Tsao TW, Czajkowski C. A chimeric prokaryotic-eukaryotic pentameric ligand gated ion channel reveals interactions between the extracellular and transmembrane domains shape neurosteroid modulation. *Neuropharmacology.* (2017) 125:343–52. doi: 10.1016/j.neuropharm.2017.08.007
150. Jiang X, Shu HJ, Krishnan K, Qian M, Taylor AA, Covey DF, et al. Clickable neurosteroid photolabel reveals selective Golgi compartmentalization with preferential impact on proximal inhibition. *Neuropharmacology.* (2016) 108:193–206. doi: 10.1016 j.neuropharm.2016.04.031
151. Wagner TF, Loch S, Lambert S, Straub I, Mannebach S, Mathar I, et al. Transient receptor potential M3 channels are ionotropic steroid receptors in pancreatic beta cells. *Nat Cell Biol.* (2008) 10:1421–30. doi: 10.1038/ncb1801
152. Harteneck, C. Pregnenolone sulfate: from steroid metabolite to TRP channel ligand. *Molecules.* (2013) 18:12012–28. doi: 10.3390/molecules181012012
153. Chen SC, Wu FS. Mechanism underlying inhibition of the capsaicin receptor-mediated current by pregnenolone sulfate in rat dorsal root ganglion neurons. *Brain Res.* (2004) 1027:196–200. doi: 10.1016/j.brainres.2004.08.053
154. Zamudio-Bulcock PA, Everett J, Harteneck C, Valenzuela CF. Activation of steroid-sensitive TRPM3 channels potentiates glutamatergic transmission at cerebellar Purkinje neurons from developing rats. *J Neurochem.* (2011) 119:474–85. doi: 10.1111/j.1471-4159.2011.07441.x
155. Zamudio-Bulcock PA, Valenzuela CF. Pregnenolone sulfate increases glutamate release at neonatal climbing fiber-to-Purkinje cell synapses. *Neuroscience.* (2011) 175:24–36. doi: 10.1016/j.neuroscience.2010.11.063
156. Valenzuela CF, Partridge LD, Mameli M, Meyer DA. Modulation of glutamatergic transmission by sulfated steroids: role in fetal alcohol spectrum disorder. *Brain Res Rev.* (2008) 57:506–19. doi: 10.1016/j.brainresrev.2007.04.009
157. Yamamoto S, Wajima T, Hara Y, Nishida M, Mori Y. Transient receptor potential channels in Alzheimer's disease. *Biochim Biophys Acta.* (2007) 1772:958–67. doi: 10.1016/j.bbadis.2007.03.006
158. Shigetomi E, Tong X, Kwan KY, Corey DP, Khakh BS. TRPA1 channels regulate astrocyte resting calcium and inhibitory synapse efficacy through GAT-3. *Nat Neurosci.* (2011) 15:70–80. doi: 10.1038/nn.3000
159. Bosson A, Paumier A, Boisseau S, Jacquier-Sarlin M, Buisson A, Albrieux M. TRPA1 channels promote astrocytic Ca^{2+} hyperactivity and synaptic dysfunction mediated by oligomeric forms of amyloid-β peptide. *Mol Neurodegener.* (2017) 12:53. doi: 10.1186/s13024-017-0194-8
160. Bianchi BR, Zhang XF, Reilly RM, Kym PR, Yao BB, Chen J. Species comparison and pharmacological characterization of human, monkey, rat,

and mouse TRPA1 channels. *J Pharmacol Exp Ther.* (2012) 341:360–8. doi: 10.1124/jpet.111.189902

161. Nagatomo K, Kubo Y. Caffeine activates mouse TRPA1 channels but suppresses human TRPA1 channels. *Proc Natl Acad Sci USA.* (2008) 105:17373–8. doi: 10.1073/pnas.0809769105
162. Whittaker MT, Gibbs TT, Farb DH. Pregnenolone sulfate induces NMDA receptor dependent release of dopamine from synaptic terminals in the striatum. *J Neurochem.* (2008) 107:510–21. doi: 10.1111/j.1471-4159.2008.05627.x
163. Sadler SE, Maller JL. Identification of a steroid receptor on the surface of Xenopus oocytes by photoaffinity labeling. *J Biol Chem.* (1982) 257:355–61.
164. Sadler SE, Bower MA, Maller JL. Studies of a plasma membrane steroid receptor in Xenopus oocytes using the synthetic progestin RU 486. *J Steroid Biochem.* (1985) 22:419–26.
165. Micevych PE, Mermelstein PG. Membrane estrogen receptors acting through metabotropic glutamate receptors: an emerging mechanism of estrogen action in brain. *Mol Neurobiol.* (2008) 38:66–77. doi: 10.1007/s12035-008-8034-z
166. Storman EM, Liu NJ, Wessendorf MW, Gintzler AR. Physical linkage of estrogen receptor α and aromatase in rat: oligocrine and endocrine actions of CNS-produced estrogens. *Endocrinology.* (2018) 159:2683–97. doi: 10.1210/en.2018-00319
167. McEwen BS, Gould E, Orchinik M, Weiland NG, Woolley CS. Oestrogens and the structural and functional plasticity of neurons: implications for memory, ageing and neurodegenerative processes. *Ciba Found Symp.* (1995) 191:52–66; discussion 66–73.
168. Abrahám IM, Todman MG, Korach KS, Herbison AE. Critical *in vivo* roles for classical estrogen receptors in rapid estrogen actions on intracellular signaling in mouse brain. *Endocrinology.* (2004) 145:3055–61. doi: 10.1210/en.2003-1676
169. Mukai H, Kimoto T, Hojo Y, Kawato S, Murakami G, Higo S, et al. Modulation of synaptic plasticity by brain estrogen in the hippocampus. *Biochim Biophys Acta.* (2010) 1800:1030–44. doi: 10.1016/j.bbagen.2009.11.002
170. Ooishi Y, Kawato S, Hojo Y, Hatanaka Y, Higo S, Murakami G, et al. Modulation of synaptic plasticity in the hippocampus by hippocampus-derived estrogen and androgen. *J Steroid Biochem Mol Biol.* (2012) 131:37–51. doi: 10.1016/j.jsbmb.2011.10.004
171. Tabatadze N, Smejkalova T, Woolley CS. Distribution and posttranslational modification of synaptic ERα in the adult female rat hippocampus. *Endocrinology.* (2013) 154:819–30. doi: 10.1210/en.2012-1870
172. Gibbs TT, Russek SJ, Farb DH. Sulfated steroids as endogenous neuromodulators. *Pharmacol Biochem Behav.* (2006) 84:555–67. doi: 10.1016/j.pbb.2006.07.031
173. Asaba H, Hosoya K, Takanaga H, Ohtsuki S, Tamura E, Takizawa T, Terasaki T. Blood-brain barrier is involved in the efflux transport of a neuroactive steroid, dehydroepiandrosterone sulfate, via organic anion transporting polypeptide 2. *J Neurochem.* (2000) 75:1907–16. doi: 10.1046/j.1471-4159.2000.0751907.x
174. Suzuki M, Suzuki H, Sugimoto Y, and Sugiyama Y. ABCG2 transports sulfated conjugates of steroids and xenobiotics. *J. Biol.Chem.* (2003) 278:22644–9. doi: 10.1074/jbc.M212399200
175. Miyajima M, Kusuhara H, Fujishima M, Adachi Y, Sugiyama Y. Organic anion transporter 3 mediates the efflux transport of an amphipathic organic anion, dehydroepiandrosterone sulfate, across the blood-brain barrier in mice. *Drug Metab Dispos.* (2011) 39:814–9. doi: 10.1124/dmd.110.036863
176. Qaiser MZ, Dolman DEM, Begley DJ, Abbott NJ, Cazacu-Davidescu M, Corol DI, et al. Uptake and metabolism of sulphated steroids by the blood-brain barrier in the adult male rat. *J Neurochem.* (2017) 142:672–85. doi: 10.1111/jnc.14117
177. Grube M, Hagen P, Jedlitschky G. Neurosteroid transport in the brain: role of ABC and SLC transporters. *Front Pharmacol.* (2018) 9:354. doi: 10.3389/fphar.2018.00354
178. Vallée M, Vitiello S, Bellocchio L, Hébert-Chatelain E, Monlezun S, Martin-Garcia E, et al. Pregnenolone can protect the brain from cannabis intoxication. *Science.* (2014) 343:94–8. doi: 10.1126/science.1243985
179. Wang W, Jia Y, Pham DT, Palmer LC, Jung KM, Cox CD, et al. Atypical endocannabinoid signaling initiates a new form of memory-related plasticity at a cortical input to hippocampus. *Cereb Cortex.* (2018) 28:2253–66. doi: 10.1093/cercor/bhx126
180. Knapstein P, David A, Wu CH, Archer DF, Flickinger GL, Touchstone JC. Metabolism of free and sulfoconjugated DHEA in brain tissue *in vivo* and *in vitro. Steroids.* (1968) 11:885–96. doi: 10.1016/S0039-128X(68)80102-3
181. Mayo W, Dellu F, Robel P, Cherkaoui J, Le Moal M, Baulieu EE, et al. Infusion of neurosteroids into the nucleus basalis magnocellularis affects cognitive processes in the rat. *Brain Res.* (1993) 607:324–8. doi: 10.1016/0006-8993(93)91524-V
182. Wong M, Moss RL. Patch-clamp analysis of direct steroidal modulation of glutamate receptor-channels. *J Neuroendocrinol.* (1994) 6:347–55. doi: 10.1111/j.1365-2826.1994.tb00592.x
183. Higashi T, Sugitani H, Yagi T, Shimada K. Studies on neurosteroids XVI. Levels of pregnenolone sulfate in rat brains determined by enzyme-linked immunosorbent assay not requiring solvolysis. *Biol Pharm Bull.* (2003) 26:709–711. doi: 10.1248/bpb.26.709
184. Schumacher M, Liere P, Akwa Y, Rajkowski K, Griffiths W, Bodin K, et al. Pregnenolone sulfate in the brain: a controversial neurosteroid. *Neurochem Int.* (2008) 52:522–40. doi: 10.1016/j.neuint.2007.08.022
185. Nanfaro F, Cabrera R, Bazzocchini V, Laconi M, Yunes R. Pregnenolone sulfate infused in lateral septum of male rats impairs novel object recognition memory. *Pharmacol Rep.* (2010) 62:265–72. doi: 10.1016/S1734-1140(10)70265-6
186. Steckelbroeck S, Nassen A, Ugele B, Ludwig M, Watzka M, Reissinger A, et al. Steroid sulfatase (STS) expression in the human temporal lobe: enzyme activity, mRNA expression and immunohistochemistry study. *J Neurochem.* (2004) 89:403–17. doi: 10.1046/j.1471-4159.2004.02336.x
187. Bruins Slot LA, Piazza PV, Colpaert FC. Neuroactive steroids and the constraint of memory. *Eur J Neurosci.* (1999) 11:4081–8. doi: 10.1046/j.1460-9568.1999.00824
188. Matthews DB, Morrow AL, Tokunaga S, McDaniel JR. Acute ethanol administration and acute allopregnanolone administration impair spatial memory in the Morris water task. *Alcohol Clin Exp Res.* (2002) 26:1747–51. doi: 10.1097/01.ALC.0000037219.79257.17
189. Johansson IM, Birzniece V, Lindblad C, Olsson T, Bäckström T. Allopregnanolone inhibits learning in the Morris water maze. *Brain Res.* (2002) 934:125–31. doi: 10.1016/S0006-8993(02)02414-9
190. Wiltgen BJ, Sanders MJ, Ferguson C, Homanics GE, Fanselow MS. Trace fear conditioning is enhanced in mice lacking the delta subunit of the GABAA receptor. *Learn Mem.* (2005) 12:327–33. doi: 10.1101/lm.89705
191. Amato RJ, Moerschbaecher JM, Winsauer PJ. Effects of pregnanolone and flunitrazepam on the retention of response sequences in rats. *Pharmacol Biochem Behav.* (2011) 99:391–8. doi: 10.1016/j.pbb.2011.05.023
192. Sripada RK, Marx CE, King AP, Rampton JC, Ho SS, Liberzon I. Allopregnanolone elevations following pregnenolone administration are associated with enhanced activation of emotion regulation neurocircuits. *Biol Psychiatry.* (2013) 73:1045–53. doi: 10.1016/j.biopsych.2012.12.008
193. van Doren MJ, Matthews DB, Janis GC, Grobin AC, Devaud LL, Morrow AL. Neuroactive steroid 3alpha-hydroxy-5alpha-pregnan-20-one modulates electrophysiological and behavioral actions of ethanol. *J Neurosci.* (2000) 20:1982–9. doi: 10.1523/JNEUROSCI.20-05-01982.2000
194. Gorin RE, Crabbe JC, Tanchuck MA, Long SL, Finn DA. Effects of finasteride on chronic and acute ethanol withdrawal severity in the WSP and WSR selected lines. *Alcohol Clin Exp Res.* (2005) 29:939–48. doi: 10.1097/01.ALC.0000167742.11566.01
195. Ardeshiri A, Kelley MH, Korner IP, Hurn PD, Herson PS. Mechanism of progesterone neuroprotection of rat cerebellar Purkinje cells following oxygen-glucose deprivation. *Eur J Neurosci.* (2006) 24:2567–74. doi: 10.1111/j.1460-9568.2006.05142.x
196. Pallarés M, Darnaudéry M, Day J, Le Moal M, Mayo W. The neurosteroid pregnenolone sulfate infused into the nucleus basalis increases both acetylcholine release in the frontal cortex or amygdala and spatial memory. *Neuroscience.* (1998) 87:551–8. doi: 10.1016/S0306-4522(98)00174-2
197. Wang JM, Singh C, Liu L, Irwin RW, Chen S, Chung EJ, et al. Allopregnanolone reverses neurogenic and cognitive deficits in mouse model

of Alzheimer's disease. *Proc Natl Acad Sci USA.* (2010) 107:6498–503. doi: 10.1073/pnas.1001422107

198. Bengtsson SK, Johansson M, Bäckström T, Wang M. Chronic allopregnanolone treatment accelerates Alzheimer's disease development in AβPP(Swe)PSEN1(ΔE9) mice. *J Alzheimers Dis.* (2012) 31:71–84. doi: 10.3233/JAD-2012-120268
199. Bengtsson SK, Johansson M, Backstrom T, Nitsch RM, Wang M. Brief but chronic increase in allopregnanolone cause accelerated AD pathology differently in two mouse models. *Curr Alzheimer Res.* (2013) 10:38–47. doi: 10.2174/1567205011310010006
200. Bengtsson SK, Johansson M, Bäckström T. Long-term continuous allopregnanolone elevation causes memory decline and hippocampus shrinkage, in female wild-type B6 mice. *Horm Behav.* (2016) 78:160–7. doi: 10.1016/j.yhbeh.2015.10.010
201. Irwin RW, Solinsky CM, Loya CM, Salituro FG, Rodgers KE, Bauer G, et al. Allopregnanolone preclinical acute pharmacokinetic and pharmacodynamic studies to predict tolerability and efficacy for Alzheimer's disease. *PLoS ONE.* (2015) 10:e0128313. doi: 10.1371/journal.pone.0128313
202. Genazzani AR, Petraglia F, Bernardi F, Casarosa E, Salvestroni C, Tonetti A, et al. Circulating levels of allopregnanolone in humans: gender, age, and endocrine influences. *J Clin Endocrinol Metab.* (1998) 83:2099–103. doi: 10.1210/jcem.83.6.4905
203. Kask K, Bäckström T, Nilsson LG, Sundström-Poromaa I. Allopregnanolone impairs episodic memory in healthy women. *Psychopharmacology (Berl).* (2008) 199:161–8. doi: 10.1007/s00213-008-1150-7
204. Rabinowitz A, Cohen SJ, Finn DA, Stackman RW Jr. The neurosteroid allopregnanolone impairs object memory and contextual fear memory in male C57BL/6J mice. *Horm Behav.* (2014) 66:238–46. doi: 10.1016/j.yhbeh.2014.05.005
205. Cohen SJ, Stackman RW Jr. Assessing rodent hippocampal involvement in the novel object recognition task. A review. *Behav Brain Res.* (2015) 285:105–17. doi: 10.1016/j.bbr.2014.08.002
206. Mòdol L, Darbra S, Pallarès M. Neurosteroids infusion into the CA1 hippocampal region on exploration, anxiety-like behaviour and aversive learning. *Behav Brain Res.* (2011) 222:223–9. doi: 10.1016/j.bbr.2011.03.058
207. Ertman N, Andreano JM, Cahill L. Progesterone at encoding predicts subsequent emotional memory. *Learn Mem.* (2011) 18:759–63. doi: 10.1101/lm.023267.111
208. Nielsen SE, Ertman N, Lakhani YS, Cahill L. Hormonal contraception usage is associated with altered memory for an emotional story. *Neurobiol Learn Mem.* (2011) 96:378–84. doi: 10.1016/j.nlm.2011.06.013
209. Locci A, Porcu P, Talani G, Santoru F, Berretti R, Giunti E, et al. Neonatal estradiol exposure to female rats changes GABAA receptor expression and function, and spatial learning during adulthood. *Horm Behav.* (2017) 87:35–46. doi: 10.1016/j.yhbeh.2016.10.005
210. Paris JJ, Brunton PJ, Russell JA, Walf AA, Frye CA. Inhibition of 5α-reductase activity in late pregnancy decreases gestational length and fecundity and impairs object memory and central progestogen milieu of juvenile rat offspring. *J Neuroendocrinol.* (2011) 23:1079–90. doi: 10.1111/j.1365-2826.2011.02219.x
211. Porcu P, Lallai V, Locci A, Catzeddu S, Serra V, Pisu MG, et al. Changes in stress-stimulated allopregnanolone levels induced by neonatal estradiol treatment are associated with enhanced dopamine release in adult female rats: reversal by progesterone administration. *Psychopharmacology (Berl).* (2017) 234:749–60. doi: 10.1007/s00213-016-4511-7
212. Fadalti M, Petraglia F, Luisi S, Bernardi F, Casarosa E, Ferrari E, et al. Changes of serum allopregnanolone levels in the first 2 years of life and during pubertal development. *Pediatr Res.* (1999) 46:323–7. doi: 10.1203/00006450-199909000-00013
213. Grosso S, Luisi S, Mostardini R, Matera M, Barlocco EG, Casarosa E, et al. Circulating levels of allopregnanolone, a neuroactive steroid, and leptin during treatment with valproic acid in children with epilepsy. *Neuroendocrinology.* (2011) 93:159–64. doi: 10.1159/000321664
214. Andréen L, Sundström-Poromaa I, Bixo M, Nyberg S, Bäckström T. Allopregnanolone concentration and mood–a bimodal association in postmenopausal women treated with oral progesterone. *Psychopharmacology (Berl).* (2006) 187:209–21. doi: 10.1007/s00213-006-0417-0
215. Wang M, Seippel L, Purdy RH, Bãckström T. Relationship between symptom severity and steroid variation in women with premenstrual syndrome: study on serum pregnenolone, pregnenolone sulfate, 5 alpha-pregnane-3,20-dione and 3 alpha-hydroxy-5 alpha-pregnan-20-one. *J Clin Endocrinol Metab.* (1996) 81:1076–82.
216. Ottander U, Poromaa IS, Bjurulf E, Skytt A, Bäckström T, Olofsson JI. Allopregnanolone and pregnanolone are produced by the human corpus luteum. *Mol Cell Endocrinol.* (2005) 239:37–44. doi: 10.1016/j.mce.2005.04.007
217. Bixo M, Andersson A, Winblad B, Purdy RH, Bäckström T. Progesterone, 5alpha-pregnane-3,20-dione and 3alpha-hydroxy-5alpha-pregnane-20-one in specific regions of the human female brain in different endocrine states. *Brain Res.* (1997) 764:173–8. doi: 10.1016/S0006-8993(97)00455-1
218. Hedström H, Bäckström T, Bixo M, Nyberg S, Wang M, Gideonsson I, Turkmen S. Women with polycystic ovary syndrome have elevated serum concentrations of and altered GABA(A) receptor sensitivity to allopregnanolone. *Clin Endocrinol (Oxf).* (2015) 83:643–50. doi: 10.1111/cen.12809
219. Soleman RS, Kreukels BPC, Veltman DJ, Cohen-Kettenis PT, Hompes PGA, Drent ML, et al. Does polycystic ovary syndrome affect cognition? A functional magnetic resonance imaging study exploring working memory. *Fertil Steril.* (2016) 105:1314–21.e1. doi: 10.1016/j.fertnstert.2016.01.034
220. Schmidt PJ, Purdy RH, Moore PH Jr, Paul SM, Rubinow DR. Circulating levels of anxiolytic steroids in the luteal phase in women with premenstrual syndrome and in control subjects. *J Clin Endocrinol Metab.* (1994) 79:1256–60. doi: 10.1210/jcem.79.5.7962316
221. Bicíková M, Lapcík O, Hampl R, Stárka L, Knuppen R, Haupt O, et al. A novel radioimmunoassay of allopregnanolone. *Steroids.* (1995) 60:210–3. doi: 10.1016/0039-128X(94)00039-F
222. Innala E, Bäckström T, Poromaa IS, Andersson C, Bixo M. Women with acute intermittent porphyria have a defect in 5α-steroid production during the menstrual cycle. *Acta Obstet Gynecol Scand.* (2012) 91:1445–52. doi: 10.1111/j.1600-0412.2012.01536.x
223. Nyberg S, Bäckström T, Zingmark E, Purdy RH, Poromaa IS. Allopregnanolone decrease with symptom improvement during placebo and gonadotropin-releasing hormone agonist treatment in women with severe premenstrual syndrome. *Gynecol Endocrinol.* (2007) 23:257–66. doi: 10.1080/09513590701253511
224. Ferree NK, Kamat R, Cahill L. Influences of menstrual cycle position and sex hormone levels on spontaneous intrusive recollections following emotional stimuli. *Conscious Cogn.* (2011) 20:1154–62. doi: 10.1016/j.concog.2011.02.003
225. Ferree NK, Wheeler M, Cahill L. The influence of emergency contraception on post-traumatic stress symptoms following sexual assault. *J Forensic Nurs.* (2012) 8:122–30. doi: 10.1111/j.1939-3938.2012.01134.x
226. Shen H, Gong QH, Yuan M, Smith SS. Short-term steroid treatment increases delta GABAA receptor subunit expression in rat CA1 hippocampus: pharmacological and behavioral effects. *Neuropharmacology.* (2005) 49:573–86. doi: 10.1016/j.neuropharm.2005.04.026
227. Smith CC, Vedder LC, McMahon LL. Estradiol and the relationship between dendritic spines, NR2B containing NMDA receptors, and the magnitude of long-term potentiation at hippocampal CA3-CA1 synapses. *Psychoneuroendocrinology.* (2009) 34(Suppl. 1):S130–42. doi: 10.1016/j.psyneuen.2009.06.003
228. Shen H, Sabaliauskas N, Sherpa A, Fenton AA, Stelzer A, Aoki C, Smith SS. A critical role for alpha4betadelta GABAA receptors in shaping learning deficits at puberty in mice. *Science.* (2010) 327:1515–8. doi: 10.1126/science.1184245
229. Afroz S, Shen H, Smith SS. α4βδ GABAA receptors reduce dendritic spine density in CA1 hippocampus and impair relearning ability of adolescent female mice: effects of a GABA agonist and a stress steroid. *Neuroscience.* (2017) 347:22–35. doi: 10.1016/j.neuroscience.2017.01.051
230. Sabaliauskas N, Shen H, Molla J, Gong QH, Kuver A, Aoki C, Smith SS. Neurosteroid effects at α4βδ GABAA receptors alter spatial learning and synaptic plasticity in CA1 hippocampus across the estrous cycle of the mouse. *Brain Res.* (2015) 1621:170–86. doi: 10.1016/j.brainres.2014.12.026
231. Ferando I, Mody I. Altered gamma oscillations during pregnancy through loss of δ subunit-containing GABA(A) receptors on

parvalbumin interneurons. *Front Neural Circuits.* (2013) 7:144. doi: 10.3389/fncir.2013.00144
232. Müller C, Remy S. Septo-hippocampal interaction. *Cell Tissue Res.* (2018) 373:565–75. doi: 10.1007/s00441-017-2745-2
233. Muzzio IA, Kentros C, Kandel E. What is remembered? Role of attention on the encoding and retrieval of hippocampal representations. *J Physiol.* (2009) 587:2837–54. doi: 10.1113/jphysiol.2009.172445
234. Andreescu CE, Milojkovic BA, Haasdijk ED, Kramer P, De Jong FH, Krust A, et al. Estradiol improves cerebellar memory formation by activating estrogen receptor beta. *J Neurosci.* (2007) 27:10832–9. doi: 10.1523/JNEUROSCI.2588-07.2007
235. Konrad C, Engelien A, Schöning S, Zwitserlood P, Jansen A, Pletziger E, et al. The functional anatomy of semantic retrieval is influenced by gender, menstrual cycle, and sex hormones. *J Neural Transm (Vienna).* (2008) 115:1327–37. doi: 10.1007/s00702-008-0073-0
236. Easton A, Webster LA, Eacott MJ. The episodic nature of episodic-like memories. *Learn Mem.* (2012) 19:146–50. doi: 10.1101/lm.025676.112
237. Roberts E. Pregnenolone from Selye to Alzheimer and a model of the pregnenolone sulfate binding site on the GABAA receptor. *Biochem Pharmacol.* (1995) 49:1–16. doi: 10.1016/0006-2952(94)00258-N
238. Ritsner MS, Gibel A, Shleifer T, Boguslavsky I, Zayed A, Maayan R, et al. Pregnenolone and dehydroepiandrosterone as an adjunctive treatment in schizophrenia and schizoaffective disorder: an 8-week, double-blind, randomized, controlled, 2-center, parallel-group trial. *J Clin Psychiatry.* (2010) 71:1351–62. doi: 10.4088/JCP.09m05031yel
239. Nagaya N, Acca GM, Maren S. Allopregnanolone in the bed nucleus of the stria terminalis modulates contextual fear in rats. *Front Behav Neurosci.* (2015) 9:205. doi: 10.3389/fnbeh.2015.00205
240. Sierra-Mercado D, Padilla-Coreano N, Quirk GJ. Dissociable roles of prelimbic and infralimbic cortices, ventral hippocampus, and basolateral amygdala in the expression and extinction of conditioned fear. *Neuropsychopharmacology.* (2011) 36:529–38. doi: 10.1038/npp.2010.184
241. Sakamoto H, Ukena K, Tsutsui K. Effects of progesterone synthesized *de novo* in the developing Purkinje cell on its dendritic growth and synaptogenesis. *J Neurosci.* (2001) 21:6221–32. doi: 10.1523/JNEUROSCI.21-16-06221.2001
242. Tsutsui K, Sakamoto H, Ukena K. Biosynthesis and action of neurosteroids in the cerebellar Purkinje neuron. *J Steroid Biochem Mol Biol.* (2003) 85:311–21. doi: 10.1016/S0960-0760(03)00229-2
243. Wulff P, Schonewille M, Renzi M, Viltono L, Sassoe-Pognetto M, Badura A. et al. Synaptic inhibition of Purkinje cells mediates consolidation of vestibulo-cerebellar motor learning. *Nat Neurosci.* (2009) 12:1042–9. doi: 10.1038/nn.2348
244. Dieni CV, Sullivan JA, Faralli M, Contemori S, Biscarini A, Pettorossi VE, et al. 17 beta-estradiol synthesis modulates cerebellar dependent motor memory formation in adult male rats. *Neurobiol Learn Mem.* (2018) 155:276–86. doi: 10.1016/j.nlm.2018.08.011
245. Gonzalez-Usano A, Cauli O, Agusti A, Felipo V. Pregnenolone sulfate restores the glutamate-nitric-oxide-cGMP pathway and extracellular GABA in cerebellum and learningand motor coordination in hyperammonemic rats. *ACS Chem Neurosci.* (2014) 5:100–5. doi: 10.1021/cn400168y
246. Acca GM, Mathew AS, Jin J, Maren S, Nagaya N. Allopregnanolone induces state-dependent fear via the bed nucleus of the stria terminalis. *Horm Behav.* (2017) 89:137–44. doi: 10.1016/j.yhbeh.2017.01.002
247. Mayo W, George O, Darbra S, Bouyer JJ, Vallée M, Darnaudéry M, et al. Individual differences in cognitive aging: implication of pregnenolone sulfate. *Prog Neurobiol.* (2003) 71:43–8. doi: 10.1016/j.pneurobio.2003.09.006
248. George O, Vallée M, Vitiello S, Le Moal M, Piazza PV, Mayo W. Low brain allopregnanolone levels mediate flattened circadian activity associated with memory impairments in aged rats. *Biol Psychiatry.* (2010) 68:956–63. doi: 10.1016/j.biopsych.2010.03.022
249. Caruso D, Barron AM, Brown MA, Abbiati F, Carrero P, Pike CJ, et al. Age-related changes in neuroactive steroid levels in 3xTg-AD mice. *Neurobiol Aging.* (2013) 34:1080–9. doi: 10.1016/j.neurobiolaging.2012.10.007
250. Klöppel S, Kotschi M, Peter J, Egger K, Hausner L, Frölich L, et al. Separating symptomatic Alzheimer's disease from depression based on structural MRI. *J Alzheimers Dis.* (2018) 63:353–63. doi: 10.3233/JAD-170964
251. Rosario ER, Chang L, Head EH, Stanczyk FZ, Pike CJ. Brain levels of sex steroid hormones in men and women during normal aging and in Alzheimer's disease. *Neurobiol Aging.* (2011) 32:604–13. doi: 10.1016/j.neurobiolaging.2009.04.008
252. Hogervorst E, Bandelow S, Combrinck M, Smith AD. Low free testosterone is an independent risk factor for Alzheimer's disease. *Exp Gerontol.* (2004) 39:1633–9. doi: 10.1016/j.exger.2004.06.019
253. Resnick SM, Matsumoto AM, Stephens-Shields AJ, Ellenberg SS, Gill TM, Shumaker SA, et al. Testosterone treatment and cognitive function in older men with low testosterone and age-associated memory impairment. *JAMA.* (2017) 317:717–27. doi: 10.1001/jama.2016.21044
254. Darbra S, George O, Bouyer JJ, Piazza PV, Le Moal M, Mayo W. Sleep-wake states and cortical synchronization control by pregnenolone sulfate into the pedunculopontine nucleus. *J Neurosci Res.* (2004) 76:742–7. doi: 10.1002/jnr.20074
255. George O, Vallée M, Le Moal M, Mayo W. Neurosteroids and cholinergic systems: implications for sleep and cognitive processes and potential role of age-related changes. *Psychopharmacology (Berl).* (2006) 186:402–13. doi: 10.1007/s00213-005-0254-6
256. Mayo W, Le Moal M, Abrous DN. Pregnenolone sulfate and aging of cognitive functions: behavioral, neurochemical, and morphological investigations. *Horm Behav.* (2001) 40:215–7. doi: 10.1006/hbeh.2001.1677
257. Darnaudéry M, Bouyer JJ, Pallarés M, Le Moal M, Mayo W. The promnesic neurosteroid pregnenolone sulfate increases paradoxical sleep in rats. *Brain Res.* (1999) 818:492–8. doi: 10.1016/S0006-8993(98)01338-9
258. Darnaudéry M, Koehl M, Piazza PV, Le Moal M, Mayo W. Pregnenolone sulfate increases hippocampal acetylcholine release and spatial recognition. *Brain Res.* (2000) 852:173–9. doi: 10.1016/S0006-8993(99)01964-2
259. Riemann D, Hohagen F, Krieger S, Gann H, Müller WE, Olbrich R, et al. Cholinergic REM induction test: muscarinic supersensitivity underlies polysomnographic findings in both depression and schizophrenia. *J Psychiatr Res.* (1994) 28:195–210. doi: 10.1016/0022-3956(94)90006-X
260. Baran B, Correll D, Vuper TC, Morgan A, Durrant SJ, Manoach DS, et al. Spared and impaired sleep-dependent memory consolidation in schizophrenia. *Schizophr Res.* (2018) S0920-9964:30231-7. doi: 10.1016/j.schres.2018.04.019
261. Waterhouse RN, Chang RC, Atuehene N, Collier TL. *In vitro* and *in vivo* binding of neuroactive steroids to the sigma-1 receptor as measured with the positron emission tomography radioligand [18F]FPS. *Synapse.* (2007) 61:540–6. doi: 10.1002/syn.20369
262. Maurice T, Roman FJ, Privat A. Modulation by neurosteroids of the *in vivo* (+)-[3H]SKF-10,047 binding to sigma 1 receptors in the mouse forebrain. *J Neurosci Res.* (1996) 46:734–43. doi: 10.1002/(SICI)1097-4547(19961215)46:6<734::AID-JNR10>3.0.CO;2-U
263. Gibbs TT, Farb DH. Dueling enigmas: neurosteroids and sigma receptors in the limelight. *Sci STKE.* (2000) 2000:pe1. doi: 10.1126/stke.2000.60.pe1
264. Maurice T, Strehaiano M, Duhr F, Chevallier N. Amyloid toxicity is enhanced after pharmacological or genetic invalidation of the σ1 receptor. *Behav Brain Res.* (2018) 339:1–10. doi: 10.1016/j.bbr.2017.11.010
265. Lanzenberger R, Mitterhauser M, Kranz GS, Spindelegger C, Wadsak W, Stein P, et al. Progesterone level predicts serotonin-1a receptor binding in the male human brain. *Neuroendocrinology.* (2011) 94:84–8. doi: 10.1159/000328432
266. Stein P, Baldinger P, Kaufmann U, Christina RM, Hahn A, Höflich A, et al. Relation of progesterone and DHEAS serum levels to 5-HT1A receptor binding potential in pre- and postmenopausal women. *Psychoneuroendocrinology.* (2014) 46:52–63. doi: 10.1016/j.psyneuen.2014.04.008
267. Vidal B, Sebti J, Verdurand M, Fieux S, Billard T, Streichenberger N, et al. Agonist and antagonist bind differently to 5-HT1A receptors during Alzheimer's disease: a post-mortem study with PET radiopharmaceuticals. *Neuropharmacology.* (2016) 109:88–95. doi: 10.1016/j.neuropharm.2016.05.009
268. Koh MT, Haberman RP, Foti S, McCown TJ, Gallagher M. Treatment strategies targeting excess hippocampal activity benefit aged rats with

cognitive impairment. *Neuropsychopharmacology.* (2010) 35:1016–25. doi: 10.1038/npp.2009.207
269. Yassa MA, Mattfeld AT, Stark SM, Stark CE. Age-related memory deficits linked to circuit-specific disruptions in the hippocampus. *Proc Natl Acad Sci USA.* (2011) 108:8873–8. doi: 10.1073/pnas.1101567108
270. Bakker A, Krauss GL, Albert MS, Speck CL, Jones LR, Stark CE, et al. Reduction of hippocampal hyperactivity improves cognition in amnestic mild cognitive impairment. *Neuron.* (2012) 74:467–74. doi: 10.1016/j.neuron.2012.03.023
271. Wu JW, Hussaini SA, Bastille IM, Rodriguez GA, Mrejeru A, Rilett K, et al. Neuronal activity enhances tau propagation and tau pathology *in vivo*. *Nat Neurosci.* (2016) 19:1085–92. doi: 10.1038/nn.4328
272. Nuriel T, Angulo SL, Khan U, Ashok A, Chen Q, Figueroa HY, et al. Neuronal hyperactivity due to loss of inhibitory tone in APOE4 mice lacking Alzheimer's disease-like pathology. *Nat Commun.* (2017) 8:1464. doi: 10.1038/s41467-017-01444-0
273. Shetty AK, Turner DA. Hippocampal interneurons expressing glutamic acid decarboxylase and calcium-binding proteins decrease with aging in Fischer 344 rats. *J Comp Neurol.* (1998) 394:252–69. doi: 10.1002/(SICI)1096-9861(19980504)394:2<252::AID-CNE9>3.0.CO;2-1
274. Stanley EM, Fadel JR, Mott DD. Interneuron loss reduces dendritic inhibition and GABA release in hippocampus of aged rats. *Neurobiol Aging.* (2012) 33:431.e1–13. doi: 10.1016/j.neurobiolaging.2010.12.014
275. Kwakowsky A, Calvo-Flores Guzmán B, Pandya M, Turner C, Waldvogel HJ, Faull RL. GABAA receptor subunit expression changes in the human Alzheimer's disease hippocampus, subiculum, entorhinal cortex and superior temporal gyrus. *J Neurochem.* (2018) 145:374–92. doi: 10.1111/jnc.14325
276. Reddy DS, Estes WA. Clinical potential of neurosteroids for CNS disorders. *Trends Pharmacol Sci.* (2016) 37:543–61. doi: 10.1016/j.tips.2016.04.003
277. Chen S, Wang JM, Irwin RW, Yao J, Liu L, Brinton RD. Allopregnanolone promotes regeneration and reduces β-amyloid burden in a preclinical model of Alzheimer's disease. *PLoS ONE.* (2011) 6:e24293. doi: 10.1371/journal.pone.0024293
278. Brinton RD. Neurosteroids as regenerative agents in the brain: therapeutic implications. *Nat Rev Endocrinol.* (2013) 9:241–50. doi: 10.1038/nrendo.2013.31
279. Zhang P, Xie MQ, Ding YQ, Liao M, Qi SS, Chen SX, et al. Allopregnanolone enhances the neurogenesis of midbrain dopaminergic neurons in APPswe/PSEN1 mice. *Neuroscience.* (2015) 290:214–26. doi: 10.1016/j.neuroscience.2015.01.019
280. Pereira AC, Gray JD, Kogan JF, Davidson RL, Rubin TG, Okamoto M, et al. Age and Alzheimer's disease gene expression profiles reversed by the glutamate modulator riluzole. *Mol Psychiatry.* (2017) 22:296–305. doi: 10.1038/mp.2016.33
281. Girard C, Liu S, Cadepond F, Adams D, Lacroix C, Verleye M, et al. Etifoxine improves peripheral nerve regeneration and functional recovery. *Proc Natl Acad Sci USA.* (2008) 105:20505–10. doi: 10.1073/pnas.0811201106
282. Kreisl WC, Lyoo CH, McGwier M, Snow J, Jenko KJ, Kimura N, et al. *In vivo* radioligand binding to translocator protein correlates with severity of Alzheimer's disease. *Brain.* (2013) 136:2228–38. doi: 10.1093/brain/awt145
283. Setiawan E, Wilson AA, Mizrahi R, Rusjan PM, Miler L, Rajkowska G, et al. Role of translocator protein density, a marker of neuroinflammation, in the brain during major depressive episodes. *JAMA Psychiatry.* (2015) 72:268–275. doi: 10.1001/jamapsychiatry.2014.2427
284. Brown RC, Cascio C, Papadopoulos V. Pathways of neurosteroid biosynthesis in cell lines from human brain: regulation of dehydroepiandrosterone formation by oxidative stress and beta-amyloid peptide. *J Neurochem.* (2000) 74:847–59. doi: 10.1046/j.1471-4159.2000.740847.x
285. Aly HF, Metwally FM, Ahmed HH. Neuroprotective effects of dehydroepiandrosterone (DHEA) in rat model of Alzheimer's disease. *Acta Biochim Pol.* (2011) 58:513–20. doi: 10.18388/abp.2011_2218
286. Menon V. Large-scale brain networks and psychopathology: a unifying triple network model. *Trends Cogn Sci.* (2011) 15:483–506. doi: 10.1016/j.tics.2011.08.003
287. Hodgetts CJ, Shine JP, Williams H, Postans M, Sims R, Williams J, et al. Increased posterior default mode network activity and structural connectivity in young adult APOE-ε4 carriers: a multimodal imaging investigation. *Neurobiol Aging.* (2019) 73:82–91. doi: 10.1016/j.neurobiolaging.2018.08.026
288. Ofer I, LeRose C, Mast H, LeVan P, Metternich B, Egger K, et al. Association between seizure freedom and default mode network reorganization in patients with unilateral temporal lobe epilepsy. *Epilepsy Behav.* (2018) S1525-5050:30822–3. doi: 10.1016/j.yebeh.2018.10.025
289. White TP, Joseph V, Francis ST, Liddle PF. Aberrant salience network (bilateral insula and anterior cingulate cortex) connectivity during information processing in schizophrenia. *Schizophr Res.* (2010) 123:105–15. doi: 10.1016/j.schres.2010.07.020
290. Sripada RK, King AP, Garfinkel SN, Wang X, Sripada CS, Welsh RC, et al. Altered resting-state amygdala functional connectivity in men with posttraumatic stress disorder. *J Psychiatry Neurosci.* (2012) 37:241–9. doi: 10.1503/jpn.110069
291. Sripada RK, King AP, Welsh RC, Garfinkel SN, Wang X, Sripada CS, et al. Neural dysregulation in posttraumatic stress disorder: evidence for disrupted equilibrium between salience and default mode brain networks. *Psychosom Med.* (2012) 74:904–11. doi: 10.1097/PSY.0b013e318273bf33
292. Sripada RK, Welsh RC, Marx CE, Liberzon I. The neurosteroids allopregnanolone and dehydroepiandrosterone modulate resting-state amygdala connectivity. *Hum Brain Mapp.* (2014) 35:3249–61. doi: 10.1002/hbm.22399
293. Canteras NS, Swanson LW. Projections of the ventral subiculum to the amygdala, septum, and hypothalamus: a PHAL anterograde tract-tracing study in the rat. *J Comp Neurol.* (1992) 324:180–94. doi: 10.1002/cne.903240204
294. Li S, Kirouac GJ. Projections from the paraventricular nucleus of the thalamus to the forebrain, with special emphasis on the extended amygdala. *J Comp Neurol.* (2008) 506:263–87. doi: 10.1002/cne.21502
295. Li S, Kirouac GJ. Sources of inputs to the anterior and posterior aspects of the paraventricular nucleus of the thalamus. *Brain Struct Funct.* (2012) 217:257–73. doi: 10.1007/s00429-011-0360-7
296. Penzo MA, Robert V, Tucciarone J, De Bundel D, Wang M, Van Aelst L, et al. The paraventricular thalamus controls a central amygdala fear circuit. *Nature.* (2015) 519:455–9. doi: 10.1038/nature13978
297. Uzunova V, Sheline Y, Davis JM, Rasmusson A, Uzunov DP, Costa E, et al. Increase in the cerebrospinal fluid content of neurosteroids in patients with unipolar major depression who are receiving fluoxetine or fluvoxamine. *Proc Natl Acad Sci USA.* (1998) 95:3239–44. doi: 10.1073/pnas.95.6.3239
298. Khisti RT, Chopde CT, Jain SP. Antidepressant-like effect of the neurosteroid 3alpha-hydroxy-5alpha-pregnan-20-one in mice forced swim test. *Pharmacol Biochem Behav.* (2000) 67:137–43. doi: 10.1016/S0091-3057(00)00300-2
299. Pinna G, Dong E, Matsumoto K, Costa E, Guidotti A. In socially isolated mice, the reversal of brain allopregnanolone down-regulation mediates the anti-aggressive action of fluoxetine. *Proc Natl Acad Sci USA.* (2003) 100:2035–40. doi: 10.1073/pnas.0337642100
300. Pinna G, Costa E, Guidotti A. Fluoxetine and norfluoxetine stereospecifically facilitate pentobarbital sedation by increasing neurosteroids. *Proc Natl Acad Sci USA.* (2004) 101:6222–5. doi: 10.1073/pnas.0401479101
301. Devall AJ, Santos JM, Fry JP, Honour JW, Brandão ML, Lovick TA. Elevation of brain allopregnanolone rather than 5-HT release by short term, low dose fluoxetine treatment prevents the estrous cycle-linked increase in stress sensitivity in female rats. *Eur Neuropsychopharmacol.* (2015) 25:113–23. doi: 10.1016/j.euroneuro.2014.11.017
302. Morrow AL, Janis GC, VanDoren MJ, Matthews DB, Samson HH, Janak PH, Grant KA. Neurosteroids mediate pharmacological effects of ethanol: a new mechanism of ethanol action? *Alcohol Clin Exp Res.* (1999) 23:1933–40. doi: 10.1111/j.1530-0277.1999.tb04094.x
303. Cagetti E, Pinna G, Guidotti A, Baicy K, Olsen RW. Chronic intermittent ethanol (CIE) administration in rats decreases levels of neurosteroids in hippocampus, accompanied by altered behavioral responses to neurosteroids and memory function. *Neuropharmacology.* (2004) 46:570–9. doi: 10.1016/j.neuropharm.2003.10.001

304. Finn DA, Jimenez VA. Dynamic adaptation in neurosteroid networks in response to alcohol. *Handb Exp Pharmacol.* (2017). doi: 10.1007/164_2017_82. [Epub ahead of print].
305. Mantella RC, Butters MA, Dew MA, Mulsant BH, Begley AE, Tracey B, et al. Cognitive impairment in late-life generalized anxiety disorder. *Am J Geriatr Psychiatry.* (2007) 15:673–9. doi: 10.1097/JGP.0b013e31803111f2
306. Lee BK, Glass TA, McAtee MJ, Wand GS, Bandeen-Roche K, Bolla KI, et al. Associations of salivary cortisol with cognitive function in the Baltimore memory study. *Arch Gen Psychiatry.* (2007) 64:810–8. doi: 10.1001/archpsyc.64.7.810
307. Lenze EJ, Mantella RC, Shi P, Goate AM, Nowotny P, Butters MA, et al. Elevated cortisol in older adults with generalized anxiety disorder is reduced by treatment: a placebo-controlled evaluation of escitalopram. *Am J Geriatr Psychiatry.* (2011) 19:482–90. doi: 10.1097/JGP.0b013e3181ec806c
308. Singh C, Liu L, Wang JM, Irwin RW, Yao J, Chen S, et al. Allopregnanolone restores hippocampal-dependent learning and memory and neural progenitor survival in aging 3xTgAD and nonTg mice. *Neurobiol Aging.* (2012) 33:1493–506. doi: 10.1016/j.neurobiolaging.2011.06.008
309. Loi SM, Eratne D, Kelso W, Velakoulis D, Looi JC. Alzheimer disease: non-pharmacological and pharmacological management of cognition and neuropsychiatric symptoms. *Australas Psychiatry.* (2018) 26:358–65. doi: 10.1177/1039856218766123
310. Soravia LM, Heinrichs M, Winzeler L, Fisler M, Schmitt W, Horn H, et al. Glucocorticoids enhance *in vivo* exposure-based therapy of spider phobia. *Depress Anxiety.* (2014) 31:429–35. doi: 10.1002/da.22219
311. Li S, Graham BM. Estradiol is associated with altered cognitive and physiological responses during fear conditioning and extinction in healthy and spider phobic women. *Behav Neurosci.* (2016) 130:614–23. doi: 10.1037/bne0000166
312. Kirkby LA, Luongo FJ, Lee MB, Nahum M, Van Vleet TM, Rao VR, etal. An amygdala-hippocampus subnetwork that encodes variation in human mood. *Cell.* (2018) 175:1688–700.e14. doi: 10.1016/j.cell.2018.10.005
313. Alfano J, Pedersen RC, Kramer RE, Brownie AC. Cholesterol metabolism in the rat adrenal cortex: acute temporal changes following stress. *Can J Biochem Cell Biol.* (1983) 61:708–13. doi: 10.1139/o83-089
314. Aguilera G, Kiss A, Lu A, Camacho C. Regulation of adrenal steroidogenesis during chronic stress. *Endocr Res.* (1996) 22:433–43. doi: 10.1080/07435809609043729
315. do Vale S, Selinger L, Martins JM, Gomes AC, Bicho M, do Carmo I, et al. The relationship between dehydroepiandrosterone (DHEA), working memory and distraction–a behavioral and electrophysiological approach. *PLoS ONE.* (2014) 9:e104869. doi: 10.1371/journal.pone.0104869
316. Shia RM, Hagen JA, McIntire LK, Goodyear CD, Dykstra LN, Narayanan L. Individual differences in biophysiological toughness: sustaining working memory during physical exhaustion. *Mil Med.* (2015) 180:230–6. doi: 10.7205/MILMED-D-14-00363
317. Diamond DM, Fleshner M, Rose GM. The enhancement of hippocampal primed burst potentiation by dehydroepiandrosterone sulfate (DHEAS) is blocked by psychological stress. *Stress.* (1999) 3:107–21. doi: 10.3109/10253899909001116
318. Castanho TC, Moreira PS, Portugal-Nunes C, Novais A, Costa PS, Palha JA, et al. The role of sex and sex-related hormones in cognition, mood and well-being in older men and women. *Biol Psychol.* (2014) 103:158–66. doi: 10.1016/j.biopsycho.2014.08.015
319. Dalla C, Whetstone AS, Hodes GE, Shors TJ. Stressful experience has opposite effects on dendritic spines in the hippocampus of cycling versus masculinized females. *Neurosci Lett.* (2009) 449:52–6. doi: 10.1016/j.neulet.2008.10.051
320. Hayward C, Sanborn K. Puberty and the emergence of gender differences in psychopathology. *J Adolesc Health.* (2002) 30:49–58. doi: 10.1016/S1054-139X(02)00336-1
321. Kessler RC, Berglund P, Demler O, Jin R, Merikangas KR, Walters EE. Lifetime prevalence and age-of-onset distributions of DSM-IV disorders in the National Comorbidity Survey Replication. *Arch Gen Psychiatry.* (2005) 62:593–602. doi: 10.1001/archpsyc.62.6.593
322. Reardon LE, Leen-Feldner EW, Hayward C. A critical review of the empirical literature on the relation between anxiety and puberty. *Clin Psychol Rev.* (2009) 29:1–23. doi: 10.1016/j.cpr.2008.09.005
323. Van Oort FV, Greaves-Lord K, Verhulst FC, Ormel J, Huizink AC. The developmental course of anxiety symptoms during adolescence: the TRAILS study. *J Child Psychol Psychiatry.* (2009) 50:1209–17. doi: 10.1111/j.1469-7610.2009.02092.x
324. Merikangas KR, Nakamura EF, Kessler RC. Epidemiology of mental disorders in children and adolescents. *Dialogues Clin Neurosci.* (2009) 11:7–20.
325. Merikangas KR, He JP, Brody D, Fisher PW, Bourdon K, Koretz DS. Prevalence and treatment of mental disorders among US children in the 2001-2004 NHANES. *Pediatrics.* (2010) 125:75–81. doi: 10.1542/peds.2008-2598
326. Merikangas KR, He JP, Burstein M, Swanson SA, Avenevoli S, Cui L, et al. Lifetime prevalence of mental disorders in U.S. adolescents: results from the National Comorbidity Survey Replication–Adolescent Supplement (NCS-A). *J Am Acad Child Adolesc Psychiatry.* (2010) 49:980–9. doi: 10.1016/j.jaac.2010.05.017
327. Leikanger E, Ingul JM, Larsson, B. Sex and age-related anxiety in a community sample of Norwegian adolescents. *Scand J Psychol.* (2012) 53:150–7. doi: 10.1111/j.1467-9450.2011.00915.x
328. Legerstee JS, Verhulst FC, Robbers SC, Ormel J, Oldehinkel AJ, van Oort FV. Gender-specific developmental trajectories of anxiety during adolescence: determinants and outcomes. the TRAILS study. *J Can Acad Child Adolesc Psychiatry.* (2013) 22:26–34.
329. Purdy RH, Morrow AL, Moore PH Jr, Paul SM. Stress-induced elevations of gamma-aminobutyric acid type A receptor-active steroids in the rat brain. *Proc Natl Acad Sci USA.* (1991) 88:4553–7. doi: 10.1073/pnas.88.10.4553
330. Darbra S, Pallarès M. Neonatal allopregnanolone increases novelty-directed locomotion and disrupts behavioural responses to GABA(A) receptor modulators in adulthood. *Int J Dev Neurosci.* (2009) 27:617–25. doi: 10.1016/j.ijdevneu.2009.05.008
331. Mòdol L, Darbra S, Vallèe M, Pallarès M. Alteration of neonatal Allopregnanolone levels affects exploration, anxiety, aversive learning and adult behavioural response to intrahippocampal neurosteroids. *Behav Brain Res.* (2013) 241:96–104. doi: 10.1016/j.bbr.2012.11.043
332. Darbra S, Mòdol L, Llidó A, Casas C, Vallée M, Pallarès M. Neonatal allopregnanolone levels alteration: effects on behavior and role of the hippocampus. *Prog Neurobiol.* (2014) 113:95–105. doi: 10.1016/j.pneurobio.2013.07.007
333. Ansseau M, von Frenckell R, Cerfontaine JL, Papart P. Pilot study of PK 11195, a selective ligand for the peripheral-type benzodiazepine binding sites, in inpatients with anxious or depressive symptomatology. *Pharmacopsychiatry.* (1991) 24:8–12. doi: 10.1055/s-2007-1014425
334. Ströhle A, Romeo E, di Michele F, Pasini A, Hermann B, Gajewsky G, et al. Induced panic attacks shift gamma-aminobutyric acid type A receptor modulatory neuroactive steroid composition in patients with panic disorder: preliminary results. *Arch Gen Psychiatry.* (2003) 60:161–8. doi: 10.1001/archpsyc.60.2.161
335. Merritt P, Stangl B, Hirshman E, Verbalis J. Administration of dehydroepiandrosterone (DHEA) increases serum levels of androgens and estrogens but does not enhance short-term memory in post-menopausal women. *Brain Res.* (2012) 1483:54–62. doi: 10.1016/j.brainres.2012.09.015
336. Irwin RW, Wang JM, Chen S, Brinton RD. Neuroregenerative mechanisms of allopregnanolone in Alzheimer's disease. *Front Endocrinol.* (2012) 2:117. doi: 10.3389/fendo.2011.00117
337. Frye CA, Paris JJ, Walf AA, Rusconi JC. Effects and mechanisms of 3α,5α,-THP on emotion, motivation, and reward functions involving pregnane xenobiotic receptor. *Front Neurosci.* (2012) 5:136. doi: 10.3389/fnins.2011.00136
338. Moguilevsky JA, Wuttke W. Changes in the control of gonadotrophin secretion by neurotransmitters during sexual development in rats. *Exp Clin Endocrinol Diabetes.* (2001) 109:188–95. doi: 10.1055/s-2001-15105
339. Calogero AE, Palumbo MA, Bosboom AM, Burrello N, Ferrara E, Palumbo G, et al. The neuroactive steroid allopregnanolone suppresses hypothalamic gonadotropin-releasing hormone release through a mechanism mediated by

the gamma-aminobutyric acidA receptor. *J Endocrinol.* (1998) 158:121–5. doi: 10.1677/joe.0.1580121

340. Sim JA, Skynner MJ, Herbison AE. Direct regulation of postnatal GnRH neurons by the progesterone derivative allopregnanolone in the mouse. *Endocrinology.* (2001) 142:4448–53. doi: 10.1210/endo.142.10.8451
341. Wisden W, Laurie DJ, Monyer H, Seeburg PH. The distribution of 13 GABAA receptor subunit mRNAs in the rat brain. I. Telencephalon, diencephalon, mesencephalon. *J Neurosci.* (1992) 12:1040–62. doi: 10.1523/JNEUROSCI.12-03-01040.1992
342. Staley KJ, Mody I. Shunting of excitatory input to dentate gyrus granule cells by a depolarizing GABAA receptor-mediated postsynaptic conductance. *J Neurophysiol.* (1992) 68:197–212. doi: 10.1152/jn.1992.68.1.197
343. Gulledge AT, Stuart GJ. Excitatory actions of GABA in the cortex. *Neuron.* (2003) 37:299–309. doi: 10.1016/S0896-6273(02)01146-7
344. Alger BE, Nicoll RA. Pharmacological evidence for two kinds of GABA receptor on rat hippocampal pyramidal cells studied *in vitro*. *J Physiol.* (1982) 328:125–41. doi: 10.1113/jphysiol.1982.sp014256
345. Shen H, Gong QH, Aoki C, Yuan M, Ruderman Y, Dattilo M, et al. Reversal of neurosteroid effects at alpha4beta2delta GABAA receptors triggers anxiety at puberty. *Nat Neurosci.* (2007) 10:469–77. doi: 10.1038/nn1868
346. Kuver A, Smith SS. Flumazenil decreases surface expression of α4β2δ GABAA receptors by increasing the rate of receptor internalization. *Brain Res Bull.* (2016) 120:131–43. doi: 10.1016/j.brainresbull.2015.11.015
347. Vashchinkina E, Manner AK, Vekovischeva O, den Hollander B, Uusi-Oukari M, Aitta-Aho T, et al. Neurosteroid Agonist at GABAA receptor induces persistent neuroplasticity in VTA dopamine neurons. *Neuropsychopharmacology.* (2014) 39:727–37. doi: 10.1038/npp.2013.258
348. Khisti RT, Chopde CT. Serotonergic agents modulate antidepressant-like effect of the neurosteroid 3alpha-hydroxy-5alpha-pregnan-20-one in mice. *Brain Res.* (2000) 865:291–300. doi: 10.1016/S0006-8993(00)02373-8
349. Nelson M, Pinna G. S-norfluoxetine microinfused into the basolateral amygdala increases allopregnanolone levels and reduces aggression in socially isolated mice. *Neuropharmacology.* (2011) 60:1154–9. doi: 10.1016/j.neuropharm.2010.10.011
350. Samardzic J, Hencic B, Jancic J, Jadzic D, Djuric M, Obradovic DI, et al. Neurosteroid dehydroepiandrosterone improves active avoidance retrieval and induces antidepressant-like behavior in rats. *Neurosci Lett.* (2017) 660:17–21. doi: 10.1016/j.neulet.2017.09.013
351. Lu CY, Liu X, Jiang H, Pan F, Ho CS, Ho RC. Effects of traumatic stress induced in the juvenile period on the expression of gamma-aminobutyric acid receptor type A subunits in adult rat brain. *Neural Plast.* (2017) 2017:5715816. doi: 10.1155/2017/5715816
352. Brown ES, Park J, Marx CE, Hynan LS, Gardner C, Davila D, et al. A randomized, double-blind, placebo-controlled trial of pregnenolone for bipolar depression. *Neuropsychopharmacology.* (2014) 39:2867–73. doi: 10.1038/npp.2014.138
353. Lisman JE, Coyle JT, Green RW, Javitt DC, Benes FM, Heckers S, et al. Circuit-based framework for understanding neurotransmitter and risk gene interactions in schizophrenia. *Trends Neurosci.* (2008) 31:234–42. doi: 10.1016/j.tins.2008.02.005
354. Murray JD, Anticevic A, Gancsos M, Ichinose M, Corlett PR, Krystal JH, et al. Linking microcircuit dysfunction to cognitive impairment: effects of disinhibition associated with schizophrenia in a cortical working memory model. *Cereb Cortex.* (2014) 24:859–72. doi: 10.1093/cercor/bhs370
355. de Jonge JC, Vinkers CH, Hulshoff Pol HE, Marsman A. GABAergic mechanisms in schizophrenia: linking postmortem and *in vivo* studies. *Front Psychiatry.* (2017) 8:118. doi: 10.3389/fpsyt.2017.00118
356. Möhler H, Rudolph U. Disinhibition, an emerging pharmacology of learning and memory. *F1000Res.* (2017) 6:F1000 Faculty Rev-101. doi: 10.12688/f1000research.9947.1
357. Billingslea EN, Tatard-Leitman VM, Anguiano J, Jutzeler CR, Suh J, Saunders JA, et al. Parvalbumin cell ablation of NMDA-R1 causes increased resting network excitability with associated social and self-care deficits. *Neuropsychopharmacology.* (2014) 39:1603–13. doi: 10.1038/npp.2014.7
358. Coyle JT, Tsai G, Goff D. Converging evidence of NMDA receptor hypofunction in the pathophysiology of schizophrenia. *Ann N Y Acad Sci.* (2003) 1003:318–27. doi: 10.1196/annals.1300.020
359. Pilowsky LS, Bressan RA, Stone JM, Erlandsson K, Mulligan RS, Krystal JH, et al. First *in vivo* evidence of an NMDA receptor deficit in medication-free schizophrenic patients. *Mol Psychiatry.* (2006) 11:118–9. doi: 10.1038/sj.mp.4001751
360. Sohal VS, Zhang F, Yizhar O, Deisseroth K. Parvalbumin neurons and gamma rhythms enhance cortical circuit performance. *Nature.* (2009) 459:698–702. doi: 10.1038/nature07991
361. Fazzari P, Paternain AV, Valiente M, Pla R, Luján R, Lloyd K, et al. Control of cortical GABA circuitry development by Nrg1 and ErbB4 signalling. *Nature.* (2010) 464:1376–80. doi: 10.1038/nature08928
362. Balu DT, Coyle JT. Glutamate receptor composition of the post-synaptic density is altered in genetic mouse models of NMDA receptor hypo- and hyperfunction. *Brain Res.* (2011) 1392:1–7. doi: 10.1016/j.brainres.2011.03.051
363. Pitcher GM, Kalia LV, Ng D, Goodfellow NM, Yee KT, Lambe EK, et al. Schizophrenia susceptibility pathway neuregulin 1-ErbB4 suppresses Src upregulation of NMDA receptors. *Nat Med.* (2011) 17:470–8. doi: 10.1038/nm.2315
364. Gonzalez-Burgos G, Lewis DA. NMDA receptor hypofunction, parvalbumin-positive neurons, and cortical gamma oscillations in schizophrenia. *Schizophr Bull.* (2012) 38:950–7. doi: 10.1093/schbul/sbs010
365. Forrest AD, Bang J, Featherstone RE, Bloom JH, Luminais MS, Zhang RV, et al. Pyramidal cell-selective GluN1 knockout causes impairments in salience attribution and related EEG activity. *Exp Brain Res.* (2018) 236:837–46. doi: 10.1007/s00221-017-5152-8
366. Rotaru DC, Lewis DA, Gonzalez-Burgos G. The role of glutamatergic inputs onto parvalbumin-positive interneurons: relevance for schizophrenia. *Rev Neurosci.* (2012) 23:97–109. doi: 10.1515/revneuro-2011-0059
367. Chung DW, Wills ZP, Fish KN, Lewis DA. Developmental pruning of excitatory synaptic inputs to parvalbumin interneurons in monkey prefrontal cortex. *Proc Natl Acad Sci USA.* (2017) 114:E629–37. doi: 10.1073/pnas.1610077114
368. Verret L, Mann EO, Hang GB, Barth AM, Cobos I, Ho K, et al. Inhibitory interneuron deficit links altered network activity and cognitive dysfunction in Alzheimer model. *Cell.* (2012) 149:708–21. doi: 10.1016/j.cell.2012.02.046
369. Palop JJ, Mucke L. Network abnormalities and interneuron dysfunction in Alzheimer disease. *Nat Rev Neurosci.* (2016) 17:777–92. doi: 10.1038/nrn.2016.141
370. Carlén M, Meletis K, Siegle JH, Cardin JA, Futai K, Vierling-Claassen D, et al. A critical role for NMDA receptors in parvalbumin interneurons for gamma rhythm induction and behavior. *Psychiatry.* (2012) 17:537–48. doi: 10.1038/mp.2011.31
371. Iwata Y, Nakajima S, Suzuki T, Keefe RS, Plitman E, Chung JK, et al. Effects of glutamate positive modulators on cognitive deficits in schizophrenia: a systematic review and meta-analysis of double-blind randomized controlled trials. *Mol Psychiatry.* (2015) 20:1151–60. doi: 10.1038/mp.2015.68
372. Marx CE, Shampine LJ, Duncan GE, VanDoren MJ, Grobin AC, Massing MW, et al. Clozapine markedly elevates pregnenolone in rat hippocampus, cerebral cortex, and serum: candidate mechanism for superior efficacy? *Pharmacol Biochem Behav.* (2006) 84:598–608. doi: 10.1016/j.pbb.2006.07.026
373. Wong P, Sze Y, Chang CC, Lee J, Zhang X. Pregnenolone sulfate normalizes schizophrenia-like behaviors in dopamine transporter knockout mice through the AKT/GSK3β pathway. *Transl Psychiatry.* (2015) 5:e528. doi: 10.1038/tp.2015.21
374. Ramsey TL, Liu Q, Brennan MD. Replication of SULT4A1-1 as a pharmacogenetic marker of olanzapine response and evidence of lower weight gain in the high response group. *Pharmacogenomics.* (2014) 15:933–9. doi: 10.2217/pgs.14.54
375. Marx CE, Duncan GE, Gilmore JH, Lieberman JA, Morrow AL. Olanzapine increases allopregnanolone in the rat cerebral cortex. *Biol Psychiatry* (2000) 47:1000–4. doi: 10.1016/S0006-3223(99)00305-4
376. Ugale RR, Hirani K, Morelli M, Chopde CT. Role of neuroactive steroid allopregnanolone in antipsychotic-like action of olanzapine in rodents. *Neuropsychopharmacology.* (2004) 29:1597–609. doi: 10.1038/sj.npp.1300460
377. Marx CE, VanDoren MJ, Duncan GE, Lieberman JA, Morrow AL. Olanzapine and clozapine increase the GABAergic neuroactive steroid

allopregnanolone in rodents. *Neuropsychopharmacology.* (2003) 28:1–13. doi: 10.1038/sj.npp.1300015
378. Grimes KM, Zanjani A, Zakzanis KK. Memory impairment and the mediating role of task difficulty in patients with schizophrenia. *Psychiatry Clin Neurosci.* (2017) 71:600–11. doi: 10.1111/pcn.12520
379. Kapur S, Remington G, Jones C, Wilson A, DaSilva J, Houle S, et al. High levels of dopamine D2 receptor occupancy with low-dose haloperidol treatment: a PET study. *Am J Psychiatry.* (1996) 153:948–50. doi: 10.1176/ajp.153.7.948
380. Dougherty DD, Bonab AA, Spencer TJ, Rauch SL, Madras BK, Fischman AJ. Dopamine transporter density in patients with attention deficit hyperactivity disorder. *Lancet.* (1999) 354:2132–3. doi: 10.1016/S0140-6736(99)04030-1
381. Efimova EV, Gainetdinov RR, Budygin EA, Sotnikova TD. Dopamine transporter mutant animals: a translational perspective. *J Neurogenet.* (2016) 30:5–15. doi: 10.3109/01677063.2016.1144751
382. Reith ME, Xu C, Chen NH. Pharmacology and regulation of the neuronal dopamine transporter. *Eur J Pharmacol.* (1997) 324:1–10. doi: 10.1016/S0014-2999(97)00065-4
383. Amara SG, Kuhar MJ. Neurotransmitter transporters: recent progress. *Annu Rev Neurosci.* (1993) 16:73–93. doi: 10.1146/annurev.ne.16.030193.000445
384. Giros B, Jaber M, Jones SR, Wightman RM, Caron MG. Hyperlocomotion and indifference to cocaine and amphetamine in mice lacking the dopamine transporter. *Nature.* (1996) 379:606–12. doi: 10.1038/379606a0
385. Madras BK, Fahey MA, Miller GM, De La Garza R, Goulet M, Spealman RD, et al. Non-amine-based dopamine transporter (reuptake) inhibitors retain properties of amine-based progenitors. *Eur J Pharmacol.* (2003) 479:41–51. doi: 10.1016/j.ejphar.2003.08.055
386. Gainetdinov RR. Dopamine transporter mutant mice in experimental neuropharmacology. *Naunyn Schmiedebergs Arch Pharmacol.* (2008) 377:301–13. doi: 10.1007/s00210-007-0216-0
387. Gainetdinov RR, Caron MG. Monoamine transporters: from genes to behavior. *Annu Rev Pharmacol Toxicol.* (2003) 43:261–84. doi: 10.1146/annurev.pharmtox.43.050802.112309
388. Gasior M, Carter RB, Witkin JM. Neuroactive steroids: potential therapeutic use in neurological and psychiatric disorders. *Trends Pharmacol Sci.* (1999) 20:107–12. doi: 10.1016/S0165-6147(99)01318-8
389. Parésys L, Hoffmann K, Froger N, Bianchi M, Villey I, Baulieu EE, et al. Effects of the synthetic neurosteroid: 3β-methoxypregnenolone (MAP4343) on behavioral and physiological alterations provoked by chronic psychosocial stress in tree shrews. *Int J Neuropsychopharmacol.* (2016) 19:pyv119. doi: 10.1093/ijnp/pyv119
390. Carter RB, Wood PL, Wieland S, Hawkinson JE, Belelli D, Lambert JJ, et al. Characterization of the anticonvulsant properties of ganaxolone (CCD 1042; 3α-hydroxy-3β-methyl-5α-pregnan-20-one), a selective, high-affinity, steroid modulator of the γ-aminobutyric acidA receptor. *J Pharmacol Exp Ther.* (1997) 280:1284–95.
391. Pinna G, Rasmusson AM. Ganaxolone improves behavioral deficits in a mouse model of post-traumatic stress disorder. *Front Cell Neurosci.* (2014) 8:256. doi: 10.3389/fncel.2014.00256
392. Rasmusson AM, Marx CE, Jain S, Farfel GM, Tsai J, Sun X, et al. A randomized controlled trial of ganaxolone in posttraumatic stress disorder. *Psychopharmacology (Berl).* (2017) 234:2245–57. doi: 10.1007/s00213-017-4649-y
393. Ciarlone SL, Wang X, Rogawski MA, Weeber EJ. Effects of the synthetic neurosteroid ganaxolone on seizure activity and behavioral deficits in an Angelman syndrome mouse model. *Neuropharmacology.* (2017) 116:142–50. doi: 10.1016/j.neuropharm.2016.12.009
394. Wieland S, Belluzzi J, Hawkinson JE, Hogenkamp D, Upasani R, Stein L, et al. Anxiolytic and anticonvulsant activity of a synthetic neuroactive steroid Co 3-0593. *Psychopharmacology (Berl).* (1997) 134:46–54. doi: 10.1007/s002130050424
395. Ferree NK, Cahill L. Post-event spontaneous intrusive recollections and strength of memory for emotional events in men and women. *Conscious Cogn.* (2009) 18:126–34. doi: 10.1016/j.concog.2008.11.008
396. Mohedano-Moriano A, Martinez-Marcos A, Pro-Sistiaga P, Blaizot X, Arroyo-Jimenez MM, Marcos P, et al. Convergence of unimodal and polymodal sensory input to the entorhinal cortex in the fascicularis monkey. *Neuroscience.* (2008) 151:255–71. doi: 10.1016/j.neuroscience.2007.09.074
397. Sripada RK, Marx CE, King AP, Rajaram N, Garfinkel SN, Abelson JL, et al. DHEA enhances emotion regulation neurocircuits and modulates memory for emotional stimuli. *Neuropsychopharmacology.* (2013) 38:1798–807. doi: 10.1038/npp.2013.79
398. Wahlstrom KL, Huff ML, Emmons EB, Freeman JH, Narayanan NS, McIntyre CK, et al. Basolateral amygdala inputs to the medial entorhinal cortex selectively modulate the consolidation of spatial and contextual learning. *J Neurosci.* (2018) 38:2698–712. doi: 10.1523/JNEUROSCI.2848-17.2018
399. Lussier AL, Romay-Tallón R, Caruncho HJ, Kalynchuk LE. Altered GABAergic and glutamatergic activity within the rat hippocampus and amygdala in rats subjected to repeated corticosterone administration but not restraint stress. *Neuroscience.* (2013) 231:38–48. doi: 10.1016/j.neuroscience.2012.11.037
400. Lee V, MacKenzie G, Hooper A, Maguire J. Reduced tonic inhibition in the dentate gyrus contributes to chronic stress-induced impairments in learning and memory. *Hippocampus.* (2016) 26:1276–90. doi: 10.1002/hipo.22604
401. Pineles SL, Nillni YI, Pinna G, Irvine J, Webb A, Arditte Hall KA, et al. PTSD in women is associated with a block in conversion of progesterone to the GABAergic neurosteroids allopregnanolone and pregnanolone measured in plasma. *Psychoneuroendocrinology.* (2018) 93:133–41. doi: 10.1016/j.psyneuen.2018.04.024
402. Lee AL, Ogle WO, Sapolsky RM. Stress and depression: possible links to neuron death in the hippocampus. *Bipolar Disord.* (2002) 4:117–28. doi: 10.1034/j.1399-5618.2002.01144.x
403. Nishimura KJ, Ortiz JB, Conrad CD. Antagonizing the GABAA receptor during behavioral training improves spatial memory at different doses in control and chronically stressed rats. *Neurobiol Learn Mem.* (2017) 145:114–8. doi: 10.1016/j.nlm.2017.09.002

6

Biomarkers for PTSD at the Interface of the Endocannabinoid and Neurosteroid Axis

*Graziano Pinna**

The Psychiatric Institute, Department of Psychiatry, College of Medicine, University of Illinois at Chicago, Chicago, IL, United States

Keywords: allopregnanolone, biomarkers, N-palmitoylethanolamine, PPAR-α, endocannabinoids, 5α-reductase, contextual fear responses, PTSD

***Correspondence:**
Graziano Pinna
gpinna@uic.edu;
graziano_pinna@yahoo.com

INTRODUCTION

In the search for reliable and, possibly, specific biomarkers for neuropsychiatric disorders, growing evidence has demonstrated that biosynthesis of neuroactive steroids and the endocannabinoid system are involved in the neuropathology of post-traumatic stress disorder (PTSD) and major depressive disorder (Uzunova et al., 1998; Rasmusson et al., 2006; reviewed in Locci and Pinna, 2017a). Although, undisputable progress has been made to assess validity of biomarkers for psychiatric disorders, the topic still remains underdeveloped as compared to other fields of neuroscience (Fernandes et al., 2017). The diagnosis of psychiatric disorders still relies on subjective measures centered on the DSM-5 criteria which have several shortcomings (Brewin et al., 2017). Psychiatric conditions are poorly understood and there is a wide heterogeneity in how illness manifests in several individuals. Furthermore, self-assessment of one's own feelings can be biased, ill-defined, and difficult, making psychological diagnoses unreliable and may lead to treatment inefficacy. Biomarkers discovery would significantly improve treatment matching. Thus, searching for potential biomarkers to guide precision medicine in the treatment of PTSD, and to increase the success of clinical trials and prompt the development of novel and specific treatments, is required. To aid this search, more sophisticated methodological tools and validated animal models has also become essential to reliably correlate behavioral changes with neurochemical alterations (reviewed in Ngounou Wetie et al., 2013). The overlap of symptoms and the comorbidity with other psychiatric disorders such as major depressive disorder, anxiety spectrum disorders, and even suicidal ideation (Franklin et al., 2017), suggest a bio-signature for PTSD should include the relation of numerous biomarkers rather than having only a few (Locci and Pinna, 2017a). A refined approach to more specifically "bio-define" PTSD can be to establish a *biomarker axis* or in other words, to assess the relation of various biomarkers, which fluctuate in concert and correlate uniquely with PTSD behavioral modifications. Insofar, a *biomarker axis* may provide a higher accuracy in the diagnosis of the disorder with benefits for prediction in PTSD treatment response and relapse (Locci et al., 2018; Pinna and Izumi, 2018). As a matter of fact, the "gold standard" treatment for PTSD and depression, the selective serotonin reuptake inhibitors (SSRIs), improve only half of the treatment-seeking patients and they are associated with severe side-effects (Golden et al., 2002; Rush et al., 2006; Kemp et al., 2008; reviewed in Bernardy and Friedman, 2017). This also suggests these psychiatric disorders are complex, multifaceted diseases arising from multiple and diverse neurobiological backgrounds and therefore, symptoms may not always recapitulate to a serotonergic deficit and administering an SSRI may not always improve symptoms. Unveiling reliable biomarkers is also a necessity for patient stratification in treatment selection as well as for drug development through clinical trials. The development of state-of-the-art technologies and methodological rigor are essential to allow for the discovery of more reliable biomarkers in psychiatry. Employing the gas chromatography-mass spectrometry (GC-MS) to achieve this goal is highly innovative and provides reliable information based on a powerful technology with high sensitivity and unsurpassed structure selectivity (Uzunov et al., 1996; Pinna et al., 2000). Hence, by applying the GC-MS measurements of neuroactive steroids in serum, plasma, CSF and post-mortem brain, in the past decade, we have shed light in the fundamental role of neuroactive steroids in patients with neuropsychiatric disorders (Rasmusson et al., 2006, 2017; Agis-Balboa et al., 2014; Pineles et al., 2018; reviewed in Locci and Pinna, 2017a).

The biosynthesis of allopregnanolone, a positive allosteric modulator of GABA's action at $GABA_A$ receptors has been found deficient in a number of neuropsychopathologies, including epilepsy (e.g., PHDH19), major depression, PTSD, perceived social isolation, post-partum depression, premenstrual syndrome, and anorexia nervosa or obesity complicated by anxiety and depression symptoms in women (Romeo et al., 1998; Uzunova et al., 1998; Rasmusson et al., 2006, 2018; Nemeroff, 2008; Lovick, 2013; Trivisano et al., 2017; Dichtel et al., 2018; Pineles et al., 2018). Therapeutic measures aimed at reinstating normal allopregnanolone levels in deficient-patients correlates with improved symptoms (Kanes et al., 2017). The question arises as to whether allopregnanolone biosynthesis *per se* is a reliable biomarker to predict, diagnose and instruct treatment selection of patients or whether its relation with neurotransmitter systems ($GABA_A$ and NMDA receptors), stimulation of neurotropic factors (e.g., BDNF), and/or crosstalk with the endocannabinoid system (e.g., PPAR-α) may provide a valuable *biomarker axis* with a higher disorder-selectivity. This analysis includes both neurosteroids that are positive allosteric modulators of $GABA_A$ receptors (Pinna et al., 2000; Belelli and Lambert, 2005), such as allopregnanolone and pregnanolone and their sulfated forms that are inhibitors of NMDA-mediated tonic neurotransmission, which results in neuroprotection (Vyklicky et al., 2016).

The novel discovery that the endocannabinoid system regulates the biosynthesis of neurosteroids, including allopregnanolone has recently opened the field for assessing valuable PTSD biomarkers at the interface of these neuronal systems. In recent years, cannabinoid-based agents have become an integral part of drug discovery for PTSD treatment (Ruehle et al., 2012; Neumeister et al., 2014). The impact of the endocannabinoid system is under-scored by the density of receptors in glutamatergic neurons of emotion-relevant areas, including the the amygdaloid complex, the hippocampus and the frontal cortex (Katona, 2009). Synthetic cannabinoid receptor antagonists or knockouts enhance fear acquisition and impair fear extinction, a core feature of PTSD (Reich et al., 2008; Papini et al., 2015). In addition to the well assessed role of the endocannabinoid, anandamide (AEA) or 2-arachidonoyl-glycerol (2-AG) both in neuropsychiatric disorders and animal models of stress (Chhatwal et al., 2005; Umathe et al., 2011; Dubreucq et al., 2012), compelling evidence indicates stimulation of the intracellular endocannabinoid target, peroxisome-proliferator activated receptor (PPAR)-α by its endogenous neuromodulator, N-palmitoylethanolamine (PEA) engages the biosynthesis of neurosteroids to modulate emotional behavior (Locci and Pinna, 2017b; Locci et al., 2018) (please see **Figure 1** for a graphic representation).

This unforeseen behavioral and neurosteroidogenic function of PPAR-α, formally known to regulate pathophysiological functions, including inflammation and oxidative stress, opens the field for potential novel biomarkers for PTSD.

This article will discuss whether new discoveries in the field support a biomarker role for allopregnanolone biosynthesis and the endocannabinoid system for stress-induced disorders with focus on PTSD. The strategy of assessing a *biomarker axis*, which indicates the relation of various inter-related neurobiological deficits for one disorder (**Figure 2**), may help for diagnosis accuracy and for designing successful individualized treatments.

NEUROSTEROID ACTION AT $GABA_A$ AND NMDA RECEPTORS

Sulfated or unconjugated neuroactive steroids modulate ionotropic amino acid neurotransmitter receptors, including $GABA_A$ and NMDA receptors. The $GABA_A$ receptor offers two binding residues that express affinity for allopregnanolone and unconjugated congeners (e.g., pregnanolone) that act as potent positive allosteric modulators of the action of GABA at $GABA_A$ receptors. One is located at the interface of the α/β subunits, and the other is within the cavity of α subunits (Hosie et al., 2006). The α,β,γ $GABA_A$ receptor subtype is the most frequent synaptic configuration and is highly sensitive to benzodiazepines but shows lower sensitivity to GABA and neurosteroids (Nusser and Mody, 2002). The α,β,δ $GABA_A$ receptor subtype expressed in the extrasynaptic region is benzodiazepine-insensitive, show low efficacy for GABA, but neurosteroids increase its agonist efficacy (Stell et al., 2003; Shu et al., 2012). This receptor combination shows high efficacy for neurosteroids (Brown et al., 2002; Nusser and Mody, 2002; Wohlfarth et al., 2002; **Figure 1**). Sulfated neurosteroids such as pregnenolone sulfate, dehydroepiandrosterone sulfate, pregnanolone sulfate, and allopregnanolone sulfate may function as endogenous neuromodulators by inhibiting $GABA_A$ receptors, or depending on the receptor conformation and the sulfated neuroactive steroid examined, by activating or inhibiting NMDA-mediated neurotransmission (Park-Chung et al., 1999). Sulfation at C3 is essential to reverse the direction of modulation from positive to negative in $GABA_A$ receptors. Steroid negative and positive modulators act through distinct sites, which implies that steroid negative and positive modulators can act independently or coordinately to modulate the flavor of GABAergic-mediated inhibitory neurotransmission (reviewed in Smith et al., 2014). While, micromolar concentrations of pregnenolone sulfate negatively modulate $GABA_A$ receptors, pregnenolone sulfate can negatively or positively modulate NMDA receptors, depending on the receptor subunits expressed (Malayev et al., 2002; Smith et al., 2014). For instance, pregnenolone sulfate potentiates NMDA receptors that contain NR2A and NR2B subunits, but negatively modulates NR2C and NR2D-containing receptors (Malayev et al., 2002). Recent studies showed that pregnanolone

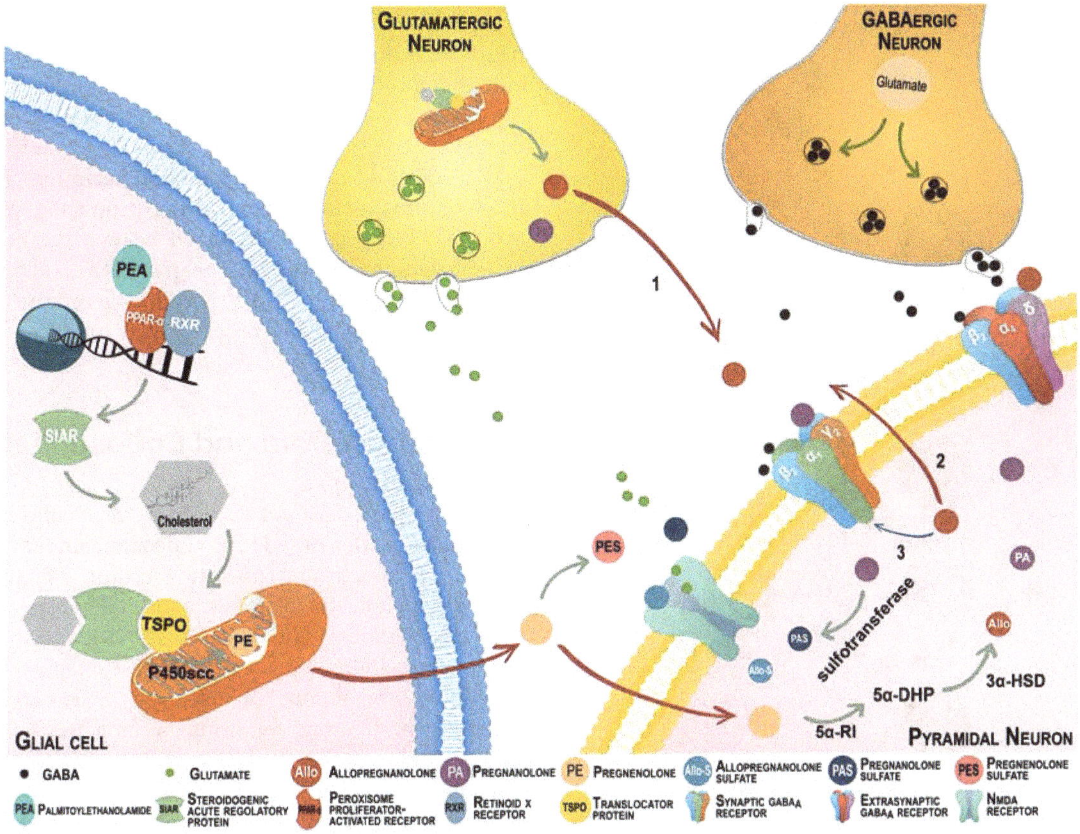

FIGURE 1 | The endocannabinoid and neurosteroid systems cross-talk regulates emotional behavior. The neurosteroids, allopregnanolone (Allo) and its equipotent isomer pregnanolone (PA) are primarily synthesized in glutamatergic corticolimbic neurons and upon secretion; they may act at $GABA_A$ receptors located on cell bodies or dendrites of distal pyramidal neurons (Arrow 1). They may also act at $GABA_A$ receptors located on glutamatergic neurons' dendrites or cell bodies by an autocrine mechanism (Arrow 2), or may access and act at the intracellular sites of $GABA_A$ receptors located in glutamatergic neurons that produced allopregnanolone itself (Arrow 3) (Agís-Balboa et al., 2006, 2007; Pinna et al., 2008). Allopregnanolone plays a central neuromodulatory role in facilitating the action of GABA at $GABA_A$ receptors (a primary target of anxiolytics) and in the fine-tuning of the receptor for agonists and GABAmimetic agents (Pinna et al., 2000). The finding that allopregnanolone facilitates the efficacy of $GABA_A$ receptor allosteric modulators substantiates its endogenous physiological relevance (Pinna et al., 2000, 2008; Guidotti et al., 2001). Importantly, $GABA_A$ receptors composed by α,β,γ subunits are the most common configuration in the synaptic membranes and they are responsible for the inhibitory *phasic* currents. These receptors are benzodiazepine-sensitive but show lower sensitivity to GABA and allopregnanolone (Nusser and Mody, 2002). The $GABA_A$ receptors including α,β,δ subtypes are mostly extrasynaptic and mediate inhibitory *tonic* currents. Of note, they are not sensitive to benzodiazepines and show low efficacy for GABA, however, allopregnanolone increase their efficacy (Stell et al., 2003; Shu et al., 2012). The efficacy of GABAergic neurosteroids is greatly enhanced for this receptor combination (Brown et al., 2002; Nusser and Mody, 2002; Wohlfarth et al., 2002). Remarkably, protracted stress favors a $GABA_A$ receptor composition with high sensitivity for allopregnanolone and its analogs (Locci and Pinna, 2017a). Following the action of sulphotransferase, allopregnanolone, and pregnanolone can be transformed into allopregnanolone sulfate (Allo-S) and pregnanolone sulfate (PAS). These sulfated steroids can be measured by gas chromatography-mass spectrometry in serum, CSF, and brain of patients or rodents in concentrations consistent with a physiological role in modulating neurotransmitter systems (Smith et al., 2014; Locci and Pinna, 2017b). Recently, pregnanolone sulfate has been shown to inhibit NMDA receptors. Pregnanolone sulfate can accumulate in plasma membranes and may accesses binding sites that are located at NMDA receptors (Borovska et al., 2012). Importantly, pregnanolone sulfate, and probably allopregnanolone sulfate, is highly potent at inhibiting tonic rather than synaptically mediated NMDA receptor neurotransmissions. While synaptic NMDA receptors play a pivotal role in synaptic plasticity, learning and memory, as well as in synaptogenesis, tonic-mediated NMDA receptor neurotransmission is mostly involved with excitotoxicity. Thus, the effects of pregnanolone sulfate negative modulation of tonic-mediated NMDA receptor neurotransmission have relevance for neuroprotection (Vyklicky et al., 2016). By this mechanism, these allopregnanolone and pregnanolone sulfated derivatives may play a role in the regulation of cognitive processes and of emotional behavior (reviewed in Locci and Pinna, 2017a). There is growing evidence that the intracellular peroxisome proliferator-activated receptor (PPAR-α) is also a cannabinoid target (depicted on the bottom right). PPAR-α heterodimerize with the retinoid X receptor (RXR) and binds to the consensus regions on the target gene promoters and initiates transcription (Neumeister, 2013). Given that endoannabinoids activate PPAR-α (Marsicano et al., 2002; Pistis and Melis, 2010), the activation of these nuclear receptors represents a novel mechanism by which cannabinoids may modulate behavior. The endocannabinoid congener, N-palmitoylethanolamine (PEA) is a PPAR-α endogenous agonist, which is decreased in PTSD patients (Wilker et al., 2016). Recent preclinical findings showed that supplementing PEA in rodent PTSD models improves emotional behavior by enhancing allopregnanolone biosynthesis in corticolimbic glutamatergic neurons. This effect is mimicked by PPAR-α agonists and prevented by allopregnanolone biosynthetic enzyme blockers and by deletion of the PPAR-α gene (Locci and Pinna, 2017b). Thus, anxiolytic, anti-aggressive and anti-fear effects of PEA and synthetic PPAR-α agonists may relate to an induction of corticolimbic allopregnanolone's biosynthetic enzymes. This may result in potentiation of $GABA_A$ receptor and, possibly, in an inhibition of tonic-mediated NMDA signal transduction associated with improved behavioral dysfunction. Stress effects on PEA levels and probably expression of PPAR-α may result in the downregulation of allopregnanolone's biosynthetic enzyme expression and allopregnanolone levels. The interface of the endocannabinoid and neurosteroid systems may provide an important *biomarker axis* to selectively predict, diagnose, and establish the best individualized treatment selection for PTSD patients.

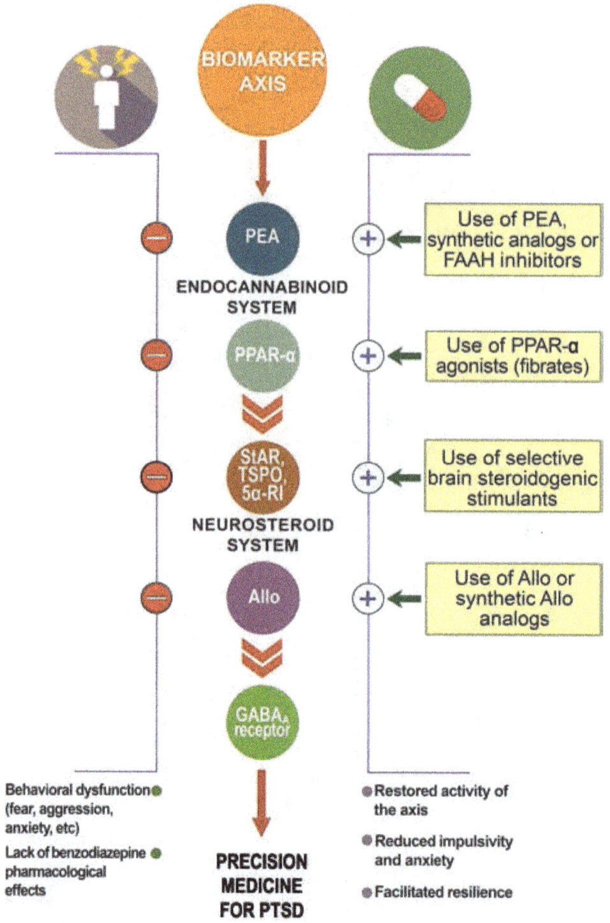

FIGURE 2 | Biomarker axis at the interface of the endocannabinoid and neurosteroid systems. In animal models of PTSD, protracted stress results in the downregulation of allopregnanolone biosynthetic enzymes (e.g., 5α-reductase type I, 5α-RI) and allopregnanolone concentrations in corticolimbic glutamatergic neurons of the frontal cortex, hippocampus, and basolateral amygdala. This allopregnanolone decrease correlates with behavioral dysfunction, such as increased aggression, enhanced contextual fear responses and anxiety-like behavior (Pinna et al., 2003; Pibiri et al., 2008). Supplying allopregnanolone or stimulating its biosynthesis decreases anxiety-like behavior, aggression and fear responses (Pinna, 2013; Pinna and Rasmusson, 2014). Stress may also result in changes in $GABA_A$ receptor subunit expression (Pinna et al., 2006; reviewed in Locci and Pinna, 2017a) with increased $\alpha4$, $\alpha5$, and δ subunits and decreased $\alpha1$, $\alpha2$, and $\gamma2$, which result in down-regulated benzodiazepine binding sites and inefficacy of benzodiazepine pharmacological action (Pinna et al., 2006; Nin et al., 2011b). Protracted stress results in increased $GABA_A$ receptor subunits, including $\alpha_{4-5},\beta,\delta$ highly sensitivity for allopregnanolone (Locci and Pinna, 2017a). Both allopregnanolone biosynthesis downregulation and decreased benzodiazepine binding sites have been reported in PTSD patients (Rasmusson et al., 2006, 2018; Geuze et al., 2008). Thus, the combination of downregulation of allopregnanolone biosynthesis, changes in $GABA_A$ receptor subunit expression, and lack of benzodiazepine pharmacological action are peculiar changes observed in PTSD that may provide a selective *biomarker axis* for this disorder. Stress may affect PEA levels and expression of PPAR-α, which in turn may downregulate allopregnanolone concentrations. Thus, the PPAR-α-allopregnanolone axis may provide further biomarker candidates to support selection of the best individualized precision medicine for PTSD. Allo, allopregnanolone; GABA, γ-aminobutyric acid; PEA, N-palmitoylethanolamine; PPAR-α, peroxisome-proliferator activated receptor-α; StAR, steroidogenic acute regulatory protein; TSPO, 18 kDa translocator protein.

sulfate has a potent inhibitory action at tonic rather than synaptically-activated NMDA receptors, which provides neuroprotection and possibly improves emotional behavior and cognition (Vyklicky et al., 2016). This feature is relevant for developing a novel class of steroid-based NMDA-inhibitors devoid of the psychotomimetic effects that characterize classical NMDA receptor inhibitors, including ketamine. While $GABA_A$ receptor subunit expression during protracted stress has been previously investigated (discussed below), the role and action of sulfated pregnanolone, pregnenolone, allopregnanolone, and the expression of NMDA receptor subunits in PTSD patients and in rodent stress models, still warrants elucidation.

The Neurosteroid and Endocannabinoid Crosstalk

Intriguingly, studies conducted in cell cultures, brainstem and spinal cord showed the endocannabinoid, PEA binding at the ligand-activated nuclear receptor, PPAR-α stimulates allopregnanolone biosynthesis and potentiates pentobarbital-induced sedation (Sasso et al., 2010, 2012; Raso et al., 2011). These observations suggest that PPAR-α may play a role in the regulation of emotions by inducing neurosteroidogenesis in corticolimbic neurons following binding with its endogenous ligand, PEA, or synthetic agonists. Whereas the classic cannabinoid receptor type 1 (CB1) has been shown to regulate emotions and stress responses, PPAR-α's role on emotions remains poorly understood (Riebe and Wotjak, 2011; Häring et al., 2012). The relevance of the endocannabinoid system in behavior is highlighted by expression of CB1 and PPAR-α in glutamatergic neurons of emotion-relevant areas that have been identified by brain imaging to be critical in PTSD (amygdala, hippocampus, frontal cortex) (Moreno et al., 2004; Lo Verme et al., 2005; Shin et al., 2006; D'Agostino, 2007; D'Agostino et al., 2009; Katona, 2009; Petrosino and Di Marzo, 2017). Moreover, evidence suggests CB1 disruption leads to impaired fear extinction (Reich et al., 2008), depressive- and anxiety-like behavior, while agonists, like AEA, induce anxiolysis and improve fear responses (Hill and Patel, 2013). Current thought suggests that the effects of AEA at CB1 account for the majority of anti-fear effects of endocannabinoids (Marsicano et al., 2002; Viveros et al., 2005; Kamprath et al., 2006; Thiemann et al., 2008; Jacob et al., 2012), however this view seems no longer tenable (Pistis and Melis, 2010). In addition to these cell-surface cannabinoid receptors (O'Sullivan, 2007), there is growing evidence that PPAR-α's activation represents a novel mechanism by which cannabinoids modulate behavior. Stimulation of PPAR-α by PEA or synthetic PPAR-α agonists was recently shown to elevate corticolimbic allopregnanolone levels in hippocampus, amygdala, frontal cortex and in olfactory bulb, which correlated with improvement of PTSD-like behavior in socially isolated mice (Locci and Pinna, 2017a). PEA facilitates contextual fear extinction and fear extinction retention and induces anti-aggressive, anxiolytic, and antidepressant-like effects in socially isolated mice (Locci and Pinna, 2017b; Locci et al., 2017). PPAR-α synthetic agonists normalized allopregnanolone levels and improved behavior, whereas antagonism at PPAR-α, inhibition of allopregnanolone biosynthetic enzymes, or PPAR-α KO mice prevented both PEA-induced behavior and its neurosteroidogenic effects (Locci and Pinna, 2017b). While the role of PPAR-α in neuropsychiatric disorders is just emerging, studies in the field suggest serum PEA and oleoylethanolamide (OEA) concentrations increase after acute social stressor (Dlugos, 2012) and decrease following recovery (Hill et al., 2009a). Stress evokes fast induction of fatty acid amide hydrolase (FAAH), which reduces PEA and AEA levels (Patel et al., 2005; Hill et al., 2009b). In PTSD patients, symptoms are inversely correlated with reduced hair levels of PEA, OEA and stearoylethanolamide (SEA) in both males and females (Wilker et al., 2016). PEA adjunctive therapy to citalopram improves symptoms in depressed patients (Ghazizadeh-Hashemi, 2018). Furthermore, intense workouts increase PEA and OEA levels and improve depression and PTSD (Heyman, 2012). In rodents, exposure to predator stressors reduces cardiac PEA and OEA levels (Holman et al., 2014), but, antidepressant-like effects are induced by increasing PEA and OEA (Adamczyk et al., 2008; Umathe et al., 2011; Melis et al., 2013). Collectively, the crosstalk between the endocannabinoid system and neurosteroid biosynthesis during stress may unveil *biomarker axis* uniquely altered in specific stress-induced mood disorders.

BIOMARKERS AND TREATMENT OPTIONS FOR PTSD AT THE INTERFACE OF THE ENDOCANNABINOID AND NEUROSTEROID AXIS

Psychiatric disorders, such as PTSD, are not currently amenable to objective neurobiological determinations as is routine practice in the diagnosis and treatment of other medical conditions. This is most likely due to the general complexity and multifactorial origins of these disorders and the difficulty to establish a consistent bio-signature. While no biomarkers for PTSD have to date been firmly assessed with diagnostic validity, a consistent progress in the field has been done. Biomarker candidates for PTSD have been proposed but often they share overlaps with other psychiatric disorders with similar symptoms and that are currently treated with same drugs. Indeed, the first-choice pharmacological treatments for PTSD, the SSRIs, act through multiple molecular mechanisms other than by inhibiting serotonin reuptake. These mechanisms include the stimulation of neurosteroid and endocannabinoid biosynthesis and neurotrophic factors, such as BDNF, which are found deficient in PTSD. Increasing allopregnanolone levels is also associated with increased BDNF expression (Nin et al., 2011a). Collectively, these findings have contributed to improve our understanding of the psychobiological abnormalities associated with PTSD and promote the development of novel targeted treatment options. For instance, the correlation between the impairment of neurosteroid biosynthesis and behavioral modifications in neuropsychiatric disorders has been the focus of several studies (van Broekhoven and Verkes, 2003; reviewed in Pinna, 2013; Agis-Balboa et al., 2014; Locci and Pinna, 2017a). A reduction in the content of the GABAergic modulator allopregnanolone and its equipotent isomer pregnanolone was reported in cerebrospinal fluid (CSF) and serum of major depression and PTSD patients (Romeo et al., 1998; Uzunova et al., 1998; Rasmusson et al., 2006, 2016; Pineles et al., 2018). A negative correlation between CSF allopregnanolone levels and PTSD symptoms was more recently confirmed in male patients (Rasmusson et al., 2018). Other clinical studies support the significance of allopregnanolone biosynthesis as a biomarker of mood disorders (Uzunova et al., 1998; Agis-Balboa et al., 2014; reviewed in Zorumski et al., 2013; Schüle et al., 2014; Locci and Pinna, 2017a) with finding showing decreased allopregnanolone levels in postpartum depression (Nemeroff, 2008), under treatment with finasteride, an allopregnanolone biosynthetic enzyme blocker (Altomare and Capella, 2002; Caruso, 2015; Welk et al., 2017), and with anorexia nervosa or obesity complicated by anxiety and depression (Dichtel et al., 2018). Intriguingly, SSRI treatments normalize plasma, CSF, and brain allopregnanolone content in association with improvement of symptoms in responders only (Romeo et al., 1998; Uzunova et al., 1998; Agis-Balboa et al., 2014). These findings are in support of the role of allopregnanolone in the mechanisms of SSRIs' anxiolytic effects (Pinna, 2015). The downregulation of neurosteroid levels found in PTSD and depressed patients can be modeled in rodents exposed to protracted stress, including the socially-isolated mouse. Allopregnanolone is produced in brain corticolimbic neurons (**Figure 1**) and a reduction of its levels by prolonged social isolation (Agís-Balboa et al., 2006, 2007) or exposure to single prolonged stressors, results in development of anxiety-like behavior, aggression and enhanced contextual fear conditioning responses associated with impairment of fear extinction and elevated spontaneous fear responses at recall (Pinna et al., 2003; Pibiri et al., 2008; Pinna and Rasmusson, 2014; Qiu et al., 2015). These preclinical studies further support allopregnanolone as a putative *biomarker* for stress-induced emotional modification, such as exaggerated fear responses and impaired fear extinction, a hallmark in PTSD (Pibiri et al., 2008; Pinna et al., 2008; Pinna and Rasmusson, 2012). This evidence also suggests that new therapeutic approaches should counteract the downregulation of neurosteroid biosynthesis to improve symptoms in PTSD patients. In recent phase 3 clinical trials, intravenous allopregnanolone (brexanolone or SAGE-547) or an oral analog (SAGE-217) showed a rapid and long-lasting remission of post-partum depression and major depressive disorder symptoms, conditions highly comorbid with PTSD (Kanes et al., 2017; http://investor.sagerx.com/news-releases/news-release-details/sage-announces-pivotal-phase-3-trial-status-sage-217-major). If successfully developed, SAGE-217 will be the first durable, rapid-acting, oral, short-course treatment for mood disorders with potential application for PTSD treatment. Stress tremendously affects the expression of $GABA_A$ receptor subunits (Pinna et al., 2006; reviewed in Locci and Pinna, 2017a). After social isolation, the α4, α5, and δ subunit expression was increased, and the α1, α2, and γ2 were significantly decreased in corticolimbic areas. These changes result in decreased benzodiazepine recognition sites and lower pharmacological response to benzodiazepines

(Pinna et al., 2006). Remarkably, protracted stress favors a $GABA_A$ receptor composition with high sensitivity for allopregnanolone and its analogs (Locci et al., 2017; reviewed in Locci and Pinna, 2017a). Clinical findings support lower benzodiazepine recognition site binding in brain of PTSD patients in association with benzodiazepine-insensitivity (Geuze et al., 2008). Altogether, these findings suggest that isolation stress results in: (i) changes in $GABA_A$ receptor subunit composition; (ii) downregulated neurosteroidogenesis; and (iii) lack of response to benzodiazepines, which may provide a unique *biomarker axis* for PTSD (**Figure 2**). Allopregnanolone, analogs or stimulation of allopregnanolone biosynthesis may be a valuable therapeutic strategy for stress-induced psychiatric disorders, characterized by benzodiazepine-inefficacy and poor response to SSRIs. The pharmacological profile of SSRIs on stimulation of neurotropic factors, including the brain-derived neurotrophic factor (BDNF), via stimulation of allopregnanolone biosynthesis is an additional important mechanism to consider when establishing biomarkers for PTSD. BDNF expression decrease in PTSD patients is associated with symptom severity. In the socially isolated mouse, fluoxetine improves behavior by elevating the corticolimbic levels of allopregnanolone and BDNF expression, independently from the action of these drugs on serotonin reuptake inhibition. This and other evidence suggest that neurosteroid biosynthesis and BDNF expression may be interrelated (Nin et al., 2011a; Frye et al., 2014), and this may provide further support for biomarker selection.

Hence, biomarkers that instruct which treatment would be most effective for a patient is expected to considerably reduce non-responders and non-completers rate. Discovering new targets and agents to stimulate allopregnanolone biosynthesis is pivotal in this process. While more research is required to elucidate the interaction between the endocannabinoid system and allopregnanolone biosynthesis and specifically, following activation of PPAR-α, undoubtedly their cross-talk offers a unique opportunity to assess a biomarker axis that encompasses these two systems (**Figure 2**). A better assessment can be done following clarification of how stress affects PPAR-α expression and function. The concentrations of its main endogenous modulators, PEA, OEA, and SEA, which were found decreased in hair of PTSD patients, should be confirmed systemically in serum and CSF of patients. Preclinical studies should also verify whether their biosynthesis is altered in brain of rodent models of stress-induced behavioral deficits. Furthermore, methods development to simultaneously determine both endocannabinoid (AEA), cannabinoid-like (PEA) and neurosteroid (allopregnanolone) concentrations in same samples will consistently enhance the understanding on how the two systems are coordinated in neuropsychiatric disorders.

Both endocannabinoids and neurosteroids can be measured by GC-MS, however, presently there is no method that can determine them simultaneously in the same samples. Our laboratory established GC-MS methods to determine neurosteroids and their sulfates in human and rodent samples and we are currently developing new methods to include the quantification of endocannabinoids with demonstrated involvement in the pathophysiology of PTSD. Hence, these studies will clarify whether allopregnanolone levels down-regulation is causally linked to a PPAR-α expression down-regulation and/or endocannabinoid concentrations. The goal is to provide a reliable bio-signature that may uniquely define neurobiological alteration in PTSD and shows diagnostic validity.

While many aspects that relate to the endocannabinoid and neurosteroid cross-talk remain presently obscure, our current findings highlight the potential for: (i) assessing novel biomarkers to predict, diagnose, and treat PTSD at the interface of the PPAR-α-allopregnanolone axis; and (ii) repurposing FDA-approved PPAR-α agonists for the treatment of PTSD after positive clinical trials. Very few drugs are direct agonists of PPAR-α, and none have been tested for their potential effects in fear responses. However, one class of drugs, the fibrates are fibric acid derivatives that are prescribed to lower plasma lipids and triglyceride levels and are synthetic PPAR-α agonists that may be exploited in rodent models of PTSD to improve behavioral deficits.

CONCLUSIONS

Progress in assessing biomarkers to predict PTSD and its treatment response will guide the future of novel PTSD medications that may be designed to improve neurotransmission (GABA, NMDA), and neuroendocrinologic (allopregnanolone biosynthesis) and anti-inflammatory (PPAR-α) responses. Research supports precision medicine for PTSD designed to stimulate neurosteroidogenesis after assessing in subpopulations of PTSD patients a downregulation of allopregnanolone biosynthesis. This can be achieved by acting at neurosteroidogenic targets or by mimicking allopregnanolone's function (e.g., analogs). Several neuronal targets to enhance steroidogenesis have recently been discovered and these include the endocannabinoid target PPAR-α. The crosstalk between the endocannabinoid system and the biosynthesis of neurosteroids, involving their targeted receptors or the biosynthetic enzymes promises to provide unique bio-signatures for stress-induced disorders.

Collectively, advances in the field suggest biomarker-based diagnosis and treatments for PTSD that encompass the neurosteroid and endocannabinoid systems may not be a far reach and these may provide a pivotal complement to the current practice of assessing the disorder based on self-reported symptoms and psychiatrist assessments.

AUTHOR CONTRIBUTIONS

The author confirms being the sole contributor of this work and approved it for publication.

ACKNOWLEDGMENTS

The Author wishes to thank Mr. Dario Aspesi for graphic design. This study was supported by the United States Department of Defense Grant W81XWH-15-1-0521 and Veteran Affairs Grant VA241-15-D-0041 (to GP).

REFERENCES

1. Adamczyk, P., Gołda, A., McCreary, A. C., Filip, M., and Przegalinski, E. (2008). Activation of endocannabinoid transmission induces antidepressant-like effects in rats. *J. Physiol. Pharmacol.* 59, 217–228.
2. Agis-Balboa, R. C., Guidotti, A., and Pinna, G. (2014). Allopregnanolone biosynthesis is downregulated in the prefrontal cortex/Brodmann's area 9 (BA9) of depressed patients. *Psychopharmacology* 231, 3569–3580. doi: 10.1007/s00213-014-3567-5
3. Agís-Balboa, R. C., Pinna, G., Zhubi, A., Maloku, E., Veldic, M., Costa, E. (2006). Characterization of brain neurons that express enzymes mediating neurosteroid biosynthesis. *Proc. Natl. Acad. Sci. U.S.A.* 103, 14602–14607. doi: 10.1073/pnas.0606544103
4. Agís-Balboa, R. C., Pinna, G., Pibiri, F., Kadriu, B., Costa, E., and Guidotti, A. (2007). Down-regulation of neurosteroid biosynthesis in corticolimbic circuits mediates social isolation-induced behavior in mice. *Proc. Natl. Acad. Sci. U.S.A.* 104, 18736–18741. doi: 10.1073/pnas.0709419104
5. Altomare, G., and Capella, G. L. (2002). Depression circumstantially related to the administration of finasteride for androgenetic alopecia. *J. Dermatol.* 29, 665–669. doi: 10.1111/j.1346-8138.2002.tb00200.x
6. Belelli, D., and Lambert, J. J. (2005). Neurosteroids: endogenous regulators of the GABA(A) receptor. *Nat. Rev. Neurosci.* 6, 565–575. doi: 10.1038/nrn1703
7. Bernardy, N. C., and Friedman, M. J. (2017). Pharmacological management of posttraumatic stress disorders. *Curr. Opin. Psychol.* 14, 116–121. doi: 10.1016/j.copsyc.2017.01.003
8. Borovska, J., Vyklicky, V., Stastna, E., Kapras, V., Slavikova, B., Horak, M., et al. (2012). Access of inhibitory neurosteroids to the NMDA receptor. *Br. J. Pharmacol.* 166, 1069–1083. doi: 10.1111/j.1476-5381.2011.01816.x
9. Brewin, C. R., Cloitre, M., Hyland, P., Shevlin, M., Maercker, A., and Bryant, R. A. (2017). A review of current evidence regarding the ICD-11 proposals for diagnosing PTSD and complex PTSD. *Clin. Psychol. Rev.* 58, 1–15. doi: 10.1016/j.cpr.2017.09.001
10. Brown, N., Kerby, J., Bonnert, T. P., Whiting, P. J., and Wafford, K. A. (2002). Pharmacological characterization of a novel cell line expressing human alpha(4)beta(3)delta GABA(A) receptors. *Br. J. Pharmacol.* 136, 965–974. doi: 10.1038/sj.bjp.0704795
11. Caruso, D. (2015). Patients treated for male pattern hair with finasteride show, after discontinuation of the drug, altered levels of neuroactive steroids in cerebrospinal fluid and plasma. *J. Steroid Biochem. Mol. Biol.* 146, 74–79. doi: 10.1016/j.jsbmb.2014.03.012
12. Chhatwal, J. P., Davis, M., Maguschak, K. A., and Ressler, K. J. (2005). Enhancing cannabinoid neurotransmission augments the extinction of conditioned fear. *Neuropsychopharmacology* 30, 516–524. doi: 10.1038/sj.npp.1300655
13. D'Agostino, G. (2007). Acute intracerebroventricular administration of palmitoylethanolamide, an endogenous peroxisome proliferator-activated receptor-alpha agonist, modulates carrageenan-induced paw edema in mice. *J. Pharmacol. Exp. Ther.* 322, 1137–1143. doi: 10.1124/jpet.107.123265
14. D'Agostino, G., La Rana, G., Russo, R., Sasso, O., Iacono, A., Esposito, E., et al., (2009). Central administration of palmitoylethanolamide reduces hyperalgesia in mice via inhibition of NF-κB nuclear signalling in dorsal root ganglia. *Eur. J. Pharmacol.* 613, 54–59. doi: 10.1016/j.ejphar.2009.04.022
15. Dichtel, L. E., Lawson, E. A., Schorr, M., Meenaghan, E., Paskal, M. L., Eddy, K. T., et al. (2018). Neuroactive steroids and affective symptoms in women across the weight spectrum. *Neuropsychopharmacology.* doi: 10.1038/npp.2017.269
16. Dlugos, A. (2012). Acute stress increases circulating anandamide and other N-acylethanolamines in healthy humans. *Neuropsychopharmacology* 37, 2416–2427. doi: 10.1038/npp.2012.100
17. Dubreucq, S., Matias, I., Cardinal, P., Häring, M., Lutz, B., Marsicano, G., et al. (2012). Genetic dissection of the role of cannabinoid type-1 receptors in the emotional consequences of repeated social stress in mice. *Neuropsychopharmacology* 37, 1885–1900. doi: 10.1038/npp.2012.36
18. Fernandes, B. S., Williams, L. M., Steiner, J., Leboyer, M., Carvalho, A. F., and Berk, M. (2017). The new field of 'precision psychiatry'. *BMC Med.* 15:80. doi: 10.1186/s12916-017-0849-x
19. Franklin, C. L., Raines, A. M., Cuccurullo, L. J., Chambliss, J. L., Maieritsch, K. P., and Tompkins, A. M. (2017). 27 ways to meet PTSD: using the PTSD-checklist for DSM-5 to examine PTSD core criteria. *Psychiatry Res.* 261, 504–507. doi: 10.1016/j.psychres.2018.01.021
20. Frye, C. A., Koonce, C. J., and Walf, A. A. (2014). Involvement of pregnane xenobiotic receptor in mating-induced allopregnanolone formation in the midbrain and hippocampus and brain-derived neurotrophic factor in the hippocampus among female rats. *Psychopharmacology (Berl).* 231, 3375–3390. doi: 10.1007/s00213-014-3569-3
21. Geuze, E., van Berckel, B. N., Lammertsma, A. A., Boellaard, R., de Kloet, C. S., and Vermetten, E. (2008). Reduced GABA-A benzodiazepine receptor binding in veterans with post-traumatic stress disorder. *Mol. Psychiatry* 13, 74–83. doi: 10.1038/sj.mp.4002054
22. Ghazizadeh-Hashemi, M. (2018). Palmitoylethanolamide as adjunctive therapy in major depressive disorder: a double-blind, randomized and placebo-controlled trial. *J. Affect. Disord.* 232, 127–133. doi: 10.1016/j.jad.2018.02.057
23. Golden, R. N., Nemeroff, C. B., McSorley, P., Pitts, C. D., and Dubé, E. M. (2002). Efficacy and tolerability of controlled-release and immediate-release paroxetine in the treatment of depression. *J. Clin. Psychiatry* 63, 577–584. doi: 10.4088/JCP.v63n0707
24. Guidotti, A., Dong, E., Matsumoto, K., Pinna, G., Rasmusson, A. M., and Costa, E. (2001). The socially-isolated mouse: a model to study the putative role of allopregnanolone and 5alpha-dihydroprogesterone in psychiatric disorders. *Brain Res. Brain Res. Rev.* 37, 110–115. doi: 10.1016/S0165-0173(01)00129-1
25. Häring, M., Guggenhuber, S., and Lutz, B. (2012). Neuronal populations mediating the effects of endocannabinoids on stress and emotionality. *Neuroscience* 1, 145–158. doi: 10.1016/j.neuroscience.2011.12.035
26. Heyman, E. (2012). Intense exercise increases circulating endocannabinoid and BDNF levels in humans-possible implications for reward and depression. *Psychoneuroendocrinology* 37, 844–851. doi: 10.1016/j.psyneuen.2011.09.017
27. Hill, M. N., Hillard, C. J., Bambico, F. R., Patel, S., Gorzalka, B. B., and Gobbi, (2009b). The therapeutic potential of the endocannabinoid system for the development of a novel class of antidepressants. *Trends Pharmacol. Sci.* 30, 484–493. doi: 10.1016/j.tips.2009.06.006
28. Hill, M. N., Miller, G. E., Carrier, E. J., Gorzalka, B. B., and Hillard, C. J. (2009a). Circulating endocannabinoids and N-acyl ethanolamines are differentially regulated in major depression and following exposure to social stress. *Psychoneuroendocrinology* 34, 1257–1262. doi: 10.1016/j.psyneuen.2009.03.013 Hill, M. N., and Patel, S. (2013). Translational evidence for the involvement of the endocannabinoid system in stress-related psychiatric illnesses. *Biol. Mood Anxiety Disord.* 3:19. doi: 10.1186/2045-5380-3-19
29. Holman, E. A., Guijarro, A., Lim, J., and Piomelli, D. (2014). Effects of acute stress on cardiac endocannabinoids, lipogenesis, and inflammation in rats. *Psychosom. Med.* 76, 20–28. doi: 10.1097/PSY.0000000000000025
30. Hosie, A. M., Wilkins, M. E., da Silva, H. M., and Smart, T. G. (2006). Endogenous neurosteroids regulate GABAA receptors through two discrete transmembrane sites. *Nature* 444, 486–489. doi: 10.1038/nature05324
31. Jacob, W., Marsch, R., Marsicano, G., Lutz, B., and Wotjak, C. T. (2012). Cannabinoid CB1 receptor deficiency increases contextual fear memory under highly aversive conditions and long-term potentiation *in vivo*. *Neurobiol. Learn. Mem.* 98, 47–55. doi: 10.1016/j.nlm.2012.04.008
32. Kamprath, K., Marsicano, G., Tang, J., Monory, K., Bisogno, T., Di Marzo, V., et al. (2006). Cannabinoid CB1 receptor mediates fear extinction via habituation- like processes. *J. Neurosci.* 26, 6677–6686. doi: 10.1523/JNEUROSCI.0153- 06.2006
33. Kanes, S., Colquhoun, H., Gunduz-Bruce, H., Raines, S., Arnold, R., and Schacterle, A. (2017). Brexanolone (SAGE-547 injection) in post-partum depression: a randomized controlled trial. *Lancet* 390, 480–489. doi: 10.1016/S0140-6736(17)31264-3
34. Katona, I. (2009) Endocannabinoid receptors: CNS localization of the CB1 cannabinoid receptor. *Curr. Top Behav. Neurosci.* 1, 65–86. doi: 10.1007/978-3-540-88955-7_3
35. Kemp, A. H., Gordon, E., Rush, A. J., and Williams, L. M. (2008). Improving the prediction of treatment response in depression: integration of clinical, cognitive, psychophysiological, neuroimaging, and genetic measures. *CNS Spectr.* 13, 1066–1086. doi: 10.1017/S1092852900017120

36. Lo Verme, J., Fu, J., Astarita, G., La Rana, G., Russo, R., Calignano, A., et al. (2005). The nuclear receptor peroxisome proliferator-activated receptor-alpha mediates the anti-inflammatory actions of palmitoylethanolamide. *Mol. Pharmacol.* 67, 15–19. doi: 10.1124/mol.104.006353
37. Locci, A., and Pinna, G. (2017a). Neurosteroid biosynthesis down-regulation and changes in GABAA receptor subunit composition: a biomarker axis in stress-induced cognitive and emotional impairment. *Br. J. Pharmacol.* 174, 3226–3241. doi: 10.1111/bph.13843
38. Locci, A., and Pinna, G. (2017b). "Stimulation of the endocannabinoid system by PEA engages neurosteroid biosynthesis to improve anxiety and fear in a PTSD mouse model. 165.19," in *47th Annual Meeting Society for Neuroscience* (Washington, DC).
39. Locci, A., Geoffroy, P., Miesch, M., Mensah-Nyagan, A.-G., and Pinna, G. (2017). Social isolation in early versus late adolescent mice is associated with persistent behavioral deficits that can be improved by neurosteroid-based treatment. *Front. Cell Neurosci.* 11:208. doi: 10.3389/fncel.2017.00208
40. Locci, A., Khan, F., Khan, M. A., and Pinna, G. (2018). "Neurosteroid-based biomarkers and therapeutic approaches to facilitate resilience after trauma," in *Facilitating Fear After Trauma: A Translational Approach,* eds G. Pinna and T. Izumi (New York, NY: Nova Biomedical Publication).
41. Lovick, T. (2013). SSRIs and the female brain-potential for utilizing steroid- stimulating properties to treat menstrual cycle-linked dysphorias. *J. Psychopharmacol.* 27, 1180–1185. doi: 10.1177/0269881113490327
42. Malayev, A., Gibbs, T. T., and Farb, D. H. (2002). Inhibition of the NMDA response by pregnenolone sulphate reveals subtype selective modulation of NMDA receptors by sulphated steroids. *Br. J. Pharmacol.* 135, 901–909. doi: 10.1038/sj.bjp.0704543
43. Marsicano, G., Wotjak, C. T., Azad, S. C., Bisogno, T., Rammes, G., Cascio, M. G., et al. (2002). The endogenous cannabinoid system controls extinction of aversive memories. *Nature* 418, 530–534. doi: 10.1038/nature00839
44. Melis, M., Carta, G., Pistis, M., and Banni, S. (2013). Physiological role of peroxisome proliferator-activated receptors type alpha on dopamine systems. *CNS Neurol Disord Drug Targets.* 12, 70–77. doi: 10.2174/1871527311312010012
45. Moreno, S., Farioli-Vecchioli, S., and Cer,ù, M. P. (2004). Immunolocalization of peroxisome proliferator-activated receptors and retinoid X receptors in the adult rat CNS. *Neuroscience* 123, 131–145. doi: 10.1016/j.neuroscience.2003.08.064
46. Nemeroff, C. B. (2008). Understanding the pathophysiology of postpartum depression: implications for the development of novel treatments. *Neuron* 59, 185–186. doi: 10.1016/j.neuron.2008.07.015
47. Neumeister, A. (2013). The endocannabinoid system provides an avenue for evidence-based treatment development for PTSD Depress *Anxiety.* 30, 93–96. doi: 10.1002/da.22031
48. Neumeister, A., Seidel, J., Ragen, B. J., and Pietrzak, R. H. (2014). Translational evidence for a role of endocannabinoids in the etiology and treatment of posttraumatic stress disorder. *Psychoneuroendocrinology* 51, 577–584. doi: 10.1016/j.psyneuen.2014.10.012
49. Ngounou Wetie, A. G., Sokolowska, I., Wormwood, K., Beglinger, K., Michel, T. M., Thome, J., et al. (2013). Mass spectrometry for the detection of potential psychiatric biomarkers. *J. Mol. Psychiatry* 1:8. doi: 10.1186/2049-9256-1-8
50. Nin, M. S., Martinez, L. A., Thomas, R., Nelson, M., and Pinna, G. (2011b). Allopregnanolone and S-norfluoxetine decrease anxiety-like behavior in a mouse model of anxiety/depression. *Trabajos del Instituto Cajal* 83, 215–216.
51. Nin, M. S., Martinez, L. A., Pibiri, F., Nelson, M., and Pinna, G. (2011a). Neurosteroids reduce social isolation-induced behavioral deficits: a proposed link with neurosteroid-mediated upregulation of BDNF expression. *Front. Endocrin.* 2:73. doi: 10.3389/fendo.2011.00073
52. Nusser, Z., and Mody, I. (2002). Selective modulation of tonic and phasic inhibitions in dentate gyrus granule cells. *J. Neurophysiol.* 87, 2624–2628. doi: 10.1152/jn.2002.87.5.2624
53. O'Sullivan, S. E. (2007). Cannabinoids go nuclear: evidence for activation of peroxisome proliferator-activated receptors. *Br. J. Pharmacol.* 152, 576–582. doi: 10.1038/sj.bjp.0707423
54. Papini, S., Sullivan, G. M., Hien, D. A., Shvil, E., and Neria, Y. (2015). Toward a translational approach to targeting the endocannabinoid system in posttraumatic stress disorder: a critical review of preclinical research. *Biol. Psychol.* 104, 8–18. doi: 10.1016/j.biopsycho.2014.10.010
55. Park-Chung, M., Malayev, A., Purdy, R. H., Gibbs, T. T., and Farb, D. A. (1999). Sulfated and unsulfated steroids modulate gamma-aminobutyric acidA receptor function through distinct sites. *Brain Res.* 830, 72–87. doi: 10.1016/S0006-8993(99)01381-5
56. Patel, S., Carrier, E. J., Ho, W. S., Rademacher, D. J., Cunningham, S., Reddy, D. S. et al. (2005). The postmortal accumulation of brain N-arachidonylethanolamine (anandamide) is dependent upon fatty acid amide hydrolase activity. *J. Lipid Res.* 46, 342–349. doi: 10.1194/jlr.M400377-JLR200
57. Petrosino, S., and Di Marzo, V. (2017). The pharmacology of palmitoylethanolamide and first data on the therapeutic efficacy of some of its new formulations. *Br. J. Pharmacol.* 174, 1349–1365. doi: 10.1111/bph. 13580
58. Pibiri, F., Nelson, M., Guidotti, A., Costa, E., and Pinna, G. (2008). Decreased corticolimbic allopregnanolone expression during social isolation enhances contextual fear: a model relevant for posttraumatic stress disorder. *Proc. Natl. Acad. Sci. U.S.A.* 105, 5567–5572. doi: 10.1073/pnas.0801853105
59. Pineles, S. L., Nillni, Y. I., Pinna, G., Irvine, J., Webb, A., Hall, A., et al. (2018). PTSD in women is associated with a block in conversion of progesterone to the GABAergic neurosteroids allopregnanolone and pregnanolone: confirmed in plasma. *Psychoneuroendocrinology* 93, 133–141. doi: 10.1016/j.psyneuen.2018.04.024
60. Pinna, G. (2013). Targeting neurosteroidogenesis as therapy for PTSD. *Front. Pharmacol.* 4:166. doi: 10.3389/fphar.2013.00166
61. Pinna, G. (2015). "The Neurosteroidogenic Action of Fluoxetine Unveils the Mechanism for the Anxiolytic Property of SSRIs," in *Fluoxetine: Pharmacology, Mechanisms of Action and Potential Side Effects, Pharmacology - Research, Safety Testing and Regulation Series,* ed G. Pinna (New York, NY: Nova Biomedical Publication).
62. Pinna, G., Agis-Balboa, R. C., Pibiri, F., Nelson, M., Guidotti, A., and Costa, E. (2008). Neurosteroid biosynthesis regulates sexually dimorphic fear and aggressive behavior in mice. *Neurochem. Res.* 33, 1990–2007. doi: 10.1007/s11064-008-9718-5
63. Pinna, G., Agis-Balboa, R. C., Zhubi, A., Matsumoto, K., Grayson, D. R., Costa, E., et al. (2006). Imidazenil and diazepam increase locomotor activity in mice exposed to protracted social isolation. *Proc. Natl. Acad. Sci. U.S.A.* 103, 4275–4280. doi: 10.1073/pnas.0600329103
64. Pinna, G., and Izumi, T. (2018). "Biomarkers for resilience after trauma: a translational approach," in *Preface Facilitating Fear After Trauma: A Translational Approach,* eds G. Pinna and T. Izumi (New York, NY: Nova Biomedical Publication).
65. Pinna, G., and Rasmusson, A. (2014). Ganaxolone improves behavioral deficits in a mouse model of post-traumatic stress disorder. *Front. Cell. Neurosci.* 8:256. doi: 10.3389/fncel.2014.00256
66. Pinna, G., and Rasmusson, A. M. (2012). Upregulation of neurosteroid biosynthesis as a pharmacological strategy to improve behavioral deficits in a putative mouse model of PTSD. *J. Neuroendocrinol.* 24, 102–116. doi: 10.1111/j.1365-2826.2011.02234.x
67. Pinna, G., Dong, E., Matsumoto, K., Costa, E., and Guidotti, A. (2003). In socially isolated mice, the reversal of brain allopregnanolone down-regulation mediates the anti-aggressive action of fluoxetine. *Proc. Natl. Acad. Sci. U.S.A.* 100, 2035–2040. doi: 10.1073/pnas.0337642100
68. Pinna, G., Uzunova, V., Matsumoto, K., Puia, G., Mienville, J. M., Costa, E., et al. (2000). Brain allopregnanolone regulates the potency of the GABA(A) receptor agonist muscimol. *Neuropharmacology* 39, 440–448. doi: 10.1016/S0028-3908(99)00149-5
69. Pistis, M., and Melis, M. (2010). From surface to nuclear receptors: the endocannabinoid family extends its assets. *Curr. Med. Chem.* 17, 1450–1467. doi: 10.2174/092986710790980014
70. Qiu, Z. K., Zhang, G. H., He, J. L., Ma, J. C., Zeng, J., Shen, D., et al. (2015). Free and Easy Wanderer Plus (FEWP) improves behavioral deficits in an animal model of post-traumatic stress disorder by stimulating allopregnanolone biosynthesis. *Neurosci. Lett.* 602, 162–166. doi: 10.1016/j.neulet.2015. 06.055
71. Rasmusson, A. M., King, M., Gregor, K., Scioli-Salter, E., Pineles, S., Valovski, I., et al. (2016). "Sex differences in the enzyme site at which GABAergic neuroactive steroid synthesis is blocked in PTSD: implications for targeting of PTSD therapeutics," in *Symposium: Sex Specificity in Posttraumatic Stress Disorder: From Biological Mechanisms to Treatment*

Response, eds F. K. Chair and J. T. Discussant (Dallas, TX: 32nd Annual Meeting, International Society for Traumatic Stress Studies).

72. Rasmusson, A. M., King, M., Gregor, K., Scioli-Salter, E., Pineles, S., Valovski, I., et al. (2018). GABAergic neurosteroids in cerebrospinal fluid are negatively associated with PTSD severity in men. *Biol. Psychiatry* 83, S15–S16. doi: 10.1016/j.biopsych.2018.02.055
73. Rasmusson, A. M., Marx, C. E., Pineles, S. L., Locci, A., Scioli-Salter, E. R., Nillni, Y. I., et al. (2017). Neuroactive steroids and PTSD treatment. *Neurosci. Lett.* 649, 156–163. doi: 10.1016/j.neulet.2017.01.054
74. Rasmusson, A. M., Pinna, G., Paliwal, P., Weisman, D., Gottschalk, C., Charney, D., et al. (2006). Decreased cerebrospinal fluid allopregnanolone levels in women with posttraumatic stress disorder. *Biol. Psychiatry* 60, 704–713. doi: 10.1016/j.biopsych.2006.03.026
75. Raso, G. M., Esposito, E., Vitiello, S., Iacono, A., Santoro, A., D'Agostino, G., et al. (2011). Palmitoylethanolamide stimulation induces allopregnanolone synthesis in C6 Cells and primary astrocytes: involvement of peroxisome-proliferator activated receptor-α. *J. Neuroendocrinol.* 23, 591–600. doi: 10.1111/j.1365-2826.2011.02152.x
76. Reich, C. G., Mohammadi, M. H., and Alger, B. E. (2008). Endocannabinoid modulation of fear responses: learning and state-dependent performance effects. *J. Psychopharmacol.* 22, 769–777. doi: 10.1177/0269881107083999
77. Riebe, C. J., and Wotjak, C. T. (2011). Endocannabinoids and stress. *Stress* 14, 384–397. doi: 10.3109/10253890.2011.586753
78. Romeo, E., Ströhle, A., Spalletta, G., di Michele, F., Hermann, B., Holsboer, F., et al. (1998). Effects of antidepressant treatment on neuroactive steroids in major depression. *Am. J. Psychiatry* 155, 910–913. doi: 10.1176/ajp.155. 7.910
79. Ruehle, S., Rey, A. A., Remmer, F., and Lutz, B. (2012). The endocannabinoid system in anxiety, fear memory and habituation. *J. Psychopharmacol.* 26, 23–39. doi: 10.1177/0269881111408958
80. Rush, A. J., Bernstein, I. H., Trivedi, M. H., Carmody, T. J., Wisniewski, S., Mundt, J. C., et al. (2006). An evaluation of the quick inventory of depressive symptomatology and the hamilton rating scale for depression: a sequenced treatment alternatives to relieve depression trial report. *Biol. Psychiatry* 59, 493–501. doi: 10.1016/j.biopsych.2005.08.022
81. Sasso, O., La Rana, G., Vitiello, S., Russo, R., D'Agostino, G., Iacono, A., et al. (2010). Palmitoylethanolamide modulates pentobarbital-evoked hypnotic effect in mice: involvement of allopregnanolone biosynthesis. *Eur. Neuropsychopharmacol.* 20, 195–206. doi: 10.1016/j.euroneuro.2009.09.003
82. Sasso, O., Russo, R., Vitiello, S., Raso, G. M., D'Agostino, G., Iacono, A., et al. (2012). Implication of allopregnanolone in the antinociceptive effect of N-palmitoylethanolamide in acute or persistent pain. *Pain* 153, 33–41. doi: 10.1016/j.pain.2011.08.010
83. Schüle, C., Nothdurfter, C., and Rupprecht, R. (2014). The role of allopregnanolone in depression and anxiety. *Prog. Neurobiol.* 113, 79–87. doi: 10.1016/j.pneurobio.2013.09.003
84. Shin, L. M., Rauch, S. L., and Pitman, R. K. (2006). Amygdala, medial prefrontal cortex, and hippocampal function in PTSD. *Ann. N.Y. Acad. Sci.* 1071, 67–79. doi: 10.1196/annals.1364.007
85. Shu, H. J., Bracamontes, J., Taylor, A., Wu, K., Eaton, M. M., Akk, G., et al. (2012). Characteristics of concatemeric GABA(A) receptors containing α4/δ subunits expressed in Xenopus oocytes. *Br. J. Pharmacol.* 165, 2228–2243. doi: 10.1111/j.1476-5381.2011.01690.x
86. Smith, C. C., Gibbs, T. T., and Farb, D. H. (2014). Pregnenolone sulfate as a modulator of synaptic plasticity. *Psychopharmacology (Berl)* 231, 3537–3556. doi: 10.1007/s00213-014-3643-x
87. Stell, B. M., Brickley, S. G., Tang, C. Y., Farrant, M., and Mody, I. (2003). Neuroactive steroids reduce neuronal excitability by selectively enhancing tonic inhibition mediated by delta subunit-containing GABAA receptors. *Proc. Natl. Acad. Sci. U.S.A.* 100, 14439–14444. doi: 10.1073/pnas.2435457100
88. Thiemann, G., van der Stelt, M., Petrosino, S., Molleman, A., Di Marzo, V., and Hasenöhrl, R. U. (2008). The role of the CB1 cannabinoid receptor and its endogenous ligands, anandamide and 2-arachidonoylglycerol, in amphetamine-induced behavioural sensitization. *Behav. Brain Res.* 187, 289–296. doi: 10.1016/j.bbr.2007.09.022
89. Trivisano, M., Lucchi, C., Rustichelli, C., Terracciano, A., Cusmai, R., Ubertini, G. M., et al. (2017). Reduced steroidogenesis in patients with PCDH19-female limited epilepsy. *Epilepsia* 58, e91–e95. doi: 10.1111/epi.13772
90. Umathe, S. N., Manna, S. S., and Jain, N. S. (2011). Involvment of endocannabinoids in antidepressant and anti-compulsive effect of fluoxetine in mice. *Behav. Brain. Res.* 223, 125–134. doi: 10.1016/j.bbr.2011.04.031
91. Uzunov, D. P., Cooper, T. B., Costa, E., and Guidotti, A. (1996). Fluoxetine-elicited changes in brain neurosteroid content measured by negative ion mass fragmentography. *Proc. Natl. Acad. Sci. U.S.A.* 93, 12599–12604. doi: 10.1073/pnas.93.22.12599
92. Uzunova, V., Sheline, Y., Davis, J. M., Rasmusson, A., Uzunov, D. P., Costa, E., et al. (1998). Increase in the cerebrospinal fluid content of neurosteroids in patients with unipolar major depression who are receiving fluoxetine or fluvoxamine. *Proc. Natl. Acad. Sci. U.S.A.* 95, 3239–3244. doi: 10.1073/pnas.95. 6.3239
93. van Broekhoven, F., and Verkes, R. J. (2003). Neurosteroids in depression: a review. *Psychopharmacology* 165, 97–110. doi: 10.1007/s00213-002-1257-1
94. Viveros, M. P., Marco, E. M., and File, S. E. (2005). Endocannabinoid system and stress and anxiety responses. *Pharmacol. Biochem. Behav.* 81, 331–342. doi: 10.1016/j.pbb.2005.01.029
95. Vyklicky, V., Smejkalova, T., Krausova, B., Balik, A., Korinek, M., Borovska, J., et al. (2016). Preferential Inhibition of tonically over phasically activated NMDA receptors by pregnane derivatives. *J. Neurosci.* 36, 2161–2175. doi: 10.1523/JNEUROSCI.3181-15.2016
96. Welk, B., McArthur, E., Ordon, M., Anderson, K. K., Hayward, J., and Dixon, S. (2017). Association of suicidality and expression with 5α-reductase inhibitors. *JAMA Int. Med.* 177, 683–691. doi: 10.1001/jamainternmed.2017.0089
97. Wilker, S., Pfeiffer, A., Elbert, T., Ovuga, E., Karabatsiakis, A., Krumbholz, A., et al. (2016). Endocannabinoid concentrations in hair are associated with PTSD symptom severity. *Psychoneuroendocrinology* 67, 198–206. doi: 10.1016/j.psyneuen.2016.02.010
98. Wohlfarth, K. M., Bianchi, M. T., and Macdonald, R. L. (2002). Enhanced neurosteroid potentiation of ternary GABA(A) receptors containing the delta subunit. *J. Neurosci.* 22, 1541–1549. doi: 10.1523/JNEUROSCI.22-05-01541.2002
99. Zorumski, C. F., Paul, S. M., Izumi, Y., Covey, D. F., and Mennerick, S. (2013). Neurosteroids, stress and depression: potential therapeutic opportunities. *Neurosci. Biobehav. Rev.* 37, 109–122. doi: 10.1016/j.neubiorev.2012.10.005

7

On the Role of Testosterone in Anxiety-Like Behavior Across Life in Experimental Rodents

*Emese Domonkos [1], Július Hodosy [1,2], Daniela Ostatníková [2] and Peter Celec [1,3,4]**

[1] *Faculty of Medicine, Institute of Molecular Biomedicine, Comenius University, Bratislava, Slovakia,* [2] *Faculty of Medicine, Institute of Physiology, Comenius University, Bratislava, Slovakia,* [3] *Faculty of Medicine, Institute of Pathophysiology, Comenius University, Bratislava, Slovakia,* [4] *Department of Molecular Biology, Faculty of Natural Sciences, Comenius University, Bratislava, Slovakia*

Correspondence:
Peter Celec
petercelec@gmail.com

Testosterone affects brain functions and might explain some of the observed behavioral sex differences. Animal models may help in elucidating the possible involvement of sex hormones in these sex differences. The effects of testosterone have been intensively investigated, especially in anxiety models. Numerous experiments have brought inconsistent results with either anxiolytic or anxiogenic effects. Besides methodological variations, contradictory findings might be explained by the divergent metabolism of testosterone and its recognition by neurons during prenatal and postnatal development. Gonadectomy and subsequent supplementation have been used to study the role of sex hormones. However, the variable duration of hypogonadism might affect the outcomes and the effect of long-term androgen deficiency is understudied. Testosterone can be metabolized to dihydrotestosterone strengthening the androgen signaling, but also to estradiol converting the androgen to estrogen activity. Moreover, some metabolites of testosterone can modulate γ-aminobutyric acid and serotonergic neurotransmission. Here we review the currently available experimental data in experimental rodents on the effects of testosterone on anxiety during development. Based on the experimental results, females are generally less anxious than males from puberty to middle-age. The anxiety-like behavior of females and males is likely influenced by early organizational effects, but might be modified by activational effects of testosterone and its metabolites. The effects of sex hormones leading to anxiogenesis or anxiolysis depend on factors affecting hormonal status including age. The biological and several technical issues make the study of effects of testosterone on anxiety very complex and should be taken into account when interpreting experimental results.

Keywords: anxiety-like behavior, perinatal, adolescence, puberty, aging

INTRODUCTION

Besides depression, anxiety disorders, including generalized anxiety disorder, panic disorder, phobias, social anxiety disorder, separation anxiety disorder, obsessive-compulsive disorder and post-traumatic stress disorder, are the most common of all mental disorders (1). According to a survey performed in 2010, 14% of the population in Europe suffers from an anxiety disorder each year (2). The prevalence rate of anxiety disorders is influenced by various factors, including gender (3).

It is known that sex hormones affect brain morphology as well as brain functions. Based on the sex differences in prevalence of anxiety disorders in human, the role of sex hormones has been intensively investigated. A large body of animal experiments has brought contradictory results showing either anxiolytic or anxiogenic effects of testosterone (4, 5). These inconsistent findings might be due to differences in organizational and activational actions of testosterone affecting the neuronal circuits during prenatal and postnatal development. Therefore, in the present paper, the currently available experimental data on the sex differences in anxiety-like behavior and the potential role of testosterone affecting these differences across different period of life are reviewed.

SEX DIFFERENCES IN ANXIETY-LIKE BEHAVIOR IN RODENT MODELS

Anxiety is interconnected with behavioral and brain functions such as fear response. In clinical practice, anxiety is considered to be a consequence of overestimated response to threat in uncertain situations associated with prolonged hyper-vigilance and hyper-arousal (6). In neuropsychiatric studies, rodents are the most commonly used animal models (7). While in humans, anxiety might be assessed by self-report questionnaire, in rodents anxiety is evaluated based on temporary behavioral responses to various threatening stimuli. Therefore the translational value of such evaluation is disputable. On the other hand, animal experiments are crucial to elucidate causality behind observed associations. Although mice and rats may differ in some behavioral traits, the behavioral tests assessing anxiety in rodents are based on their common innate avoidance of certain conditions, such as bright illuminations (8) or open space (9–11). Therefore the most of the anxiety tests are suitable for both, mice and rats (7). In anxiety assessment it should be also considered that anxiety is associated with other behavioral phenotypes, such as aggression and violence (12–19). These exhibit sex differences and positive correlations with testosterone concentration (20, 21). Furthermore, anxiety-related behavior assessed in experimental rodents is often related to their cognitive performance, which might be affected by sex hormones (22, 23) and dependent on androgen signaling (24).

It should be noted that some behavioral traits, including anxiety, might be influenced by estrous cycle in females. It has been shown that female rat in proestrus display more explorative behavior in a novel environment and less freezing behavior following shock in defensive burying test, they spent more time in the open arm of the elevated plus maze and interact longer with an unfamiliar social partner in comparison to males but also to females during other phases of the estrous cycle (25). Although, to cover whole estrous cycle, females in the experiments are often selected for each stages and a heterogeneous group is used, but it leads to high inter-individual variability (26–28). Therefore, the assessment of sex differences in anxiety behavior is problematic.

Women are twice more likely to experience anxiety as men (26). However, it seems that sex differences in the behavioral stress responses mostly point to the opposite direction. Despite of the evidence suggesting the effect of hormonal fluctuation, the behavior of the females is often generalized without considering the estrous cycle, especially in the earlier experiments investigating sex differences. Such results show that adult female rats move in the open field more than males (29), while male rats display more freezing behavior and defecation, longer-lasting grooming reaction, less rearing as well as less time spent in the center zone of the arena (28). Females, mice as well as rats, make more entries into the open arms and spent greater time in open arms of the elevated plus maze, interact more with a same-sex social partner in a novel environment and bury fewer marbles than males (27, 28, 30, 31). On the contrary, in the Vogel conflict test, male rats seems to be less anxious than females indicated by more licking of the drinking spout during the punish period (30). In time spent in the bright chamber of the light-dark box, contradictory results have been found. In some experiments, females show higher anxiety than males (32), in other experiments, the opposite sex difference was proved (33), while the lack of sex differences is published rarely (27). It should be noted that sex differences in experimental animals in anxiety-like behavior might depend on many factors, such as strain (34) or breeding condition (32), and other sources of inter-individual variability are likely not identified yet (35). The sex differences in frequently used behavioral tests for anxiety changing with age, as well as the short- and long-term consequences of testosterone deprivation or exposure in males in different periods of life are illustrated in **Figure 1**.

THE ROLE OF TESTOSTERONE IN ANXIETY-LIKE BEHAVIOR OF RODENTS ACROSS DIFFERENT LIFE PERIODS

The sexually dimorphic behaviors related to anxiety can be influenced by both, organizational and activational effects of gonadal hormones. Organization of the neuronal circuits by testosterone and/or its metabolites predetermines the behavioral responses to the activational effects of sex hormones later in life. Besides the sensitive period of early—prenatal and perinatal development (15, 27), increasing amount of evidence supports the hypothesis that pubertal hormones (re)organize the brain and determine a variety of adult behaviors during adolescence (36, 37) or outside of the classic critical periods of neurodevelopment (38). An overview of the results of some experiments investigating sex differences and the role of testosterone in anxiety-like behavior, with particular regard to the age of animals with hormone manipulation and analysis of the outcomes, is provided in **Table 1**.

PRENATAL AND NEONATAL PERIOD

Early development is a critical period for brain formation and also for its modulation by sex hormones contributing to sexual dimorphism. Prenatal exposure to testosterone excess is associated with impaired neural development and mental

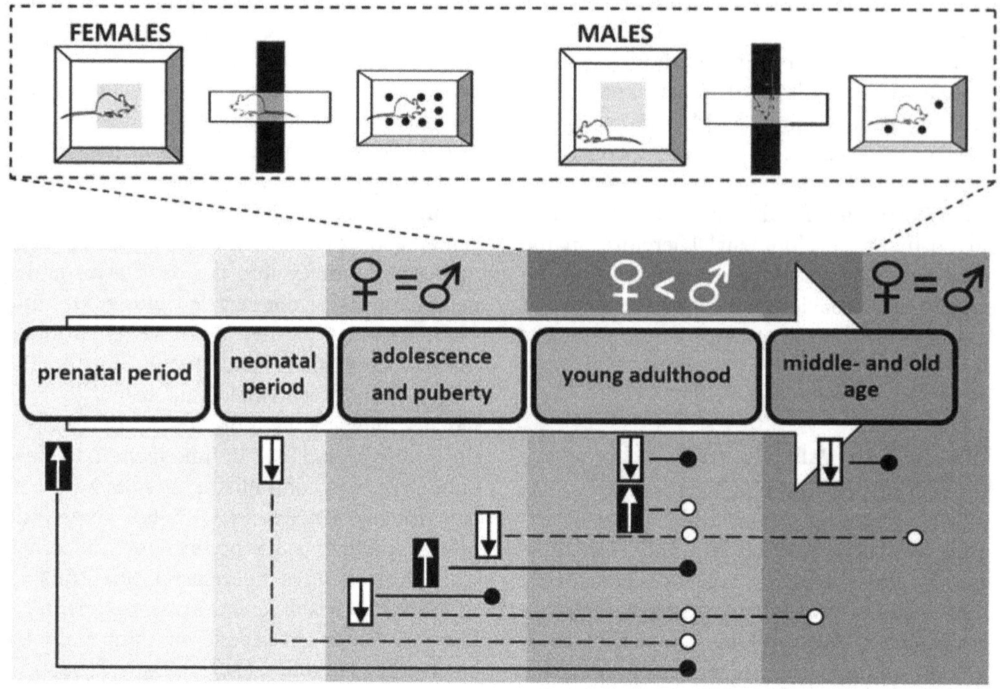

FIGURE 1 | Sex differences in anxiety-like behavior assessed using the open field, elevated plus maze and marble-burying tests. The consequences of testosterone exposure and deprivation in males are shown across the life. ↑ - testosterone exposure; ↓ - testosterone deprivation; ○ - anxiolytic effect; ● - anxiogenic effect.

functions (44, 45). Offspring of women with polycystic ovary syndrome is exposed to high concentration of androgens *in utero*. As shown in a rat model, maternal hypergonadism may result in increased risk for developing anxiety disorder in offspring, especially in female offspring (39). Inhibition of testosterone aromatization to estradiol in pregnant dams may induce increased defecation and freezing in the open field, as well as decreased number of hangings from and time spent on the open arms, pointing out an increased emotionality and anxiety in both, female and male offspring (28, 46). Accordingly, exposure to high concentration of testosterone during prenatal development leads to anxiogenesis in the adulthood, and females seems to be more sensitive to this effect of prenatal testosterone.

In addition to prenatal, also perinatal exposure to testosterone may predetermine anxiety-related behavior later during life. As found in adult rats and mice, testosterone injected on the day of birth or neonatal ovariectomy can masculinize anxiety-related behavior of females increasing the number of the marbles buried (27) and decreasing the time spent on the open arms (47). On contrary, adult male rats, castrated on the day of birth have a higher locomotor activity in the open arena, spent more time in the center zone, in the light chamber, in the open arms, and exhibit a higher number of novel object visits than their sham operated counterparts (40, 48). These results suggest that the absence of estrogens in females and testosterone in males during the perinatal period restrain the normal differentiation of gender-specific adult anxiety responses to the particular stimuli.

ADOLESCENCE

Puberty is a restricted period in adolescence characterized by a rapid elevation of circulating sex hormones accompanied by reproductive maturation. Adolescence, as the age between childhood and adulthood, represents a sensitive period in neurodevelopment as well. Numerous evidence proves that the remodeling of the adolescent brain occurs under the influence of sex hormones (36, 37). A large body of animal experiments has shown that sex differences in several anxiety tests arise from the organizational effects of testosterone at peri-pubertal age. In rats, male gonadectomy, either at puberty onset or shortly thereafter, results in lower anxiety in the open area, the behavioral response typical for females (29). Similar effects of pre-pubertal castration were found in the elevated plus maze and light-dark box, where adult male rats that had been gonadectomized prior to puberty exhibit a higher frequency of head-dipping and more time spent in the open arms or in the light part of the light-dark box (33). Environment-related social anxiety in males is organized also by pubertal sex hormones, where the aromatization of testosterone seems to be critical (49). In addition, middle- (12-months old) as well as old-aged male rats (30-months old) that have been castrated before puberty onset or at late adolescent age, respectively, display lower or similar anxiety in comparison to intact aged-matched females in a test-specific manner (41, 42). Pre-pubertal gonadectomy has anxiogenic consequences in male mice in the elevated plus maze, but anxiolytic effect in female mice in the marble-burying test (26). On the other side, testosterone exposure and social experience during adolescence

TABLE 1 | Overview of some experimental results on the effect of testosterone on anxiety-like behavior in regard to age at hormone manipulation.

References	Species/Gender	Age at intervention	Intervention	Age at anxiety examination	Anxiety examination	Outcome
PRE- UND PERINATAL PERIOD						
(39)	Rat (Wistar) Females and males	Prenatal period (GD 15–19)	Prenatal androgen exposure (PNA): pregnant dams administered with testosterone (0.5 mg/kg/d)	Young adulthood (PND 53-59)	Elevated plus maze	PNA offspring, particularly females, showed anxiety-like behavior
(28)	Rat (Wistar) Females and males	Prenatal period (GD 15–20)	Prenatal inhibition of testosterone aromatization: pregnant dams administered with 1,4,6-androstatriene-3.17-dione (ATD; aromatase inhibitor, 5 mg/rat)	Adolescence and young adulthood (1 and 3 months)	Open field, elevated cross maze	Gender differences: females were more active, less anxious and emotional than males at 3 months prenatal ATD resulted in increases in anxiety and emotionality, which in males depended on the age of examination
(27)	Mice (129:C57BL/6J) Females and males	Perinatal period (day of birth)	Testosterone injected in females (100 µg/pup)	Young adulthood (PND 67–78)	Marble-burying test, light-dark box	Gender differences: females were less anxious than males in marble-burying single injection of testosterone masculinized female anxiety-related behavior in marble-burying test
(40)	Rat (Long Evans) Males	Perinatal period (day of birth)	Gonadectomy	Young adulthood (ca. PND 120)	Open field, novel object exposure, light-dark box, elevated plus maze	Neonatal gonadectomy had anxiolytic effect in adult rats
PERIPUBERTAL AGE						
(26)	Mice (C57BL/6N) Females and males	Pre-pubertal age (PND 24-25)	Gonadectomy	Before puberty (PND 24) and late puberty (PND 40-47)	Elevated plus maze, open field, marble-burying test	Gender differences: in late adolescence males were less anxious than females, these gender differences were not found prior puberty or in young adulthood males as well as females showed an increase in anxiety-like behavior in marble-burying test from pre-pubertal to late-pubertal age; pre-pubertal gonadectomy had anxiogenic effect in males, but anxiolytic effect in females at late-pubertal age
(27)	Mice (129:C57BL/6J) Females and males	Pre-pubertal age (PND 28)	Ovariectomy + testosterone capsules implanted in females (3 mm/mouse)	Young adulthood (PND 67-78)	Marble-burying test, light-dark box	Testosterone treatment masculinized female anxiety-related behavior in marble-burying test
(41)	Rats (Lewis) Females and males	Pre-pubertal age (PND 29-31)	Gonadectomy in males	Middle-age (from 12 months)	Open field, light-dark box, elevated plus maze, PhenoTyper cage	Gender differences: females were less anxious than males in most of the conducted tests long-term androgen deficiency decreased sex differences (anxiolytic effect in males);
(33)	Rat (Lister hooded) Females and males	pre-pubertal age (PND 33-34) and post-pubertal age (PND 58-59)	Gonadectomy in males	Young adulthood (PND 101–110)	Elevated plus maze, light-dark box, open field	Gender differences: at PND 95–96, intact males were more anxious than intact females in light-dark box pre-pubertally castrated males displayed less anxious behavior than post-pubertally castrated males
(42)	Rats (Wistar) Females and males	Post-pubertal age (PND 47)	Gonadectomy in males	Old-age (30 months)	Open field, light-dark box, elevated plus maze, PhenoTyper cage	No gender differences were found in anxiety-related behavior at old age except the light-dark box (anxiolytic effects) gonadectomy had no effect on anxiety in males

(Continued)

TABLE 1 | Continued

References	Species/Gender	Age at intervention	Intervention	Age at anxiety examination	Anxiety examination	Outcome
MIDDLE- AND OLD AGE						
(22)	Rats (Fisher) Males	Young adulthood (4 months), middle-age (13 months) and old-age (24 months)	Gonadectomy + testosterone capsules implanted (10 mm/rat) in gonadally intact male rats: testosterone (1 mg/kg) 3α-diol (1 mg/kg)	Young adulthood (4 months), middle-age (13 months) and old-age (24 months)	Defensive freezing	13- and 24-months old rats displayed more freezing than 4-months old rats; gonadectomy in 4-months old rats, but not in 13- and 24-months old rats, increased freezing, which was reversed by chronic testosterone supplementation; a single injection of 3α-diol, but not testosterone, had anxiolytic effect regardless of the age
(41)	Rats (Lewis) Males	Middle-age (from 12 months)	In pre-pubertally gonadectomized rats: single injection of testosterone (1 mg/kg) single injection of estradiol (100 μg/kg) 2-week estradiol treatment (10μg/kg)	Middle-age (from 12 months)	Elevated plus maze	None of the treatment affected anxiety-related behavior in gonadectomized male rats
(23)	Mice (C57/B6) Males	Old-age (24 months)	Testosterone, 3α-diol or estradiol injected in aged intact mice (1 mg/kg)	Old-age (24 months)	Open field, light-dark box, elevated plus maze, zero maze, mirror chamber, Vogel conflict test	In gonadally intact aged testosterone and 3α-diol had anxiolytic effects in all of the conducted tests, while estradiol had anxiolytic effects in open field, light-dark box and mirror chamber only
(43)	Rats (Fisher) Females and males	Old-age (20 months)	Exposure to chronic restraint stress for 21 days	Old-age (21.5 months)	Open field, novel object exposure	Gender differences: males were generally more anxious than females stress increased male and decreased female anxiety-related behaviors, and had no effect on testosterone concentration

equally increase anxiety-like behavior, as shown in adult male hamsters (50). In females rats, single testosterone administration at the day of birth (organizational effect) as well as continual testosterone exposure from the puberty onset (activational effect) increases activity in marble-burying test of anxiety-like behavior, abolishing sex differences in adulthood (27). Furthermore, while in 1-month-old intact rats no sex differences were found in anxiety-like behavior, testing at 3 months of age revealed clear sex differences in reaction to the environmental novelty, females being more active and less anxious than males in the open field and in the elevated plus maze (28). Interestingly, in late adolescence, male mice spent more time on open arms than females. However, this sex difference in open-arm time is not present prior to puberty onset and does not persist into young adulthood (26).

ADULTHOOD

Most published experiments examine the role of testosterone in anxiety-like behavior and the underlying mechanisms in young adult animals. Unlike the anxiolytic effect of peri-pubertal castration, castration of adult males is frequently associated with increased anxiety-like behavior in a battery of behavioral tests, such as open field, elevated plus maze, and defensive-burying test (51–58). However, in some experiments in rats, no effect of adult gonadectomy was found (29, 33). Presumably, the different time interval between hormone deprivation and behavioral examination among the studies may result in these differences. The short-term effect of gonadectomy has been investigated in a large number of experiments, while the effects of the long-term hypogonadism are understudied.

The anxiogenic effect of adult castration might be reversed by hormone supplementation (52, 54, 59–63). The anxiolytic-like effect of testosterone has been revealed in gonadally intact healthy animals, as well (64–66). However, testosterone can be either reduced by 5α-reductase to the more potent androgen dihydrotestosterone, or aromatized by aromatase to estradiol converting the androgen to estrogen activity. In brain, dihydrotestosterone can be further metabolized to 5α-androstane-3α,17β-diol (3α-diol) and to 5α-androstane-3β,17β-diol (3β-diol), neuroactive steroids possessing neuromodulatory activity (67). One of the most cited study investigating the rapid effects of testosterone on anxiety-like behavior in mice has suggested that the anxiolytic effect of testosterone is mediated by its 5α-reduced metabolites (64). Likewise, it has been proved that administration of 3α-diol decreases anxiety-like behavior in male rats (52, 59, 60, 63) as well as in female rats (68), while inhibition of testosterone metabolism to 3α-diol increases anxiety in male rats (62). Similar to effect of hormone administration, sexual experience and the exposure of intact male rats or mice to female subjects may decrease anxiety-like behavior associated with increased concentration of testosterone in plasma and hippocampus, as well as increased hypothalamic testosterone and 3α-diol concentration (64, 69). On the other hand, estradiol (61) and another metabolite of testosterone, androsterone (70), may cause anxiolysis, as well. Fernández-Guasti and Martínez-Mota (54) have shown that repeated administration of testosterone, but not a single injection of testosterone, nor treatment with 3α-diol or androsterone produced anxiolysis in male gonadectomized rats (54). According to published data, the manifestation of the anxiolytic-like effect of testosterone or its metabolites is highly dependent on dose and duration of treatment (54, 58, 64, 65, 71).

Due to its complex metabolism, the effects of testosterone might be mediated through different mechanisms of action. Testosterone and dihydrotestosterone are ligands of the androgen receptor. The latter binds with a greater affinity to the receptor and activates gene transcription resulting in an increased androgen activity (72). The role of androgen signaling in the regulation of anxiety-related behavior was demonstrated by administration of the androgen receptor antagonist flutamide (52, 54, 66), but also using the animal model of testicular feminization mutation (73–76) and androgen receptor knockout mice (77). In addition, it has been shown that some selective androgen receptor modulators may exert neuroprotective effects (78) and may affect some behavioral and brain functions (79–83). However, experimental studies examining their effects on anxiety important for the deeper understanding of the association between testosterone and anxiety, but potentially also for therapeutic applications are lacking. Testosterone can exert its effects also via estrogen receptors following aromatization of testosterone to estradiol, as well as by conversion of dihydrotestosterone to 3α-diol and 3β-diol (23, 71). Furthermore, it was shown that testosterone may modulate γ-aminobutyric acid (GABA)-stimulated chloride influx (84). This might be due to the fact that 3α-diol and androsterone can bind to $GABA_A$/benzodiazepine receptor. Unlike to $GABA_C$ receptor, which seems not to be involved in the regulation of anxiety by testosterone (85), inhibition of $GABA_A$ receptor by bicucculine or picrotoxin (64), as well as by flumazenil (70) diminishes the anxiolytic effect of testosterone metabolites. In females, inhibition of $GABA_A$ and ERβ receptor diminishes the anxiolytic effect of testosterone, but not when aromatase is inhibited. Thus, the anxiolytic effect of testosterone might be mediated by its reduced metabolites via $GABA_A$ with participation of ERβ (86). On the other side, using βER-knockout mice, it has been shown that the anxiolytic effect of testosterone metabolites mediated by the $GABA_A$ receptor may be not as robust as via activation of ERβ receptor (70). In addition, it was shown that testosterone can regulate serotonin neurotransmission. Gonadectomy results in decreased expression of 5-HT_{2A} serotonergic receptors in hippocampus, testosterone replacement enhances 5-HT_{2A} expression accompanied by reduced anxiety (58). On the contrary, inhibition of 5-HT_{1A} receptor increases efficacy of testosterone treatment leading to enhanced anxiolytic-like effect (53). As shown by observation of inter-individual differences, anxious animals display higher expression of tryptophan hydroxylase—an enzyme involved in serotonin synthesis, and higher concentration of serotonin in amygdala than their non-anxious counterparts (35). Interestingly, while in gonadally intact rats, anxiety-like behavior positively correlates with the expression of tryptophan hydroxylase, this association is abolished by gonadectomy. As serotonin depletion diminishes anxiety level in anxious individuals, it also reverses the anxiogenic effect of gonadectomy (57).

AGING

Aging is associated with a progressive decline of circulating testosterone resulting from decreased function of the hypothalamo-pituitary-gonadal axis. Unlike menopause in women, andropuase in men is a long-lasting process. The age-related hypogonadism in men is considered to cause some of the senescence symptoms, including anxiety (87). This has been proved in rats. While gonadectomy in young adulthood and, partially, at middle-age induces anxiety, this effect is less apparent in aged rats (22). On the other hand, in a genetic mouse model of aging, no association was found between low testosterone and anxiety (88). It should be considered that andropause is via negative feedback associated with increased concentration of luteinizing hormone. In adult female rats, agonist of gonadotropin-releasing hormone triptorelin, which inhibits luteinizing hormone release, alone as well as in combination with estradiol treatment reduces gonadectomy-induced anxiety (89). Further experiments are needed to examine the impact of luteinizing hormone modulation on anxiety in aging males.

In our laboratory, sex differences in anxiety-like behavior of middle-aged (12-months old) rats have been shown. Aging females were less anxious than aging males in a battery of behavioral tests (41). Similarly, male rats at older age (21-months old) have proved to be generally more anxious than females. In addition, stress in males increased, while in females it decreased anxiety-like behavior (43). However, we have shown that at very old age (30-months old) female and male rats do not differ any more in anxiety-like behavior in elevated plus maze and light-dark box, or in open-field ambulation, except rearing behavior (42). These results suggest that the causal role of endogenous testosterone in anxiety-related behavior at is doubtful at least in aging animals. However, it should be considered that the anxiety-like behavior in these rats might be biased by age-related decline in locomotor activity (90). Presumably, the sex differences, observed in young and middle-aged animals, result from the organizational effect of testosterone occurring at early development and puberty. These differences, however, do not persist into the old age, which can be caused by age-related cognitive and affective decline.

There is some evidence suggesting the anti-anxiety properties of exogenous testosterone as well as its metabolites, 3α-diol and estradiol, in old gonadally intact rats (23, 91) or in rats gonadectomized at old age (22). On contrary, we have demonstrated that neither single administration of testosterone or estradiol, nor short-term treatment with estradiol affect anxiety-like behavior in middle-aged rats, when they suffer from long-term hypogonadism initiated before puberty onset (41). Therefore, it seems to be possible that the length of testosterone deficiency as well as the age of animals might determine the activational effect of supplemented hormones on anxiety-like behavior. Furthermore, the age, dose and duration of hormone replacement therapy as well as their interactions were shown to influence the action of testosterone leading to either anxiolysis or anxiogenesis (91).

CONCLUSION

Sex differences in anxiety-like behavior origin from organizational effect and might be modified by activational effect of sex hormones. There are critical periods across life that are crucial in organization of neuronal circuits and pre-programming the activational effect of testosterone on anxiety-like behavior. According to the current experimental studies, testosterone exposure during brain development predetermines higher anxiety in males. Furthermore, the absence of testosterone during the activation of neuronal circuits involved in anxiety results in anxiogenesis, as well. Although it seems that testosterone might have anxiolytic effect in adult males following short-term androgen deficiency, the impact of testosterone on anxiety-related behavior following long-term hypogonadal condition is understudied, mainly in aged animals, and needs further examinations. Based on the experimental results, age is a crucial factor that modulates the effect of both, endogenous and exogenous sex hormones. Thus, studying the expression of the various androgen receptors in different brain regions during development will be important to understand the contradictory findings from different experiments. Testosterone exposure or even deficiency in critical periods of development may have long-lasting consequences persisting into middle- or old age. This should be considered when interpreting experimental results and potentially hormonal treatments in human patients.

AUTHOR CONTRIBUTIONS

ED drafted the manuscript, prepared the table and the figure. JH corrected the draft. DO corrected the draft. PC designed the review and corrected the draft. All authors approved the final version of the manuscript.

FUNDING

The authors are supported by Slovak research and development agency (grant number APVV-15-0045).

REFERENCES

1. Kendrick T, Pilling S. Common mental health disorders — identification and pathways to care: NICE clinical guideline. *Br J Gen Pract.* (2012) 62:47–9. doi: 10.3399/bjgp12X616481
2. Wittchen HU, Jacobi F, Rehm J, Gustavsson A, Svensson M, Jönsson B, et al. The size and burden of mental disorders and other disorders of the brain in Europe 2010. *Eur Neuropsychopharmacol.* (2011) 21:655–79. doi: 10.1016/j.euroneuro.2011.07.018
3. Alonso J, Angermeyer MC, Bernert S, Bruffaerts R, Brugha TS, Bryson H, et al. Prevalence of mental disorders in Europe: results from the European Study

of the Epidemiology of Mental Disorders (ESEMeD) project. *Acta Psychiatr Scand.* (2004) 109:21–7. doi: 10.1111/j.1600-0047.2004.00327.x
4. Celec P, Ostatníková D, Hodosy J. On the effects of testosterone on brain behavioral functions. *Front. Neurosci.* (2015) 9:12. doi: 10.3389/fnins.2015.00012
5. McHenry J, Carrier N, Hull E, Kabbaj M. Sex differences in anxiety and depression: role of testosterone. *Front Neuroendocrinol.* (2014) 35:42–57. doi: 10.1016/j.yfrne.2013.09.001
6. Sylvers P, Lilienfeld SO, LaPrairie JL. Differences between trait fear and trait anxiety: Implications for psychopathology. *Clin Psychol Rev.* (2011) 31:122–37. doi: 10.1016/j.cpr.2010.08.004
7. Padurariu M, Antioch I, Balmus I, Ciobica A, El-lethey HS. Describing some behavioural animal models of anxiety and their mechanistics with special reference to oxidative stress and oxytocin relevance. *Int J Vet Sci. Med.* (2017) 5:98–104. doi: 10.1016/j.ijvsm.2017.08.003
8. Crawley J, Goodwin FK. Preliminary report of a simple animal behavior model for the anxiolytic effects of benzodiazepines. *Pharmacol Biochem Behav.* (1980) 13:167–70.
9. Pellow S, Chopin P, File SE, Briley M. Validation of open : closed arm entries in an elevated plus-maze as a measure of anxiety in the rat. *J Neurosci Methods* (1985) 14:149–67. doi: 10.1016/0165-0270(85)90031-7
10. Schmitt U, Hiemke C. Combination of open field and elevated plus-maze: a suitable test battery to assess strain as well as treatment differences in rat behavior. *Prog Neuro-Psychopharmacol Biol Psychiatry* (1998) 22:1197–215. doi: 10.1016/S0278-5846(98)00051-7
11. Seibenhener ML, Wooten MC. Use of the open field maze to measure locomotor and anxiety-like behavior in mice. *J Vis Exp.* (2015) 8. doi: 10.3791/52434
12. Bacqué-Cazenave J, Cattaert D, Delbecque JP, Fossat P. Social harassment induces anxiety-like behaviour in crayfish. *Sci Rep.* (2017) 7:1–7. doi: 10.1038/srep39935
13. Birger M, Swartz M, Cohen D, Alesh Y, Grishpan C, Kotelr M. Aggression: the testosterone-serotonin link. *Isr Med Assoc J.* (2003) 5:653–8.
14. Bondar NP, Lepeshko AA, Reshetnikov VV. Effects of early-life stress on social and anxiety-like behaviors in adult mice: sex-specific effects. *Behav Neurol.* (2018) 2018:32–4. doi: 10.1155/2018/1538931
15. Dela Cruz C, Pereira OCM. Prenatal testosterone supplementation alters puberty onset, aggressive behavior, and partner preference in adult male rats. *J Physiol Sci.* (2012) 62:123–31. doi: 10.1007/s12576-011-0190-7
16. Giammanco M, Tabacchi G, Giammanco S, Di Majo D, La Guardia M. Testosterone and aggressiveness. *Med Sci Monit.* (2005) 11:RA136–45. doi: 10.5812/ijem.3661
17. Kudryavtseva NN, Bondar NP, Avgustinovich DF. Effects of repeated experience of aggression on the aggressive motivation and development of anxiety in male mice. *Neurosci Behav Physiol.* (2004) 34:721–30. doi: 10.1023/B:NEAB.0000036013.11705.25
18. Ma XC, Jiang D, Jiang WH, Wang F, Jia M, Wu J, et al. Social isolation-induced aggression potentiates anxiety and depressive-like behavior in male mice subjected to unpredictable chronic mild stress. *PLoS ONE* (2011) 6:e20955. doi: 10.1371/journal.pone.0020955
19. Neumann ID, Veenema AH, Beiderbeck DI. Aggression and anxiety: social context and neurobiological links. *Front Behav Neurosci.* (2010) 4:12. doi: 10.3389/fnbeh.2010.00012
20. Assari S, Caldwell CH, Zimmerman MA. Sex differences in the association between testosterone and violent behaviors. *Trauma Mon.* (2014) 19:26–32. doi: 10.5812/traumamon.18040
21. Harris JA, Rushton JP, Hampson E, Jackson DN. Salivary testosterone and self report aggressive and pro social personality characteristics in men and women. *AggressBehav.* (1996) 22:321–31. doi: 10.1002/(SICI)1098-2337(1996)22:5<321::AID-AB1>3.0.CO;2-M
22. Frye C, Edinger K, Lephart E, Walf A. 3alpha-androstanediol, but not testosterone, attenuates age-related decrements in cognitive, anxiety, and depressive behavior of male rats. *Front Aging Neurosci.* (2010) 2:15. doi: 10.3389/fnagi.2010.00015
23. Frye CA, Edinger K, Sumida K. Androgen administration to aged male mice increases anti-anxiety behavior and enhances cognitive performance. *Neuropsychopharmacology* (2008) 33:1049–61. doi: 10.1038/sj.npp.1301498
24. Jones BA, Watson NV. Spatial memory performance in androgen insensitive male rats. *Physiol Behav.* (2005) 85:135–41. doi: 10.1016/j.physbeh.2005.03.023
25. Frye CA, Petralia SM, Rhodes ME. Estrous cycle and sex differences in performance on anxiety tasks coincide with increases in hippocampal progesterone and 3 alpha, 5 alpha –THP. *Pharmacol Biochem Behav.* (2000). 67:587–96. doi: 10.1016/S0091-3057(00)00392-0
26. Boivin JR, Piekarski DJ, Wahlberg JK, Wilbrecht L. Age, sex, and gonadal hormones differently influence anxiety- and depression-related behavior during puberty in mice. *Psychoneuroendocrinology* (2017) 85:78–87. doi: 10.1016/j.psyneuen.2017.08.009
27. Goel N, Bale TL. Organizational and activational effects of testosterone on masculinization of female physiological and behavioral stress responses. *Endocrinology* (2008) 149:6399–405. doi: 10.1210/en.2008-0433
28. Ordyan NÉ, Pivina SG, Akulova VK. Effects of impaired testosterone metabolism during prenatal ontogenesis on the level of anxiety and behavior of rats in a novel environment. *Neurosci Behav Physiol.* (2007) 37:435–41. doi: 10.1007/s11055-007-0032-5
29. Brand T, Slob AK. Peripubertal castration of male rats, adult open field ambulation and partner preference behavior. *Behav Brain Res.* (1988) 30:111–7. doi: 10.1016/0166-4328(88)90141-6
30. Johnston AL, File SE. Sex differences in animal tests of anxiety. *Physiol Behav.* (1991) 49:245–50. doi: 10.1016/0031-9384(91)90039-Q
31. Primus RJ, Kellogg CK. Gonadal hormones during puberty organize environment-related social interaction in the male rat. *Horm Behav.* (1990) 24:311–23. doi: 10.1016/0018-506X(90)90012-M
32. Guo M, Wu CF, Liu W, Yang JY, Chen D. Sex difference in psychological behavior changes induced by long-term social isolation in mice. *Prog Neuro Psychopharmacology Biol Psychiatry* (2004) 28:115–21. doi: 10.1016/j.pnpbp.2003.09.027
33. Brown GR, Kulbarsh KD, Spencer KA, Duval C. Peri-pubertal exposure to testicular hormones organizes response to novel environments and social behaviour in adult male rats. *Horm Behav.* (2015) 73:135–41. doi: 10.1016/j.yhbeh.2015.07.003
34. Burke NN, Coppinger J, Deaver DR, Roche M, Finn DP, Kelly J. Sex differences and similarities in depressive- and anxiety-like behaviour in the Wistar-Kyoto rat. *Physiol Behav.* (2016) 167:28–34. doi: 10.1016/j.physbeh.2016.08.031
35. Näslund J, Studer E, Pettersson R, Hagsäter M, Nilsson S, Nissbrandt H, et al. Differences in anxiety-like behavior within a batch of wistar rats are associated with differences in serotonergic transmission, enhanced by acute sri administration, and abolished by serotonin depletion. *Int J Neuropsychopharmacol.* (2015) 18:1–9. doi: 10.1093/ijnp/pyv018
36. Schulz K, Molenda-Figueira H, Sisk C. Back to the future: the organizational–activational hypothesis adapted to puberty and adolescence. *Horm Behav.* (2009) 55:597–604. doi: 10.1016/j.yhbeh.2009.03.010.Back
37. Sisk CL, Zehr JL. Pubertal hormones organize the adolescent brain and behavior. *Front Neuroendocrinol.* (2005) 26:163–74. doi: 10.1016/j.yfrne.2005.10.003
38. Palanza P. Animal models of anxiety and depression: how are females different? *Neurosci Biobehav Rev.* (2001) 25:219–33. doi: 10.1016/S0149-7634(01)00010-0
39. Hu M, Richard JE, Maliqueo M, Kokosar M, Fornes R, Benrick A, et al. Maternal testosterone exposure increases anxiety-like behavior and impacts the limbic system in the offspring. *Proc Natl Acad Sci USA.* (2015) 112:201507514. doi: 10.1073/pnas.1507514112
40. Zuloaga DG, Jordan CL, Breedlove SM. The organizational role of testicular hormones and the androgen receptor in anxiety-related behaviors and sensorimotor gating in rats. *Endocrinology* (2011a) 152:1572–81. doi: 10.1210/en.2010-1016
41. Domonkos E, Borbélyová V, Csongová M, Bosý M, Kačmárová M, Ostatníková D, et al. Sex differences and sex hormones in anxiety-like behavior of aging rats. *Horm Behav.* (2017) 93:159–65. doi: 10.1016/j.yhbeh.2017.05.019
42. Borbélyová V, Domonkos E, Bábícková J, Tóthová L, Bos? M, Hodosy J, et al. No effect of testosterone on behavior in aged Wistar rats. *Aging* (2016) 8:2848–61. doi: 10.18632/aging.101096
43. Bowman RE, Maclusky NJ, Diaz SE, Zrull MC, Luine VN. Aged rats : sex differences and responses to chronic stress. *Brain Res.* (2006) 6:156–66. doi: 10.1016/j.brainres.2006.07.047

44. Baron-Cohen S, Knickmeyer RC, Belmonte MK. Sex differences in the brain: implications for explaining autism. *Science* (2005) 310:819–23. doi: 10.1126/science.1115455
45. Xu X-J, Zhang H-F, Shou X-J, Li J, Jing W-L, Zhou Y, et al. Prenatal hyperandrogenic environment induced autistic-like behavior in rat offspring. *Physiol Behav.* (2015) 138:13–20. doi: 10.1016/j.physbeh.2014.09.014
46. Pivina SG, Akulova VK, Ordyan NÉ. Characteristics of behavior and stress reactivity of the hypophyseal-adrenocortical system in rats with prenatal inhibition of testosterone metabolism. *Neurosci Behav Physiol.* (2007) 37:53–8. doi: 10.1007/s11055-007-0149-6
47. Leret ML, Molina-Holgado F, González MI. The effect of perinatal exposure to estrogens on the sexually dimorphic response to novelty. *Physiol Behav.* (1994) 55:371–3. doi: 10.1016/0031-9384(94)90148-1
48. Lucion AB, Charchat H, Pereira GA, Rasia-Filho AA. Influence of early postnatal gonadal hormones on anxiety in adult male rats. *Physiol Behav.* (1996) 60:1419–23.
49. Kellogg CK, Lundin A. Brain androgen-inducible aromatase is critical for adolescent organization of environment-specific social interaction in male rats. *Horm Behav.* (1999) 35:155–62. doi: 10.1006/hbeh.1998.1508
50. Morris JS, Weil ZM, Nelson RJ. Sexual experience and testosterone during adolescence alter adult neuronal morphology and behavior. *Horm Behav.* (2013) 64:454–60. doi: 10.1016/j.yhbeh.2013.08.001
51. Carrier N, Saland SK, Duclot F, He H, Mercer R. The anxiolytic and antidepressant-like effects of testosterone and estrogen in gonadectomized male rats. *Biol Psychiatry* (2015) 78:259–69. doi: 10.1016/j.biopsych.2014.12.024
52. Edinger KL, Frye CA. Intrahippocampal administration of an androgen receptor antagonist, flutamide, can increase anxiety-like behavior in intact and DHT-replaced male rats. *Horm Behav.* (2006) 50:216–22. doi: 10.1016/j.yhbeh.2006.03.003
53. Fedotova J, Hritcu L. Testosterone promotes anxiolytic-like behavior in gonadectomized male rats via blockade of the 5-HT1Areceptors. *Gen Comp Endocrinol.* (2017) 254:14–21. doi: 10.1016/j.ygcen.2017.09.006
54. Fernández-Guasti A, Martínez-Mota L. Anxiolytic-like actions of testosterone in the burying behavior test: Role of androgen and GABA-benzodiazepine receptors. *Psychoneuroendocrinology* (2005) 30:762–70. doi: 10.1016/j.psyneuen.2005.03.006
55. Frye CA, Seliga AM. Testosterone increases analgesia, anxiolysis, and cognitive performance of male rats. *Cogn Affect Behav Neurosci.* (2001) 1:371–81.
56. Khakpai F. The effect of opiodergic system and testosterone on anxiety behavior in gonadectomized rats. *Behav Brain Res.* (2014) 263:9–15. doi: 10.1016/j.bbr.2014.01.013
57. Näslund J, Studer E, Johansson E, Eriksson E. Effects of gonadectomy and serotonin depletion on inter-individual differences in anxiety-like behaviour in male Wistar rats. *Behav Brain Res.* (2016) 308:160–5. doi: 10.1016/j.bbr.2016.04.015
58. Nikmahzar E, Jahanshahi M, Ghaemi A, Naseri GR, Moharreri AR, Lotfinia AA. Hippocampal serotonin-2A receptor-immunoreactive neurons density increases after testosterone therapy in the gonadectomized male mice. *Anat Cell Biol.* (2016) 49:259. doi: 10.5115/acb.2016.49.4.259
59. Edinger KL, Frye CA. Testosterone's anti-anxiety and analgesic effects may be due in part to actions of its 5alpha-reduced metabolites in the hippocampus. *Psychoneuroendocrinology* (2005) 30:418–30. doi: 10.1016/j.psyneuen.2004.11.001
60. Edinger KL, Frye CA. Testosterone's analgesic, anxiolytic, and cognitive-enhancing effects may be due in part to actions of its 5alpha-reduced metabolites in the hippocampus. *Behav Neurosci.* (2004) 118:1352–64. doi: 10.1037/0735-7044.118.6.1352
61. Filova B, Malinova M, Babickova J, Tothova L, Ostatnikova D, Celec P, et al. Effects of testosterone and estradiol on anxiety and depressive-like behavior via a non-genomic pathway. *Neurosci Bull.* (2015) 31:288–96. doi: 10.1007/s12264-014-1510-8
62. Frye CA, Edinger KL. Testosterone's metabolism in the hippocampus may mediate its anti-anxiety effects in male rats. *Pharmacol Biochem Behav.* (2004) 78:473–81. doi: 10.1016/j.pbb.2004.04.019
63. Osborne DM, Edinger K, Frye CA. Chronic administration of androgens with actions at estrogen receptor beta have anti-anxiety and cognitive-enhancing effects in male rats. *Age* (2009) 31:191–8. doi: 10.1007/s11357-009-9114-3
64. Aikey JL, Nyby JG, Anmuth DM, James PJ. Testosterone rapidly reduces anxiety in male house mice (*Mus musculus*). *Horm Behav.* (2002) 42:448–60. doi: 10.1006/hbeh.2002.1838
65. Buddenberg TE, Komorowski M, Ruocco LA, Silva MA, Topic B. Attenuating effects of testosterone on depressive-like behavior in the forced swim test in healthy male rats. *Brain Res Bull.* (2009) 79:182–6. doi: 10.1016/j.brainresbull.2009.02.008
66. Hodosy J, Zelmanová D, Majzúnová M, Filová B, Malinová M, Ostatníková D, et al. The anxiolytic effect of testosterone in the rat is mediated via the androgen receptor. *Pharmacol Biochem Behav.* (2012) 102:191–5. doi: 10.1016/j.pbb.2012.04.005
67. Durdiakova J, Ostatnikova D, Celec P. Testosterone and its metabolites–modulators of brain functions. *Acta Neurobiol Exp.* (2011) 71:434–54.
68. Frye CA, Lacey EH. Posttraining androgens' enhancement of cognitive performance is temporally distinct from androgens' increases in affective behavior. *Cogn Affect Behav Neurosci.* (2001) 1:172–82. doi: 10.3758/CABN.1.2.172
69. Edinger KL, Frye CA. Sexual experience of male rats influences anxiety-like behavior and androgen levels. *Physiol Behav.* (2007) 92:443–53. doi: 10.1016/j.physbeh.2007.04.018
70. Frye CA, Koonce CJ, Edinger KL, Osborne DM, Walf AA. Androgens with activity at estrogen receptor beta have anxiolytic and cognitive-enhancing effects in male rats and mice. *Horm Behav.* (2008) 54:726–34. doi: 10.1016/j.yhbeh.2008.07.013
71. Pak TR, Chung WCJ, Lund TD, Hinds LR, Clay CM, Handa RJ. The androgen metabolite, 5α-androstane-3β, 17β-diol, is a potent modulator of estrogen receptor-beta1-mediated gene transcription in neuronal cells. *Endocrinology* (2005) 146:147–55. doi: 10.1210/en.2004-0871
72. Brinkmann AO. Molecular mechanisms of androgen action–a historical perspective. *Methods Mol Biol.* (2011) 776:3–24. doi: 10.1007/978-1-61779-243-4_1.
73. Chen CV, Brummet JL, Lonstein JS, Jordan CL, Breedlove SM. New knockout model confirms a role for androgen receptors in regulating anxiety-like behaviors and HPA response in mice. *Horm Behav.* (2014) 65:211–8. doi: 10.3851/IMP2701.Changes
74. Hamson DK, Jones BA, Csupity AS, Ali FM, Watson NV. Androgen insensitive male rats display increased anxiety-like behavior on the elevated plus maze. *Behav Brain Res.* (2014) 259:158–63. doi: 10.1016/j.bbr.2013.11.021
75. Zuloaga DG, Poort JE, Jordan CL, Breedlove SM. Male rats with the testicular feminization mutation of the androgen receptor display elevated anxiety-related behavior and corticosterone response to mild stress. *Horm Behav.* (2011) 60:380–8. doi: 10.1016/j.yhbeh.2011.07.008
76. Zuloaga DG, Morris JA, Jordan CL, Breedlove SM. Mice with the testicular feminization mutation demonstrate a role for androgen receptors in the regulation of anxiety-related behaviors and the hypothalamic-pituitary-adrenal axis. *Horm Behav.* (2008) 54:758–66. doi: 10.1016/j.yhbeh.2008.08.004
77. Chen CV, Brummet JL, Jordan CL, Breedlove SM. Down, but not out : partial elimination of androgen receptors in the male mouse brain does not affect androgenic regulation of anxiety or HPA activity (2015) 157:764–73. doi: 10.1210/en.2015-1417
78. Jayaraman A, Christensen A, Moser VA, Vest RS, Miller CP, Hattersley G, et al. Selective androgen receptor modulator RAD140 is neuroprotective in cultured neurons and kainate-lesioned male rats. *Endocrinology* (2014) 155:1398–406. doi: 10.1210/en.2013-1725
79. Akita K, Harada K, Ichihara J, Takata N, Takahashi Y, Saito K. A novel selective androgen receptor modulator, NEP28, is efficacious in muscle and brain without serious side effects on prostate. *Eur J Pharmacol.* (2013) 720:107–14. doi: 10.1016/j.ejphar.2013.10.042
80. Hengevoss J, Piechotta M, Müller D, Hanft F, Parr MK, Schänzer W, et al. Combined effects of androgen anabolic steroids and physical activity on the hypothalamic-pituitary-gonadal axis. *J Steroid Biochem Mol Biol.* (2015) 150:86–96. doi: 10.1016/j.jsbmb.2015.03.003
81. Kudwa AE, López FJ, McGivern RF, Handa RJ. A selective androgen receptor modulator enhances male-directed sexual preference, proceptive behavior,

and lordosis behavior in sexually experienced, but not sexually naive, female rats. *Endocrinology* (2010) 151:2659–68. doi: 10.1210/en.2009-1289
82. Miner JN, Chang W, Chapman MS, Finn PD, Mei HH, López FJ, et al. An orally active selective androgen receptor modulator is efficacious on bone, muscle, and sex function with reduced impact on prostate. *Endocrinology* (2007) 148:363–73. doi: 10.1210/en.2006-0793
83. Morimoto M, Amano Y, Oka M, Harada A, Fujita H, Hikichi Y, et al. Amelioration of sexual behavior and motor activity deficits in a castrated rodent model with a selective androgen receptor modulator SARM-2f. *PLoS ONE* (2017) 12:e0189480. doi: 10.1371/journal.pone.0189480
84. Bitran D, Kellogg CK, Hilvers RJ. Treatment with an anabolic-androgenic steroid affects anxiety-related behavior and alters the sensitivity of cortical GABAA receptors in the rat. *Horm Behav.* (1993) 27:568–83. doi: 10.1006/hbeh.1993.1041
85. Roohbakhsh A, Moghaddam AH, Delfan KM. Anxiolytic-like effect of testosterone in male rats: GABAC receptors are not involved. *Iran J Basic Med Sci.* (2011) 14:376–82. doi: 10.22038/ijbms.2011.5027
86. Gutiérrez-García AG, Contreras CM, Vásquez-Hernández DI, Molina-Jiménez T, Jacome-Jacome E. Testosterone reduces cumulative burying in female Wistar rats with minimal participation of estradiol. *Pharmacol Biochem Behav.* (2009) 93:406–12. doi: 10.1016/j.pbb.2009.06.002
87. Zhang XW, Liu ZH, Hu XW, Yuan YQ, Bai WJ, Wang XF, et al. Androgen replacement therapy improves psychological distress and health-related quality of life in late onset hypogonadism patients in Chinese population. *Chin. Med. J.* (2012) 125:3806–10. doi: 10.3760/cma.j.issn.0366-6999.2012.21.011
88. Egashira N, Koushi E, Okuno R, Shirakawa A, Mishima K, Iwasaki K, et al. Depression-like behavior and reduced plasma testosterone levels in the senescence-accelerated mouse. *Behav Brain Res.* (2010) 209:142–7. doi: 10.1016/j.bbr.2010.01.030
89. Arfa-Fatollahkhani P, Nahavandi A, Abtahi H, Anjidani S, Borhani S, Jameie SB, et al. The effect of luteinizing hormone reducing agent on anxiety and novel object recognition memory in gonadectomized rats. *Basic Clin Neurosci.* (2017) 8:113–20. doi: 10.18869/nirp.bcn.8.2.113
90. Hamezah HS, Durani LW, Ibrahim NF, Yanagisawa D, Kato T, Shiino A, et al. Volumetric changes in the aging rat brain and its impact on cognitive and locomotor functions. *Exp Gerontol.* (2017) 99:69–79. doi: 10.1016/j.exger.2017.09.008
91. Onaolapo OJ, Onaolapo AY, Omololu TA, Oludimu AT, Segun-busari T, Omoleke, T. Exogenous testosterone, aging, and changes in behavioral response of gonadally intact male mice. *J Exp Neurosci.* (2016) 10:59–70. doi: 10.4137/JEN.S39042.TYPE

8

Central Nervous System Involvement in ANCA-Associated Vasculitis: What Neurologists Need to Know

Yang Zheng[1], Yinxi Zhang[1], Mengting Cai[1], Nanxi Lai[2], Zhong Chen[1,2] and Meiping Ding[1*]*

[1] Department of Neurology, Second Affiliated Hospital, School of Medicine, Zhejiang University, Hangzhou, China,
[2] Department of Pharmacology, Key Laboratory of Medical Neurobiology of the Ministry of Health of China, College of Pharmaceutical Sciences, School of Medicine, Zhejiang University, Hangzhou, China

***Correspondence:**
Zhong Chen
chenzhong@zju.edu.cn
Meiping Ding
dmp-neurology@zju.edu.cn

Objective: To provide a comprehensive review of the central nervous system (CNS) involvement in anti-neutrophil cytoplasmic antibody (ANCA)-associated vasculitis (AAV), including the pathogenesis, clinical manifestations, ancillary investigations, differential diagnosis, and treatment. Particular emphasis is placed on the clinical spectrum and diagnostic testing of AAV.

Recent Findings: AAV is a pauci-immune small-vessel vasculitis characterized by neutrophil-mediated vasculitis and granulomatousis. Hypertrophic pachymeninges is the most frequent CNS presentation. Cerebrovascular events, hypophysitis, posterior reversible encephalopathy syndrome (PRES) or isolated mass lesions may occur as well. Spinal cord is rarely involved. In addition, ear, nose and throat (ENT), kidney and lung involvement often accompany or precede the CNS manifestations. Positive ANCA testing is highly suggestive of the diagnosis, with each ANCA serotype representing different groups of AAV patients. Pathological evidence is the gold standard but not necessary. Once diagnosed, prompt initiation of induction therapy, including steroid and other immunosuppressants, can greatly mitigate the disease progression.

Conclusions and Relevance: Early recognition of AAV as the underlying cause for various CNS disorders is important for neurologists. Ancillary investigations especially the ANCA testing can provide useful information for diagnosis. Future studies are needed to better delineate the clinical spectrum of CNS involvement in AAV and the utility of ANCA serotype to classify those patients.

Evidence Review: We searched Pubmed for relevant case reports, case series, original research and reviews in English published between Sep 1st, 2001 and Sep 1st, 2018. The following search terms were used alone or in various combinations: "ANCA," "proteinase 3/PR3-ANCA," "myeloperoxidase/MPO-ANCA," "ANCA-associated vasculitis," "Wegener's granulomatosis," "microscopic polyangiitis," "Central nervous system," "brain" and "spinal cord". All articles identified were full-text papers.

Keywords: anti-neutrophil cytoplasmic antibodies, vasculitis, granulomatosis with polyangiitis, microscopic polyangiitis, central nervous system

INTRODUCTION

Central nervous system (CNS) vasculitis, with its myriad and evolving presentations, always poses a great diagnostic challenge for neurologists. It occurs either as part of a systemic vasculitis, or a primary disorder restricted to the CNS (1). Anti-neutrophil cytoplasmic antibody (ANCA) - associated vasculitis (AAV), a systemic small-vessel vasculitis, is characterized by pathogenic ANCA production (1). In the clinical practice, AAV mainly includes granulomatosis with polyangiitis (GPA), microscopic polyangiitis (MPA) and eosinophilic granulomatosis with polyangiitis (EGPA) (1). Timely recognition and diagnosis of AAV is important, since the progressive disease can be dramatically mitigated by prompt use with steroid and other immunosuppressive agents.

Neurologic involvement is not uncommon in AAV throughout the disease course, ranging from 22 to 54% in patients with GPA (2–5) and 34 to 72% in those with MPA (2–4). CNS is affected in <15% of patients with AAV (5) but accounts for much of the morbidity in those patients (1–3, 7–10). However, the heterogeneous CNS symptoms in AAV may hinder early diagnosis among neurologists, causing treatment delays and disease progression, leading to relapses, or even death.

Therefore, this review aims to increase the awareness of AAV among neurologists. We mainly focus on GPA and MPA, which have distinctive features compared with EGPA (6–10). This review comprehensively illustrates the pathogenesis, CNS manifestations, ancillary investigations, and treatment algorithms warranted for AAV patients with CNS involvement. In particular, we put a special emphasis on its clinical spectrum and the utility of ACNA testing in diagnosing and subtyping those patients.

PATHOPHYSIOLOGY

A basic understanding of how pathogenic ANCAs are induced, take effect and invade the CNS helps to understand its manifestations and illuminate potential targets for treatment in AAV. Pathogenic ANCAs, targeting mainly at proteinase 3 (PR3) and myeloperoxidase (MPO) expressed by innate immune cells, are the major contributor to the pathogenesis of AAV, according to *in vitro* and *in vivo* experimental data (11). An overview of the pathophysiology is shown in **Figure 1**. Pathogenic ANCAs are induced by the interplay of multiple environmental, genetic, and immunological factors (8, 11, 15). An encounter with the antisense peptides of PR3 or MPO triggers the immunological self-amplication network (11). The antigen-recognition capability of each individual, however, is more likely genetically determined (8). In addition, the generation of pathogenic ANCAs is further facilitated by an impaired immunological regulation, as in the pathogenesis of the few treatable neurological disorders (16–19). The function of regulatory T (T_{REG}) cells and regulatory B cells with CD5 expression are suppressed, whereas the circulating effector memory T cells (T_{EM}) (20) and ANCA-producing B cells (15) are proliferated and activated.

Following the generation of pathogenic ANCAs, different pathways lead to the two major pathological changes in AAV, namely vasculitis, and granulomatosis. Neutrophils, activated by pathogenic ANCAs and fueled by the alternative complement pathway (13), play the central role. Activated neutrophils can transmigrate the vessel wall and undergo respiratory burst, degranulation, neutrophil extracellular traps (NETs), apoptosis and necrosis (14), causing disruptions of the endothelium and thus activation of the coagulation cascade, leading to fibroid necrosis at sites of vasculitic inflammation. This neutrophil-activation process is further augmented by the complement system, especially the alternative pathway, with C5a playing a key role in-between (13). By contrast, the pathogenesis of extravascular granulomatosis is less well-understood. Current thinking holds that the chronic inflammation is initiated by the acute neutrophil-mediated necrosis (21). Subsequently, defects in the cell death machinery and aberrant reaction of monocytes and macrophages contribute to the chronic inflammation and granulomatosis formation in AAV.

CNS can be affected in AAV through one of the following pathways (22, 23): (1) inflammation, obstruction or increased permeability of the small to medium-sized cerebral vessels due to systemic vasculitis; (2) infiltration or compression of granulomatous pathology from adjacent structures; (3) granulomatous lesions developing *de novo* within the CNS. Mechanisms vary according to the specific CNS structures involved. In general, extra-axial lesions involving the dura, or pituitary gland are mainly attributed to granulomatous inflammation, while parenchyma pathologies are mediated by vasculitis and breakdown of blood brain barrier (24). However, it remains unclear whether pathogenic ANCAs are produced intrathecally or from the systemic circulation and how the two ANCA serotypes contribute to different CNS manifestations.

THE MANY FACES OF AAV WITH CNS INVOLVEMENT

Epidemiology

AAV, especially GPA and MPA, is a multisystem disease. Up to 40–50% of patients have a remitting-relapsing course (7, 12). The onset of CNS flare is mostly acute or subacute, depending on the specific neurological syndrome. CNS symptoms usually present late in the disease course (5, 25). No gender predilection is observed and most patients tend to have their first CNS flare in the middle age (5, 25, 26).

Overview of Systemic AAV

It is of great help to know the accompanying systemic symptoms at the time of or prior to CNS flare. A long-term history of constitutional symptoms like fever, weight loss, fatigue and arthralgia are often suggestive of an autoimmune etiology. In addition, organs susceptible to AAV damage include ear, nose and throat (ENT), lung and kidney (6). ENT involvement for over 3 months, presenting as chronic sinusitis, otitis media, or mastoiditis, is diagnostic of AAV, (3, 7, 24). History of renal dysfunction (proteinuria, hematuria

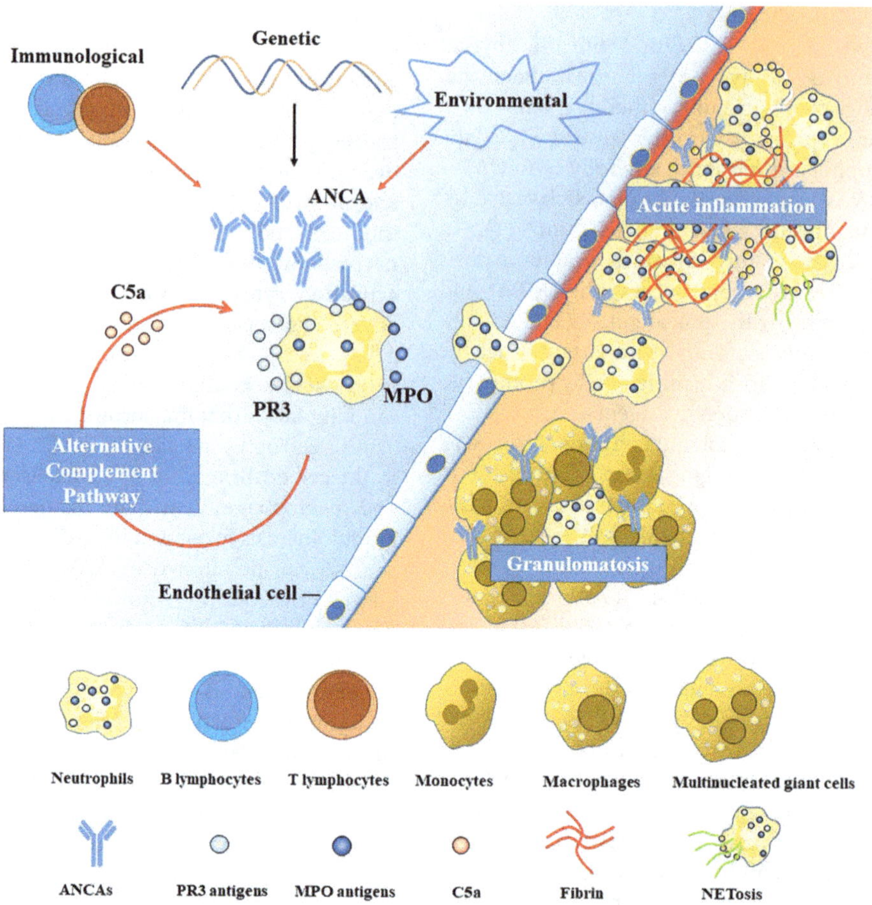

FIGURE 1 | Pathogenesis of anti-neutrophil cytoplasmic antibody (ANCA)-associated vasculitides (AAV). The left side of the diagram (with blue background) represents the blood stream and the right (with orange background) the interstitial tissue, separated by a line of endothelial cells. ANCAs are autoantibodies directed against proteins in the cytoplasmic granules of neutrophils. The two antigenic targets are proteinase 3 (PR3) and myeloperoxidase (MPO) normally expressed on the surface or inside the cytoplasm of resting neutrophils (11, 12). The interplay among genetic, environmental, and immunological factors contributes to the high membrane expression and release of PR3 and MPO, leading to the production and proliferation of pathogenic ANCAs. Primed neutrophils are activated by ANCAs and transmigrate the vessel wall, undergoing respiratory bursts, degranulation, and neutrophil extracellular traps (NETs) generation (11), which are further augmented by the alternative complement pathway (13). The neutrophil-mediated processes are the major contributor to the injury and inflammation of the endothelial cells lining the vascular wall in the early phase (14). Monocytes are subsequently recruited at sites of acute inflammation and necrosis, inducing the development of granulomatous inflammation mainly mediated by an exaggerated monocyte/macrophage reaction (11). Potential treatment targets are illustrated by red arrows in the figure, including the T-cell and B-cell dysregulation, environmental triggers (microbes, drugs), aberrant activation of alternative complement pathway and NETs. ANCA, anti-neutrophil cytoplasmic antibody; MPO, myeloperoxidase; PR3, proteinase 3; NET, neutrophil extracellular trap.

and acute kidney failure) and pulmonary problems (pulmonary nodules, infiltration, alveolar hemorrhage, chronic cough, asthma, or rarely respiratory failure) were also frequently reported. Therefore, for patients suspected with AAV, an investigation of systemic symptoms is warranted. Manifestations highly suggestive of AAV are listed in **Table 1**.

Clinical and Imaging Spectrum of CNS Involvement in AAV

CNS presentations in AAV patients vary, including headache, ischemic infarction, intracranial hemorrhage, encephalopathy (seizures, neuropsychiatric disorders, confusion, or altered consciousness), and rarely spinal cord symptoms. Those symptoms are caused by the involvement of corresponding CNS structures including the dura mater, brain parenchyma, pituitary gland, spinal cord, and leptomeninges with decreasing frequency.

Brain Parenchyma Involvement

(a) Cerebrovascular events

Ischemic infarctions and intracranial hemorrhages, though rare, can be the initial presentation of AAV and are always associated with significant morbidity (29–31). Timely recognition of AAV as the underlying cause is difficult at the first visit in the emergency room due to its rarity. Therefore, the distinguishing features of AAV-related strokes can aid in early diagnosis and improve

TABLE 1 | Systemic manifestations of AAV other than CNS#.

Involved organ	Manifestations
Constitutional symptoms	Fever, weight loss, polyarthralgia, polymyalgia, malaise, polyarthritis
Ear nose and throat (ENT)	Chronic sinusitis*, chronic otitis media*, chronic mastoiditis*, bloody nasal discharge/crusts/ulcers/granuloma*, subglottic stenosis*
Trachea and lung	Hemoptysis (due to pulmonary hemorrhage* or tracheobronchial disease), lung nodules*, cough, dyspnea, pleuritic pain
Kidney	Glomerulonephritis (especially rapidly progressive glomerulonephritis)*
Skin	Leukocytoclastic angiitis* (typically palpable purpura involving the lower extremities with focal necrosis and ulceration)
Eye and orbit	Epislceritis/scleritis*, uveitis, conjunctivitis, corneal ulceration, retinal vasculitis, optic neuropathy, retro-orbital mass or inflammation*
Peripheral nervous system	Mononeuritis multiplex*, cranial neuropathies*
Gastrointestional tract	Diarrhea, nausea, vomiting, abdominal pain, gastrointestinal hemorrhage; Elevated liver enzymes
Cardiovascular	Ischemic cardiac pain, cardiomyopathy, congestive heart failure, loss of pulses, valvular heart disease, pericarditis

#The table is adapted from previous reviews on related topics (6, 12, 27).
**Clinical features highly suggestive of AAV (6, 28).*
AAV, anti-neutrophil cytoplasmic antibody-associated vasculitis; CNS, central nervous system.

prognosis. Ischemic infarctions typically present as an isolated or multiple lesions affecting the white matter, since distal penetrating vessels are predominantly affected. Medullary and pontine infarctions were also reported in some cases (29, 30). Ischemic infarctions caused by AAV are typically resistant to antiplatelet therapy and tend to recur without proper immunosuppressive therapy. Patients with AAV are also at an increased risk of hemorrhagic transformation after reperfusion therapy of ischemic stroke (32). Hemorrhagic events occur less often. They more often affect the brain parenchyma (31), and sometimes the subarachnoid space (33). Brain Imaging findings usually correspond to the specific disease in each patient, involving ischemic, hemorrhagic lesions, or variable degrees of small-vessel diseases affecting both white and gray matter (34). Nonspecific white matter lesions with T2 hyperintensities can appear in the periventricular, subcortical regions, the basal ganglia, the mesencephalon and pons.

(b) **Posterior reversible encephalopathy syndrome**
Posterior reversible encephalopathy syndrome (PRES) is a rare yet unique complication in the late phase of AAV (35, 36). Clinically, this entity typically presents with an acute onset. Symptoms are generalized and include encephalopathy, seizures, headache and visual disturbance. Brain imaging typically reveals findings consistent with vasogenic edema, predominantly involving the bilateral parieto-occipital regions. Most patients with PRES have a dramatic improvement within days to weeks, with only the supportive therapy. Symptoms may recur when the underlying AAV is not well-controlled.

(c) **Isolated parenchymal mass lesions**
Isolated parenchymal mass lesions were very rarely reported in AAV (37–39), which often present with a discrete granuloma. Symptoms vary depending on the location of lesions, with seizures as the most frequent presentation (38). Brain magnetic resonance imaging (MRI) of isolated parenchymal granulomas reveals a well-delineated mass with a high signal intensity on T2-weighted images and enhancement on gadolinium-enhanced sequences (39).

(d) **Cognitive impairment**
Cognitive decline, though mostly subclinical and mild, can occur in AAV patients as well, with an estimated prevalence of 30% (40). According to one study of 13 AAV patients (40), the pattern of cognitive impairment, mainly affecting abstract reasoning, attention and non-verbal memory, is different from that of age-related dementia. On brain MRI, multiple white matter lesions, mainly located in the periventricular or juxtacortical areas, are often associated with the cognitive impairment (40).

Brain Meninges Involvement

Pachymeninges is affected more frequently than leptomeninges (41). The frequency of hypertrophic pachymeningitis (HP) in adult AAV ranges from 18 to 35%, depending on the methodology of studies and the sample populations selected (41, 42). Manifestations of AAV-related pachymeningitis vary depending on the location and extent of inflammation. Headache, the dominant symptom of HP, is often severe and resistant to analgesics (22). Besides, neck stiffness is not commonly seen along with headache. Cranial nerves may be compressed by the thickened dura mater and cause symptoms such as visual loss, double vision, and facial palsies. Other times the pachymeningeal inflammation may infiltrate the brain parenchyma and cause impaired consciousness and seizures (24, 42). Notably, an entity named "CNS-limited AAV" was recently proposed by Yoloseki et al. for patients with MPO-ANCA-positive hypertrophic pachymeningitis, characterized by an elderly female predominance, less severe neurological damages, and lower rates of developing into the generalized disease (24). Yet it remains unclear whether the "CNS-limited AAV" represents a novel AAV phenotype or merely a transient disease stage (24).

Imaging studies are valuable in identifying hypertrophic thickening of the dura mater, monitoring disease activity and assessing the damage of adjacent structures. On brain MRI and computed tomography (CT) scans, HP typically shows linear thickening of dura mater or a bulging mass with enhancement. Gadolinium-enhanced T1-weighted MR imaging offers certain advantages over other sequences in identifying active inflammation of the thickened dura mater with superior spatial resolution. The brain pachymeningitis can involve the tentorium cerebelli, cranial fossa, cavernous sinus, falx cerebri, or convexity with no site preference. Additionally, brain-imaging studies can help assess the potential sinonasal and orbital involvement, a common occurrence in AAV. Additionally, the damage of adjacent bone structures is prominent on brain CT scans (41, 43).

Pituitary Gland and Stalk Involvement

Inflammation of the pituitary, termed hypophysitis, is rarely seen in AAV, yet requiring special consideration (44–46). Constitutional symptoms including fatigue, lethargy, headache, weight loss, and appetite loss frequently occur. Endocrine disturbances most commonly include diabetes insipidus, and hypogonadism (45). Other less common ones include hypothyroidism, adrenocorticotropic hormone (ACTH) deficiency and growth hormone (GH) deficiency (45, 47). Pituitary stalk compression resulting from pituitary enlargement may cause hyperprolectinemia as well (22). Visual deficits result with optic chiasm compression (45). Outcome of hypopituitarism is less favorable, despite the treatment with immunosuppressive agents. Pituitary dysfunction tends to persist, even though other systemic symptoms can come to remission after standard treatment (45, 46).

Brain MRI typically shows an enlarged pituitary gland or thickened stalk with peripheral enhancement on post-contrast sequences. Other findings include the lack of posterior pituitary hyperintensity on T1 images. Normal MRI, as reported in some cases, does not exclude pituitary involvement (47).

Spinal Cord Involvement

In general, spinal cord is rarely involved in AAV (48). The three possible mechanisms underlying spinal cord involvement include necrotizing inflammation of the spinal vasculature, compression of the spinal cord by inflamed thickened meninges as well as the formation of primary spinal granulomas (48). Clinical syndromes of the spinal cord include hypertrophic pachymeningitis (41, 48) and compressive myelopathy (49). Contrast-enhanced MRI of the spinal cord is of great diagnostic value and biopsy is often warranted to confirm the diagnosis.

Non-CNS Entities Highly Associated With CNS Involvement

(a) **Cranial neuropathy**

Cranial neuropathies are rarely the only manifestation in AAV, but rather coexist with other CNS symptoms such as headache and systemic symptoms. Previous investigations found a prevalence between 2 and 10% of cranial neuropathies in patients diagnosed with GPA (50) and MPA (51, 52). Commonly affected cranial nerves in AAV include cranial nerve II–VIII (50). Bulbar palsy, by contrast, is less commonly involved (53).

(b) **Orbital disease**

Eye involvement was reported in around 30–50% of patients diagnosed with GPA (54), with the orbit and sclera most frequently involved. MPA, by contrast, rarely impair eye movement (52). Symptoms vary and typically include proptosis, diplopia, decreased vision and orbital pain (55), resulting from compressions of ocular granuloma, granulomatous inflammation of the optic nerve and ischemic optic neuropathy due to vascular occlusion (56). MR imaging and CT can help reveal mucosal and bony lesions in the orbit and rule out continuous extension.

(c) **Parasinal disease**

For patients with CNS manifestations suspected of AAV, an evaluation of paranasal sinuses is a must. Findings indicative of granulomatosis in the paranasal sinuses include a soft-tissue mass, thickening of the sinus wall, or "ground-glass" material in the lumen (34). As in orbital involvement, non-contrast CT scan has its diagnostic value in evaluating the nasal cavity, paranasal sinuses, mastoids and temporal bone, due to a better resolution of mucosal and bony pathologies compared with MRI (43). Brain MRI may also aid in the evaluation of soft tissue masses within those cavities.

Differences Between ANCA Serotypes

There is an increasing consensus that the ANCA serotype, either MPO-ANCA or PR3-ANCA, has a crucial role in AAV (12). Distinctively, previous studies revealed that the ANCA serotype represents two separate groups of patients in epidemiology, genetic background, clinical features, laboratory features as well as prognosis. We summarized the differences between MPO- and PR3-ANCA positive AAV in **Table 2**. Specifically, for AAV patients with CNS involvement, the ANCA serotype matters as well (24). Though the two serotypes tended to affect the nervous system with a similar frequency (57), they differ in the pattern and severity of CNS involvement. According to one study of patients with HP in Japan, MPO-ANCA-positive HP had an elderly female predominance, more frequently had lesions limited to the dura mater and upper airways, and was less likely to have a generalized systemic progression. On the contrary, PR3-ANCA-positive HP tended to have more severe neurological damages and a generalized disease progression (24). However, evidence remains limited to patients with HP. Extrapolation of the utility of ANCA serotype in other CNS manifestations remains to be further studied.

DIAGNOSIS

The diagnosis of CNS involvement in AAV, similar to the disease overall, requires consideration of clinical, serological, radiographic, and, when available, pathological evidence (61). In patients with established AAV, new-onset neurologic deficits with abnormal radiological and cerebrospinal fluid (CSF) findings are suggestive of CNS involvement. For patients without established underlying disease, neurologic symptoms closely compatible with CNS syndromes known to arise in AAV warrant further investigations for the systemic disease. In either case, ancillary tests are of important value in making the

TABLE 2 | Comparison of PR3- and MPO-ANCA-positive AAV.

Features	PR3-ANCA-positive AAV	MPO-ANCA-positive AAV
Pathophysiology (12, 57)	Apoptosis of endothelial cells; Release of sFlt1 by monocytes; No established mouse model	Production of intracellular oxidants; No induction of release of sFlt1 by monocytes; Pathogenicity of autoantibody proved in mouse models
Epidemiology (12, 57)	Northern Europe, America and Australia	Southern Europe and Asia
Genetic background (8, 12, 57)	HLA-DP, SERPINA1, PRTN3	HLA-DQ, CTLA4
Clinical features (12, 57–59)	More ENT involvement; Cavititating pulmonary lesions, nodules and masses; More organs involved	More often renal-limited; Fibrosing pulmonary lesions and patchy infiltrates
Pathological features (12)	Granuloma and vasculitis	Granuloma and fibrosis
Response to induction therapy (12, 60)	Better response to rituximab than cyclophosphamide	Increased risk of initial treatment failure
Long-term outcome (12)	More relapses Better prognosis	Less relapses Higher risk of long-term kidney and alveolar damage Worse prognosis

PR3, proteinase 3; MPO, myeloperoxidase; ANCA, anti-neutrophil cytoplasmic antibodies; AAV, anti-neutrophil cytoplasmic antibody-associated vasculitis; HLA, human leukocyte antigen; ENT, ear, nose and throat.

Box 1 | Investigations in AAV-related CNS involvement.

ANCA immunoassays (MPO- and PR3- ANCA testing)
CBC, CMP, CRP, ESR (to evaluate the organ functions and the state of inflammation)
Autoimmune panel, complement levels (to differentiate from other inflammatory conditions)
Endocrine panel (to evaluate the pituitary function)
Screening for HIV, hepatitis, and tuberculosis
Analysis of cerebrospinal fluid (measure inflammatory mediators and degradation proteins, assess the blood-brain barrier and exclude infection)
Chest CT
Brain imaging (CT; MRI, suggested sequences include T1/T2 weighted-imaging, FLAIR, DWI, SWI and contrast enhanced T1 sequences)
Biopsy

AAV, anti-neutrophil cytoplasmic antibody-associated vasculitis; ANCA, anti-neutrophil cytoplasmic antibodies; MPO, myeloperoxidase; PR3, proteinase 3; CBC, complete blood count; CMP, comprehensive metabolic panel; CRP, C reactive protein; ESR, erythrocyte sedimentation rate; HIV, human immunodeficiency virus; CT, computed tomography; MRI, magnetic resonance imaging; FLAIR, fluid-attenuating inversion recovery; DWI, diffusion-weighted imaging; SWI, susceptibility-weighted imaging.

diagnosis and excluding other causes of the CNS abnormalities (**Box 1**). This section describes workup that can aid in the diagnosis of AAV with CNS involvement, and with special interest, pays extra attention to the value of ANCA testing in-between.

ANCA Serology

ANCA testing is strongly recommended for patients with clinical features suggestive of AAV (**Table 1**) (6, 62). Its value lies mainly in AAV screening, and when positive, warrants further investigations for confirmative diagnosis. Positivity of the test is highly suggestive of AAV but not diagnostic by itself (6). However, the combination of ANCA positivity and certain clinical features are sufficient for AAV diagnosis, according to the widely-used classification algorithm proposed by Watts (28). A negative ANCA immunoassay, which occurs in up to half of pathologically diagnosed GPA and MPA, does not exclude AAV (6, 63). The negativity may be related to the limited sensitivity of ANCA testing, especially at the early stage of disease without systemic involvement (7). The diagnosis of AAV cannot be excluded merely based on a negative ANCA test. Therefore, biopsy of the affected organ is required for seronegative patients (6).

Regarding the testing techniques of ANCA, the most recent consensus recommended high-quality antigen-specific immunoassays for MPO- and PR3- ANCAs detection (6). ELISAs are the preferred screening methodology with a high sensitivity and specificity. Indirect immunofluorescence (IIF) for cytoplasmic ANCA (C-ANCA) and perinuclear ANCA (P-ANCA) detection is no longer prioritized as the screening test, given its large variability and poor diagnostic accuracy (6). When necessary, performing another assay or testing with another different methodology can yield higher sensitivity and specificity (6). In cases of emergency such as pulmonary-renal syndrome, rapid screening assays for ANCAs, including dot blots and biochip technology, are also available (64).

Controversy remains in the role of ANCA levels in monitoring disease activity and prediction of prognosis (63). Published studies reveal inconsistent results regarding the role of ANCA levels in predicting clinical relapse and reflecting disease activity (65–67). A meta-analysis in 2012 concluded that both a rise in ANCA and persistently positive ANCA were strongly associated with disease relapse and had a modest predictive value (66). Furthermore, results from a recent single-center study indicated that the predictive value of ANCA was only significant in renal-involved AAV, compared with those without renal involvement (68). Overall, current thinking holds that ANCA levels alone are helpful but not sufficient to determine relapse or reflect disease activity (6), and ANCA testing is not recommended to guide clinical decisions on treatment (61). Nevertheless, severe relapses are unlikely without elevated ANCA levels (69). The significance of serial monitoring remains to be proven.

Other Laboratory Investigations

A diligent workup should be ordered for patients suspected of AAV, including complete blood count (CBC), complete metabolic profile (CMP), acute phase reactants, the autoimmune panel, the endocrine panel, the complement level and investigations for potential infections. For patients with endocrine dysfunction or abnormal pituitary on MRI, levels of pituitary hormones also need to be investigated. Laboratory tests typically show elevated markers of inflammation. Leukocytosis, thrombocytosis, normochromic normocytic anemia, elevated erythrocyte sedimentation rate (ESR) and C-reactive protein (CRP) values are indicative of the diagnosis (3, 7). Kidney functions, including serum creatinine and urinalysis, are warranted for the evaluation of renal injury. Regarding the autoimmune panel, autoantibodies other than ANCAs can be present (63), including antinuclear antibodies, rheumatoid factors, IgG4, anti-glomerular basement membrane antibodies and antiphospholipid antibodies, with unknown significance (63). Lastly, for differential diagnosis, investigations for potential infections (tuberculosis, human immunodeficiency virus, hepatitis) and complement levels are also required.

Box 2 | Conditions other than AAV with positive ANCA immunoassays#.

Vasculitis of other causes
Anti-GBM disease, IgA-vasculitis*
Gastrointestinal diseases
Ulcerative colitis, Primary Sclerosing Cholangitis, Inflammatory liver disease
Systemic inflammatory conditions
IgG4-related disease, Rheumatoid arthritis, Systemic lupus erythematous
Infection
Infective endocarditis, Tuberculosis, HIV, Amoeba infection
Malignancies
Hematological neoplasia
Drugs
Hydralazine, Propylthiouracil, Levamisole, Minocycline, Cocaine.

#The box is based upon previous reviews on related topics (6, 27). Serum ANCAs should be tested according to the algorithm proposed by the 2017 consensus on testing of ANCAs (6).
*IgA-vasculitis can show positive IgA-ANCAs in the active stage of disease, but IgG-ANCAs were rarely reported (27).
AAV, anti-neutrophil cytoplasmic antibody-associated vasculitis; ANCA, anti-neutrophil cytoplasmic antibodies; GBM, glomerular basement membrane; HIV, human immunodeficiency virus.

Cerebrospinal Fluid

Lumbar puncture is warranted for suspected patients as well. CSF analysis has a high sensitivity but low specificity in the diagnosis of AAV-related CNS disease. Most had mild lymphocyte-predominant pleocytosis, elevated protein levels and normal glucose level (7, 25, 37). Therefore, a normal CSF analysis makes the diagnosis of AAV less likely. Infectious etiology and flow cytometry for atypical cancer cells should be tailored to clinical manifestations and risk factors.

Pathology

Histopathology is the gold standard for diagnosis of small vessel vasculitis. Samples can be taken from affected organs, most commonly the kidney and the skin. Lung and nasal biopsies are rarely performed, limited by the high rate of false negatives. Brain biopsies can also be taken from corresponding structures including the dura, brain parenchyma and the overlying leptomeninges. Typically two types of pathological findings have been described: (1) necrotizing vasculitis affecting small to medium vessels; (2) granulomatosis with inflammatory cell infiltration (monocytes, plasma cells, eosinophils, and polymorphonuclear leukocytes) (41). Fibrinoid necrosis and edema were also detected in some cases. In patients of HP, fibrosis of the dura mater was always present as well (24, 41). A negative yield of biopsy, however, does not exclude the diagnosis of AAV due to its segmental nature of lesions.

Differential Diagnosis

AAV must be distinguished from ANCA-positive conditions where ANCA does not exert a direct role in pathophysiology (**Box 2**). Multiple conditions other than AAV show an elevated titer of serum ANCAs. Nonetheless, ANCAs do not mediate a direct pathogenic role, but rather indicate a chronic immune response of neutrophil cell death most times (63). Compared with the mimics, a high level and affinity of ANCAs and clinical features suggestive of AAV are important clues for the correct diagnosis (6).

Differential diagnosis can be further narrowed down to entities with both similar CNS manifestations and ANCA positivity. These mainly include systemic inflammatory diseases (IgG4 related-disease, rheumatoid arthritis, systemic lupus erythematosus, Bechet syndrome), infective diseases (tuberculosis, human immunodeficiency virus) and malignancies (lymphoma).

In particular, diagnosis of AAV can be especially difficult at an early stage with only CNS presentations and a seronegative ANCA test, which may be an under-recognized common occurrence (24). Characteristics and diagnostic criteria of this entity remain to be elucidated. Differential diagnosis is therefore protean, varying according to the specific CNS manifestation of the patient. We suggest a thorough investigation of systemic involvement to exclude alternative causes including infection and malignancy. In particular, A continued monitoring of ANCA testing may be useful for those with idiopathic hypertrophic pachymeningitis (24). Most importantly, biopsy of the lesion is highly recommended in such cases to confirm the diagnosis.

TREATMENT

Treatment should be started in a timely manner for patients highly suspected of AAV, even in the absence of pathological evidence. Steroid is an essential part of therapy, with the addition of a well-chosen immunosuppressant critical to prevent relapses and achieve remission of CNS symptoms in the long run. The treatment algorithm is shown in **Figure 2**. There are two phases of treatment, namely remission-induction and remission-maintenance. The choice of regimen in each phase depends mainly on the disease stage of the

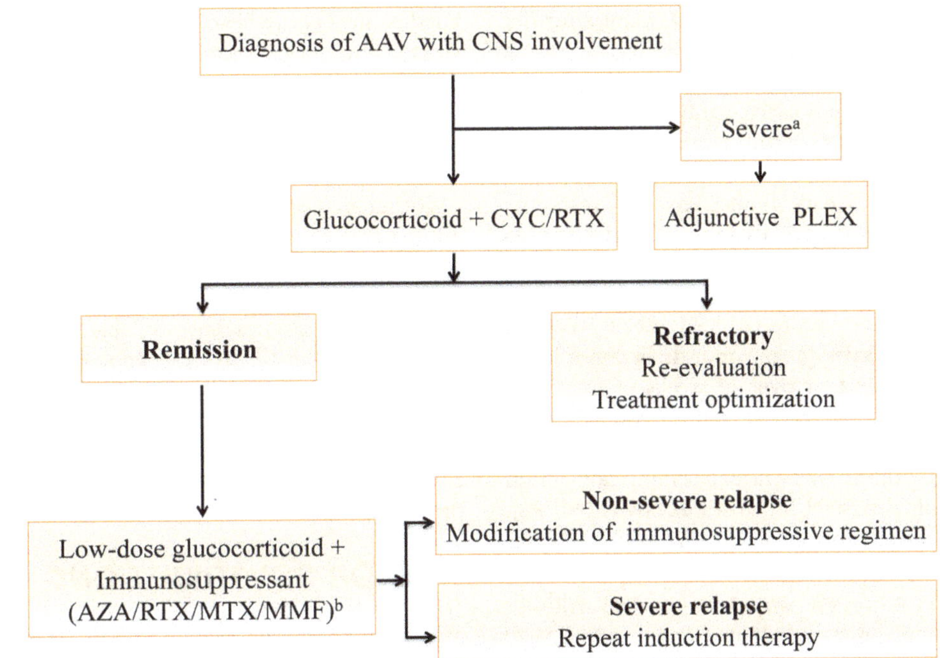

FIGURE 2 | Treatment algorithm for anti-neutrophil cytoplasmic antibody (ANCA)-associated vasculitides (AAV) with central nervous system (CNS) involvement. The algorithm is formulated and terms are defined according to the 2016 European league Against Rheumatism (EULAR)/European Renal Association-European Dialysis and Transplant Association (ERA-EDTA) recommendations (61). For AAV with CNS involvement, the remission-induction therapy mainly consists of high-dose steroids and cyclophosphamide (CYC), or rituximab (RTX) for CYC-intolerant patients. Plasma exchange should be considered for those with a serum creatine level of $\geq$500 µmol/L or diffuse alveolar hemorrhage. Once complete remission is achieved, patients should be switched to the maintenance regimen. A combination of low-dose steroid and an oral immunosuppressive agent including azathioprine (AZA), methotrexate (MTX), mycophenolate mofetil (MMF) or RTX is used for at least 24 months (61). For patients refractory to the remission-induction therapy, referral to experts for reevaluation and treatment optimization is warranted (61). Severe relapses with organ- or life-threatening conditions are treated as per new disease, while non-severe relapses are managed with modification of the previous immunosuppressive regimen (61). [a]AAV with severe renal impairment or diffuse alveolar hemorrhage; [b]Drugs are listed in order of the strength of vote. AAV, anti-neutrophil cytoplasmic antibody-associated vasculitides; ANCA, anti-neutrophil cytoplasmic antibodies; AZA, azathioprine; CNS, central nervous system; CYC, cyclophosphamide; MTX, methotrexate; MMF, mycophenolate mofetil; PLEX, plasma exchange; RTX, rituximab.

patient, as per the European Renal Association—European Dialysis and Transplant Association (ERA-EDTA) management recommendations for AAV (61). Generally, CNS involvement is regarded as an organ-threatening manifestation in AAV, especially for those with meningeal inflammation or retro-orbital disease. Remission-induction treatment for organ-threatening AAV typically consists of high-dose glucocorticoids and oral or intravenous (IV) cyclophosphamide (CYC) (1), termed CYC-based therapy. Glucocorticoids usually start with the dose of 1g intravenous methylprednisolone on 3 consecutive days, followed with 1 mg/kg daily oral corticosteroids (up to 80 mg per day), and a gradual reduction to daily dose of 7.5 to 10 mg within 3–5 months (7, 10). CYC can be given either intravenously in pulses or orally. The intravenous CYC, at a dose of 15 mg/kg (up to 1200 mg), are prescribed every 2 weeks initially and every 3 weeks from the 4th pulse. Daily oral CYC is given at a dose of 2 mg/kg/d. The CYC-based therapy is effective in 70-90% of patients (70), and the oral regimen can better prevent relapses (71). However, the daily oral regimen, compared with intravenous CYC, also poses more safety issues due to the cumulative toxicity (71, 72) including infertility, bladder hemorrhage, severe cytopenias, serious infection, and an increased risk of malignancy. Apart from the most recognized CYC-based therapy, the identification of the important role of B cells in the pathogenesis of AAV facilitated the use of rituximab (RTX) as an alternative to CYC (73). Two large randomized trials revealed RTX (375 mg/m^2, once a week for four infusions) to be equivalent to CYC in terms of efficacy and safety in remission induction for AAV among treatment-naïve patients, and likely superior for relapsing disease (74).

Once complete remission (absence of any disease activity, usually attained after 8–12 weeks of treatment) is achieved, patients should be started with maintenance therapy to prevent further relapses, which should be continued for at least 24 months (61). In the remission maintenance phase, the induction regimen is switched to a combination of low-dose glucocorticoids and an oral immunosuppressive agent such as azathioprine (AZA), methotrexate (MTX), mycophenolate mofetil (MMF), or RTX (61). AZA (2 mg/kg/day) is the most commonly used immunosuppressive agent for remission maintenance, with MTX (20–25 mg/kg/week) as a similar alternative (72). AZA, with a lower relapse rate, is generally preferred over MMF. However, the relapse rate remains as high as 40% by 2 years despite the maintenance therapy with AZA or MTX (75). RTX is a potentially safer maintenance drug with a higher efficacy (76). However, the utility and toxicity profile of RTX require further confirmation (76–80). In addition, the adjunctive use of plasma exchange (PLEX) (7 sessions over 2 weeks) in AAV patients with severe renal dysfunction and/or alveolar hemorrhage seems reasonable in the short-term, but remains elusive in the long run (81).

Another issue to tackle in AAV is the treatment response. Refractory to remission-induction treatment is defined as follows: (1) unchanged or increased disease activity after 4 weeks of treatment (2) <50% reduction in the disease score [e.g., Birmingham Vasculitis Activity Score (BVAS)] after 6 weeks of treatment (3) Presence of at least one major or three minor items on the disease activity score after over 12 weeks of treatment (61, 82). For AAV patients refractory to therapy, reevaluation and optimization of treatment, in close collaboration with experts, are recommended (61). Adjunctive intravenous immunoglobulin may help for those with persistent low disease activity (61, 83). Furthermore, relapses are not uncommon in AAV. Major relapses with organ- or life-threatening conditions are treated as per new disease, while non-severe relapses should be managed with an escalation or modification of the previous immunosuppressive regimen (61).

CONCLUSION AND FUTURE PERSPECTIVES

For neurologists, prompt diagnosis of AAV in patients with CNS presentations allows timely treatment and thus a dramatic improvement in prognosis. A myriad of CNS presentations including hypertrophic pachymeningitis, ischemic stroke, intracranial hemorrhage and pituitary dysfunction, combined with certain systemic symptoms, raise the suspicion of AAV. Further ancillary tests are required, among which ANCA testing yields a great diagnostic value. ANCA positivity strongly suggests the diagnosis of AAV but ANCA negativity does not rule out the diagnosis. Once diagnosed, early treatment with steroid and immunosuppressant is essential to prevent neurological relapses and sequelae.

Recent evidence suggests the presence of "CNS-limited AAV" as a distinct subset in AAV. Efforts to better elucidate its phenotypic features, optimal treatment and long-term outcome are an important focus of future research. Furthermore, accumulating studies suggest that PR3-ANCAs and MPO-ANCAs define distinctive conditions among patients with AAV. Whether the same rule applies to the neurological conditions in CNS-involved AAV, however, remains unknown. Continued attempts are needed to validate the utility of ANCA specificity in classifying CNS manifestations, guiding treatment decisions, and predicting prognosis.

AUTHOR CONTRIBUTIONS

YZ: contributed to data collection, conception of the work and drafting the manuscript. YxZ: conception of the work and revising the manuscript. MC: revising the manuscript and figures. NL: revising the manuscript and tables. ZC and MD: revising the manuscript and final approval of the version to be published.

FUNDING

This work was supported by the National Natural Science Foundation of China (grant numbers 81671283; 81872844).

REFERENCES

1. Jennette JC, Falk RJ, Bacon PA, Basu N, Cid MC, Ferrario F, et al. 2012 revised International Chapel Hill consensus conference nomenclature of vasculitides. *Arthritis Rheum.* (2013) 65:1–11. doi: 10.1002/art.37715
2. Sada K, Yamamura M, Harigai M, Fujii T, Dobashi H, Takasaki Y, et al. Classification and characteristics of Japanese patients with antineutrophil cytoplasmic antibody-associated vasculitis in a nationwide prospective, inception cohort study. *Arthritis Res Ther.* (2014) 16: R101. doi: 10.1186/ar4550
3. Zhang W, Zhou G, Shi Q, Zhang X, Zeng XF, Zhang FC. Clinical analysis of nervous system involvement in ANCA-associated systemic vasculitides. *Clin Exp Rheumatol.* (2009) 27(1 Suppl 52):S65–9.
4. Agard C, Mouthon L, Mahr A, Guillevin Lc. Microscopic polyangiitis and polyarteritis nodosa: how and when do they start? *Arthrit Rheum.* (2003) 49:709–15. doi: 10.1002/art.11387
5. Graf J. Central nervous system disease in antineutrophil cytoplasmic antibodies-associated vasculitis. *Rheum Dis Clin North Am.* (2017) 43:573–8. doi: 10.1016/j.rdc.2017.06.006
6. Bossuyt X, Cohen Tervaert JW, Arimura Y, Blockmans D, Flores-Suarez LF, Guillevin L, et al. Position paper: Revised 2017 international consensus on testing of ANCAs in granulomatosis with polyangiitis and microscopic polyangiitis. *Nat Rev Rheumatol.* (2017) 13:683–92. doi: 10.1038/nrrheum.2017.140
7. Kallenberg CG. Key advances in the clinical approach to ANCA-associated vasculitis. *Nat Rev Rheumatol.* (2014) 10:484–93. doi: 10.1038/nrrheum.2014.104
8. Lyons PA, Rayner TF, Trivedi S, Holle JU, Watts RA, Jayne DR, et al. Genetically distinct subsets within ANCA-associated vasculitis. *N Engl J Med.* (2012) 367:214–23. doi: 10.1056/NEJMoa1108735
9. van der Geest KSM, Brouwer E, Sanders JS, Sandovici M, Bos NA, Boots AMH, et al. Towards precision medicine in ANCA-associated vasculitis. *Rheumatology* (2018) 57:1332–9. doi: 10.1093/rheumatology/kex367
10. Sznajd J, Mukhtyar C. How to treat ANCAassociated vasculitis: practical messages from 2016 EULAR/ERAEDTA recommendations. *Pol Arch Med Wewn* (2016) 126:781–8. doi: 10.20452/pamw.3598
11. Jennette JC, Falk RJ. Pathogenesis of antineutrophil cytoplasmic autoantibody-mediated disease. *Nat Rev Rheumatol.* (2014) 10:463–73. doi: 10.1038/nrrheum.2014.103
12. Cornec D, Gall EC-L, Fervenza FC, Specks U. ANCA-associated vasculitis — clinical utility of using ANCA specificity to classify patients. *Nat Rev Rheumatol.* (2016) 12:570–9. doi: 10.1038/nrrheum.2016.123
13. Chen M, Jayne DRW, Zhao M-H. Complement in ANCA-associated vasculitis: mechanisms and implications for management. *Nat Rev Nephrol.* (2017) 13:359–67. doi: 10.1038/nrneph.2017.37
14. Soderberg D, Segelmark M. Neutrophil extracellular traps in ANCA-Associated Vasculitis. *Front Immunol.* (2016) 7:256. doi: 10.3389/fimmu.2016.00256
15. Dumoitier N, Terrier B, London J, Lofek S, Mouthon L. Implication of B lymphocytes in the pathogenesis of ANCA-associated vasculitides. *Autoimmun Rev.* (2015) 14:996–1004. doi: 10.1016/j.autrev.2015.06.008
16. Feng B, Tang Y, Chen B, Xu C, Wang Y, Dai Y, et al. Transient increase of interleukin-1beta after prolonged febrile seizures promotes

adult epileptogenesis through long-lasting upregulating endocannabinoid signaling. *Sci Rep.* (2016) 6:21931. doi: 10.1038/srep21931

17. Zhao J, Wang Y, Xu C, Liu K, Wang Y, Chen L, et al. Therapeutic potential of an anti-high mobility group box-1 monoclonal antibody in epilepsy. *Brain Behav Immun.* (2017) 64:308–19. doi: 10.1016/j.bbi.2017.02.002
18. Crisp SJ, Kullmann DM, Vincent A. Autoimmune synaptopathies. *Nat Rev Neurosci.* (2016) 17:103–17. doi: 10.1038/nrn.2015.27
19. Berlit P. Diagnosis and treatment of cerebral vasculitis. *Ther Adv Neurol Disord.* (2010) 3:29–42. doi: 10.1177/1756285609347123
20. Morgan MD, Day CJ, Piper KP, Khan N, Harper L, Moss PA, et al. Patients with Wegener's granulomatosis demonstrate a relative deficiency and functional impairment of T-regulatory cells. *Immunology* (2010) 130:64–73. doi: 10.1111/j.1365-2567.2009.03213.x
21. Petersen HJ, Smith AM. The role of the innate immune system in granulomatous disorders. *Front Immunol.* (2013) 4:120. doi: 10.3389/fimmu.2013.00120
22. Holle JU, Gross WL. Neurological involvement in Wegener's granulomatosis. *Curr Opin Rheumatol.* (2011) 23:7–11. doi: 10.1097/BOR.0b013e32834115f9
23. Drachman DA. Neurological Complications of Wegener's Granulomatosis. *Arch Neurol.* (1963) 8:145–55. doi: 10.1001/archneur.1963.00460020045003
24. Yokoseki A, Saji E, Arakawa M, Kosaka T, Hokari M, Toyoshima Y, et al. Hypertrophic pachymeningitis: significance of myeloperoxidase anti-neutrophil cytoplasmic antibody. *Brain* (2014) 137(Pt 2):520–36. doi: 10.1093/brain/awt314
25. Fragoulis GE, Lionaki S, Venetsanopoulou A, Vlachoyiannopoulos PG, Moutsopoulos HM, Tzioufas AG. Central nervous system involvement in patients with granulomatosis with polyangiitis: a single-center retrospective study. *Clin Rheumatol.* (2018) 37:737–47. doi: 10.1007/s10067-017-3835-y
26. Seror R, Mahr A, Ramanoelina J, Pagnoux C, Cohen P, Guillevin L. Central nervous system involvement in Wegener granulomatosis. *Medicine* (2006) 85:54–65. doi: 10.1097/01.md.0000200166.90373.41
27. Weiner M, Segelmark M. The clinical presentation and therapy of diseases related to anti-neutrophil cytoplasmic antibodies (ANCA). *Autoimmun Rev.* (2016) 15:978–82. doi: 10.1016/j.autrev.2016.07.016
28. Watts R, Lane S, Hanslik T, Hauser T, Hellmich B, Koldingsnes W, et al. Development and validation of a consensus methodology for the classification of the ANCA-associated vasculitides and polyarteritis nodosa for epidemiological studies. *Ann Dis.* (2006) 66:222–7. doi: 10.1136/ard.2006.054593
29. Yanagiha K, Ishii K, Ueno T, Marushima A, Tamaoka A. Medial medullary infarction caused by antineutrophil cytoplasmic antibody-related vasculitis: Case report and review of the literature. *Medicine* (2017) 96:e7722. doi: 10.1097/MD.0000000000007722
30. Chen NC, Lai PH, Fang HC, Chou KJ, Chen CL. Microscopic polyangiitis with an initial presentation of pontine infarction. *Am J Med Sci.* (2012) 344:163–5. doi: 10.1097/MAJ.0b013e3182536789
31. Iglesias E, Eleftheriou D, Mankad K, Prabhakar P, Brogan PA. Microscopic polyangiitis presenting with hemorrhagic stroke. *J Child Neurol.* (2014) 29:NP1–4. doi: 10.1177/0883073813488661
32. Ito Y, Suzuki K, Yamazaki T, Yoshizawa T, Ohkoshi N, Matsumura A. ANCA-associated vasculitis (AAV) causing bilateral cerebral infarction and subsequent intracerebral hemorrhage without renal and respiratory dysfunction. *J Neurol Sci.* (2006) 240(1–2):99–101. doi: 10.1016/j.jns.2005.07.003
33. Aratani S, Sakai Y, Tsuruoka S. A case of microscopic polyangiitis with subarachnoid hemorrhage and cardiovascular complications. *J Nippon Med Sch.* (2017) 84:251–5. doi: 10.1272/jnms.84.251
34. Abdel Razek AA, Alvarez H, Bagg S, Refaat S, Castillo M. Imaging spectrum of CNS vasculitis. *Radiographics* (2014) 34:873–94. doi: 10.1148/rg.344135028
35. Fuentes AG, Komarla A, Gomez JI. Posterior reversible encephalopathy syndrome in a patient with ANCA-associated vasculitis. *Rheumatol Int.* (2012) 32:2529–30. doi: 10.1007/s00296-010-1367-8
36. Patel UV, Patel NJ. Posterior reversible leukoencephalopathy syndrome as a presenting manifestation of p-ANCA-associated vasculitis. *BMJ Case Rep.* (2014) 2014:bcr2013202022. doi: 10.1136/bcr-2013-202022
37. De Luna G, Terrier B, Kaminsky P, Le Quellec A, Maurier F, Solans R, et al. Central nervous system involvement of granulomatosis with polyangiitis: clinical-radiological presentation distinguishes different outcomes. *Rheumatology* (2015) 54:424–32. doi: 10.1093/rheumatology/keu336
38. Spisek R, Kolouchova E, Jensovsky J, Rusina R, Fendrych P, Plas J, et al. Combined CNS and pituitary involvement as a primary manifestation of Wegener granulomatosis. *Clin Rheumatol.* (2006) 25:739–42. doi: 10.1007/s10067-005-0065-5
39. Berlis A, Petschner F, Botefur IC, Spreer J. Wegener granuloma in the fourth ventricle. *AJNR Am J Neuroradiol.* (2003) 24:523–5.
40. Mattioli F, Capra R, Rovaris M, Chiari S, Codella M, Miozzo A, et al. Frequency and patterns of subclinical cognitive impairment in patients with ANCA-associated small vessel vasculitides. *J Neurol Sci.* (2002) 195:161–6. doi: 10.1016/S0022-510X(02)00015-1
41. Yonekawa T, Murai H, Utsuki S, Matsushita T, Masaki K, Isobe N, et al. A nationwide survey of hypertrophic pachymeningitis in Japan. *J Neurol Neurosurg Psychiatry* (2013) 85:732–9. doi: 10.1136/jnnp-2013-306410
42. Choi HA, Lee MJ, Chung CS. Characteristics of hypertrophic pachymeningitis in patients with granulomatosis with polyangiitis. *J Neurol.* (2017) 264:724–32. doi: 10.1007/s00415-017-8416-0
43. Pakalniskis MG, Berg AD, Policeni BA, Gentry LR, Sato Y, Moritani T, et al. The many faces of granulomatosis with polyangiitis: a review of the head and neck imaging manifestations. *Am J Roentgenol.* (2015) 205:W619–29. doi: 10.2214/AJR.14.13864
44. Kapoor E, Cartin-Ceba R, Specks U, Leavitt J, Erickson B, Erickson D. Pituitary dysfunction in granulomatosis with polyangiitis: the mayo clinic experience. *J Clin Endocrinol Metab.* (2014) 99:3988–94. doi: 10.1210/jc.2014-1962
45. Esposito D, Trimpou P, Giugliano D, Dehlin M, Ragnarsson O. Pituitary dysfunction in granulomatosis with polyangiitis. *Pituitary* (2017) 20:594–601. doi: 10.1007/s11102-017-0811-0
46. Yong TY, Li JY. Pituitary involvement in granulomatosis with polyangiitis. *J Clin Rheumatol.* (2014) 20:123–4. doi: 10.1097/RHU.0000000000000092
47. De Parisot A, Puechal X, Langrand C, Raverot G, Gil H, Perard L, et al. Pituitary involvement in granulomatosis with polyangiitis: report of 9 patients and review of the literature. *Medicine* (2015) 94:e748. doi: 10.1097/MD.0000000000000748
48. Decker ML, Emery DJ, Smyth PS, Lu J-Q, Lacson A, Yacyshyn E. Microscopic polyangiitis with spinal cord involvement: a case report and review of the literature. *J Stroke Cereb Dis.* (2016) 25:1696–704. doi: 10.1016/j.jstrokecerebrovasdis.2016.01.034
49. Nair RP, Kongwad LI. Nontuberculous antineutrophil cytoplasmic antibody-positive pachymeningitis presenting as high cervical myelopathy. *World Neurosurg.* (2017) 107:1042 e1– 1042.e5. doi: 10.1016/j.wneu.2017.08.035
50. Soderstrom A, Revaz S, Dudler J. Cranial neuropathies in granulomatosis with polyangiitis (Wegener's): a case-based review. *Clin Rheumatol.* (2015) 34:591–6. doi: 10.1007/s10067-013-2420-2
51. Gwathmey KG, Burns TM, Collins MP, Dyck PJ. Vasculitic neuropathies. *Lancet Neurol.* (2014) 13:67–82. doi: 10.1016/S1474-4422(13)70236-9
52. Guillevin L, Durand-Gasselin B, Cevallos R, Gayraud M, Lhote F, Callard P, et al. Microscopic polyangiitis: clinical and laboratory findings in eighty-five patients. *Arthritis Rheum.* (1999) 42:421–30.
53. Nowack R, Wachtler P, Kunz J, Rasmussen N. Cranial nerve palsy in Wegener's granulomatosis–lessons from clinical cases. *J Neurol.* (2009) 256:299–304. doi: 10.1007/s00415-009-0121-1
54. Kubaisi B, Abu Samra K, Foster CS. Granulomatosis with polyangiitis (Wegener's disease): An updated review of ocular disease manifestations. *Intractable Rare Dis Res.* (2016) 5:61–9. doi: 10.5582/irdr.2016.01014
55. Papaliodis GN. Ophthalmologic manifestations of systemic vasculitis. *Curr Opin Ophthalmol.* (2017) 28:613–6. doi: 10.1097/ICU.0000000000000422
56. Vodopivec I, Lobo AM, Prasad S. Ocular inflammation in neurorheumatic disease. *Semin Neurol.* (2014) 34:444–57. doi: 10.1055/s-0034-1390393
57. Hilhorst M, van Paassen P, Tervaert JW, Limburg Renal R. Proteinase 3-ANCA Vasculitis versus Myeloperoxidase-ANCA Vasculitis. *J Am Soc Nephrol.* (2015) 26:2314–27. doi: 10.1681/ASN.2014090903
58. Lionaki S, Blyth ER, Hogan SL, Hu Y, Senior BA, Jennette CE, et al. Classification of antineutrophil cytoplasmic autoantibody vasculitides: the role of antineutrophil cytoplasmic autoantibody specificity for myeloperoxidase or proteinase 3 in disease recognition and prognosis. *Arthritis Rheum.* (2012) 64:3452–62. doi: 10.1002/art.34562

59. Mahr A, Katsahian S, Varet H, Guillevin L, Hagen EC, Hoglund P, et al. Revisiting the classification of clinical phenotypes of anti-neutrophil cytoplasmic antibody-associated vasculitis: a cluster analysis. *Ann Rheum Dis.* (2013) 72:1003–10. doi: 10.1136/annrheumdis-2012-201750
60. Unizony S, Villarreal M, Miloslavsky EM, Lu N, Merkel PA, Spiera R, et al. Clinical outcomes of treatment of anti-neutrophil cytoplasmic antibody (ANCA)-associated vasculitis based on ANCA type. *Ann Rheum Dis.* (2016) 75:1166–9. doi: 10.1136/annrheumdis-2015-208073
61. Yates M, Watts RA, Bajema IM, Cid MC, Crestani B, Hauser T, et al. EULAR/ERA-EDTA recommendations for the management of ANCA-associated vasculitis. *Ann Rheum Dis.* (2016) 75:1583–94. doi: 10.1136/annrheumdis-2016-209133
62. Basu N, Watts R, Bajema I, Baslund B, Bley T, Boers M, et al. EULAR points to consider in the development of classification and diagnostic criteria in systemic vasculitis. *Ann Rheum Dis.* (2010) 69:1744–50. doi: 10.1136/ard.2009.119032
63. Wiik AS. Autoantibodies in ANCA-associated vasculitis. *Rheum Dis Clin North Am.* (2010) 36:479–89. doi: 10.1016/j.rdc.2010.05.001
64. Csernok E, Moosig F. Current and emerging techniques for ANCA detection in vasculitis. *Nat Rev Rheumatol.* (2014) 10:494–501. doi: 10.1038/nrrheum.2014.78
65. Segelmark M, Phillips BD, Hogan SL, Falk RJ, Jennette JC. Monitoring proteinase 3 antineutrophil cytoplasmic antibodies for detection of relapses in small vessel vasculitis. *Clin Diagn Lab Immunol.* (2003) 10:769–74. doi: 10.1128/CDLI.10.5.769-774.2003
66. Tomasson G, Grayson PC, Mahr AD, Lavalley M, Merkel PA. Value of ANCA measurements during remission to predict a relapse of ANCA-associated vasculitis–a meta-analysis. *Rheumatology* (2012) 51:100–9. doi: 10.1093/rheumatology/ker280
67. Morgan MD, Szeto M, Walsh M, Jayne D, Westman K, Rasmussen N, et al. Negative anti-neutrophil cytoplasm antibody at switch to maintenance therapy is associated with a reduced risk of relapse. *Arthritis Res Ther.* (2017) 19:129. doi: 10.1186/s13075-017-1321-1
68. Kemna MJ, Damoiseaux J, Austen J, Winkens B, Peters J, van Paassen P, et al. ANCA as a predictor of relapse: useful in patients with renal involvement but not in patients with nonrenal disease. *J Am Soc Nephrol.* (2015) 26:537–42. doi: 10.1681/ASN.2013111233
69. Specks U. Accurate relapse prediction in ANCA-associated vasculitis-the search for the Holy Grail. *J Am Soc Nephrol.* (2015) 26:505–7. doi: 10.1681/ASN.2014080817
70. Jones RB, Tervaert JW, Hauser T, Luqmani R, Morgan MD, Peh CA, et al. Rituximab versus cyclophosphamide in ANCA-associated renal vasculitis. *N Engl J Med.* (2010) 363:211–20. doi: 10.1056/NEJMoa0909169
71. Harper L, Morgan MD, Walsh M, Hoglund P, Westman K, Flossmann O, et al. Pulse versus daily oral cyclophosphamide for induction of remission in ANCA-associated vasculitis: long-term follow-up. *Ann Rheum Dis.* (2012) 71:955–60. doi: 10.1136/annrheumdis-2011-200477
72. Pagnoux C, Mahr A, Hamidou MA, Boffa JJ, Ruivard M, Ducroix JP, et al. Azathioprine or Methotrexate Maintenance for ANCA-Associated Vasculitis. *N Engl J Med.* (2008) 359:2790–803. doi: 10.1056/NEJMoa0802311
73. Jennette JC, Falk RJ. B cell-mediated pathogenesis of ANCA-mediated vasculitis. *Semin Immunopathol.* (2014) 36:327–38. doi: 10.1007/s00281-014-0431-y
74. Stone JH, Merkel PA, Spiera R, Seo P, Langford CA, Hoffman GS, et al. Rituximab versus cyclophosphamide for ANCA-associated vasculitis. *N Engl J Med.* (2010) 363:221–32. doi: 10.1056/NEJMoa0909905
75. Tanna A, Pusey C. Clinical trials. Rituximab for maintenance of remission in AAV. *Nat Rev Nephrol.* (2015) 11:131–2. doi: 10.1038/nrneph.2014.254
76. Pendergraft WF, Cortazar FB, Wenger J, Murphy AP, Rhee EP, Laliberte KA, et al. Long-term maintenance therapy using rituximab-induced continuous B-cell depletion in patients with ANCA vasculitis. *Clin J Am Soc Nephrol.* (2014) 9:736–44. doi: 10.2215/CJN.07340713
77. Cartin-Ceba R, Golbin JM, Keogh KA, Peikert T, Sanchez-Menendez M, Ytterberg SR, et al. Rituximab for remission induction and maintenance in refractory granulomatosis with polyangiitis (Wegener's): ten-year experience at a single center. *Arthritis Rheum.* (2012) 64:3770–8. doi: 10.1002/art.34584
78. Rhee EP, Laliberte KA, Niles JL. Rituximab as maintenance therapy for anti-neutrophil cytoplasmic antibody-associated vasculitis. *Clin J Am Soc Nephrol.* (2010) 5:1394–400. doi: 10.2215/CJN.08821209
79. Besada E, Koldingsnes W, Nossent JC. Long-term efficacy and safety of pre-emptive maintenance therapy with rituximab in granulomatosis with polyangiitis: results from a single centre. *Rheumatology* (2013) 52:2041–7. doi: 10.1093/rheumatology/ket257
80. Guillevin L, Pagnoux C, Karras A, Khouatra C, Aumaitre O, Cohen P, et al. Rituximab versus azathioprine for maintenance in ANCA-associated vasculitis. *N Engl J Med.* (2014) 371:1771–80. doi: 10.1056/NEJMoa1404231
81. Matthew J. Koster KJW. Recent advances in understanding and treating vasculitis. *F1000Research* (2016) 5:1436. doi: 10.12688/f1000research.8403.1
82. Hellmich B, Flossmann O, Gross WL, Bacon P, Cohen-Tervaert JW, Guillevin L, et al. EULAR recommendations for conducting clinical studies and/or clinical trials in systemic vasculitis: focus on anti-neutrophil cytoplasm antibody-associated vasculitis. *Ann Rheum Dis.* (2007) 66:605–17. doi: 10.1136/ard.2006.062711
83. Fortin PM, Tejani AM, Bassett K, Musini VM. Intravenous immunoglobulin as adjuvant therapy for Wegener's granulomatosis. *Cochrane Database Syst Rev.* (2013) CD007057. doi: 10.1002/14651858.CD007057

9

Estradiol and the Development of the Cerebral Cortex: An Unexpected Role?

Matthew C. S. Denley[1], *Nicholas J. F. Gatford*[1], *Katherine J. Sellers*[1*] *and Deepak P. Srivastava*[1,2*]

[1] *Department of Basic and Clinical Neuroscience, Maurice Wohl Clinical Neuroscience Institute, London, United Kingdom,*
[2] *MRC Centre for Neurodevelopmental Disorders, King's College London, London, United Kingdom*

Correspondence:
Katherine J. Sellers
katherine.sellers@kcl.ac.uk
Deepak P. Srivastava
deepak.srivastava@kcl.ac.uk

The cerebral cortex undergoes rapid folding in an "inside-outside" manner during embryonic development resulting in the establishment of six discrete cortical layers. This unique cytoarchitecture occurs via the coordinated processes of neurogenesis and cell migration. In addition, these processes are fine-tuned by a number of extracellular cues, which exert their effects by regulating intracellular signaling pathways. Interestingly, multiple brain regions have been shown to develop in a sexually dimorphic manner. In many cases, estrogens have been demonstrated to play an integral role in mediating these sexual dimorphisms in both males and females. Indeed, 17β-estradiol, the main biologically active estrogen, plays a critical organizational role during early brain development and has been shown to be pivotal in the sexually dimorphic development and regulation of the neural circuitry underlying sex-typical and socio-aggressive behaviors in males and females. However, whether and how estrogens, and 17β-estradiol in particular, regulate the development of the cerebral cortex is less well understood. In this review, we outline the evidence that estrogens are not only present but are engaged and regulate molecular machinery required for the fine-tuning of processes central to the cortex. We discuss how estrogens are thought to regulate the function of key molecular players and signaling pathways involved in corticogenesis, and where possible, highlight if these processes are sexually dimorphic. Collectively, we hope this review highlights the need to consider how estrogens may influence the development of brain regions directly involved in the sex-typical and socio-aggressive behaviors as well as development of sexually dimorphic regions such as the cerebral cortex.

Keywords: aromatase, subventricular zone, cortical plate, neurogenesis, migration, sexual dimorphism, 17β-estradiol, brain synthesized

INTRODUCTION

The complex neuronal organization and architecture of the cerebral cortex is thought to be responsible for the higher cognitive function bestowed upon mammals. The unique anatomical compartmentalization and lamination of discrete neurons arranges into horizontal layer identifiable with specific molecular markers (Kriegstein and Parnavelas, 2006; Molyneaux et al., 2007; Greig et al., 2013). This organization is established during embryonic development, and is achieved in an "inside-outside" fashion, with the "deep" or "inner" layers developing first and the outer layers developing last. Critically, this unique cytoarchitecture is the basis by which the correct assembly of synaptic connectivity and therefore, functional cortical circuitry is established (Marín et al., 2010). Mechanistically, the inside-outside organization of the cerebral cortex is established throughout development and controlled by coordinating processes in neurogenesis, cell migration (Götz and Huttner, 2005; Taverna et al., 2014) as well as responses to extracellular cues and activation of intracellular signaling pathways (Hippenmeyer, 2014; Hansen et al., 2017). The phenotypic display of this coordination can be seen in **Figure 1**. Whilst our understanding of the molecular events that underlie these processes is ever growing, understanding the mechanisms and signals that exert influences over corticogenesis remains a major challenge. This is particularly emphasized by increasing evidence that abnormal corticogenesis may contribute to a range of neurodevelopment and psychiatric disorders (Hoerder-Suabedissen et al., 2013; Ishii et al., 2016).

BACKGROUND

Neurons forming the basic unit of nervous tissue architecture was a notion first proposed and described by Ramón y Cajal (1911). Connectivity between these units underlies the normal brain functions of neural circuitry in cognition and behavior. Therefore, understanding the developmental formation of neural circuitry is vital to understanding how these structures respond to environmental, physiological and pathological stimuli. Steroid hormones, such as estrogen, have long been the focus of research and review (Alcaraz et al., 1969; Dominique Toran-Allerand, 1976; Hammond and Rowe, 1976), and have long been suggested to be key signals orchestrating the development of sexual dimorphism of many cerebral regions. However, previous research has also indicated that estrogen can have wildly polarized effects in terms of behavior and physiology (Alcaraz et al., 1969; Gillies and McArthur, 2010). Research has also suggested that this response is due to specific estrogen receptor

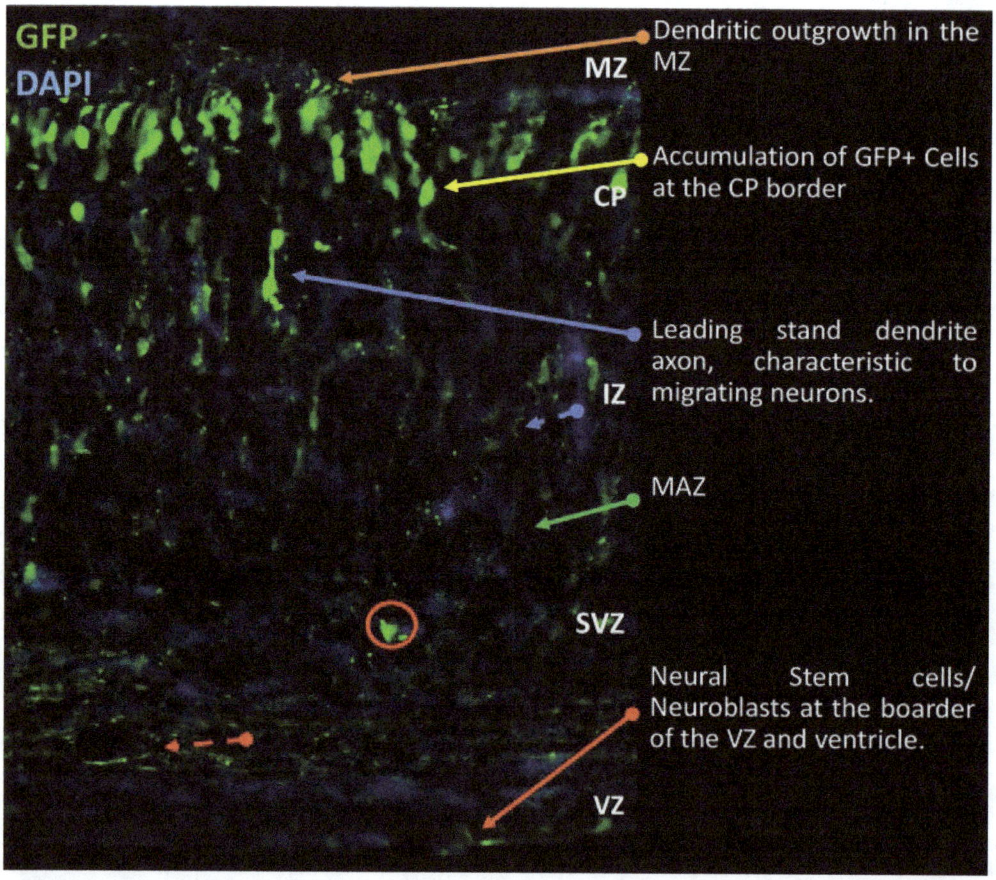

FIGURE 1 | Gross morphological schematic of sub-compartments in the developing rodent cortex. Representative image of developing cortex. Electroporation of eGFP was performed at E14.5 and brains collected at P0 as previously described (Srivastava et al., 2012a,b). The cortex is comprised of four morphologically distinct regions, the VZ, SVZ, IZ, and CP. Further to this there are the MAZ and MZ, located in the IZ and CP respectively. Located on the basal surface of the cortex proximal to the cerebral ventricles is the VZ responsible for generation of NSCs. Beyond the VZ, the SVZ contains proliferating and early differentiating neural progenitors. Between the SVZ and IZ, the MAZ is a point of accumulation of polarizing cells. After which the cells migrate through the IZ to the CP where terminal translocation takes place. This brief outline is the general schematic throughout development of the cortex. Cells migrate to the outmost layer and continually build on top of each other in a sedimentary manner. IZ, intermediate zone; MAZ, multipolar cell accumulation zone; CP, cortical plate; GFP, green fluorescence; NSCs, Neural Stem Cells; VZ, ventricular zone; SVZ, subventricular zone; MZ, marginal zone.

subtypes and, thus, is dependent on the expression in the discrete location of the receptor in specific brain regions. However, response to estrogen exposure is impeccably sensitive to factors such as dose and stage of life cycle (Katzenellenbogen et al., 2000; Sánchez-Criado et al., 2004). More recent research has made attempts to explain the mechanism behind sexual dimorphic response to estrogen during development (Grassi D. et al., 2012; Grassi S. et al., 2012; Liu et al., 2017). Interest in estrogen is further emphasized because of the demonstrable ability to affect psychiatric and neurodegenerative disorders (Arevalo et al., 2011; Srivastava et al., 2013b; Gobinath et al., 2017). This includes, for example, Autism Spectrum Disorder, which shows a strong male bias (Werling and Geschwind, 2013) and therefore suggests sexual dimorphic underlying physiology (Adhya et al., 2018).

Sexual dimorphism is not wholly dependent on the action and mechanism of hormones. Indeed, sex hormones and other gonadal secretions do have sex-specific effects on the brain, but gene expression in individual cells may have a larger role in the dimorphic phenotype. Increasing evidence has suggested a role for developmental mediation by X and Y chromosome-linked genes (Arnold, 2004). These revelations have led to a neurodevelopmental debate: epigenetics or genetics? This debate suggested that development of specific areas in the brain may be hormone-dependent, whilst others are hormone-independent (Reisert and Pilgrim, 1991). Here, we specifically discuss the hormone-dependent roles in neurodevelopment.

Estrogens are a class of steroids of which 17β-estradiol (often referred to as estradiol or just E2) is the main biologically active form (Blaustein, 2008). This class of steroid has long been known to exert powerful effects on development of the nervous system, as well as its function and plasticity (McEwen and Alves, 1999; McCarthy, 2008; Brinton, 2009; Srivastava et al., 2013b). Importantly, increasing evidence suggests that in addition to their actions within the hypothalamus (Kelly et al., 2005), estrogens exert effects within the neocortex and hippocampus (McEwen and Alves, 1999; Srivastava et al., 2013b). Moreover, the actions of estrogens during development and in the mature brain are not limited to those described in females. Effects of estrogens have also been consistently reported in males, albeit in a sexually dimorphic manner in many cases (Gillies and McArthur, 2010; McCarthy and Nugent, 2013; Gobinath et al., 2017). However, our current understanding of the role estrogens such as estradiol play in regulating the cellular or molecular processes critical for corticogenesis is limited. In this review, we will discuss the evidence that implicate a role for estrogens during the development of the cortex. Furthermore, we will highlight specific molecular pathways involved in developing the complex neuronal organization of the neocortex and emphasize how estrogens, particularly, estradiol signaling, interacts with these processes.

THE CASE FOR ESTROGEN IN THE DEVELOPING CORTEX

Canon has long established that the main source of estrogen production is the female sex organs. However, there is growing evidence that the key enzyme that converts androgens into estrogens, aromatase, is highly expressed in nervous tissue (Yague et al., 2006; Ish et al., 2007; Hojo et al., 2009; Boon et al., 2010; Saldanha et al., 2013). Aromatase has been identified in the hypothalamus, hippocampus, visual cortex, and temporal cortex in avian, mammalian, and human brain (Rune and Frotscher, 2005; Yague et al., 2006; Boon et al., 2010; Azcoitia et al., 2011; Saldanha et al., 2011).

The abundance of information on aromatase expression hints toward its fundamental importance. Aromatase expression has been evolutionarily conserved in nervous tissue, from chordates and early teleost. Complete removal of sex organs demonstrates that the expression is indeed sourced from within the nervous tissue, as removal does not lead to a complete loss-of-function (Yague et al., 2006; Ish et al., 2007; Hojo et al., 2009; Boon et al., 2010; Konkle and McCarthy, 2011; Saldanha et al., 2011). Indeed, Callard et al. (1978) highlighted that aromatase expression is highly concentrated to the forebrain in vertebrates. Furthermore, goldfish and toadfish demonstrate a high concentration of aromatase in the hypothalamus and preoptic areas (Pasmanik and Callard, 1985). Interestingly, work in toadfish demonstrated that expression of aromatase in certain neural areas accounted for sexually dimorphic behaviors (Pasmanik and Callard, 1985). Estrogens and aromatase expression in the limbic system as an evolutionarily conserved "ancient" function is further reinforced by the presence of both steroid and enzyme in non-mammalian vertebrate reptiles (Callard et al., 1977).

The evolutionary conservation model fits within the evolution of "higher cognition" in mammals, such as humans. Humans express aromatase and estrogens in the limbic system, and frontal cortex where they play roles in cognitive ability (Sasano et al., 1998). As the human neocortex has develop, so too has our ability to utilize estrogens and the "Aromadition—the system under aromatase control" to alter structures depending on stress/learning interactions, exploiting a combination of rapid and sustained cellular mechanisms (Konkle and McCarthy, 2011; Saldanha et al., 2011; Srivastava et al., 2011). Furthermore, the discovery of neuroactive steroidal involvement in clinical investigation has highlighted a very real application of estrogens as pharmaceutical agents (Stoffel-Wagner, 2001).

Estrogens have shown the ability to enact change in a very short time scale. Through modulation of spinogenesis, synaptogenesis, and synaptic connectivity, estrogen is able to enact these rapid changes in neural circuits (Saldanha et al., 2011; Srivastava et al., 2013b; Sellers et al., 2015a,b). For examples, when rat cortical neurons were treated with 10 nM Estradiol, structural changes (spinogenesis) were observed within 30 min. Studies into the ability of estrogens to influence behavior also demonstrate a rapid influence of estradiol and estrogen receptor agonists (Srivastava et al., 2013b; Luine, 2014; Sellers et al., 2015a; Gobinath et al., 2017). However, these studies present a clear inverted U-shaped curve. Previous studies have suggested that either 1–2 or 5 μg/kg dose of estradiol receives a better effect (Inagaki et al., 2010), reflecting the optimal level of receptor dynamic activation (Srivastava et al., 2013b; Luine, 2014). However, this dose response may be limited to enhancement of behavioral and cognitive tasks.

Studies *in vivo* have shown that estrogen receptors have an integral function in the development of cerebral architecture. Specifically, the pyramidal cells of the hippocampus and the cortical laminae II-VI demonstrate expression of ER mRNA and ER protein (Shughrue and Merchenthaler, 2000). Studies in this area began to elucidate further evidence of the large scale of nuclear ERs spread across the cortex, particularly in laminae III-V (Shughrue et al., 1999). Evidence for the implication of estrogen receptors in organization of the cortex has been the discovery of extra-nuclear ERα in dendritic spines and astrocytes (Milner et al., 2000). ERß mRNA and protein has also been detected in the cortex of rats (Shughrue and Merchenthaler, 2001).

These data indicate that ERs are indeed expressed through the cortical laminae of rodents. However, much less is known about the expression of ERs and estrogen-related genes, transcription factors and proteins during development. Our preliminary studies examining the expression of aromatase has begun to illuminate potential pathways linking estrogen and development, particularly sexually dimorphic development.

Aromatase has been found to be highly expressed in pyramidal neurons as well as glial cells (Kretz et al., 2004; Yague et al., 2006, 2008). Consistent with this, there is increasing evidence that estradiol is produced within the neocortex even in the absence of sex organs in both male and female animals (Ish et al., 2007; Hojo et al., 2009). Critically, estradiol, as well as other steroids, have been measured in embryonic brains of male and female rats within the cortex (Konkle and McCarthy, 2011). These findings are mirrored by previous findings of aromatase activity in the cortex and hippocampus in perinatal animals (Tobet et al., 1985; MacLusky et al., 1994). These studies highlight the possibility that the *de novo* synthesis of estradiol, mediated by aromatase, represents a major source of estrogens within the brain (Cornil et al., 2006; Azcoitia et al., 2011; Saldanha et al., 2011; Srivastava et al., 2013b; Balthazart and Ball, 2017), and may influence the development of the cortex (Tobet et al., 1985; MacLusky et al., 1994; Konkle and McCarthy, 2011). It is also important to note that the three major estrogen receptors (ERs): ERα, ERβ, and G-protein coupled estrogen receptor 1 (GPER1), were found to be expressed in multiple brain regions, including the cortex (Mitra et al., 2003; Milner et al., 2005). Using the BrainSpan transcriptomic atlas of the developing brain (http://www.brainspan.org/), we found several of the key molecular players involved in estrogenic signaling are expressed in the developing human brain, namely *CY19A1* (aromatase), ESR1 (ERα), ESR2 (ERβ), and GPER1 (GPER1). Specifically, these genes were found to be expressed during the developmental period spanning embryonic to late prenatal in the dorsal frontal cortex (DFC), ventral frontal cortex (VFC), and the hippocampus (HIP). CYP19A1 expression was found to increase throughout development, within these regions. Similarly, ESR1 trends toward an increase during over development, whereas ESR2 seems to be highly expressed during early corticogenesis before decreasing slightly then plateauing until late prenatal stage (Gatford, Denley and Srivastava, unpublished observations). Interestingly, the recently identified estrogen sensitive G-protein coupled receptor, GPER1 (also known as GPR30) (Srivastava and Evans, 2013) increases in its expression throughout corticogenesis. Combined, these data support the notion that the molecular machinery required for estrogenic signaling is expressed throughout early development within the cortex, and further suggests that estrogens may play a role during corticogenesis. Consistent with these data, we find that aromatase is expressed in multiple cell types within the brain of post-natal day 0 mice (Bakker et al., 2002; Karolczak et al., 2008). It should be noted that during brain development, estradiol has an organizational role and is central to the sexually dimorphic development and regulation of the neural circuitry underlying sex-typical and socio-aggressive behaviors in males and females (Nelson and Trainor, 2007; McCarthy and Arnold, 2011; Ubuka and Tsutsui, 2014). Interestingly, these effects seem to be in part mediated by the active repression of DNA methylation in the POA and hypothalamic ventromedial nucleus (Nugent et al., 2015; Mosley et al., 2017). Ultimately, whether such mechanisms are also important for the development of cortical circuitry is currently unknown. Nevertheless, taken together, these data suggest that estrogens, and aromatase, are not only present, but also actively regulated during key phases of the developing cerebral cortex.

Another line of evidence that estrogens play an important role in the development of the cortex in a sex specific manner comes from studies examining the detrimental effects of Bisphenol A (BPA). BPA is a Xenobiotic∗ and antagonist to estrogens via ERs. It has been noted that BPA alters sexual differentiation in early development. Males, but not females, exposed to BPA at 400 μg/kg altered the number of neurons and glial cells in the deep layers of the medial prefrontal cortex (Sadowski et al., 2014). Altered expression of ERs, which has shown to be sex-specific may account for this biased and unexpected mechanism (Kundakovic et al., 2013). It should be noted that BPA also binds androgen receptors (Kuiper et al., 1998; Sohoni and Sumpter, 1998), which may confer some of these effects. Sexually dimorphic neuron progeny may be attributed to the divisive effects of BPA among sexes, as specific neurons comprising sexually dimorphic regions are produced at markedly different timespans (Jacobson and Gorski, 1981). Nevertheless, the effects of BPA on neuronal and glial cell volumes within the cortex (Kubo et al., 2003) provides a strong case for estrogenic signaling in cortical development, and suggests that the steroid hormone may account for some sexual dimorphism seen in this area. However, one additional caveat of using BPA as an example to demonstrate a role for estrogens during corticogenesis, is its universal effects on other tissues in the body. The thyroid is one such example; environmental contamination by BPA results in up-regulation of thyroid hormone-responsive genes in the dentate gyrus (Zoeller et al., 2005), which is an area that has shown sexual dimorphic characteristics (Roof, 1993; Tabibnia et al., 1999). As highlighted above, BPA also strongly inhibits the activity of androgen receptors (Sohoni and Sumpter, 1998), which will have a considerable impact on the development and function of the cerebral cortex (Clark et al., 1988; Nuñez et al., 2003). A more comprehensive summary of BPAs effects can be found in Wetherill et al. (2007).

Maternal consumption and/or exposure to xenobiotic compounds can enter into the amniotic environment of the fetus and effect neurodevelopment. Exposure to xenobiotic compounds at physiological levels and from the environment can be detected in the amniotic fluid, which introduces it to the fetus (Nikaido et al., 2004; Engel et al., 2006). An area of increasing concern is that regarding dietary phytoestrogens. This area also provides further evidence to support the argument of estrogen and aromatase as key regulators of cortical development. In numerous animal models, manipulation of estrogen function by dietary phytoestrogens during gestation can lead to disrupted brain organization (Gorski, 1985; Lindzey and Korach, 1997). It has been suggested that dietary phytoestrogens are easily diffusible across the placenta and may then interfere with development (Patisaul and Jefferson, 2010). One must be cautious to draw conclusions from this, as absorption and concentration may differ wildly, especially, considering other dietary factors. In rodent studies, phytoestrogens such as polyphenols, flavonoids, and isoflavonoids have been shown to readily cross into the placenta and into the fetus brain (Doerge et al., 2001). Furthermore, during the prenatal period, systemic circulation of phytoestrogens is considerably more efficient compared to adults (Chang et al., 2000). Three anatomical locations have been particularly prominent in researching estrogen and epigenetics, the preoptic area (POA), locus coeruleus (LC), and the hypothalamic-pituitary axis (HPA), specifically the ventromedial nucleus. The POA and LC show sexual dimorphic areas, with ERα playing the more dominant role over ERß in both cases (Shughrue et al., 1997; Pérez et al., 2003; Patchev et al., 2004). Yet this raises the question, whether there are sexual dimorphic areas, hitherto undiscovered, that ERß maintains dominance?

The rodent POA has shown to be heavily sensitive to estradiol aromatized from gonadal androgens (Gorski, 1985). This is reflected in the greater volume of the male POA in comparison to the female POA. Furthermore, the expression of aromatase is variable not just in areas of sexual dimorphism, but also in response to testosterone and estrogen exposure (Roselli and Stormshak, 2010). Within the POA, the phytoestrogen genistein acts as an agonist to estrogen receptors. Exposure to genistein results in increased volumes in male but not female calbindin labeled sexually dimorphic areas (Scallet et al., 2004). This particular example highlights the importance of androgen synthesis and pharmacological dynamics, which are unfortunately beyond the scope of this literature review. Conversely, in the pre- and postnatal LC, exposure to the phytoestrogen resveratrol demasculinizes the male brain resulting in sexual dimorphism to volume and cell density (Kubo et al., 2003). It is pertinent to add that androgens are chiefly responsible for masculinizing the male brain. However, it would be irresponsible to not give weight to the estrogen (perhaps more so of ERα) mediated changes in organizational structure of the brain, with this example showing the ability of estrogen and aromatase to change both cerebral volume and cell densities in discrete areas.

CORTICAL DEVELOPMENT

Episodic processes of progenitor proliferation, neural differentiation, polarization, neuronal migration and lamination underpin the cortical development pattern (Ohtaka-Maruyama and Okado, 2015). Through selective expression of transcription factors and interaction with extra-cellular protein receptors, cortical layers are formed "inside-outside" (**Figure 1**; Angevine Jun and Sidman, 1961). Late-borne progenitors will ascend to the pial layers, whereas early-borne progenitors remain in deeper layers, which is modulated and regulated through transcription at the various episodes. Below, we highlight some of the key cell types and events that are critical for normal corticogenesis.

Proliferation and Progenitor Maintenance

In proliferative and neurogenic states during development, progenitors are produced through division and proliferation of neural stem cells (NSCs) in the ventricular zone (VZ) (**Figure 2**) and sub-ventricular zone (SVZ) (**Figure 3**). Basal progenitors of the SVZ, identified by the expression of Svetl and Tbr2, of the SVZ undergo symmetrical division and produce two neurons. Vimentin and Sox2 staining can highlight radial glial cell (RGC) (**Figure 2**) progenitors of the outer SVZ (Lancaster et al., 2013). Ngn3 contributes to maintaining progenitor oligodendrocytes in the SVZ (Ivanova et al., 2003) (**Figure 3**). Only progenitors of the VZ expressed Par complex rich domains, which develop into apical progenitors (express: Hesl, Pax6, Ki67, Phospho-vimentin, and Sox2; Knoblich, 2008) (**Figures 2, 3**). RC2, GLAST, BLBP, Nestin, and GFAP staining can also highlight RGC progenitors of the VZ (Rakic, 1971; Hartfuss et al., 2001; Liu et al., 2017; **Figure 2**). Hesl gene transcription regulates VZ progenitor pools and proliferation. However, RGCs typically divide asymmetrically, and thus, increase the diversity of daughter cells (Noctor et al., 2004). However, during highly proliferative episodes, symmetrical division is favored to increase the progenitor supply pool. Mechanistically, this process is mediated through Wnt signaling, leading to an increase in progenitor pool (ß-catenin-dependent) (Galceran et al., 2000). Interestingly, Par inheritance is directly linked to inherited Notch signaling capability (Kon et al., 2017; Bultje et al., 2018), furthermore, Notch signaling is required for neurogenesis and the maintenance of VZ NSCs (Imayoshi et al., 2010). Progenitors in the SVZ inherit or express high levels of Cuxl and Cux2, which signals them as apical progenitors (Nieto et al., 2004; **Figure 3**). G1 phase mitosis is a key regulatory point in proliferation (Dehay and Kennedy, 2007). CDK inhibitors, p27 and p57 coordinate corticogenesis and cell cycle exit. Prior to differentiation, p57 is responsible for cell cycling (Bilodeau et al., 2009). BM88 influences NSCs to exit the cell cycle and is expressed by RGCs (Koutmani et al., 2004).

Asymmetric inheritance is also seen in Pax6 and Ngn2 positive RGCs (Kawaguchi et al., 2004). Pax6 regulates neurogenesis and proliferation in the VZ and SVZ (Gan et al., 2014) and maintains the SVZ progenitor pool (Wong et al., 2015). Pax6 activity has shown to be ß-catenin-dependent. A dynamic relationship between Soxl and Pax6 controls transgression through periodical cortical development states (Suter et al., 2009; Wong et al., 2015). EphA4 binds to fibroblast growth factor (FGF), which is a potent stimulator of cortical proliferation (Collette et al., 2017). EphA4 regulates FRS2α (Yokote et al., 2005), which activates downstream RAS-MAPK and PI3K signaling pathways (Ornitz and Itoh, 2015).

Differentiation and Polarization

Differentiation of progenitors causes morphological changes, which allows migration and maturation. Differentiation and migration require dynamic cytoskeleton changes; extracellular and intrinsic signaling tightly regulates these events. For example, cadherins alter cellular dynamics (Nagafuchi et al., 1987). N-glycan-dependent attachment of cells recruits cadherin, causing greater cell-cell interaction (Hall et al., 2014). Nestin signals morphological changes within RGCs localized to axonal projections extending from the VZ (Xu et al., 2015; Vinci et al., 2016). Tbr2 generates transcriptional changes to cause cell to select a leading (axonal) strand (Sessa et al., 2008) (**Figure 2**). Ngn2 is downregulated by Hesl, which shifts a cell toward differentiation by modulating Notch signaling (Niwa et al., 2009; **Figures 2**, **3**). Ngn3 is upregulated to stimulate dendritogenesis and synaptogenesis. CRM1 mediates the nucleo-cytoplasmic shuttling of Ngn3, allowing transcriptional change (Simon-Areces et al., 2013) (**Figures 2**, **3**). In addition to its effect on proliferation, Wnt signaling utilizes ß-catenin-dependent pathways to differentiate intermediate progenitors into neurons (Clevers, 2018). Interestingly, cadherins also employ this pathway to mediate cell cycling (Zhang et al., 2013). Indeed, cadherins activate Wnt and Akt to switch from proliferation to migration (Ajioka and Nakajima, 2005).

Switching mechanisms and alterations in morphology are crucial to poising the cell to undergo polarization. The subplate of the IZ is a multipolar cell accumulation zone (MAZ) (**Figure 4**). Beyond the MAZ cells are mostly bipolar or unipolar neurons. Ngn2 regulates the transition of polarity (Ohtaka-Maruyama and Okado, 2015). Ngn2 inhibits RhoA, causing a cascade that downregulates MAPK (Zeidan et al., 2014) (**Figure 4**). RP58 regulates Ngn2-mediated morphological changes (Ohtaka-Maruyama et al., 2018). Interaction between ABP/cofilin/myosin inhibits RhoA through Rnd3 causing filopodial and lamellipodial growth and retraction (Pacary et al., 2011; Gomez and Letourneau, 2014). GDP-bound and GTP-bound oscillation regulates lamellipodium formation that orientates cells within the MAZ (Sailland et al., 2014). Par complex proteins (Par3, Par6, aPKC) cause apical base neurons to undergo polarization through Cdc42 coupling (Cappello et al., 2006). A compressive review of polarization can be found in Polleux and Snider's paper Polleux and Snider.

Migration and Lamination

Glial-guided neurons use cellular locomotion to migrate to the CP. Once in position, neurons attach their leading strand to the marginal zone (MZ) and switch to somal translocation.

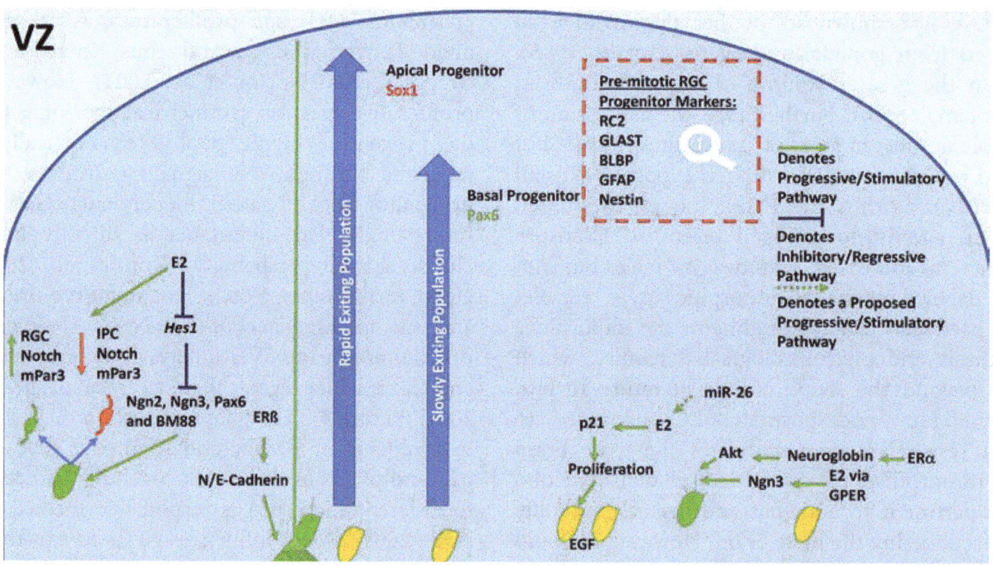

FIGURE 2 | General schematic diagram of molecular events that regulate neurogenesis and proliferation in the VZ. Neuroblasts, or NSCs divide asymmetrically, their progeny inherits either high notch and mPar3 or low notch and mPar3. RGCs receive higher notch signaling, their counterpart receives lower notch signaling and becomes an IPC. E2 inhibits Hes1 expression, resulting in increased division by inhibition of neurogenins, Pax6, and BM88. ERß is able to modulate N and E-Cadherin levels, which stabilizes end-feet of radial scaffolds and mediates adhesion. Depending on the expression of Sox1 or Pax6 a progenitor will join the rapidly or slowly ascending pool. Sox1-expressing populations (Apical progenitors) are released rapidly but remaining in the deeper layers of the CP. Pax6-expressing populations (Basal progenitors) are released slowly and comprise the superficial neurons of the CP. E2 has also shown to increase proliferation of NSCs through stimulation of p21 and increasing EGF expression. miR-26 may increase E2 synthesis or ER expression to meet this end. E2 is also able to increase neuritogenesis, leading to the formation of an axon. It accomplishes this via GPER and ERα, which are able to stimulate neuritogenesis through Ngn3 and Neuroglobin/Akt, respectively. E2, Estradiol; VZ, ventricular zone; RGC, radial glial cell; NSCs, neural stem cells; IPC, intermediate progenitor cell; Ngn, neurogenin; GLAST, astrocyte-specific glutamate transporter; BLBP, brain-lipid binding protein; GFAP, glial fibrillary acidic protein; ERα, estrogen receptor alpha; ERß, estrogen receptor beta; GPER, G-protein estrogen receptor; EGF, epidermal growth factor; CP, cortical plate.

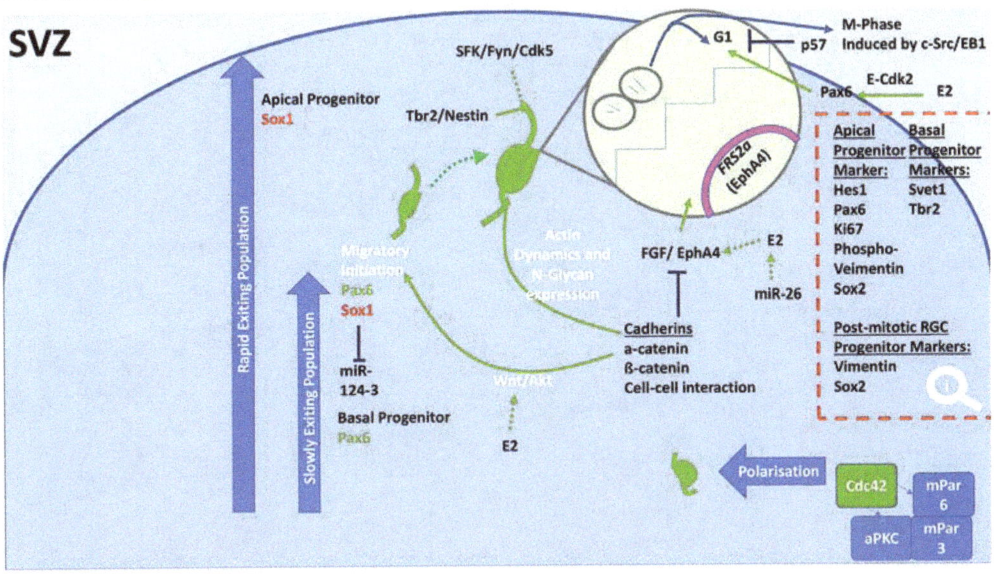

FIGURE 3 | General schematic diagram of molecular events that regulate proliferation, differentiation and the initiation of migration in the SVZ. Progenitor populations in the SVZ and outer SVZ undergo proliferation, differentiation, polarization, which are controlled to achieve either neural population increases or migration. In both these populations, collections of cellular processes are regulated to shift balance between proliferation and differentiation. Cadherins cause cell-cell interactions through Wnt/Akt signaling, which result in altered levels of Pax6 or Sox1 expression. Cadherins increase expression of actin dynamic molecules and N-glycan. Resulting in axonal growth and migration, which involves incorporation of Tbr2, Nestin, and the SFK/Fyn/Cdk5 pathway. Cadherins influence the cell cycle through inhibition of the growth factor FGF and EphA4, which results in decreased proliferation and increased differentiation to allow migration. E2 is able to increase FGF/EphA4 action leading to greater proliferation. This action is achieved through E2 stimulating Pax6 through E-Cdk2. Polarization of migrating neurons in the SVZ can be accomplished by the coupling of Cdc42 to an aPKC/mPar6/mPar3 complex. SVZ, subventricular zone; miR, microRNA; E2, Estradiol; ERα, estrogen receptor alpha; ERß, estrogen receptor beta; GPER, G-protein estrogen receptor; aPKC, atypical protein kinase C; FGF, fibroblast growth factor; FRS2a, fibroblast growth factor receptor substrate 2a; G1, Gap 1 phase; SFK, Src family kinase; EphA4, Ephrin type-A receptor 4; Fyn, Src tyrosine-protein kinase fyn; NSCs, neural stem cells.

Chemotaxis is mediated through membrane-bound receptors and extracellular matrix proteins, including Rac, brain-derived neurotropic factor (BDNF) and TrkB signaling (**Figure 4**; Zhou et al., 2018). Calcium-dependent mechanisms recruit BDNF (Zhou et al., 2018). BDNF binding to TrkB stimulates axonal growth and dendritic morphological change (Cohen-Cory and Fraser, 1995; Wang et al., 2015) (**Figure 4**). The selection and elongation of a leading (axonal) strand stimulates migration. Migration can be induced by Tiam1/Rac1/ERK signaling (Xiao et al., 2013). Interaction between the SFK Fyn and serine/threonine kinase family member Cdk5 are evidenced to play a leading role in progenitor cell axon guidance and dendritic orientation (Sasaki et al., 2002; **Figure 4**). Reelin and Dab1 alter cytoskeleton morphology through CLASP2 (Dillon et al., 2017). Cux1 and Cux2 regulate dendritic morphology through Pax6 and p27 in pyramidal neurons (Nieto et al., 2004).

The lamination process relies on signaling pathways that halt migration and trigger neuronal maturation through terminal and somal translocation. Reelin, Dab1, Wnt/Fizzled, and SPARC-like1 (SC1) are essential for this process. Wnt/Frizzled and reelin signaling regulates boundary formation during lamination (Augustine et al., 2001; Brault et al., 2001; Franco et al., 2018). SPARC-like1 (SC1) signals detachment of RGCs from the membrane. Terminal translocation in neurons is signaled by Dab1 and Cullin5 interaction (Feng et al., 2007; **Figure 5**). Migrating neurons interact with reelin through RapGEF2 (Ye et al., 2014). Neurons extend dendrites into the CP, which requires elongator to acetylate α-tubulin resulting in microtubule reassembly (Creppe et al., 2009; Heng et al., 2010). Interaction between reelin and VLDLR and ApoER2 causes Dab1 phosphorylation, which recruits PI3K and Lis1 (Bock et al., 2003; Chai and Frotscher, 2016; Lane-Donovan and Herz, 2017). Nectin1 and Nectin3 show capability of facilitating and mediating somal translocation (Hirota and Nakajima, 2017; **Figure 5**). N-cadherin interacts through the Nectin's cytoplasmic domain region.

CYTOARCHITECTURE-SPECIFIC MECHANISM INVOLVED IN SEXUAL DIFFERENTIATION

Sexual differentiation in the central nervous systems occurs throughout vertebrate evolution, including human beings (Jazin and Cahill, 2010). Hypothalamic nuclei are profoundly sensitive to sex-dependent change. The anteroventral periventricular (AVPV) nuclei in the hypothalamus is typical of the sexual dimorphism. Due to caspase-dependent apoptotic signaling induced by perinatal exposure to estradiol (Waters and Simerly, 2009), males typically have a smaller AVPV than their female peers (Simerly et al., 1985). The phenotype of this is a decreased cellular volume (Forger et al., 2004). Estradiol has shown to be a

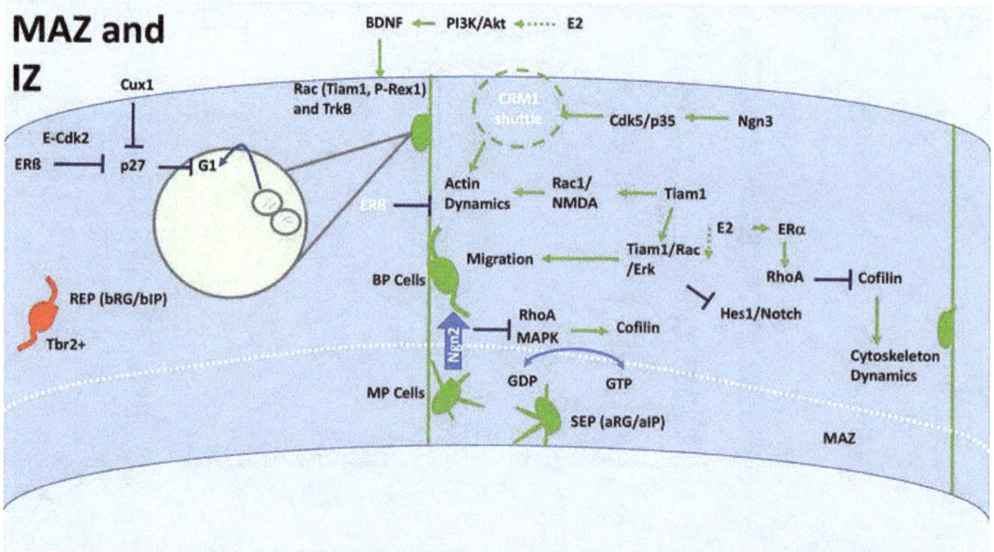

FIGURE 4 | General schematic of corticogenesis in the IZ and MAZ, including differentiation and migration. The IZ facilitates cytoskeleton changes that affect the morphology of the migrating cell, much of this will occur in the MAZ. The MAZ is an accumulation ground for multipolar cells that are forming into mature bipolar neurons, which can then enter into the CP. The MAZ is comprised of two populations SEP and REP. Whereas the REP population passes straight through the MAZ, the SEP remains in the MAZ for much longer. Ultimately, the SEP forms the more superficial layer of the CP. REP can be distinguished from SEPs as they are Tbr2+. Crossing from the MAZ to IZ requires a transition from MP to BP, which is initiated by Ngn2, which inhibits RhoA and MAPK that have a downstream effect on Cofilin. Cofilin interacts with RGCs to increase cytoskeleton dynamics and affect a neuronal morphology. Cofilin can also be inhibited by RhoA, which is modulated through ERα. Oscillation between GDP and GTP control orientation and polarization of cells within the MAZ. This is achieved through lamellipodium formation and interaction with the cofilin system. Upregulation of Tiam1 or E2 can result in activation of Tiam1/Rac/Erk signaling, which stimulates BP cells to migrate through the IZ. Tiam1 also activates Rac1/NMDA to alter actin dynamics, which results in increased elongation, synaptogenesis and dendritogenesis. This process can be negatively regulated by ERβ or actively upregulated by Ngn3 through Cdk5/p35 activating a CRM1 shuttle. RGCs are stimulated to move toward the CP by interaction with BDNF. E2 stimulation via PI3K/Akt signaling can cause BDNF expression. BDNF binds to TrkB and upregulates Rac/Tiam1/P-Rex1 activity. Through Cux1 and E2 (ERβ), proliferation is inhibited at this stage allowing for migration to take place. Both Cux1 and E2 inhibit p27, which stops proliferating cells at the G1 phase. E2, estradiol; IZ, intermediate zone; MAZ multipolar cell accumulation zone; CP, cortical plate; RGC, Radial glial cell; ERα, estrogen receptor alpha; ERβ, estrogen receptor beta; BP, bipolar; MP, multipolar; SEP, slow exiting population; REP, rapidly exiting population; BDNF, brain-derived neurotrophic factor; NMDA, N-methyl-D-aspartate; TrkB, Tropomyosin receptor kinase B; MAPK, mitogen-activated protein kinase; PI3K, Phosphoinositide 3 kinase; Akt, Protein Kinase B; bRG/bIP, basal radial glia/intermediate progenitor; aRG/aIP, apical radial glia/intermediate progenitor; G(D/T)P, guanosine (di/tri)-phosphate; CRM1, chromosomal maintenance 1/exportin 1; Cux1, cut like homeobox 1; RhoA, Ras homolog gene family, A; EphA4, Ephrin type-A receptor 4; Tiam1, T-cell lymphoma Invasion And Metastasis 1; Erk, extracellular signal-regulated kinases; Tbr2, T-box brain 2; E-Cdk2, G1 phase specific Cyclin E, Cyclin-dependent kinase 2; NSCs, neural stem cells.

crucial hormone in regulating and mediating the development of the neocortex (Beyer, 1999; McEwen and Alves, 1999). For example, ERß knockout mice (ERβKO) have revealed that ERβ is necessary for cortical lamination, which indicates a potential role for estradiol in orientation through actin dynamics (Wang et al., 2003), although the mechanisms by which this occurs is poorly understood. Ultimately, it is not clear if this mechanism may lead to sexually dimorphic phenotypes. A number of studies have shown that estradiol increases the proliferative status in embryonic NSCs (Fried et al., 2004), which involves ERs but is limited to neurogenesis in embryonic development (Brännvall et al., 2002). Estradiol-induced proliferation of NSCs is mediated through the classic estradiol receptors, ERα and ERβ (Okada et al., 2010). Hitherto, the literature has not provided a comprehensive summary of the finer biochemical interactions of estradiol, which can be seen in many pathways mentioned above and throughout the cortex. In the proceeding sections, we review the evidence that indicates specific molecular players involved in corticogenesis and how these may be regulated in a sexually dimorphic manner. In addition, data that link estradiol-signaling with the regulation of key molecular players involved in the distinct and carefully orchestrated events described in the previous sections (**Figure 6**).

Markers of Proliferation in Sexual Dimorphic Areas

Sexual dimorphism during development can be attributed to physiological factors such as hormonal exposure, as well as cell-intrinsic mechanisms that lead to differentiation (Swaab et al., 1995; Tsukahara, 2009). Cell-specific differentiation can be met through numerous factors, some of which will be discussed here.

The cellular state of neural progenitors can provide a comprehensive depiction on the condition of neurogenesis. As a marker of proliferation Ki67 expression in the discrete developing areas, can provide evidence to draw conclusions about total cell volumes at maturity. Infant rat preoptic area and hypothalamus show higher expression of Ki67, when compared to adults (He et al., 2013). Furthermore, colocalisation of

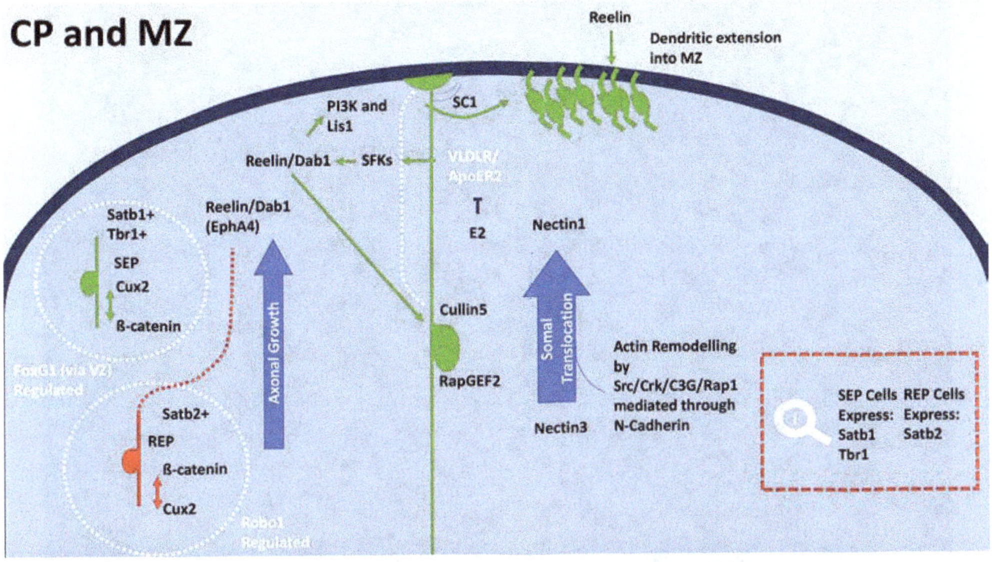

FIGURE 5 | General schematic of terminal translocation and differentiation in the CP during development. Within the CP SEP neurons (green) have high expression of Cux2 and low expression of β-catenin, whereas REP neurons (red) have high expression of β-catenin and low expression of Cux2. Satb1 positive cells express in the superficial layers of the MZ, which overlap with Tbr1 expression. Terminal translocation and therefore lamination rely on regulation by FoxG1 for the SEP neurons and radial distribution of Satb2 expressing REP neurons is regulated by Robo1. FoxG1 on deep-layer progenitors through transcription switches their progeny to upper-layer neurons through repression of Tbr1. After exiting the cell cycle, Satb2-expressing cells immediately migrate to the upper layers of the cortical plate. Satb2 expressing cells are much more reliant on the reelin/Dab1 and Ephrin-A pathways for cortical migration. Reelin binds to the RGCs by VLDLR and Apoer2 receptors (Lane-Donovan and Herz, 2017), which causes the adaptor protein Dab1 to become phosphorylated. Upon phosphorylation by SFKs, Dab1 recruits various downstream molecules including PI3K and Lis1. E2 is able to inhibit VLDLR/ApoER, modulates reelin's mechanisms in cortical migration. Reelin's interaction with cadherin is also essential for the termination of migration. Through regulating terminal translocation, the reelin/Dab1/Rap1/N-Cadherin signaling pathway leads to the inside-out lamination of the cortex. Nectin molecules expressed in the Cajal-Retzius cell (Nectin1) and the migrating neuron (Nectin3) are also necessary for somal translocation. The initiation of detachment is signaled by SC1, which is expressed on the surface at the top and bottom of RGCs surfaces. The anti-adhesive signal is crucial to proper cortical development, as the absence of SC1 results in failure of neurons to detach and properly position. Dab1 interacts with Cullin5 in the migrating cell to accumulate in the appropriate cortical layer. Termination of polarization upon reaching the appropriate location is met by the degradation of reelin receptors, N-cadherin and Dab1 by exocytosis and endocytosis. E2, Estradiol; IZ, intermediate zone; MAZ, multipolar cell accumulation zone; CP, cortical plate; RGC, Radial glial cell; ERα, estrogen receptor alpha; ERβ, estrogen receptor beta; BP, bipolar; MP, multipolar; SEP, slow exiting population; REP, rapidly exiting population; SFK, Src family kinases; PI3K, Phosphoinositide 3 kinase; SC1, SPARC-like1; VLDLR, very low-density lipoprotein receptor; ApoER2, apolipoprotein E receptor 2; Cux2, cut like homeobox 2; FoxG1, Forkhead Box G1; Dab1, Disabled-1; Tbr1, T-box brain 1; Lis-1, Lissencephaly-1; Crk, (p38/adaptor molecule crk); C3G, CRK SH3-binding GNRP; Rap1, Ras-like GTPase; Satb(1/2) Special At-rich sequence binding protein (1/2); Robo1, Roundabout Guidance Receptor 1; EphA4, Ephrin type-A receptor 4; NSCs, neural stem cells.

Ki67+ cells and estradiol is noted in the preoptic area and hypothalamus.

Nestin has also been implicated in generating larger cells volumes in sexually dimorphic ventricular areas, such as the POA (He et al., 2013). Estradiol treatment on rat telencephalon cultures did not have an effect on the proportion of nestin-positive cells (Okada et al., 2010). However, estradiol did affect the cell fate of progenitor cells from the telencephalon of rats, which caused an increase in the ratio of oligodendrocytes being produced (Okada et al., 2008). The rostral third ventricle is the site of stem cell niches that strongly express nestin, which supplies the frontal and medial neocortex with neuroblasts (He et al., 2013). Estradiol has significantly strong proliferation-promoting effects in the 3rd ventricle stem cell niche (He et al., 2015). The effect of estradiol on nestin-expressing stem cell niches may serve to further reinforce the proliferative proprieties of estradiol in the developing cortex.

Ki67 and nestin expression colocalized with estradiol in sexually dimorphic areas is suggestive of a possible mechanism. The inclusion of a proliferative marker and intermediate filament protein is suggestive that estradiol increases the proliferative state and leads to greater migration through radial axon growth (Scholzen and Gerdes, 2000; Xu et al., 2015).

Glial Fibrillary Acidic Protein (GFAP)

GFAP is a robust astrocytic marker of RGC progeny (Berman et al., 1997). Immunoreactive GFAP has been detected in neural circuits that display sexual dimorphism. These circuitries can be manipulated through introduction of exogenous steroid hormones (Martinez et al., 2006). In studies primarily focusing on the cortex, ovariectomised rats showed higher rates of cortical proliferation resulting from treatment with estradiol (Malinowska-Kolodziej et al., 2009). The study also noted co-localization of nestin and GFAP in the cortex, which can be suggested as a mark of increased radial glial migration resulting from estradiol treatment. The substantia nigra of ovariectomised parkinsonian model mice did not respond to estradiol in the same manner, with GFAP remaining unchanged (Yi et al., 2016).

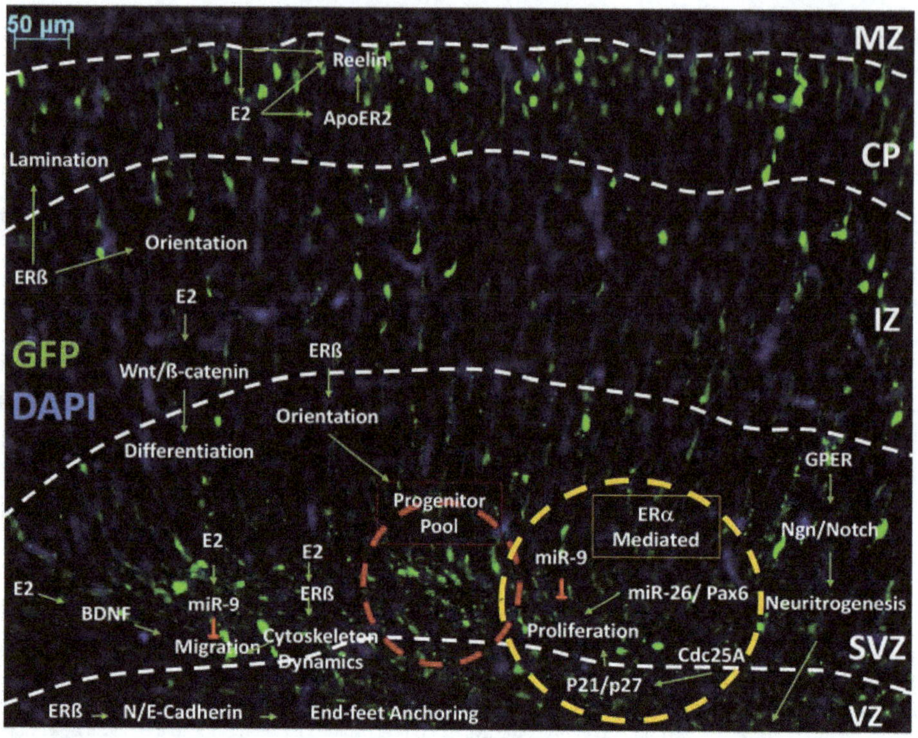

FIGURE 6 | An outline of the pathways influenced by estrogenic signaling to drive cortical development. Representative image of developing cortex. Electroporation of eGFP was performed at E14.5 and brains collected at P0 as previously described (Srivastava et al., 2012a,b). Representative image of a coronal rodent brain slice at P0 during cortical development. Estrogen (Estradiol/17ß-estradiol) is shown interacting in pathways outlined in **Figures 1–4**. that are involved in neurogenesis, proliferation, differentiation and migration. We propose that Estradiol may be able to affect the proliferative status of the progenitor pool through Pax6 and kinase inhibitors through ERß or ER. Through ERß, Estradiol can affect migration by marking terminal translocation points, therefore setting lamination boundaries. Estradiol is able to influence orientation through a number of mechanisms, which has been shown specifically in GFAP+ RGCs and mediated through ERß. Through ERß, Estradiol also alters the cytoskeleton dynamics to initiate migration. Cytoskeleton dynamics are also affected by GPER to increase neuritogenesis, which will later form axons and dendrites. Estradiol also alters differentiation state by increasing Wnt/ß-catenin signaling, which furthers dendritogenesis. Estradiol is able to negatively regulate migration and proliferation by increasing miR-9, which inhibits these processes. In regards to proliferation, it is hypothesized that ERα is primarily responsible for mediating the action of estrogenic signaling. Estradiol also interacts with reelin signaling in the CP and MZ, both directly by increasing expression and indirectly by stimulation of ApoE gene expression, which increases the activity of ApoER to affect the morphology of the cortex and cytoarchitecture of the CP. E2, estradiol; IZ, intermediate zone; MAZ, multipolar cell accumulation zone; CP, cortical plate; ERß, estrogen receptor beta; ERα, estrogen receptor alpha; GPER, G-protein estrogen receptor; miR-x, microRNA; ApoER2, apolipoprotein E receptor 2; Wnt, Wingless-type; BDNF, brain-derived neurotropic factor; p21, cyclin-dependent kinase inhibitor 1A/Cip1; p27, cyclin-dependent kinase inhibitor 1B/Kip1; Ngn, neurogenin; Cdc25A, Cell division cycle 25 homolog A; VZ, ventricular zone; SVZ, subventricular zone.

However, Yi et al.'s team used BDNF as a marker to show an estradiol-dependent increase in net migration of neurons in the midbrain. These results suggest that estradiol within the cerebral cortex is able to increase proliferative status. The interaction between GFAP and estradiol is likely mediated through ERß. Indeed, Zsarnovszky et al. (2002) showed that estradiol via ERß is able to directly regulate GFAP expression in the interpeduncular nucleus, an important component of the limbic midbrain circuitry. Furthermore, agonists of ERß, namely LY3201, caused immunoreactive GFAP in hippocampal and cortical astrocytes to increase (Tan et al., 2012). This study also found that dendritic spines could be reduced using an ERß agonist (Tan et al., 2012). This suggests the mechanism is a result of downstream ER signaling and not directly related to estradiol expression. Taken together, these data suggest interaction between GFAP and estrogen results in altered astrocytic expression and has implications in the proliferation of RGCs.

Paired Box Protein—Pax-6

The transcription factor Pax-6 is essential in neurogenesis. Mutations in the *PAX6* gene can cause serious developmental disorders such as aniridia, autism spectrum disorder, and intellectual disability (Davis et al., 2008). Pax-6 and estradiol have been targeted in a large portion of breast cancer research. Concordantly, suppression of *PAX6* gene expression inhibits cell growth, which appeared to have a knock-on effect from or to ERK1/2, p38 and cyclin D1 (Zhao et al., 2014). In ER-positive cancer cell lines, MCF-7, Pax-6 knock-down interrupts cell cycling at G1 phase and reduced proliferation (Zong et al., 2011). Estradiol's stimulation of *PAX6* has been noted in MCF7 cell lines. Estradiol is able to stimulate the transcription activity of 187 transcription factors (Li et al., 2014b), which impresses its involvement in proliferation, migration and cell cycle regulation. Based on these data, it is plausible that Pax-6 may be the facilitator for estradiol-mediated proliferation, which can be seen in the increased proliferative status of GFAP+ NSCs (**Figure 6**).

One might expect that Pax-6 knockdown models may be rescued by simulation of ERß during neurodevelopment. However, one must be cautious about the interpretation of this data. Purely due to the availability the authors have used evidence and data from MCF7 (Cancer) cultures, which are not directly comparable to neural circuits and cultures. However, it is the opinion of the authors that the MCF7 lines still suggest an interesting case for the interaction of estrogen and Pax-6.

Neurogenin (Ngn)

Intracellular progenitor Notch signaling plays a pivotal role in progenitor maintenance, cell fate and differentiation (Ohtaka-Maruyama and Okado, 2015). Balancing between Hedgehog and Notch signaling maintains correct cortical formation (Dave et al., 2011). Estradiol is able to mediate the regulators of Notch signaling via ERs (Bender et al., 2010). Through the utilization of Ngn3 and GPER1, estradiol promotes neuritogenesis in the mouse hippocampus (**Figure 6**), which also incurred the activation of PI3K signaling (Ruiz-Palmero et al., 2013). Ngn3 is promoted through downregulation of Notch signaling (Arevalo et al., 2011). Furthermore, neurogenins could be partially responsible for sex-dependent dimorphisms. Ngn3 activity has been suggested to influence sex-dependent differentiation in neurons, which may result from epigenetic regulation of sex-linked genes (Scerbo et al., 2014). Ngn3 is also repressed by estradiol-mediated inhibition of Hes-1, which is regulated through Notch signaling (Salama-Cohen et al., 2006). Ngn2 and Ngn3 have a role in division within the VZ, which is mediated by *Hes-1*. Through which, estradiol may act as a mediator control asymmetric division. Furthermore, as Ngn3 is able to stimulate the growth and migration of cells toward the CP, it is plausible that estradiol works through Ngn3 during neurodevelopment.

Kinases

Estradiol targets CDK Cdc25A to promote growth during cell cycling, which also influences expression of p21 and p27 (Foster et al., 2001). In cultured cortical neurons, activation of ERβ resulted in the phosphorylation of kinase proteins: p21-activated kinase and ERK1/2 Kinase proteins are responsible for regulation of actin cytoskeleton dynamics (Srivastava et al., 2010). Rapid estrogenic signaling mediated through ERα (Sanchez et al., 2009) activates Src/Rho/Cdk5, WAVE1 pathway and a RhoA/ROCK-2/Moesin cascade, which cause the protrusion of dendritic spines (Polleux and Snider, 2010; Srivastava et al., 2013b). It has been suggested that estradiol is a modulator of these processes (Srivastava et al., 2010; Sellers et al., 2015b; Zhao et al., 2017). Other CDKs have been implicated in cell cycle regulation. E-Cdk2 has been identified as a central component of estradiol's regulatory system during G1 to S phase of the cell cycle progression (Doisneau-Sixou et al., 2003). Upregulation of CDK inhibitor p21 can stimulate proliferation of embryonic stem cells induced by epidermal growth factor, which is activated by estradiol (Brännvall et al., 2002). Interaction with CDK inhibitors such as p27 can regulate ERs and *vice versa* to mediate transcription and gene expression (Prall et al., 1997). In the MCF-7 cell line ERα is mediated by p27 to regulate nuclear localisation and therefore transcription (Jeon et al., 2012). Estradiol is also able to utilize the ubiquitin proteasome system (UPS) to degrade p27, after phosphorylation by MAPK/ERK (Singer et al., 1999; Huang et al., 2012). This may serve as a regulatory mechanism for proliferation. Estradiol elicits rapid responses, which can be attributed to kinase phosphorylation (Srivastava et al., 2013b). These rapid actions can be attributed to involvement of tyrosine kinases (Karthikeyan and Thampan, 1996). Furthermore, by binding to cytoplasmic or membrane-bound receptors, estradiol is able to activate phosphorylation cascades by ERK, PI3K and MAPK (Singh et al., 1999; Fox et al., 2009).

Small Non-coding RNAs

In MCF-7 cell lines, estradiol's influence on small non-coding microRNA (miR) is well documented (Klinge, 2009; Jiang et al., 2016). Estradiol-stimulated proliferation can be induced by miR-26 in MCF-7 cell lines (Tan et al., 2014). Conversely, this process can be negatively regulated by estradiol through upregulation of miR-9, which inhibits proliferation and migration (Fang et al., 2015). Interestingly, whereas Tan's group (Tan et al., 2014) showed miR-26 was ER-dependent to induce proliferation, Fang et al.'s group (2015) showed miR-9 inhibited proliferation and migration independently of ERs (**Figure 6**). Current literature shows ERα induces proliferation and ERß induces apoptosis, which is reflected in miR interaction with ERα and ERß leading to polarizing effect (Helguero et al., 2005). miR-22 (Pandey and Picard, 2009), miR-221-222 (Di Leva et al., 2010), miR-206 (Adams et al., 2007; Kondo et al., 2008) are generally correlated with a reduction or inhibition of ERα and its effects. However, some miRNAs have shown to be an exception to this. miR-342 (He et al., 2013) overexpression upregulated MCF-7 cells to induce apoptosis and inhibited proliferation, which possibly highlights the interdependence of the two ERs in conditions such as extreme overexpression, which would coincide with the "ying-yang" relationship ERs have been suggested to possess (Lindberg et al., 2003).

In a clinical setting, estradiol may act on miR to account for the gender disparity seen in the diagnosis of schizophrenia (Mellios et al., 2012). Specifically, in the frontal cortex of schizophrenic male mice, miR-30b was expressed in greater quantity than in females. Many of the studies cited in this section are from cancer cell lines, which leave conclusions drawn little more than conjecture. The strength of the individual results coupled with the correlative observations, implicate miR as a player during cortical development.

Using miRs in studying cortical development will require further development of laboratory techniques. Currently, processes involved in analyzing miRs are costly and the literature has shown to be divided in agreeing upon various sequences and expression patterns (Guo et al., 2016).

Wnt

Wnt signaling coordinates the progeny of progenitor cells during differentiation (Kriska et al., 2016), which could serve as a mechanism used by estradiol to mediate differentiation. Through Wnt3A, estradiol receptor signaling is able to promote differentiation in mesenchymal progenitor cells (Gao et al., 2013). Wnt signaling is also known to regulate neuronal differentiation of cortical intermediate progenitors (Munji et al., 2011). Cross talk between Wnt and estradiol is facilitated by interaction with ß-catenin (Kouzmenko et al., 2004). A recent review highlights the importance of estradiol in Wnt signaling as a chief mediator in maintaining the balance of Wnt antagonist Dkk1 and Wnt/ß-catenin (Scott and Brann, 2013).

RhoA

As a key regulator of cell orientation in the cortex, RhoA activity is essential in cellular migration. Consequently, excess and deficit can cause impairment, however, ERα may serve as a regulator to RhoA activity and stability. Inactivation of ERα by siRNA increased RhoA protein expression, which resulted in decreased migration (Sailland et al., 2014). It is worth noting that PCR showed this process was independent of Wnt11 and N-Cadherin expression, which are established mechanisms leading to ERα activation (Dwyer et al., 2010). RhoA was also shown to decrease the transcriptional activity of ERα via RhoGDI increasing transactivation by Rho GTPase (Su et al., 2001).

Cadherin

Cadherins are used to anchor the end-feet of RGCs to the ventricular surface, which is a key aspect of maintaining polarization in the developing cortex (**Figure 6**). In ERßKO mice, migration, morphology and polarization are defective. Furthermore, it was shown that these processes could occur as ERßKO lacked the modulation of ERß over E-Cadherin and N-Cadherin (Xu et al., 2015).

BDNF and TrkB

The steroid hormone estrogen and the neurotrophin BDNF have been observed sharing mutual functions, in a co-dependent or even synergistic manner (Scharfman and Maclusky, 2005; Numakawa et al., 2010; Srivastava et al., 2013a). Respectively, they are established as two extracellular signaling molecules that work to meet numerous physiological functions. Estrogen and BDNF are both able to influence signaling cascades, synaptic structures and neuronal physiology in multiple and mutually inclusive areas (Greenberg et al., 2009; Waterhouse and Xu, 2009; Srivastava et al., 2010, 2011).

The connection between BDNF and estrogen is likely through a novel signaling system completely removed from the traditional trkB pathway. This is evidenced by no significant change in trkB mRNA or protein noted in gonadectomized or estrogen-replaced animals (Solum and Handa, 2002). Solum and Handa (2002) concluded that due to co-localisation of ERα and BDNF in pyramidal cells of the CA1 and CA3 hippocampal sub-regions. Since the publication of the Solum paper, other teams have uncovered a similar mechanism using GPER in the same cerebral region (Briz et al., 2015). Both groups concluded that estrogen and BDNF are in some way used to regulate cerebral function.

A possible mechanism for the interaction between BDNF and estrogen could be met through intracellular phosphorylation cascades. Estrogen has been documented providing restorative effects to ovariectomised mice. Estrogen (0.1 mg/kg) worked through PI3K/Akt signaling pathway to provide short-term neuroprotection of neurons in the midbrain by upregulating BDNF (Yi et al., 2016). Cultured dentate gyrus neurons *in vitro* reacted in comparable manner, as significant BDNF upregulation occurred after pharmacological exposure to estradiol (100 mM−1 μM) (Sato et al., 2007).

A comprehensive review of the literature in this area can be found in the references list (Srivastava et al., 2013a).

Neuroglobin

ERα regulates neuroglobin expression through genomic transcript region regulation (Guglielmotto et al., 2016). Estradiol is capable of upregulating neuroglobin through activation of ERß (De Marinis et al., 2013; Fiocchetti et al., 2015). Estradiol may utilize neuroglobin to regulate the formation of neurites during migration. Neuroglobin is found within the SVZ and IZ (Shang et al., 2006) and increases the phosphorylative state of Akt leading to neurite outgrowth (Li et al., 2014a).

Reelin and Dab1

In hippocampal slice cultures, exogenous application of estradiol causes reelin expression to increase from Cajal-Retzius cells, which is facilitated by ERs. Furthermore, aromatase activity contributes to reelin expression. Impairment of aromatase activity causes reelin expression to reduce (Bender et al., 2010). If the aromatase gene is knocked out in male mice, specific areas in the brain have been shown to change in size (Pierman et al., 2008). Moreover, this morphological impairment can somewhat be saved through estrogen and testosterone treatments. As shown in reeler mice, estradiol upregulates reelin mRNA in the Purkinje cells (PC) of the cerebellum, with a particularly notable effect in males. Reelin protein bands (420, 310, and 180 kDa) were also shown to be upregulated. Furthermore, *reeler* mice show an abnormal steroid hormone profile with testosterone and estradiol increased but dihydrotesterone decreased (Biamonte et al., 2009).

Apolipoprotein

Estradiol down-regulates ApoER2 in differentiating osteoblasts, which is reflected in other LDLR family members. Leading to the promotion of differentiation in osteoclasts (Gui et al., 2016). Estradiol may alter apolipoprotein expression through genomic transcript mediation. Estradiol is able to upregulate ApoE gene expression in BL6 mice (Srivastava et al., 1997). ERα mRNA expression during development correlates with regulation of differentiation of osteoblasts (Bodine et al., 1998). Differentiation of apical papilla stem cells is also regulated by estradiol via the activation of MAPK signaling (Li et al., 2014c). Furthermore, ApoER2 interacts with reelin to govern morphology and cytoarchitecture (Stranahan et al., 2013).

Estradiol and Gene Expression

The cortical transcriptome can be manipulated epigenetically by estradiol, including functions ranging from memory (Frick et al., 2011), transcription factor regulation (Jadhav et al., 2015), and cell cycling (Couse et al., 1995). Estradiol has shown to significantly alter at least 88 genes in relation to the control of the cortex (Humphreys et al., 2014). Genes associated with synaptic activity, myelination, synthesis and metabolism, neurotransmission and kinase signaling were all shown to alter expression following introduction of estradiol after ovariectomy. Removing the expression and synthesis of extra-nervous estrogen in males, would likely further exacerbate the effects and may highlight sex-dependent gene expression in cortical development. Introduction of estradiol in ovariectomised rats induces genomic changes that influence the dopaminergic and peptidergic neural networks (Sárvári et al., 2010). This may be as a result of estradiol's role in neurotransmission. It is known that aromatase is localized to the synapse and can be activated by calcium phosphorylation (Balthazart and Ball, 2017).

ERα has also shown to mediate subtle epigenetic mechanism that result in sex-specific differences in the prefrontal cortex in adulthood (Westberry and Wilson, 2012). It is plausible that this sex-specific difference is met through alteration in the inhibitory GABAergic signaling pathway. Pyramidal neurons of the prefrontal cortex rely on phosphorylation-dependent mechanisms for cellular trafficking and signaling. G protein-gated inwardly rectifying potassium channels modulate excitability and were shown to be susceptible to sex-specific neurochemistry (Marron Fernandez de Velasco et al., 2015). The extent to which estradiol is able to regulate these mechanisms remains to be seen. Estradiol affects the genetic transcriptome of 88 genes (likely more) within the cerebral cortex. However, questions remain: which mechanisms does estradiol utilize to interact with these genes and are these genes affected in different sexes? Are males more susceptible to estrogen transcriptome deficits during cortical development? Does the knockout of aromatase impact estrogenic signaling? Does aromatase knockout affect males and females unequally? Does the aromatase knockout affect the transcriptome? Answering these questions would prove to further elucidate the pathways involved in cortical development. Furthermore, answering these questions would further elucidate the mechanisms estrogen adopts to control sexual dimorphism and to what extent it is able to control sexual dimorphism. Delivering a clear mechanism for sexual dimorphism would also aid in better understanding of neurodevelopmental disorders that show biased sexual distribution, such as autism spectrum disorder.

SUMMARY AND CONCLUSIONS

In summary, many lines of evidence exist that suggest estradiol has many critical roles in corticogenesis (**Figure 6**). Hitherto, no clear mechanism has been established. Substantial evidence purports to show a connection between estradiol, migration, and neurogenesis. A strong body of evidence exists showing that estradiol influences the proliferative body within the subventricular zone, which increases the availability of NSCs. The mechanism underlying this action has not been established but may be associated with Pax-6, neurogenins, and nestin. Estradiol influences many regulators of estrogenic-signaling, which suggests that this maybe a primary function. Mechanisms underlying estradiol's influence in regulating migration has been discussed in detail. The interaction with Wnt, Cadherin as well as various kinases produce dynamic actin changes, which has been suggested as mechanism for migration. Estradiol has also shown to associate greatly with the reelin/Dab1 system. Collectively, this investigation suggests estradiol as a proliferative regulator and migratory stimulator. Disruption to estrogenic signaling may result in an enlarged SVZ from impaired migration and un-regulated proliferative cycle. Alternatively, cells may accumulate within the CP after being ejected too early from the cell cycle. Understanding these mechanisms will further benefit developmental disorders.

AUTHOR CONTRIBUTIONS

MCSD and DPS wrote the manuscript. NJFG and KJS edited and contributed to the writing of the manuscript. KJS and DPS oversaw the project.

FUNDING

This study was funded by the Medical Research Council (MRC) grant MR/L021064/1 awarded to DPS.

ACKNOWLEDGMENTS

We thank Dr. George Chennell and the Wohl Cellular Imaging Centre for help with image acquisition.

REFERENCES

1. Adams, B. D., Furneaux, H., and White, B. A. (2007). The Micro-Ribonucleic Acid (miRNA) miR-206 targets the Human Estrogen Receptor-α (ERα) and Represses ERα Messenger, RNA., and protein expression in breast cancer cell lines. *Mol. Endocrinol.* 21, 1132–1147. doi: 10.1210/me.2007-0022
2. Adhya, D., Annuario, E., Lancaster, M. A., Price, J., Baron-Cohen, S., and Srivastava, D. P. (2018). Understanding the role of steroids in typical and atypical brain development: advantages of using a "brain in a dish" approach. *J. Neuroendocrinol.* 30:e12547. doi: 10.1111/jne.12547
3. Ajioka, I., and Nakajima, K. (2005). Switching of α-catenin from αE-catenin in the cortical ventricular zone to αN-catenin II in the intermediate zone. *Dev. Brain Res.* 160, 106–111. doi: 10.1016/j.devbrainres.2005.08.004
4. Alcaraz, M., Guzmán-Flores, C., Salas, M., and Beyer, C. (1969). Effect of estrogen on the responsivity of hypothalamic and mesencephalic neurons in the female cat. *Brain Res.* 15, 439–446. doi: 10.1016/0006-8993(69)90166-8
5. Angevine Jun, J. B., and Sidman, R. L. (1961). Autoradiographic study of cell migration during histogenesis of cerebral cortex in the mouse. *Nature* 192, 766–768. doi: 10.1038/192766b0
6. Arevalo, M. A., Ruiz-Palmero, I., Simon-Areces, J., Acaz-Fonseca, E., Azcoitia, I., and Garcia-Segura, L. M. (2011). Estradiol meets notch signaling in developing neurons. *Front. Endocrinol.* 2:21. doi: 10.3389/fendo.2011.00021
7. Arnold, A. P. (2004). Sex chromosomes and brain gender. *Nat. Rev. Neurosci.* 5, 701. doi: 10.1038/nrn1494
8. Augustine, C., Gunnersen, J., Spirkoska, V., and Tan, S.-S. (2001). Place- and time-dependent expression of mouse sFRP-1 during development of the cerebral neocortex. *Mech. Dev.* 109, 395–397. doi: 10.1016/S0925-4773(01)00533-0
9. Azcoitia, I., Yague, J. G., and Garcia-Segura, L. M. (2011). Estradiol synthesis within the human brain. *Neuroscience* 191, 139–147. doi: 10.1016/j.neuroscience.2011.02.012
10. Bakker, J., Honda, S.-I., Harada, N., and Balthazart, J. (2002). The aromatase knock-out mouse provides new evidence that estradiol is required during development in the female for the expression of

sociosexual behaviors in adulthood. *J. Neurosci.* 22, 9104–9112. doi: 10.1523/JNEUROSCI.22-20-09104.2002

11. Balthazart, J., and Ball, G. F. (2017). Is brain Estradiol a hormone or a neurotransmitter? *Trends Neurosci.* 29, 241–249. doi: 10.1016/j.tins.2006.03.004
12. Bender, R. A., Zhou, L., Wilkars, W., Fester, L., Lanowski, J.-S., Paysen, D., et al. (2010). Roles of 17β-estradiol involve regulation of reelin expression and synaptogenesis in the dentate gyrus. *Cereb. Cortex* 20, 2985–2995. doi: 10.1093/cercor/bhq047
13. Berman, N. E. J., Johnson, J. K., and Klein, R. M. (1997). Early generation of glia in the intermediate zone of the developing cerebral cortex. *Dev. Brain Res.* 101, 149–164. doi: 10.1016/S0165-3806(97)00060-6
14. Beyer, C. (1999). Estrogen and the developing mammalian brain. *Anat. Embryol.* 199, 379–390. doi: 10.1007/s004290050236
15. Biamonte, F., Assenza, G., Marino, R., DAmelio, M., Panteri, R., Caruso, D., et al. (2009). Interactions between neuroactive steroids and reelin haploinsufficiency in Purkinje cell survival. *Neurobiol. Dis.* 36, 103–115. doi: 10.1016/j.nbd.2009.07.001
16. Bilodeau, S., Roussel-Gervais, A., and Drouin, J. (2009). Distinct developmental roles of cell cycle inhibitors p57Kip2 and p27Kip1 distinguish pituitary progenitor cell cycle exit from cell cycle reentry of differentiated cells. *Mol. Cell. Biol.* 29, 1895–1908. doi: 10.1128/MCB.01885-08
17. Blaustein, J. D. (2008). An estrogen by any other name. *Endocrinology* 149, 2697–2698. doi: 10.1210/en.2008-0396
18. Bock, H. H., Jossin, Y., Liu, P., Förster, E., May, P., Goffinet, A. M., et al. (2003). Phosphatidylinositol 3-Kinase interacts with the adaptor protein Dab1 in response to reelin signaling and is required for normal cortical lamination. *J. Biol. Chem.* 278, 38772–38779. doi: 10.1074/jbc.M3064 16200
19. Bodine, P. V. N., Henderson, R. A., Green, J., Aronow, M., Owen, T., Stein, G. S., et al. (1998). Estrogen receptor-α is developmentally regulated during osteoblast differentiation and contributes to selective responsiveness of gene expression. *Endocrinology* 139, 2048–2057. doi: 10.1210/endo.139.4.5897
20. Boon, W. C., Chow, J. D. Y., and Simpson, E. R. (2010). "Chapter 12-The multiple roles of estrogens and the enzyme aromatase," in *Neuroendocrinology: the Normal Neuroendocrine System*, ed L. B. Martini (Elsevier), 209–232.
21. Brännvall, K., Korhonen, L., and Lindholm, D. (2002). Estrogen-receptor-dependent regulation of neural stem cell proliferation and differentiation. *Mol. and Cell. Neurosci.* 21, 512–520. doi: 10.1006/mcne.2002.1194
22. Brault, V., Moore, R., Kutsch, S., Ishibashi, M., Rowitch, D. H., McMahon, A. P., et al. (2001). Inactivation of the (β)-catenin gene by Wnt1-Cre-mediated deletion results in dramatic brain malformation and failure of craniofacial development. *Development* 128, 1253–1264.
23. Brinton, R. D. (2009). Estrogen-induced plasticity from cells to circuits: predictions for cognitive function. *Trends Pharmacol. Sci.* 30, 212–222. doi: 10.1016/j.tips.2008.12.006
24. Briz, V., Liu, Y., Zhu, G., Bi, X., and Baudry, M. (2015). A novel form of synaptic plasticity in field CA3 of hippocampus requires GPER1 activation and BDNF release. *J. Cell Biol.* 210, 1225–1237. doi: 10.1083/jcb.201504092
25. Bultje, R. S., Castaneda-Castellanos, D. R., Jan, L. Y., Jan, Y.-N., Kriegstein, A. R., and Shi, S.-H. (2018). Mammalian Par3 regulates progenitor cell asymmetric division via notch signaling in the developing neocortex. *Neuron* 63, 189–202. doi: 10.1016/j.neuron.2009.07.004
26. Callard, G. V., Petro, Z., and Ryan, K. J. (1977). Identification of aromatase in the reptilian brain. *Endocrinology* 100, 1214–1218. doi: 10.1210/endo-100-4-1214
27. Callard, G. V., Petro, Z., and Ryan, K. J. (1978). Phylogenetic distribution of aromatase and other androgen-converting enzymes in the central nervous system. *Endocrinology* 103, 2283–2290. doi: 10.1210/endo-103-6-2283
28. Cappello, S., Attardo, A., Wu, X., Iwasato, T., Itohara, S., Wilsch-Bräuninger, M., et al. (2006). The Rho-GTPase cdc42 regulates neural progenitor fate at the apical surface. *Nat. Neurosci.* 9, 1099–1107. doi: 10.1038/nn1744
29. Chai, X., and Frotscher, M. (2016). How does Reelin signaling regulate the neuronal cytoskeleton during migration? *Neurogenesis* 3:e1242455. doi: 10.1080/23262133.2016.1242455
30. Chang, H. C., Churchwell, M. I., Delclos, K. B., Newbold, R. R., and Doerge, D. R. (2000). Mass spectrometric determination of Genistein tissue distribution in diet-exposed sprague-dawley rats. *J. Nutr.* 130, 1963–1970. doi: 10.1093/jn/130.8.1963
31. Clark, A. S., Maclusky, N. J., and Goldman-Rakic, P. (1988). Androgen binding and metabolism in the cerebral cortex of the developing rhesus monkey. *Endocrinology* 123, 932–940. doi: 10.1210/endo-123-2-932
32. Clevers, H. (2018). Wnt/ß-catenin signaling in development and disease. *Cell.* 127, 469–480. doi: 10.1016/j.cell.2006.10.018
33. Cohen-Cory, S., and Fraser, S. E. (1995). Effects of brain-derived neurotrophic factor on optic axon branching and remodelling *in vivo*. *Nature* 378, 192–196. doi: 10.1038/378192a0
34. Collette, J. C., Choubey, L., and Smith, K. M. (2017). Glial and stem cell expression of murine fibroblast growth factor receptor 1 in the embryonic and perinatal nervous system. *PeerJ.* 5:e3519. doi: 10.7717/peerj.3519
35. Cornil, C. A., Ball, G. F., and Balthazart, J. (2006). Functional significance of the rapid regulation of brain estrogens: where do the estrogens come from? *Brain Res.* 1126, 2–26. doi: 10.1016/j.brainres.2006.07.098
36. Couse, J. F., Curtis, S. W., Washburn, T. F., Lindzey, J., Golding, T. S., Lubahn, D. B., et al. (1995). Analysis of transcription and estrogen insensitivity in the female mouse after targeted disruption of the estrogen receptor gene. *Mol. Endocrinol.* 9, 1441–1454.
37. Creppe, C., Malinouskaya, L., Volvert, M.-L., Gillard, M., Close, P., Malaise, O., et al. (2009). Elongator controls the migration and differentiation of cortical neurons through acetylation of α-tubulin. *Cell* 136, 551–564. doi: 10.1016/j.cell.2008.11.043
38. Dave, R. K., Ellis, T., Toumpas, M. C., Robson, J. P., Julian, E., Adolphe, C., et al. (2011). Sonic hedgehog and notch signaling can cooperate to regulate neurogenic divisions of neocortical progenitors. *PLoS ONE* 6:e14680. doi: 10.1371/journal.pone.0014680
39. Davis, L. K., Meyer, K. J., Rudd, D. S., Librant, A. L., Epping, E. A., Sheffield, V. C., et al. (2008). Pax6 3 deletion results in aniridia, autism and mental retardation. *Hum. Genet.* 123, 371–378. doi: 10.1007/s00439-008-0484-x
40. Dehay, C., and Kennedy, H. (2007). Cell-cycle control and cortical development. *Nat. Rev. Neurosci.* 8, 438–450. doi: 10.1038/nrn2097
41. De Marinis, E., Acaz-Fonseca, E., Arevalo, M. A., Ascenzi, P., Fiocchetti, M., Marino, M., et al. (2013). 17b-oestradiol anti-inflammatory effects in primary astrocytes require oestrogen receptor b-mediated neuroglobin up-regulation. *J. Neuroendocrinol.* 25, 260–270. doi: 10.1111/jne.12007
42. Di Leva, G., Gasparini, P., Piovan, C., Ngankeu, A., Garofalo, M., Taccioli, C., et al. (2010). MicroRNA cluster 221-222 and estrogen receptor α interactions in breast cancer. *J. Natl. Cancer Inst.* 102, 706–721. doi: 10.1093/jnci/djq102
43. Dillon, G. M., Tyler, W. A., Omuro, K. C., Kambouris, J., Tyminski, C., Henry, S., et al. (2017). CLASP2 links reelin to the cytoskeleton during neocortical development. *Neuron* 93, 1344.e5-1358.e5. doi: 10.1016/j.neuron.2017. 02.039
44. Doerge, D. R., Churchwell, M. I., Chang, H. C., Newbold, R. R., and Delclos, K. B. (2001). Placental transfer of the soy isoflavone genistein following dietary and gavage administration to Sprague Dawley rats. *Reprod. Toxicol.* 15, 105–110. doi: 10.1016/S0890-6238(01)00108-3
45. Doisneau-Sixou, S. F., Sergio, C. M., Carroll, J. S., Hui, R., Musgrove, E. A., and Sutherland, R. L. (2003). Estrogen and antiestrogen regulation of cell cycle progression in breast cancer cells. *Endocr. Relat. Cancer.* 10, 179–186. doi: 10.1677/erc.0.0100179
46. Dominique Toran-Allerand, C. (1976). Sex steroids and the development of the newborn mouse hypothalamus and preoptic area *in vitro*: implications for sexual differentiation. *Brain Res.* 106, 407–412. doi:10.1016/0006-8993(76)91038-6
47. Dwyer, M. A., Joseph, J. D., Wade, H. E., Eaton, M. L., Kunder, R. S., Kazmin, D., et al. (2010). WNT11 expression is induced by estrogen-related receptor α and β-catenin and acts in an autocrine manner to increase cancer cell migration. *Cancer Res.* 70, 9298–9308. doi: 10.1158/0008-5472.CAN-10-0226
48. Engel, S. M., Levy, B., Liu, Z., Kaplan, D., and Wolff, M. S. (2006). Xenobiotic phenols in early pregnancy amniotic fluid. *Reprod. Toxicol.* 21, 110–112. doi: 10.1016/j.reprotox.2005.07.007
49. Fang, D., Yang, H., Lin, J., Teng, Y., Jiang, Y., Chen, J., et al. (2015). 17β-Estradiol regulates cell proliferation, colony formation, migration, invasion and promotes apoptosis by upregulating miR-9 and thus degrades MALAT- 1 in osteosarcoma cell MG-63 in an estrogen receptor-independent manner. *Biochem. Biophys. Res. Commun.* 457, 500–506. doi: 10.1016/j.bbrc.2014.12.114
50. Feng, L., Allen, N. S., Simo, S., and Cooper, J. A. (2007). Cullin 5 regulates Dab1 protein levels and neuron positioning during cortical development. *Genes Dev.* 21, 2717–2730. doi: 10.1101/gad.1604207
51. Fiocchetti, M., Camilli, G., Acconcia, F., Leone, S., Ascenzi, P., and Marino, M. (2015). ERβ-dependent neuroglobin up-regulation impairs 17β-

estradiol-induced apoptosis in DLD-1 colon cancer cells upon oxidative stress injury. *J. Steroid Biochem. Mol. Biol.* 149(Suppl. C), 128–137. doi: 10.1016/j.jsbmb.2015.02.005

52. Forger, N. G., Rosen, G. J., Waters, E. M., Jacob, D., Simerly, R. B., and de Vries, G. J. (2004). Deletion of bax eliminates sex differences in the mouse forebrain. *Proc. Natl. Acad. Sci. U.S.A.* 101, 13666–13671. doi: 10.1073/pnas.040 4644101
53. Foster, J. S., Henley, D. C., Bukovsky, A., Seth, P., and Wimalasena, J. (2001). Multifaceted regulation of cell cycle progression by estrogen: regulation of Cdk inhibitors and Cdc25A independent of Cyclin D1-Cdk4 function. *Mol. Cell. Biol.* 21, 794–810. doi: 10.1128/MCB.21.3.794-810.2001
54. Fox, E. M., Andrade, J., and Shupnik, M. A. (2009). Novel actions of estrogen to promote proliferation: integration of cytoplasmic and nuclear pathways. *Steroids* 74, 622–627. doi: 10.1016/j.steroids.2008.10.014
55. Franco, S. J., Martinez-Garay, I., Gil-Sanz, C., Harkins-Perry, S. R., and Müller, U. (2018). Reelin regulates cadherin function via Dab1/Rap1 to control neuronal migration and lamination in the neocortex. *Neuron* 69, 482–497. doi: 10.1016/j.neuron.2011.01.003
56. Frick, K. M., Zhao, Z., and Fan, L. (2011). The epigenetics of estrogen: epigenetic regulation of hormone-induced memory enhancement. *Epigenetics* 6, 675–680. doi: 10.4161/epi.6.6.16177
57. Fried, G., Andersson, E., Csöregh, L., Enmark, E., Gustafsson, J., Aanesen, A., and Österlund, C. (2004), Estrogen receptor beta is expressed in human embryonic brain cells and is regulated by 17β-estradiol. *Eur. J. Neurosci.* 20, 2345–2354. doi: 10.1111/j.1460-9568.2004.03693.x
58. Galceran, J., Miyashita-Lin, E. M., Devaney, E., Rubenstein, J. L., and Grosschedl, R. (2000). Hippocampus development and generation of dentate gyrus granule cells is regulated by LEF1. *Development* 127, 469–482.
59. Gan, Q., Lee, A., Suzuki, R., Yamagami, T., Stokes, A., Nguyen, B. C., et al. (2014), Pax6 mediates ß-catenin signaling for self-renewal and neurogenesis by neocortical radial glial stem cells. *Stem Cells* 32, 45–58. doi: 10.1002/stem.1561
60. Gao, Y., Huang, E., Zhang, H., Wang, J., Wu, N., Chen, X., et al. (2013). Crosstalk between Wnt/β-catenin and estrogen receptor signaling synergistically promotes osteogenic differentiation of mesenchymal progenitor cells. *PLoS ONE* 8:e82436. doi: 10.1371/journal.pone.0082436
61. Gillies, G. E., and McArthur, S. (2010). Estrogen actions in the brain and the basis for differential action in men and women: a case for sex-specific medicines. *Pharmacol. Rev,* 62, 155–198. doi: 10.1124/pr.109.002071
62. Gobinath, A. R., Choleris, E., and Galea, L. A. M. (2017). Sex, hormones, and genotype interact to influence psychiatric disease, treatment, and behavioral research. *J. Neurosci. Res.* 95, 50–64. doi: 10.1002/jnr.23872
63. Gomez, T. M., and Letourneau, P. C. (2014). Actin dynamics in growth cone motility and navigation. *J. Neurochem.* 129, 221–234. doi: 10.1111/jnc.12506 Gorski, R. A. (1985). Sexual dimorphisms of the brain. *J. Anim, Sci,* 61(Suppl. 3), 38–61. doi: 10.1093/ansci/61.Supplement_3.38
64. Götz, M., and Huttner, W. B. (2005). The cell biology of neurogenesis. *Nat. Rev. Mol. Cell Biol.* 6, 777. doi: 10.1038/nrm1739
65. Grassi, D., Lagunas N., Amorim M., Pinos H., Panzica G., Garcia-Segura L. M., et al. (2012). Role of oestrogen receptors on the modulation of NADPH-diaphorase-positive cell number in supraoptic and paraventricular nuclei of ovariectomised female rats. *J. Neuroendocrinol.* 25, 244–250. doi: 10.1111/j.1365-2826.2012.02387.x
66. Grassi, S., Frondaroli, A., Scarduzio, M., Dieni, C. V., Brecchia, G., Boiti, C., et al. (2012). Influence of sex and estrous cycle on synaptic responses of the medial vestibular nuclei in rats: role of circulating 17β-estradiol. *Brain Res. Bull.* 87, 319–327. doi: 10.1016/j.brainresbull.2011.11.008
67. Greenberg, M. E., Xu, B., Lu, B., and Hempstead, B. L. (2009). New insights in the biology of BDNF synthesis and release: implications in CNS function. *J. Neurosci.* 29, 12764–12767. doi: 10.1523/JNEUROSCI.3566-09.2009
68. Greig, L. C., Woodworth, M. B., Galazo, M. J., Padmanabhan, H., and Macklis, J. D. (2013). Molecular logic of neocortical projection neuron specification, development and diversity. *Nat. Rev. Neurosci.* 14, 755. doi: 10.1038/nrn3586
69. Guglielmotto, M., Reineri, S., Iannello, A., Ferrero, G., Vanzan, L., Miano, V., et al. (2016). E2 regulates epigenetic signature on neuroglobin enhancer-promoter in neuronal cells. *Front. Cell. Neurosci.* 10:147. doi: 10.3389/fncel.2016.00147
70. Gui, Y., Chu, N., Qiu, X., Tang, W., Gober, H.-J., Li, D., et al. (2016). 17-β-estradiol up-regulates apolipoprotein genes expression during osteoblast differentiation *in vitro*. *Biosci. Trends.* 10, 140–151. doi: 10.5582/bst.2016.01007
71. Guo, L., Yu, J., Liang, T., and Zou, Q. (2016). miR-isomiRExp: a web-server for the analysis of expression of miRNA at the miRNA/isomiR levels. *Sci. Rep.* 6, 23700. doi: 10.1038/srep23700
72. Hall, M. K., Weidner, D. A., Dayal, S., and Schwalbe, R. A. (2014). Cell surface N- glycans influence the level of functional E-cadherin at the cell-cell border. *FEBS Open Bio* 4, 892–897. doi: 10.1016/j.fob.2014.10.006
73. Hammond, M. A., and Rowe, F. A. (1976). Medial preoptic and anterior hypothalamic lesions: influences on aggressive behavior in female hamsters. *Physiol. Behav.* 17, 507–513. doi: 10.1016/0031-9384(76)90115-3
74. Hansen, A. H., Duellberg, C., Mieck, C., Loose, M., and Hippenmeyer, S. (2017). Cell polarity in cerebral cortex development—cellular architecture shaped by biochemical networks. *Front. Cell. Neurosci.* 11, 176. doi: 10.3389/fncel.2017.00176
75. Hartfuss, E., Galli, R., Heins, N., and Götz, M. (2001). Characterization of CNS precursor subtypes and radial glia. *Dev. Biol.* 229, 15–30. doi: 10.1006/dbio.2000.9962
76. He, S., Li, Z., Ge, S., Yu, Y. C., and Shi, S. H. (2015). Inside-out radial migration facilitates lineage-dependent neocortical microcircuit assembly. *Neuron* 86, 159–166. doi: 10.1016/j.neuron.2015.05.002
77. He, Y., Wu, J., Ji, M., Ma, T., Qiao, E., Ma, R., et al. (2013). miR-342 is associated with estrogen receptor-α expression and response to tamoxifen in breast cancer. *Exp. Ther. Med.* 5, 813–818. doi: 10.3892/etm.2013.915
78. Helguero, L. A., Faulds, M. H., Gustafsson, J.-A., and Haldosen, L.-A. (2005). Estrogen receptors α (ERα) and β (ERß) differentially regulate proliferation and apoptosis of the normal murine mammary epithelial cell line HC11. *Oncogene* 24, 6605–6616. doi: 10.1038/sj.onc.1208807
79. Heng, J. I.-T., Chariot, A., and Nguyen, L. (2010). Molecular layers underlying cytoskeletal remodelling during cortical development. *Trends Neurosci.* 33, 38–47. doi: 10.1016/j.tins.2009.09.003
80. Hippenmeyer, S. (2014). "Molecular pathways controlling the sequential steps of cortical projection neuron migration BT," in *Cellular and Molecular Control of Neuronal Migration*, eds L. Nguyen, and S. Hippenmeyer (Dordrecht: Springer Netherlands), 1–24.
81. Hirota, Y., and Nakajima, K. (2017). Control of neuronal migration and aggregation by reelin signaling in the developing cerebral cortex. *Front. Cell Devel. Biol.* 5:40. doi: 10.3389/fcell.2017.00040
82. Hoerder-Suabedissen, A., Oeschger, F. M., Krishnan, M. L., Belgard, T. G., Wang, W. Z., Lee, S., et al. (2013). Expression profiling of mouse subplate reveals a dynamic gene network and disease association with autism and schizophrenia. *Proc. Natl. Acad. Sci. U.S.A.* 110, 3555–3560. doi: 10.1073/pnas.1218510110
83. Hojo, Y., Higo, S., Ishii, H., Ooishi, Y., Mukai, H., Murakami, G., et al. (2009). Comparison between hippocampus-synthesized and circulation-derived sex steroids in the hippocampus. *Endocrinology* 150, 5106–5112. doi: 10.1210/en.2009-0305
84. Huang, K.-T., Pavlides, S. C., Lecanda, J., Blank, S. V., Mittal, K. R., and Gold, L. I. (2012). Estrogen and progesterone regulate p27kip1 levels via the ubiquitin-proteasome system: pathogenic and therapeutic implications for endometrial cancer. *PLoS ONE* 7:e46072. doi: 10.1371/journal.pone.0046072
85. Humphreys, G. I., Ziegler, Y. S., and Nardulli, A. M. (2014). 17β-estradiol modulates gene expression in the female mouse cerebral cortex. *PLoS ONE* 9:e111975. doi: 10.1371/journal.pone.0111975
86. Imayoshi, I., Sakamoto, M., Yamaguchi, M., Mori, K., and Kageyama, R. (2010). Essential roles of notch signaling in maintenance of neural stem cells in developing and adult brains. *J. Neurosci.* 30, 3489–3498. doi: 10.1523/JNEUROSCI.4987-09.2010
87. Inagaki, T., Gautreaux, C., and Luine, V. (2010). Acute estrogen treatment facilitates recognition memory consolidation and alters monoamine levels in memory-related brain areas. *Horm. Behav.* 58, 415–426. doi: 10.1016/j.yhbeh.2010.05.013
88. Ish, H., Tsurugizawa, T., Ogiue-Ikeda, M., Asashima, M., Mukai, H., Murakami, G., et al. (2007). Local production of sex hormones and their modulation of hippocampal synaptic plasticity. *Neuroscientist* 13, 323–334. doi: 10.1177/10738584070130040601
89. Ishii, K., Kubo, K., and Nakajima, K. (2016). Reelin and neuropsychiatric disorders. *Front. Cell. Neurosci.* 10:229. doi: 10.3389/fncel.2016.00229
90. Ivanova, A., Nakahira, E., Kagawa, T., Oba, A., Wada, T., Takebayashi, H., et al. (2003). Evidence for a second wave of oligodendrogenesis in the postnatal cerebral cortex of the mouse. *J. Neurosci. Res.* 73, 581–592. doi: 10.1002/jnr.10717
91. Jacobson, C. D., and Gorski, R. A. (1981). Neurogenesis of the sexually

dimorphic nucleus of the preoptic area in the rat. *J. Comp. Neurol.* 196, 519–529. doi:10.1002/cne.901960313

92. Jadhav, R. R., Ye, Z., Huang, R.-L., Liu, J., Hsu, P.-Y., Huang, Y.-W., et al. (2015). Genome-wide DNA methylation analysis reveals estrogen-mediated epigenetic repression of metallothionein-1 gene cluster in breast cancer. *Clin. Epigenet.* 7, 13. doi: 10.1186/s13148-015-0045-9
93. Jazin, E., and Cahill, L. (2010). Sex differences in molecular neuroscience: from fruit flies to humans. *Nat. Rev. Neurosci.* 11, 9–17. doi: 10.1038/nrn2754
94. Jeon, M. J., Yang, W., Seo, H.-S., Wang, E. S., and Shin, I. (2012). Down-regulation of estrogen receptor α (ERα) transcriptional activity by p27 is mediated by inhibition of ERα nuclear localization and modulation of the ERα transcriptional complex. *Cell. Signal.* 24, 2249–2258. doi: 10.1016/j.cellsig.2012.07.011
95. Jiang, C.-F., Li, D.-M., Shi, Z.-M., Wang, L., Liu, M.-M., Ge, X., et al. (2016). Estrogen regulates miRNA expression: implication of estrogen receptor and miR-124/AKT2 in tumor growth and angiogenesis. *Oncotarget* 7, 36940–36955. doi: 10.18632/oncotarget.9230
96. Karolczak, M., Küppers, E., and Beyer, C. (2008). Developmental expression and regulation of aromatase- and 5α-reductase type 1 mRNA in the male and female mouse hypothalamus. *J. Neuroendocrinol.* 10, 267–274. doi: 10.1046/j.1365-2826.1998.00200.x
97. Karthikeyan, N., and Thampan, R. V. (1996). Plasma membrane is the primary site of localization of the nonactivated estrogen receptor in the goat uterus: hormone binding causes receptor internalization. *Arch. Biochem. Biophys.* 325, 47–57. doi: 10.1006/abbi.1996.0006
98. Katzenellenbogen, B. S., Choi, I., Delage-Mourroux, R., Ediger, T. R., Martini, P. G. V., Montano, M., et al. (2000). Molecular mechanisms of estrogen action: selective ligands and receptor pharmacology. *J. Steroid Biochem. Mol. Biol.* 74, 279–285. doi: 10.1016/S0960-0760(00)00104-7
99. Kawaguchi, A., Ogawa, M., Saito, K., Matsuzaki, F., Okano, H., and Miyata, T. (2004), Differential expression of Pax6 and Ngn2 between pair-generated cortical neurons. *J. Neurosci. Res.* 78, 784–795. doi: 10.1002/jnr.20347
100. Kelly, M. J., Qiu, J., and Rønnekleiv, O. K. (2005). Estrogen signaling in the hypothalamus. *Vitam. Horm.* 71, 123–145. doi:10.1016/S0083-6729(05)71005-0
101. Klinge, C. M. (2009). Estrogen regulation of MicroRNA expression. *Curr. Genomics* 10, 169–183. doi: 10.2174/138920209788185289
102. Knoblich, J. A. (2008). Mechanisms of asymmetric stem cell division. *Cell* 132, 583–597. doi: 10.1016/j.cell.2008.02.007
103. Kon, E., Cossard, A., and Jossin, Y. (2017). Neuronal polarity in the embryonic mammalian cerebral cortex. *Front. Cell. Neurosci.* 11:163. doi: 10.3389/fncel.2017.00163
104. Kondo, N., Toyama, T., Sugiura, H., Fujii, Y., and Yamashita, H. (2008). miR-206 Expression is down-regulated in estrogen receptor α-positive human breast cancer. *Cancer Res.* 68, 5004–5008. doi: 10.1158/0008-5472.CAN-08-0180
105. Konkle, A. T. M., and McCarthy, M. M. (2011). Developmental time course of estradiol, testosterone, and dihydrotestosterone levels in discrete regions of male and female rat brain. *Endocrinology* 152, 223–235. doi: 10.1210/en.2010-0607
106. Koutmani, Y., Hurel, C., Patsavoudi, E., Hack, M., Gotz, M., Thomaidou, D., et al. (2004). BM88 is an early marker of proliferating precursor cells that will differentiate into the neuronal lineage. *Eur. J. Neurosci.* 20, 2509–2523. doi:10.1111/j.1460-9568.2004.03724.x
107. Kouzmenko, A. P., Takeyama, K., Ito, S., Furutani, T., Sawatsubashi, S., Maki, A., et al. (2004). Wnt/β-catenin and estrogen signaling converge *in vivo*. *J. Biol. Chem.* 279, 40255–40258. doi: 10.1074/jbc.C400331200
108. Kretz, O., Fester, L., Wehrenberg, U., Zhou, L., Brauckmann, S., Zhao, S., et al. (2004). Hippocampal synapses depend on hippocampal estrogen synthesis. *J. Neurosci.* 24, 5913–5921. doi: 10.1523/JNEUROSCI.5186-03.2004
109. Kriegstein, A., and Parnavelas, J. G. (2006). Progress in corticogenesis. *Cereb. Cortex* 16(Suppl. 1), i1–i2. doi: 10.1093/cercor/bhk041
110. Kriska, J., Honsa, P., Dzamba, D., Butenko, O., Kolenicova, D., Janeckova, L., et al. (2016). Manipulating Wnt signaling at different subcellular levels affects the fate of neonatal neural stem/progenitor cells. *Brain Res.* 1651(Suppl. C), 73–87. doi: 10.1016/j.brainres.2016.09.026
111. Kubo, K., Arai, O., Omura, M., Watanabe, R., Ogata, R., and Aou, S. (2003). Low dose effects of bisphenol A on sexual differentiation of the brain and behavior in rats. *Neurosci. Res.* 45, 345–356. doi: 10.1016/S0168-0102(02)00251-1
112. Kuiper, G. G. J. M., Lemmen, J. G., Carlsson, B., Corton, J. C., Safe, S. H., van der Saag, P. T., et al. (1998). Interaction of estrogenic chemicals and phytoestrogens with estrogen receptor β. *Endocrinology* 139, 4252–4263. doi: 10.1210/endo.139.10.6216
113. Kundakovic, M., Gudsnuk, K., Franks, B., Madrid, J., Miller, R. L., Perera, F. P., et al. (2013). Sex-specific epigenetic disruption and behavioral changes following low-dose in utero bisphenol A exposure. *Proc. Natl. Acad. Sci. U.S.A.* 110, 9956–9961. doi: 10.1073/pnas.1214056110
114. Lancaster, M. A., Renner, M., Martin, C.-A., Wenzel, D., Bicknell, L. S., Hurles, M. E., et al. (2013). Cerebral organoids model human brain development and microcephaly. *Nature* 501, 373–379. doi: 10.1038/nature12517
115. Lane-Donovan, C., and Herz, J. (2017). The ApoE receptors Vldlr and Apoer2 in central nervous system function and disease. *J. Lipid Res.* 58, 1036–1043. doi: 10.1194/jlr.R075507
116. Li, L., Liu, Q. R., Xiong, X. X., Liu, J. M., Lai, X. J., Cheng, C., et al. and Chen, X. Q. (2014a). Neuroglobin promotes neurite outgrowth via differential binding to PTEN and Akt. *Mol. Neurobiol.* 49, 149–162. doi: 10.1007/s12035-013- 8506-7
117. Li, Q., Wang, H., Yu, L., Zhou, J., Chen, J., Zhang, X., et al. (2014b). ChIP-seq predicted estrogen receptor biding sites in human breast cancer cell line MCF7. *Tumor Biol.* 35, 4779–4784. doi: 10.1007/s13277-014-1627-4
118. Li, Y., Yan, M., Wang, Z., Zheng, Y., Li, J., Ma, S., et al. (2014c). 17β-estradiol promotes the odonto/osteogenic differentiation of stem cells from apical papilla via mitogen-activated protein kinase pathway. *Stem Cell Res. Ther.* 5, 125. doi: 10.1186/scrt515
119. Lindberg, M. K., Movérare, S., Skrtic, S., Gao, H., Dahlman-Wright, K., Gustafsson, J.-A. et al. (2003). Estrogen receptor (ER)-β reduces ERα-regulated gene transcription, supporting a "Ying Yang" relationship between ERα and ERβ in mice. *Mol. Endocrinol.* 17, 203–208. doi: 10.1210/me.2002-0206
120. Lindzey, J., and Korach, K. S. (1997). Developmental and physiological effects of estrogen receptor gene disruption in mice. *Trends Endocrinol. Metab.* 8, 137–145. doi: 10.1016/S1043-2760(97)00007-6
121. Liu, J., Wang, D., Li, X., and Ningyu, W. (2017). Association between sex and speech auditory brainstem responses in adults, and relationship to sex hormone levels. *Med. Sci. Monitor* 23, 2275–2283. doi: 10.12659/MSM.904651
122. Luine, V. N. (2014). Estradiol and cognitive function: past, present and future. *Horm. Behav.* 66, 602–618. doi: 10.1016/j.yhbeh.2014.08.011
123. MacLusky, N. J., Walters, M. J., Clark, A. S., and Toran-Allerand, C. D. (1994). Aromatase in the cerebral cortex, hippocampus, and mid-brain: ontogeny and developmental implications. *Mol. Cell. Neurosci.* 5, 691–698. doi: 10.1006/mcne.1994.1083
124. Malinowska-Kolodziej, I., Larysz-Brysz, M., Jedrzejowska-Szypulka, H., Marcol, W., Wlaszczuk, A., and Lewin-Kowalik, J. (2009). 17β-estradiol and predegenerated nerve graft effect on hippocampal neurogenesis in adult female rats. *Neuro Endocrinol. Lett.* 30, 195–203.
125. Marín, O., Valiente, M., Ge, X., and Tsai, L.-H. (2010). Guiding neuronal cell migrations. *Cold Spring Harb. Perspect. Biol.* 2:a001834. doi: 10.1101/cshperspect.a001834
126. Marron Fernandez de Velasco, E., Hearing, M., Xia, Z., Victoria, N. C., Luján, R., and Wickman, K. (2015). Sex differences in GABA(B)R-GIRK signaling in layer 5/6 pyramidal neurons of the mouse prelimbic cortex. *Neuropharmacology* 95, 353–360. doi: 10.1016/j.neuropharm.2015.03.029
127. Martinez, F. G., Hermel, E. E. S., Xavier, L. L., Viola, G. G., Riboldi, J., Rasia-Filho, A. A., et al. (2006). Gonadal hormone regulation of glial fibrillary acidic protein immunoreactivity in the medial amygdala subnuclei across the estrous cycle and in castrated and treated female rats. *Brain Res.* 1108, 117–126. doi: 10.1016/j.brainres.2006.06.014
128. McCarthy, M. M. (2008). Estradiol and the developing brain. *Physiol. Rev.* 88, 91–124. doi: 10.1152/physrev.00010.2007
129. McCarthy, M. M., and Arnold, A. P. (2011). Reframing sexual differentiation of the brain. *Nat. Neurosci.* 14, 677–683. doi: 10.1038/nn.2834
130. McCarthy, M. M., and Nugent, B. M. (2013). Epigenetic contributions to hormonally-mediated sexual differentiation of the brain. *J. Neuroendocrinol.* 25, 1133–1140. doi: 10.1111/jne.12072
131. McEwen, B. S., and Alves, S. E. (1999). Estrogen actions in the central nervous system. *Endocr. Rev.* 20, 279–307. doi: 10.1210/er.20.3.279
132. Mellios, N., Galdzicka, M., Ginns, E., Baker, S. P., Rogaev, E., Xu, J., et al. (2012). Gender-specific reduction of estrogen-sensitive small, RNA., miR-30b, in subjects with schizophrenia. *Schizophrenia Bull.* 38, 433–443. doi: 10.1093/schbul/sbq091
133. Milner, T. A., Ayoola, K., Drake, C. T., Herrick, S. P., Tabori, N. E.,

McEwen, B. S., et al. (2005). Ultrastructural localization of estrogen receptor β immunoreactivity in the rat hippocampal formation. *J. Comp. Neurol.* 491, 81–95. doi: 10.1002/cne.20724

134. Milner, T. A., McEwen, B. S., Hayashi, S., Li, C. J., Reagan, L. P., and Alves, S. E. (2000). Ultrastructural evidence that hippocampal α estrogen receptors are located at extranuclear sites. *J. Comp. Neurol.* 429, 355–371. doi: 10.1002/1096- 9861(20010115)429:3<355::AID-CNE1>3.0.CO;2-#

135. Mitra, S. W., Hoskin, E., Yudkovitz, J., Pear, L., Wilkinson, H. A., Hayashi, S., et al. (2003). Immunolocalization of estrogen receptor β in the mouse brain: comparison with estrogen receptor α. *Endocrinology* 144, 2055–2067. doi:10.1210/en.2002-221069

136. Molyneaux, B. J., Arlotta, P., Menezes, J. R. L., and Macklis, J. D. (2007). Neuronal subtype specification in the cerebral cortex. *Nat. Rev. Neurosci.* 8, 427. doi:10.1038/nrn2151

137. Mosley, M., Weathington, J., Cortes, L. R., Bruggeman, E., Castillo-Ruiz, A., Xue, B., et al. (2017). Neonatal inhibition of DNA methylation alters cell phenotype in sexually dimorphic regions of the mouse brain. *Endocrinology* 158, 1838–1848. doi: 10.1210/en.2017-00205

138. Munji, R. N., Choe, Y., Li, G., Siegenthaler, J. A., and Pleasure, S. J. (2011). Wnt signaling regulates neuronal differentiation of cortical intermediate progenitors. *J. Neurosci.* 31, 1676–1687. doi: 10.1523/JNEUROSCI.5404-10.2011

139. Nagafuchi, A., Shirayoshi, Y., Okazaki, K., Yasuda, K., and Takeichi, M. (1987). Transformation of cell adhesion properties by exogenously introduced E- cadherin cDNA. *Nature* 329, 341–343. doi: 10.1038/329341a0

140. Nelson, R. J., and Trainor, B. C. (2007). Neural mechanisms of aggression. *Nat. Rev. Neurosci.* 8, 536. doi: 10.1038/nrn2174

141. Nieto, M., Monuki, E. S., Tang, H., Imitola, J., Haubst, N., Khoury, S. J., et al. (2004). Expression of Cux-1 and Cux-2 in the subventricular zone and upper layers II- IV of the cerebral cortex. *J. Comp. Neurol.* 479, 168–180. doi: 10.1002/cne.20322

142. Nikaido, Y., Yoshizawa, K., Danbara, N., Tsujita-Kyutoku, M., Yuri, T., Uehara, N., et al. (2004). Effects of maternal xenoestrogen exposure on development of the reproductive tract and mammary gland in female CD-1 mouse offspring. *Reprod. Toxicol.* 18, 803–811. doi: 10.1016/j.reprotox.2004.05.002

143. Niwa, Y., Shimojo, H., and Kageyama, R. (2009). "Ultradian oscillation networks in somite segmentation and other biological events BT - systems biology," in *The Challenge of Complexity*, eds S. Nakanishi, R. Kageyama, and D. Watanabe (Tokyo: Springer), 199–207.

144. Noctor, S. C., Martinez-Cerdeno, V., Ivic, L., and Kriegstein, A. R. (2004). Cortical neurons arise in symmetric and asymmetric division zones and migrate through specific phases. *Nat. Neurosci.* 7, 136–144. doi: 10.1038/nn1172

145. Nuñez, J., Huppenbauer, C., McAbee, M., Juraska, J., and DonCarlos, L. (2003). Androgen receptor expression in the developing male and female rat visual and prefrontal cortex. *J. Neurobiol.* 56, 293–302. doi: 10.1002/neu.10236

146. Nugent, B. M., Wright, C. L., Shetty, A. C., Hodes, G. E., Lenz, K. M., Mahurkar, A., et al. (2015). Brain feminization requires active repression of masculinization via DNA methylation. *Nat. Neurosci.* 18, 690–697. doi: 10.1038/ nn.3988

147. Numakawa, T., Yokomaku, D., Richards, M., Hori, H., Adachi, N., and Kunugi, H. (2010). Functional interactions between steroid hormones and neurotrophin BDNF. *World J. Biol. Chem.* 1, 133–143. doi: 10.4331/wjbc.v1.i5.133

148. Ohtaka-Maruyama, C., and Okado, H. (2015). Molecular pathways underlying projection neuron production and migration during cerebral cortical development. *Front. Neurosci.* 9:447. doi: 10.3389/fnins.2015.00447

149. Ohtaka-Maruyama, C., Hirai, S., Miwa, A., Heng, J. I.-T., Shitara, H., Ishii, R., et al. (2018). RP58 regulates the multipolar-bipolar transition of newborn neurons in the developing cerebral cortex. *Cell Rep.* 3, 458–471. doi:10.1016/j.celrep.2013.01.012

150. Okada, M., Makino, A., Nakajima, M., Okuyama, S., Furukawa, S., and Furukawa, Y. (2010). Estrogen stimulates proliferation and differentiation of neural stem/progenitor cells through different signal transduction pathways. *Int. J. Mol. Sci. Mol. Divers. Preserv. Int.* 11, 4114–4123. doi: 10.3390/ijms111 04114

151. Okada, M., Murase, K., Makino, A., Nakajima, M., Kaku, T., Furukawa, S., et al. (2008). Effects of estrogens on proliferation and differentiation of neural stem/progenitor cells. *Biomed. Res.* 29, 163–170. doi: 10.2220/biomedres.29.163

Ornitz, D. M., and Itoh, N. (2015). The fibroblast growth factor signaling pathway. *Wiley Interdiscip. Rev. Dev. Biol.* 4, 215–266. doi: 10.1002/wdev.176

152. Pacary, E., Heng, J., Azzarelli, R., Riou, P., Castro, D., Lebel-Potter, M., et al. (2011). Proneural transcription factors regulate different steps of cortical neuron migration through Rnd-mediated inhibition of RhoA signaling. *Neuron* 69, 1069–1084. doi: 10.1016/j.neuron.2011.02.018

153. Pandey, D. P., and Picard, D. (2009). miR-22 inhibits estrogen signaling by directly targeting the estrogen receptor α mRNA. *Mol. Cell. Biol.* 29, 3783–3790. doi: 10.1128/MCB.01875-08

154. Pasmanik, M., and Callard, G. V. (1985). Aromatase and 5α-reductase in the teleost brain, spinal cord, and pituitary gland. *Gen. Comp. Endocrinol.* 60, 244–251. doi:10.1016/0016-6480(85)90320-X

155. Patchev, A. V., Gotz, F., and Rohde, W. (2004). Differential role of estrogen receptor isoforms in sex-specific brain organization. *FASEB J.* 18, 1568–1570. doi: 10.1096/fj.04-1959fje

156. Patisaul, H. B., and Jefferson, W. (2010). The pros and cons of phytoestrogens. *Front. Neuroendocrinol.* 31, 400–419. doi: 10.1016/j.yfrne.2010.03.003

157. Pérez, S. E., Chen, E.-Y., and Mufson, E. J. (2003). Distribution of estrogen receptor alpha and beta immunoreactive profiles in the postnatal rat brain. *Dev. Brain Res.* 145, 117–139. doi: 10.1016/S0165-3806(03)00223-2

158. Pierman, S., Sica, M., Allieri, F., Viglietti-Panzica, C., Panzica, G. C., and Bakker, J. (2008). Activational effects of estradiol and dihydrotestosterone on social recognition and the arginine-vasopressin immunoreactive system in male mice lacking a functional aromatase gene. *Horm. Behav.* 54, 98–106. doi: 10.1016/j.yhbeh.2008.02.001

159. Polleux, F., and Snider, W. (2010). Initiating and growing an axon. *Cold Spring Harb. Perspect. Biol.* 2:a001925. doi: 10.1101/cshperspect.a001925

160. Prall, O. W., Sarcevic, B., Musgrove, E. A., Watts, C. K., and Sutherland, R. L. (1997). Estrogen-induced activation of Cdk4 and Cdk2 during G1-S phase progression is accompanied by increased cyclin D1 expression and decreased cyclin-dependent kinase inhibitor association with cyclin E-Cdk2. *J. Biol. Chem.* 272, 10882–10894.

161. Rakic, P. (1971). Guidance of neurons migrating to the fetal monkey neocortex. *Brain Res.* 33, 471–476. doi: 10.1016/0006-8993(71)90119-3

162. Ramón y Cajal, S. (1911). *Histology of the Nervous System of Man and Vertebrates.* New Yor, NY: Oxford University Press.

163. Reisert, I., and Pilgrim, C. (1991). Sexual differentiation of monoaminergic neurons - genetic or epigenetic? *Trends Neurosci.* 14, 468–473. doi: 10.1016/0166-2236(91)90047-X

164. Roof, R. L. (1993). The dentate gyrus is sexually dimorphic in prepubescent rats: testosterone plays a significant role. *Brain Res.* 610, 148–151. doi: 10.1016/0006-8993(93)91228-K

165. Roselli, C. E., and Stormshak, F. (2010). The ovine sexually dimorphic nucleus, aromatase, and sexual partner preferences in sheep. *J. Steroid Biochem. Mol. Biol.* 118, 252–256. doi: 10.1016/j.jsbmb.2009.10.009

166. Ruiz-Palmero, I., Hernando, M., Garcia-Segura, L. M., and Arevalo, M.-A. (2013). G protein-coupled estrogen receptor is required for the neuritogenic mechanism of 17β-estradiol in developing hippocampal neurons. *Mol. Cell. Endocrinol.* 372, 105–115. doi: 10.1016/j.mce.2013.03.018

167. Rune, G. M., and Frotscher, M. (2005). Neurosteroid synthesis in the hippocampus: role in synaptic plasticity. *Neuroscience* 136, 833–842. doi: 10.1016/j.neuroscience.2005.03.056

168. Sadowski, R. N., Wise, L. M., Park, P. Y., Schantz, S. L., and Juraska, J. M. (2014). Early exposure to bisphenol A alters neuron and glia number in the rat prefrontal cortex of adult males, but not females. *Neuroscience* 279, 122–131. doi: 10.1016/j.neuroscience.2014.08.038

169. Sailland, J., Tribollet, V., Forcet, C., Billon, C., Barenton, B., Carnesecchi, J., et al. (2014). Estrogen-related receptor α decreases RHOA stability to induce orientated cell migration. *Proc. Natl. Acad. Sci. U.S.A.* 111, 15108–15113. doi:10.1073/pnas.1402094111

170. Salama-Cohen, P., Arévalo, M.-Á., Grantyn, R., and Rodríguez-Tébar, A. (2006). Notch and NGF/p75NTR control dendrite morphology and the balance of excitatory/inhibitory synaptic input to hippocampal neurones through neurogenin 3. *J. Neurochem.* 97, 1269–1278. doi: 10.1111/j.1471-4159.2006.03783.x

171. Saldanha, C. J., Burstein, S. R., and Duncan, K. A. (2013). Induced synthesis of oestrogens by glia in the songbird brain. *J. Neuroendocrinol.* 25, 1032–1038. doi:10.1111/jne.12067

172. Saldanha, C. J., Remage-Healey, L., and Schlinger, B. A. (2011). Synaptocrine signaling: steroid synthesis and action at the synapse. *Endocr. Rev.* 32, 532–549. doi: 10.1210/er.2011-0004

173. Sanchez, A. M., Flamini, M. I., Fu, X. D., Mannella, P., Giretti, M. S., Goglia, L., et al. (2009). Rapid signaling of estrogen to WAVE1 and moesin controls

neuronal spine formation via the actin cytoskeleton. *Mol. Endocrinol.* 23, 1193–1202. doi: 10.1210/me.2008-0408

174. Sánchez-Criado, J. E., Martín de las Mulas, J., Bellido, C., Tena-Sempere, M., Aguilar, R., and Blanco, A. (2004). Biological role of pituitary estrogen receptors erα and erβ on progesterone receptor expression and action and on gonadotropin and prolactin secretion in the rat. *Neuroendocrinology* 79, 247–258. doi: 10.1159/000079100

175. Sárvári, M., Kalló, I., Hrabovszky, E., Solymosi, N., Tóth, K., Likó, Z., et al. (2010). Estradiol replacement alters expression of genes related to neurotransmission and immune surveillance in the frontal cortex of middle-aged, ovariectomized rats. *Endocrinology* 151, 3847–3862. doi: 10.1210/en.2010-0375

176. Sasaki, Y., Cheng, C., Uchida, Y., Nakajima, O., Ohshima, T., Yagi, T., et al. (2002). Fyn and Cdk5 mediate semaphorin-3A signaling, which is involved in regulation of dendrite orientation in cerebral cortex. *Neuron* 35, 907–920. doi: 10.1016/S0896-6273(02)00857-7

177. Sasano, H., Takahashi, K., Satoh, F., Nagura, H., and Harada, N. (1998). Aromatase in the human central nervous system. *Clin. Endocrinol.* 48, 325–329. doi: 10.1046/j.1365-2265.1998.00390.x

178. Sato, K., Akaishi, T., Matsuki, N., Ohno, Y., and Nakazawa, K. (2007). β-Estradiol induces synaptogenesis in the hippocampus by enhancing brain-derived neurotrophic factor release from dentate gyrus granule cells. *Brain Res.* 1150(Suppl. C), 108–120. doi: 10.1016/j.brainres.2007. 02.093

179. Scallet, A. C., Divine, R. L., Newbold, R. R., and Delclos, K. B. (2004). Increased volume of the calbindin D28k-labeled sexually dimorphic hypothalamus in genistein and nonylphenol-treated male rats. *Toxicol. Sci.* 82, 570–576. doi: 10.1093/toxsci/kfh297

180. Scerbo, M. J., Freire-Regatillo, A., Cisternas, C. D., Brunotto, M., Arevalo, M. A., Garcia-Segura, L. M., et al. (2014). Neurogenin 3 mediates sex chromosome effects on the generation of sex differences in hypothalamic neuronal development. *Front. Cell. Neurosci.* 8:188. doi: 10.3389/fncel.2014. 00188

181. Scharfman, H. E., and Maclusky, N. J. (2005). Similarities between actions of estrogen and BDNF in the hippocampus: coincidence or clue? *Trends Neurosci.* 28, 79–85. doi: 10.1016/j.tins.2004.12.005

182. Scholzen, T., and Gerdes, J. (2000). The Ki-67 protein: from the known and the unknown. *J. Cell. Physiol.* 182, 311–322. doi: 10.1002/(SICI)1097-4652(200003)182:3<311::AID-JCP1>3.0.CO;2-9

183. Scott, E. L., and Brann, D. W. (2013). Estrogen regulation of Dkk1 and Wnt/β-catenin signaling in neurodegenerative disease. *Brain Res.* 1514, 63–74. doi: 10.1016/j.brainres.2012.12.015

184. Sellers, K. J., Erli, F., Raval, P., Watson, I. A., Chen, D., and Srivastava, D. P. (2015a). Rapid modulation of synaptogenesis and spinogenesis by 17β-estradiol in primary cortical neurons. *Front. Cell. Neurosci.* 9:137. doi: 10.3389/fncel.2015.00137

185. Sellers, K. J., Raval, P., and Srivastava, D. P. (2015b). Molecular signature of rapid estrogen regulation of synaptic connectivity and cognition *Front. Neuroendocrinol.* 36, 72–89. doi: 10.1016/j.yfrne.2014. 08.001

186. Sessa, A., Mao, C., Hadjantonakis, A.-K., Klein, W. H., and Broccoli, V. (2008). Tbr2 directs conversion of radial glia into basal precursors and guides neuronal amplification by indirect neurogenesis in the developing neocortex. *Neuron* 60, 56–69. doi: 10.1016/j.neuron.2008.09.028

187. Shang, A., Zhou, D., Wang, L., Gao, Y., Fan, M., Wang, X., et al. (2006). Increased neuroglobin levels in the cerebral cortex and serum after ischemia-reperfusion insults. *Brain Res.* 1078, 219–226. doi: 10.1016/j.brainres.2006.01.064

188. Shughrue, P. J., and Merchenthaler, I. (2000). Estrogen is more than just a "Sex Hormone": novel sites for estrogen action in the hippocampus and cerebral cortex. *Front. Neuroendocrinol.* 21, 95–101. doi: 10.1006/frne.19 99.0190

189. Shughrue, P. J., and Merchenthaler, I. (2001). Distribution of estrogen receptor β immunoreactivity in the rat central nervous system. *J. Comp. Neurol.* 436, 64–81. doi: 10.1002/cne.1054

190. Shughrue, P. J., Lane, M. V., and Merchenthaler, I. (1997). Comparative distribution of estrogen receptor-α and -β mRNA in the rat central nervous system. *J. Comp. Neurol.* 388, 507–525. doi: 10.1002/(SICI)1096-9861(19971201)388:4<507::AID-CNE1>3.0.CO;2-6

191. Shughrue, P. J., Lane, M. V., and Merchenthaler, I. (1999). Localization of 125I- estrogen binding sites in the rat cerebral cortex and hippocampus: an *in vivo* autoradiographic study. *Soc. Neurosci. Abstr.* 25, 2613–2620.

192. Simerly, R. B., Swanson, L. W., Handa, R. J., and Gorski, R. A. (1985). Influence of perinatal androgen on the sexually dimorphic distribution of tyrosine hydroxylase-immunoreactive cells and fibers in the anteroventral periventricular nucleus of the rat. *Neuroendocrinology* 40, 501–510. doi: 10.1159/000124122

193. Simon-Areces, J., Acaz-Fonseca, E., Ruiz-Palmero, I., Garcia-Segura, L.-M., and Arevalo, M.-A. (2013). A CRM1-mediated nuclear export signal is essential for cytoplasmic localization of neurogenin 3 in neurons. *PLoS ONE* 8:e55237. doi: 10.1371/journal.pone.0055237

194. Singer, C. A., Figueroa-Masot, X. A., Batchelor, R. H., and Dorsa, D. M. (1999). The mitogen-activated protein kinase pathway mediates estrogen neuroprotection after glutamate toxicity in primary cortical neurons. *J. Neurosci.* 19, 2455–2463.

195. Singh, M., Sétáló, G., Guan, X., Warren, M., and Toran-Allerand, C. D. (1999). Estrogen-induced activation of mitogen-activated protein kinase in cerebral cortical explants: convergence of estrogen and neurotrophin signaling pathways. *J. Neurosci.* 19, 1179–1188.

196. Sohoni, P., and Sumpter, J. P. (1998). Several environmental oestrogens are also anti-androgens. *J. Endocrinol.* 158, 327–339. doi: 10.1677/joe.0.1580327

197. Solum, D. T., and Handa, R. J. (2002). Estrogen regulates the development of brain-derived neurotrophic factor mRNA and protein in the rat hippocampus. *J. Neurosci.* 22, 2650–2659. doi: 10.1523/JNEUROSCI.22-07-026 50.2002

198. Srivastava, D. P., and Evans, P. D. (2013). G-Protein oestrogen receptor 1: trials and tribulations of a membrane oestrogen receptor. *J. Neuroendocrinol.* 25, 1219–1230. doi: 10.1111/jne.12071

199. Srivastava, D. P., Jones, K. A., Woolfrey, K. M., Burgdorf, J., Russell, T. A., Kalmbach, A., et al. (2012a). Social, communication, and cortical structural impairments in Epac2-deficient mice. *J. Neurosci.* 32, 11864–11878. doi: 10.1523/JNEUROSCI.1349-12.2012

200. Srivastava, D. P., Waters, E. M., Mermelstein, P. G., Kramár, E. A., Shors, T. J., and Liu, F. (2011). Rapid estrogen signaling in the brain: implications for the fine-tuning of neuronal circuitry. *J. Neurosci.* 31, 16056–16063. doi: 10.1523/JNEUROSCI.4097-11.2011

201. Srivastava, D. P., Woolfrey, K. M., and Evans, P. D. (2013a). Mechanisms underlying the interactions between rapid estrogenic and BDNF control of synaptic connectivity. *Neuroscience* 239, 17–33. doi: 10.1016/j. neuroscience.2012.12.004

202. Srivastava, D. P., Woolfrey, K. M., and Penzes, P. (2013b). Insights into rapid modulation of neuroplasticity by brain estrogens. *Pharmacol. Rev..* 65, 1318–1350. doi: 10.1124/pr.111.005272

203. Srivastava, D. P., Woolfrey, K. M., Jones, K., a, Anderson, C. T., Smith, K. R., Russell, T., et al. Penzes, P. (2012b). An autism-associated variant of Epac2 reveals a role for Ras/Epac2 signaling in controlling basal dendrite maintenance in mice. *PLoS Biol.* 10:e1001350. doi: 10.1371/journal.pbio.1001350

204. Srivastava, D. P., Woolfrey, K. M., Liu, F., Brandon, N. J., and Penzes, P. (2010). Estrogen receptor β (ERβ) activity modulates synaptic signaling and structure. *J. Neurosci.* 30, 13454–13460. doi: 10.1523/JNEUROSCI.3264-10.2010

205. Srivastava, R. A., Srivastava, N., Averna, M., Lin, R. C., Korach, K. S., Lubahn, D. B., et al. (1997). Estrogen up-regulates apolipoprotein E (ApoE) gene expression by increasing ApoE mRNA in the translating pool via the estrogen receptor alpha-mediated pathway. *J. Biol. Chem.* 272, 33360–33366. doi: 10.1074/JBC.272.52.33360

206. Stoffel-Wagner, B. (2001). Neurosteroid metabolism in the human brain. *Eur. J. Endocrinol.* 145, 669–679. doi: 10.1530/eje.0.1450669

207. Stranahan, A. M., Erion, J. R., and Wosiski-Kuhn, M. (2013). Reelin signaling in development, maintenance, and plasticity of neural networks. *Ageing Res. Rev.* 12, 815–822. doi: 10.1016/j.arr.2013.01.005

208. Su, L. F., Knoblauch, R., and Garabedian, M. J. (2001). Rho GTPases as modulators of the estrogen receptor transcriptional response. *J. Biol. Chem.* 276, 3231–3237. doi: 10.1074/jbc.M005547200

209. Suter, D. M., Tirefort, D., Julien, S., and Krause, K. (2009). A Sox1 to Pax6 switch drives neuroectoderm to radial glia progression during differentiation of mouse embryonic stem cells. *Stem Cells* 27, 49–58. doi: 10.1634/stemcells.2008-0319

210. Swaab, D. F., Gooren, L. J., and Hofman, M. A. (1995). Brain research, gender and sexual orientation. *J. Homosex.* 28, 283–301. doi: 10.1300/J082v28n03_07

211. Tabibnia, G., Cooke, B. M., and Breedlove, S. M. (1999). Sex difference and laterality in the volume of mouse dentate gyrus granule cell layer. *Brain Res.* 827, 41–45. doi: 10.1016/S0006-8993(99)01262-7

212. Tan, S., Ding, K., Li, R., Zhang, W., Li, G., Kong, X., et al. (2014). Identification of miR-26 as a key mediator of estrogen stimulated cell proliferation by targeting CHD1, GREB1 and KPNA2. *Breast Cancer Res.* 16, R40. doi: 10.1186/bcr3644

213. Tan, X., Dai, Y., Wu, W., Kim, H.-J., Barros, R. P. A., Richardson, T. I., et al.

(2012). Reduction of dendritic spines and elevation of GABAergic signaling in the brains of mice treated with an estrogen receptor β ligand. *Proc. Natl. Acad. Sci. U.S.A.* 109, 1708–1712. doi: 10.1073/pnas.1121162109

214. Taverna, E., Götz, M., and Huttner, W. B. (2014). The cell biology of neurogenesis: toward an understanding of the development and evolution of the neocortex. *Annu. Rev. Cell Dev. Biol.* 30, 465–502. doi: 10.1146/annurev-cellbio-101011-155801

215. Tobet, S. A., Baum, M. J., Tang, H. B., Shim, J. H., and Canick, J. A. (1985). Aromatase activity in the perinatal rat forebrain: effects of age, sex and intrauterine position. *Brain Res.* 355, 171–178. doi: 10.1016/0165-3806(85)90038-0

216. Tsukahara, S. (2009). Sex differences and the roles of sex steroids in apoptosis of sexually dimorphic nuclei of the preoptic area in postnatal rats. *J. Neuroendocrinol.* 21, 370–376. doi: 10.1111/j.1365-2826.2009.01855.x

217. Ubuka, T., and Tsutsui, K. (2014). Review: neuroestrogen regulation of socio-sexual behavior of males. *Front. Neurosci.* 8:323. doi: 10.3389/fnins.2014.00323

218. Vinci, L., Ravarino, A., Fanos, V., Naccarato, A. G., Senes, G., Gerosa, C., et al. (2016). Immunohistochemical markers of neural progenitor cells in the early embryonic human cerebral cortex. *Eur. J. Histochem.* 60:2563. doi: 10.4081/ejh.2016.2563

219. Wang, L., Andersson, S., Warner, M., and Gustafsson, J.-Å. (2003). Estrogen receptor (ER)β knockout mice reveal a role for ERβ in migration of cortical neurons in the developing brain. *Proc. Natl. Acad. Sci. U.S.A.* 100, 703–708. doi: 10.1073/pnas.242735799

220. Wang, L., Chang, X., She, L., Xu, D., Huang, W., and Poo, M. (2015). Autocrine action of BDNF on dendrite development of adult-born hippocampal neurons. *J. Neurosci.* 35, 8384–8393. doi: 10.1523/JNEUROSCI.4682-14.201

221. Waterhouse, E. G., and Xu, B. (2009). New insights into the role of brain-derived neurotrophic factor in synaptic plasticity. *Mol. Cell. Neurosci.* 42, 81–89. doi: 10.1016/j.mcn.2009.06.009

222. Waters, E. M., and Simerly, R. B. (2009). Estrogen induces caspase-dependent cell death during hypothalamic development. *J. Neurosci.* 29, 9714–9718. doi: 10.1523/JNEUROSCI.0135-09.2009

223. Werling, D. M., and Geschwind, D. H. (2013). Sex differences in autism spectrum disorders. *Curr. Opin. Neurol.* 26, 146–153. doi: 10.1097/WCO.0b013e32835ee548

224. Westberry, J. M., and Wilson, M. E. (2012). Regulation of estrogen receptor alpha gene expression in the mouse prefrontal cortex during early postnatal development. *Neurogenetics* 13, 159–167. doi: 10.1007/s10048-012-0323-z

225. Wetherill, Y. B., Akingbemi, B. T., Kanno, J., McLachlan, J. A., Nadal, A., Sonnenschein, C., et al. (2007). *In vitro* molecular mechanisms of bisphenol A action. *Reprod, Toxicol.* 24, 178–198. doi: 10.1016/j.reprotox.2007.05.010

226. Wong, F. K., Fei, J.-F., Mora-Bermúdez, F., Taverna, E., Haffner, C., Fu, J., et al. (2015). Sustained Pax6 expression generates primate-like basal radial glia in developing mouse neocortex. *PLoS Biol.* 13:e1002217. doi: 10.1371/journal.pbio.1002217

227. Xiao, L., Hu, C., Yang, W., Guo, D., Li, C., Shen, W., et al. (2013). NMDA receptor couples Rac1-GEF Tiam1 to direct oligodendrocyte precursor cell migration. *Glia* 61, 2078–2099. doi: 10.1002/glia.22578

228. Xu, C., Funahashi, Y., Watanabe, T., Takano, T., Nakamuta, S., Namba, T., et al. (2015). Radial glial cell–neuron interaction directs axon formation at the opposite side of the neuron from the contact site. *J. Neurosci.* 43, 14517–14532. doi: 10.1523/JNEUROSCI.1266-15.2015

229. Yague, J. G., Mu-oz, A., de Monasterio-Schrader, P., DeFelipe, J., Garcia-Segura, L. M., and Azcoitia, I. (2006). Aromatase expression in the human temporal cortex. *Neuroscience*, 138, 389–401. doi: 10.1016/j.neuroscience.2005.11.054

230. Yague, J. G., Wang, A. C.-J., Janssen, W. G. M., Hof, P. R., Garcia- Segura, L. M., Azcoitia, I., et al. (2008). Aromatase distribution in the monkey temporal neocortex and hippocampus. *Brain Res.*, 1209, 115–127. doi: 10.1016/j.brainres.2008.02.061

231. Ye, T., Ip, J. P., Fu, A. K., and Ip, N. Y. (2014). Cdk5-mediated phosphorylation of RapGEF2 controls neuronal migration in the developing cerebral cortex. *Nat. Commun.* 5, 4826. doi: 10.1038/ncomms5826

232. Yi, H., Bao, X., Tang, X., Fan, X., and Xu, H. (2016). Estrogen modulation of calretinin and BDNF expression in midbrain dopaminergic neurons of ovariectomised mice. *J. Chem. Neuroanat.* 77(Suppl. C), 60–67. doi: 10.1016/j.jchemneu.2016.05.005

233. Yokote, H., Fujita, K., Jing, X., Sawada, T., Liang, S., Yao, L., et al. (2005). Trans-activation of EphA4 and FGF receptors mediated by direct interactions between their cytoplasmic domains. *Proc. Natl. Acad. Sci. U.S.A.* 102, 18866–18871. doi: 10.1073/pnas.0509741102

234. Zeidan, A., Gan, X. T., Thomas, A., and Karmazyn, M. (2014). Prevention of RhoA activation and cofilin-mediated actin polymerization mediates the antihypertrophic effect of adenosine receptor agonists in angiotensin II- and endothelin-1-treated cardiomyocytes. *Mol. Cell. Biochem.* 385, 239–248. doi: 10.1007/s11010-013-1832-2

235. Zhang, J., Shemezis, J. R., McQuinn, E. R., Wang, J., Sverdlov, M., and Chenn, A. (2013). AKT activation by N-cadherin regulates beta-catenin signaling and neuronal differentiation during cortical development. *Neural Dev.* 8:7. doi: 10.1186/1749-8104-8-7

236. Zhao, X., Yue, W., Zhang, L., Ma, L., Jia, W., Qian, Z., et al. (2014). Downregulation of PAX6 by shRNA inhibits proliferation and cell cycle progression of human non-small cell lung cancer cell lines. *PLoS ONE* 9:e85738. doi: 10.1371/journal.pone.0085738

237. Zhao, Y., Yu, Y., Zhang, Y., He, L., Qiu, L., Zhao, J., et al. (2017). Letrozole regulates actin cytoskeleton polymerization dynamics in a SRC-1 dependent manner in the hippocampus of mice. *J. Steroid Biochem. Mol. Biol.* 167, 86–97. doi: 10.1016/j.jsbmb.2016.11.013

238. Zhou, P., Porcionatto, M., Pilapil, M., Chen, Y., Choi, Y., Tolias, K. F., et al. (2018). Polarized signaling endosomes coordinate BDNF-induced chemotaxis of cerebellar precursors. *Neuron* 55, 53–68. doi: 10.1016/j.neuron.2007.05.030

239. Zoeller, R. T., Bansal, R., and Parris, C. (2005). Bisphenol-A, an environmental contaminant that acts as a thyroid hormone receptor antagonist *in vitro*, increases serum thyroxine, and alters RC3/neurogranin expression in the developing rat brain. *Endocrinology* 146, 607–612. doi: 10.1210/en.2004-1018

240. Zong, X., Yang, H., Yu, Y., Zou, D., Ling, Z., He, X., et al. (2011). Possible role of Pax-6 in promoting breast cancer cell proliferation and tumorigenesis. *BMB Rep.* 44, 595–600. doi: 10.5483/BMBRep.2011.44.9.595

241. Zsarnovszky, A., Smith, T., Hajos, F., and Belcher, S. M. (2002). Estrogen regulates GFAP-expression in specific subnuclei of the female rat interpeduncular nucleus: a potential role for estrogen receptor β. *Brain Res.* 958, 488–496. doi: 10.1016/S0006-8993(02)03771-X

10

Adverse Effects of Immunoglobulin Therapy

Yi Guo[1†], Xin Tian[1†], Xuefeng Wang[1,2] and Zheng Xiao[1]*

[1] Department of Neurology, The First Affiliated Hospital of Chongqing Medical University, Chongqing Key Laboratory of Neurology, Chongqing, China, [2] Center of Epilepsy, Beijing Institute for Brain Disorders, Beijing, China

***Correspondence:**
Zheng Xiao
xiaozhenghf@126.com

†These authors have contributed equally to this work and share first authorship.

Immunoglobulin has been widely used in a variety of diseases, including primary and secondary immunodeficiency diseases, neuromuscular diseases, and Kawasaki disease. Although a large number of clinical trials have demonstrated that immunoglobulin is effective and well tolerated, various adverse effects have been reported. The majority of these events, such as flushing, headache, malaise, fever, chills, fatigue and lethargy, are transient and mild. However, some rare side effects, including renal impairment, thrombosis, arrhythmia, aseptic meningitis, hemolytic anemia, and transfusion-related acute lung injury (TRALI), are serious. These adverse effects are associated with specific immunoglobulin preparations and individual differences. Performing an early assessment of risk factors, infusing at a slow rate, premedicating, and switching from intravenous immunoglobulin (IVIG) to subcutaneous immunoglobulin (SCIG) can minimize these adverse effects. Adverse effects are rarely disabling or fatal, treatment mainly involves supportive measures, and the majority of affected patients have a good prognosis.

Keywords: immunoglobulin, adverse effects, risk factors, preventive measures, premedication

INTRODUCTION

Immunoglobulin, also known as gamma globulin, is a therapeutic preparation comprising pooled blood donated from large numbers of healthy people. IgG is the main component of immunoglobulin, but it also contains small amounts of IgA and varying trace amounts of auxiliary materials (maltose, sucrose, etc.) (1). Applications involving immunoglobulin have expanded to include treatment for immunodeficiency diseases, idiopathic thrombocytopenic purpura (ITP), Kawasaki disease, and neurologic disorders (including Guillain–Barre syndrome, chronic inflammatory demyelinating polyneuropathy, myasthenia gravis, multiple myositis, multiple sclerosis, and autoimmune encephalitis) (2–8). Although immunoglobulin is well tolerated, adverse effects do occur. The majority of these adverse effects are mild and alleviated after infusion withdrawal, but some rare side effects are serious, including aseptic meningitis, renal impairment, thrombosis, and hemolytic anemia (9). In this paper, we reviewed the incidence, risk factors, clinical manifestations of and preventive measures for adverse effects related to immunoglobulin. The processes employed to minimize adverse reactions are briefly addressed in **Figure 1**.

HISTORICAL PERSPECTIVE

In 1890, the German scholar Behring won the 1901 Nobel Prize in medicine for developing a serum therapy for diphtheria, representing a new chapter in the search for immunotherapies (10). In 1941, Cohn et al. (11) successfully developed a process for the large-scale production of human immunoglobulin. Next, immunoglobulin was widely used during World War II. In 1952, Bruton

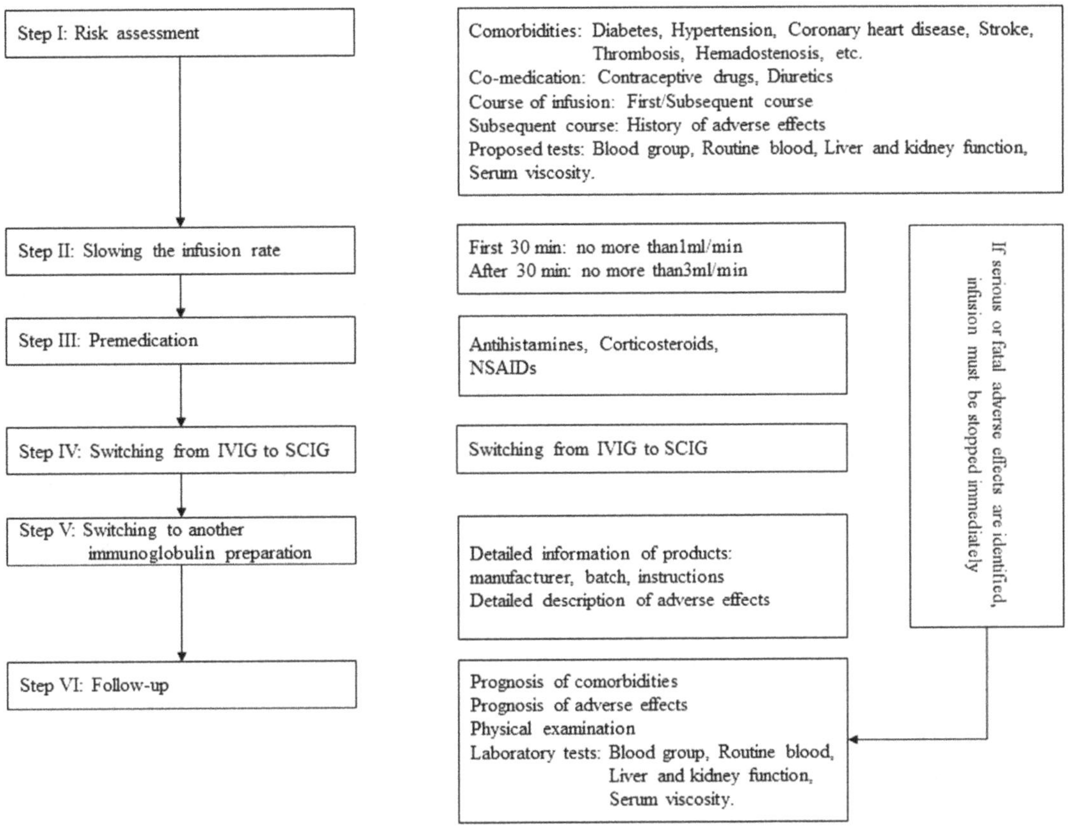

FIGURE 1 | Process that minimizes or prevents immunoglobulin-associated adverse reactions.

(12) was the first to use immunoglobulin to treat a patient identified as immunodeficient, and it later became a standard therapy for immunodeficiency diseases. Intramuscular immunoglobulin preparations were not widely applied because of their poor tolerance. Hence, many scholars began to explore intravenous immunoglobulin (IVIG) preparations. Until 1979, IVIG was approved to treat immunodeficiency disease by the American Food and Drug Administration (13). Imbach et al. (14) then introduced IVIG as a treatment for ITP, with desirable effects. Since then, IVIG has been widely used for an increasing number of diseases.

INCIDENCE OF ADVERSE EFFECTS

Patients who receive immunoglobulin therapy are often treated with immunoglobulin in repeated infusions over a long period of time, and the incidence of adverse effects related to immunoglobulin varies across a wide range. For example, in the study by Matsumoto et al. (15), 14 of 567 (2.5%) patients experienced adverse effects during infusion with IVIG. However, another study reported that 87.5% (14/16) of patients had adverse effects during treatment with repeated infusions of IVIG (16). The majority of studies have focused on the rate of adverse effects in patients receiving multiple infusions over time; however, information regarding the rate of a single infusion is scarce. For subcutaneous immunoglobulin (SCIG) preparations, many studies suggested that the adverse effects of SCIG were much lower than those of IVIG, and the incidence varied across a wide range. However, these studies cannot reveal the occurrence of adverse effects due to multiple interfering factors, such as differences in immunoglobulin preparations, individual differences, or study design variations.

Variations in immunoglobulin brands used may be the main cause for this lack of information regarding the occurrence of adverse effects, considering that different immunoglobulin formulations can have different adverse event profiles. Many clinical trials aimed to evaluate the safety of investigational immunoglobulin products that were not standardized with respect to data collection and provide a definition for adverse effect. Different studies focused on various segments of the population, and these patients had many diseases and fluctuating risk factors. Furthermore, patients who tolerated the infusions may have been shifted from the hospital to home-based infusion therapy, thereby explaining the broad range of adverse effects.

Study design variations also affected the rate of adverse effects. Most trials have involved a limited sample size, and few trials that were performed to support licensed marketed products included a control group. The lack of a control group increases the difficulty involved in unambiguously ascribing causality, and some studies did not report the frequency. In the study design, we advised investigators to predefine the time frame over which adverse effects are considered temporally associated with the infusion of the product (i.e., within 24, 48, or 72 h of the end of the infusion) in the protocol. Based on prior experience with the same products and to include all the adverse effects, *a priori* algorithm for assigning causality was developed to observe adverse effects and preidentify a list of these adverse events, which are presumed to be related to the administration of the test products.

Analyzing the epidemiology of adverse effects in clinical research is important. For patients receiving long-term IVIG replacement, the rate of adverse effects should be calculated according to the infusion times (per infusion, not per patient). Furthermore, a nationwide database for immunoglobulin-related adverse effects should be created, but the following factors that affected the passive reporting of post-marketing surveillance data in this database should be taken into consideration: (1) Some adverse effects occurring during the IVIG infusion may not be associated with IVIG; (2) some adverse events can be duplicated and result in double counting, especially adverse events that last over an extended period of time; and (3) substantial underreporting is likely to occur as it is a voluntary system.

GENERAL RISK FACTORS

Immunoglobulin Preparation-Related Risk Factors

A high concentration of IgA and anti-Rh blood group, D antigen (RhD) increases the occurrence of immunoglobulin-related adverse effects. Manlhiot et al. (17) found that adverse effects were reported more often in patients treated with immunoglobulin products that contained a concentration of IgA higher than 15 μg/ml (15 VS 8%). Similarly, a high titer of anti-RhD also increased the occurrence of adverse effects; therefore, the level of anti-RhD should be maintained as low as possible (18, 19). However, preparations produced by different manufacturers have different excipients that may increase the rates of specific adverse reactions (20) (**Table 1**).

Patient-Related Risk Factors

Patients who developed adverse effects during a previous course and those receiving a first infusion are at an increased risk of adverse effects. Sherer et al. (21) found that 9 of 10 (90%) patients who experienced an adverse effect during the first treatment course also had adverse effects during subsequent courses. A survey conducted in Iran verified that the risk was higher in patients receiving a first course than in those receiving subsequent treatment courses (16.2 VS 6.9%, respectively) (22).

Some studies have suggested that IgA-deficient patients may be at a higher risk of adverse effects. Iranian researchers found that the incidence of immunoglobulin-induced adverse effects was higher in patients with primary antibody defects, especially those with low levels of IgA (22, 23). In contrast, Rachid and colleagues found that the role of IgA-deficiency in anaphylaxis in patients during immunoglobulin therapy remains controversial (24, 25). Therefore, immunoglobulin infusion should never be withheld from IgA-deficient patients.

TABLE 1 | Components of immunoglobulin products associated with adverse effects.

Component	Patients with increased risk
Sucrose	Patients with renal failure
Glucose	Patients with diabetes
Maltose	Patients with glucose fluctuation
Sorbitol	Patients with hereditary fructose intolerance
High IgA	Patients with risk of anaphylaxis

CLASSIFICATION OF ADVERSE EFFECTS

Adverse effects are classified as immediate or delayed depending on the time of occurrence. Immediate adverse effects mainly include flu-like syndrome, dermatologic side effects, arrhythmia, hypotension, and transfusion-related acute lung injury (TRALI). Immediate side effects are categorized as mild, moderate, and severe. Mild adverse effects include light headache, fever, chills, and fatigue; they are alleviated when the infusion is slowed down or when antihistamines and nonsteroidal anti-inflammatory drugs (NSAIDs) are administered. Moderate adverse effects include chest pain, anhelation, vomiting, arthralgia, and severe headache; these effects require the infusion to be discontinued or antihistamines and NSAIDs to be administered. Severe adverse effects include hypertension, anaphylaxis, bronchospasm, and altered consciousness; these adverse effects require the infusion to be stopped immediately and for corresponding medical attention to be provided (22).

Immediate Adverse Effects

Flu-Like Symptoms

Flu-like symptoms are the most frequent adverse effects. These include flushing, nausea, fatigue, fever, chills, malaise, and lethargy. One retrospective study showed that 14 of 16 (87.5%) patients developed flu-like symptoms during immunoglobulin administration (16). Bichuetti-Silva et al. (26) found that flu-like symptoms account for more than 80% of immunoglobulin-induced adverse effects. These symptoms always occur within the first hour of infusion, and some adverse effects (such as fever or fatigue) may also arise within 24 h. The mechanism underlying these symptoms remains unclear, but it may be associated with the presence of cytokines, such as IL-6, TNF-α, prekallikrein activator, and kallikrein, in immunoglobulin products. The solution media and complement activation of an immunoglobulin preparation may also represent causes of these effects (27, 28). The majority of these symptoms are associated with rapid infusion and develop during the initial period of infusion. Hence, it is recommended that infusion should start at a slow rate for the first 30 min (29).

Dermatological Adverse Effects

The incidence of immunoglobulin-related dermatological adverse effects is nearly 6% (30, 31). The manifestations of dermatological adverse effects vary among individuals and can include urticaria, spot papules, eczema, pompholyx, lichenoid dermatitis, and desquamation. Epidermolysis is observed in some severe cases, and all of these skin lesions can occur in all parts of the body, although the hands and feet are the most common sites. Gerstenblith et al. (32) found that 62.5% of patients had pompholyx alone or a combination including pompholyx on the hands or feet. The mechanism underlying these dermatological adverse effects is unclear. Most of these reactions develop within 2 weeks of immunoglobulin administration. Interestingly, a significant number of patients with skin lesions had neurological disorders, and the repeated administration of a high-dose immunoglobulin infusion within a short period of time may be the cause of this high preponderance (32, 33). Dermatological adverse effects can be successfully treated with corticosteroids. Some severe cases require hospitalization for further management, but there are no reports of deaths resulting from severe adverse reactions of the skin in immunoglobulin-treated patients. Switching to another batch of immunoglobulin product may also reduce adverse effects to some extent (33).

Arrhythmia and Hypotension

Arrhythmia occurring during or after immunoglobulin infusion has been reported in several studies and can include supraventricular tachycardia and bradycardia, while most of the cases had a history of heart disease. In 1997, Savasan et al. (34) showed that arrhythmia developed during IVIG in two children with thrombocytopenia who both had a history of arrhythmia, and the condition was resolved in both cases with antiarrhythmic therapy. In 2015, Tufekci et al. (35) reported that supraventricular tachycardia occurred during IVIG administration in two newborn infants with immune hemolysis. Raheja et al. (36) described a case of asymptomatic bradycardia that occurred after IVIG administration in a female with ITP who reached a lowest heart rate of 30 bpm before returning to baseline levels without any therapy. Although it is not fully understood whether arrhythmia is directly related to immunoglobulin infusion, cardiac monitoring during IVIG infusion is recommended in patients with a history of cardiac disorders.

Hypotension is a rare symptom related to immunoglobulin. Some patients with hypotension also experience anaphylactic shock. Dashti-Khavidaki et al. (22) reported 216 patients who developed adverse effects, and only one of these patients developed hypotension combined with allergy and bronchospasm. Charhon et al. (37) later described a case with hypotension (a decrease in systolic blood pressure from 130–60 mmHg) and an altered mental state during immunoglobulin therapy.

Transfusion-Related Acute Lung Injury

Transfusion-related acute lung injury, a serious blood transfusion-related adverse effect with high mortality, manifests with acute respiratory distress and noncardiac pulmonary edema within 6 h of transfusion and is the main cause of blood transfusion-related death. Immunoglobulins are blood products and may also be associated with TRALI. In 2001, Risk (38) first reported a 23-year-old male with multifocal motor neuropathy who developed TRALI following IVIG therapy; the patient's condition resolved in 5 days with only nasal oxygen and bed rest. In 2008, Ahituv et al. (39) presented an adolescent patient with ITP who developed TRALI during immunoglobulin infusion. In several cases, patients with Sjögren's syndrome, Guillain–Barre syndrome, lung transplantation, immunodeficiency, or myasthenia gravis have reportedly developed TRALI after immunoglobulin infusion (40–44). Akin to blood-infusion TRALI, immune-mediated processes and the neutrophil-priming hypothesis have been proposed as possible mechanisms (45). TRALI following IVIG is a serious complication that requires urgent treatment. Diagnosing TRALI depends mainly on clinical symptoms that present after blood products are infused in the absence of other evident causes of respiratory insufficiency; a chest radiogram showing diffuse bilateral pulmonary edema is also needed (46). Patients with TRALI often require adjuvant ventilatory therapy and will recover with proper ventilation.

Delayed Adverse Effects

Delayed adverse effects can be severe or even lethal and affect less than 1% of patients. These events include thrombotic events, neurological disorders, renal impairment, hematologic disorders, electrolyte disturbance, and transfusion-related infection.

Thrombotic Events

Thrombotic events are serious adverse effects of immunoglobulin treatment with an estimated incidence of 1–16.9% (47). Daniel et al. (48) reviewed thrombotic adverse events recorded in a large administrative database from 2008 to 2010 and found that 1% (122/11785) of the patients developed immunoglobulin-induced thrombotic events. Ramírez et al. (49) found that thrombotic events affected up to 16.9% of 303 patients who received immunoglobulin infusion. The manifestations of thrombosis, which can occur in arteries, veins, and intracranial vein sinuses, are varied, and arterial thrombotic events (such as stroke, myocardial infarction, and pulmonary embolism) are the most common. A recent review identified 100 cases of thrombotic events related to the administration of immunoglobulin that occurred from 2006 to 2011; among this cohort, 80% of the thrombotic events were stroke and myocardial infarction that occurred within 24 h of completing immunoglobulin administration (50). Risk factors for thrombosis include a first infusion consisting of a large dose, oral contraceptive use, advanced age, prior/current thrombosis, preexisting atherosclerotic disease, elevated serum viscosity, a hereditary hypercoagulable state or ITP. Rajabally et al. (51) found that patients with coronary disease and prior thrombosis who were administered a daily dose ≥35 g of IVIG had a higher risk of thrombotic events. Daniel et al. (48) also found that advanced age (>45years old), prior thrombotic events, and a hypercoagulable state were risk factors for the development of thrombotic events. Moreover, an increasing number of studies have confirmed that patients with ITP are more likely to develop thrombosis when receiving IVIG (52–55). The presence of four or more risk factors seems to be significantly associated with the onset of immunoglobulin-related thrombotic events (51, 56).

Mechanisms that could potentially trigger thrombotic events include an increase in plasma viscosity, the activation of procoagulant factors, vasospasm, autoimmune vasculitis, and an increased platelet count. Increased plasma viscosity contributes most to the occurrence of thrombotic events. Bentley et al. (57) showed that IVIG can cause plasma viscosity to acutely and cumulatively rise across the complete treatment course. Similarly, Baba et al. (58) also found that increased plasma viscosity was associated with IgG concentrations during or after immunoglobulin infusion.

In addition, the average IgG half-life among individuals varied from 23 to 30 days and could be even longer in some cases (59, 60). Thrombotic complications can be prevented or minimized by early assessment in patients suspected of being at high risk, and anti-thrombus treatment is needed in patients with thrombotic complications.

Neurological Disorders

Neurological disorders associated with immunoglobulin treatment include headache, aseptic meningitis, posterior reversible encephalopathy syndrome (PRES), seizure, and abducens nerve palsy.

Headache post IVIG is a common adverse effect. More than half of patients develop headaches after immunoglobulin administration. Many studies have reported headache as an immunoglobulin-related adverse effect, while no studies have described the characteristics of immunoglobulin-related headache in detail. Headache also has a delayed onset of 6–12 h after an infusion and can last between 24 and 72 h. High-dose immunoglobulin infusion is the main risk factor for headache. Some studies have found that patients with a history of migraine are prone to developing headaches after IVIG infusion (61, 62). Among these studies, the overall incidence of IVIG-related headache in patients with a history of migraine was small, which may be due to the small sample size and patient selection bias. Prophylactic treatment used in several studies included acetaminophen, aspirin, opioids, NSAIDs, propranolol, sumatriptan, and corticosteroids alone or in combination, and all the protocols seemed to be fairly effective in the recruited individuals; however, the best drug for the treatment of immunoglobulin-related headache remains unknown (63). Alternatively, non-pharmacotherapy-related approaches, including a reduction in the infusion rate and switching to an alternative brand of IVIG or SCIG, can also reduce headache to some extent. When a headache lasts for a long time or is resistant to drug therapy, the possibility of aseptic meningitis should not be ignored.

Aseptic meningitis has been identified as an adverse effect of IVIG and affects 0.6–1% of patients. Kemmotsu et al. (64) retrospectively examined 384 patients with Kawasaki disease who received immunoglobulin infusion during 2000–2009 and identified four patients who developed aseptic meningitis, suggesting an overall incidence of 1%. In another retrospectively study, Bharath et al. (65) found that 0.6% (8/1324) of patients developed immunoglobulin-related aseptic meningitis. Several studies have reported that aseptic meningitis appears within 48 h of the initiation of IVIG therapy (64, 66, 67). The most common presenting symptoms of this condition are persistent headache, nausea, vomiting, photophobia, fever, chills, and positive Kernig's and Brudzinski's signs. In addition, in affected patients, lumbar puncture typically produces clear cerebral spinal fluid with an increased level of nucleated cells, high protein content and negative culture results (64, 66). Contributing factors include a large cumulative IVIG dose and a history of migraines. Previous studies have suggested that most patients who develop aseptic meningitis receive 1–2 g/kg immunoglobulin therapy (64, 65). Sekul et al. (66) found that patients with a history of migraines are particularly susceptible to developing aseptic meningitis.

Posterior reversible encephalopathy syndrome is another neurological disorder that can develop following immunoglobulin therapy. In 2005, Nakajia (68) reported a patient with Miller–Fisher syndrome who developed PRES following IVIG therapy. Stetefeld et al. (69) and Ribeiro et al. (70) later reported additional patients with Miller–Fisher syndrome who developed PRES during immunoglobulin infusion. The clinical manifestations in these patients include an acute onset characterized by headache, generalized seizure, visual impairment, and an altered mental state (69–71). In all of these cases, complete resolution was achieved after immunoglobulin administration ceased. While PRES is a rare complication of IVIG treatment, it should be considered in all cases with disease-typical MRI findings and clinical manifestations.

Few case reports have described patients with IVIG-associated seizures. In 2003, Kao et al. (72) reported a 37-year-old male with myelopathy who developed repetitive generalized tonic-clonic seizures following IVIG therapy. Later, aseptic meningitis was considered the cause of the seizures, and the patient's condition was controlled with valproate. In 2014, Bichuetti-Silva et al. (26) identified a separate case of seizure in a patient with common variable immunodeficiency disease following IVIG infusion, and a history of herpetic encephalitis was later recorded.

Immunoglobulin infusion may rarely be the underlying etiology of abducens nerve palsy. Wright et al. (73) reported a patient with renal transplantation who developed abducens nerve palsy during high-dose IVIG infusion. The patient recovered completely after 2 weeks, and aseptic meningitis was considered the underlying cause. Furthermore, two case reports described patients with Kawasaki disease who developed abducens nerve palsy after IVIG therapy (74, 75). However, whether abducens nerve palsy was directly related to immunoglobulin therapy in these cases is unclear.

Renal Impairment

Renal impairment following immunoglobulin treatment is a rare but dangerous adverse effect. The incidence of immunoglobulin-associated renal impairment has not been accurately determined. The FDA received information related to 114 cases of immunoglobulin-associated renal impairment or acute renal failure that occurred between 1981 and 1998 (76). Moreover, from 1999 to 2005, the French National Security Agency of Medicines and Health Products recorded 91 cases of renal impairment associated with immunoglobulin infusion (77). The precise mechanism underlying IVIG-related renal impairment remains unclear. Potential mechanisms include the precipitation of immune complexes in the glomeruli, osmotic nephritis, immunological hemolysis-associated acute tubular obstruction, and transient vascular ischemia due to a reduction in renal perfusion (78–80).

Patients with advanced age, diabetes, preexisting renal dysfunction, and dehydration have an increased risk of developing renal impairment following immunoglobulin administration. Renal impairment typically develops within 10 days after the start of immunoglobulin infusion. Oliguria, hematuria, a decreased glomerular filtration rate, and elevated serum creatinine levels are typical manifestations of renal impairment. Serum creatinine levels usually peak around day 5, and oliguric renal failure is more common than other types of renal dysfunction (9, 81, 82).

Renal function usually returns to normal after IVIG infusion is discontinued or short-term hemodialysis is performed, but a few patients with immunoglobulin-related renal impairment have developed chronic renal insufficiency or died (83, 84). Previous studies have shown that death occurs in 8–15% of these patients, but the majority of patients who die have severe underlying conditions, such as advanced age, uncontrolled diabetes, or prior renal dysfunction; therefore, the cause of this effect needs further study (83, 85, 86). In patients with renal insufficiency, renal function should be closely monitored both before and after treatment (including serum creatinine, blood urea nitrogen levels, and glomerular filtration rate). If renal function progressively declines, the rate of infusion should be reduced or treatment should be discontinued. Epstein et al. (76) verified that sucrose-containing preparations should be avoided because they are associated with a risk of osmotic nephritis. However, Kim et al. (87) found that sucrose-free IVIG could also result in renal impairment.

Hematologic Disorders: Hemolysis and Neutropenia

Hemolysis is an adverse effect related to IVIG administration that occurs in approximately 1.6% of patients but is usually neither recognized nor treated because it lacks clinical symptoms. Hemolysis can result in acute renal failure and thrombosis. In 2008, a case series conducted at Ottawa Hospital identified 16 cases of hemolysis among approximately 1,000 patients who received IVIG infusion (resulting in an incidence of 1.6%) (88). Most cases with hemolysis present no obvious clinical symptoms and are diagnosed with low hemoglobin levels on a blood examination. IVIG infusion-associated hemolysis was observed from 12 h to 10 days after the first infusion of IVIG, with the lowest hemoglobin level occurring between 1 day and 2 weeks after the last IVIG infusion. Hemolysis is a common complication of high-dose IVIG derived from non-group O blood. In a systematic review conducted by Desborough and colleagues, 62 cases of hemolysis were identified, and 97% of those patients had received a high dose of IVIG (at least 2 g/kg). Of those 62 cases, IVIG-induced hemolysis was most common in patients with type A (65%) or AB (26%) blood (89). Several more recent studies have also verified that administration of a high dose of IVIG is a contributing factor in hemolysis (90–92). This effect may be associated with the presence of A and B isoagglutinin (anti-A and anti-B antibodies) in the IVIG product. A recent cohort study found that the risk of hemolysis was lower when donors with high plasma titers of anti-A antibodies were excluded, especially in patients requiring $\geq$1.75 g IVIG/kg (93). Abnormal laboratory tests that may indicate hemolysis include decreased hemoglobin and haptoglobin levels, increased lactate dehydrogenase levels, and increased hemobilirubin and reticulocyte counts (94). The management plans generally proposed in affected patients aim to slow down the rate of infusion, switch to another IVIG product, or check the blood type for potential indications for hemolysis. Hemolysis is self-limiting in the majority of mild and moderate cases. However, proper blood transfusion is needed in severe cases when a Coombs test or a direct or indirect antiglobulin test is negative (89, 95, 96).

Immunoglobulin therapy can cause hemolysis, but it can also cause neutropenia (97). In 1998, Majer et al. (98) first described neutropenia as a complication of IVIG therapy in children with ITP. Veys et al. (99) also reported two cases of neutropenia following IVIG infusion for ITP. In addition, Matsuda et al. (100) and Bajaj et al. (101) reported that patients with neurological disorders could develop neutropenia with IVIG administration. Currently, immunoglobulin-induced neutrophils have been reported only in case reports. This condition usually occurs within 4 days after infusion and recovers spontaneously without infection in 2 weeks. However, premedication with corticosteroids may be an effective measure to prevent neutropenia (98–103).

Electrolyte Disturbance

Electrolyte disturbance is a rare adverse effect of immunoglobulin administration. In 1997, a study that examined variations in serum chemistry among 46 patients receiving IVIG infusion found that sodium and magnesium levels were significantly lower in infused patients (4 and 7% below baseline, respectively) (104). Daphnis et al. (105) retrospectively evaluated a cohort of 66 patients with ITP who received repeated IVIG infusions and found that serum sodium levels fell by 2.7 mmol/l in patients with normal renal dysfunction and 5.7 mmol/l in patients with acute renal failure. These electrolyte disturbances usually have no clinical symptoms, and affected patients generally recover without electrolyte supplementation. With regards to patients with severely compromised renal function, it is recommended that electrolyte levels can be monitored to identify hyponatremia and hyperkalemia.

Infection Risk

The long-term safety of immunoglobulin preparations is excellent. Until recently, the majority of physicians believed that IVIG infusion was associated with no risk of infection. Since immunoglobulins are blood products, there will always be a risk of underlying infection, which may be fatal. Until recently, the most commonly reported infection was the hepatitis C virus. In 1994, the FDA and Centers for Disease Control and Prevention received reports of over 100 cases of acute hepatitis virus infection in recipients of IVIG from several countries (Norway, United States, Europe, and Puerto Rico). The brand names Gammagard and Polygam accounted for the majority of the cases of hepatitis C in both the United States and Europe (106, 107). Razvi et al. (108) reported the outcomes of 58 cases with IVIG-transmitted hepatitis C, and the prognosis of these subjects was poor. Since then, no cases of immunoglobulin-induced hepatitis C have been reported.

Apart from immunoglobulin-transmitted hepatitis C, no cases of IVIG-related hepatitis B virus (HBV) have been reported. However, IVIG-related passive transfer of hepatitis B antibodies has also been reported. Several scholars have reported cases in which the patient developed positive HBV core antibodies and surface antibodies after IVIG infusion, and subsequent multiple tests revealed false-positive results due to immunoglobulin (109, 110). Ramsay and colleagues conducted a cross-sectional study that suggested that HBV antibodies (HBsAb and HBcAb) are common in patients receiving IVIG and who have confounding diagnostic results (111). Thus, the measurement of baseline HBV antibodies should be implemented when commencing immunoglobulin infusion. If the test results are negative, and there is an absence of hepatitis or risk factors, any future positive results in the context of ongoing immunoglobulin therapy should be considered false positives, HBV-DNA levels should be measured, and antiviral treatment should be given cautiously.

Since the introduction of adequate management and advanced testing technologies, no cases of IVIG-related prion disease or HIV transmission have been reported. Radomski et al. (112) found that two dedicated and one supplemental step [solvent/detergent (S/D) treatment and nanofiltration (20 nm) in combination with ion-exchange chromatography] could prevent pathogen transmission. Although the infection risk is much lower in IVIG than in other blood products, the possibility of infection can never be neglected.

Other Adverse Effects

Other adverse effects of immunoglobulin therapy include uveitis, passively acquired thyroid autoantibodies and reversible splenial lesion syndrome. Kocak et al. (113) reported a case in which a 44-year-old female developed bilateral uveitis following the administration of IVIG for 2 days. The patient was treated with topical corticosteroids and had achieved complete resolution at 1-month follow-up. In 2017, Uchida et al. (114) reported two cases in which thyroid autoantibodies passively acquired following IVIG administration. Finally, Uygur et al. (115) described a case of reversible splenial lesion syndrome caused by IVIG therapy.

TABLE 2 | Predisposing factors for immunoglobulin-induced adverse effects.

Adverse effect	Predisposing factors
Flu-like symptoms	High dose, rapid infusion rate, accompanying infection, previous adverse effects
Dermatological adverse effects	High dose, rapid infusion rate, accompanying infection, male patients with chronic inflammatory demyelinating polyneuropathy
Arrhythmia and hypotension	History of heart disease
Transfusion-related acute lung injury	Rapid infusion rate
Thrombotic events	High dose, rapid infusion rate, advanced age, being bedridden, diabetes mellitus, hypertension, dyslipidemia, prior/current thrombosis, preexisting atherosclerotic disease, elevated serum viscosity, oral contraceptive use, hereditary hypercoagulable state, idiopathic thrombocytopenic purpura
Aseptic meningitis	High dose
Renal impairment	Rapid infusion rate, advanced age, renal insufficiency, nephrotic syndrome, diabetes mellitus, dehydration, sepsis paraproteinemia, nephrotoxic drugs, hemolysis, sucrose-containing preparations
Hemolysis	High dose, rapid infusion rate, non-O blood group, underlying inflammatory state

PREVENTIVE MEASURES

Risk Assessment and Adequate Monitoring

Immunoglobulins cause various adverse effects; some of these effects are severe and fatal. Hence, a detailed medical history should be obtained in every patient being considered for immunoglobulin treatment. This information should include age, the infusion course of immunoglobulin, concomitant diseases (diabetes, hypertension, coronary heart disease, stroke, thrombotic events, hemadostenosis, etc.), and co-medications (e.g., contraceptive drugs and diuretics). Laboratory tests are also needed, such as a blood group test, routine blood tests, and tests of liver and kidney function. A variety of risk factors must be considered when evaluating possible adverse effects, and special precautions should be considered in patients with a history of allergies or thrombotic events. In these patients who have a heightened risk of developing adverse effects, special monitoring should be employed within the first 24 h following immunoglobulin administration in a hospital. The proposed factors that predispose a patient to immunoglobulin-induced adverse effects are shown in **Table 2**.

Slowing Down the Infusion Rate

The adverse effects described here are closely related to the rate of immunoglobulin infusion. Hence, slowing down the rate of infusion can greatly reduce the rate of adverse reactions, especially flu-like symptoms, hemolysis, thrombosis, and renal impairment (22, 63, 116). Strictly controlling the infusion rate during the first administration is recommended. During the first infusion, an initial slower rate should be implemented for the first 30 min, and then the rate may be increased if no adverse effects occur (we recommend using the infusion rate according to the instructions provided by different brands). Slowing the rate should be considered if any adverse effects occur. The infusion should be discontinued if slowing the rate does not alleviate these adverse reactions.

Premedication and Prehydration

Premedication with antihistamines, corticosteroids, or NSAIDs can markedly reduce the severity and incidence of IVIG-induced adverse effects. In 1998, Roberton et al. (117) assessed the effect of premedication with methylprednisolone in a large crossover study that included 10 patients who had previously experienced frequent adverse reactions. Methylprednisolone was administered at a dose of 1 mg/kg 20 min prior to IVIG infusion, and the pretreated patients exhibited a marked decrease in the severity of IVIG-induced immediate adverse events ($P < 0.01$), with only one patient discontinuing IVIG infusion, whereas IVIG was interrupted in 8 of the 10 patients who were not pretreated with methylprednisolone. Souayah et al. (118) examined the safety profile of home infusion of IVIG in patients with neuroimmunologic disorders. In all, 276 patients were premedicated with antihistamines, corticosteroids, or NSAIDs, and the incidence of IVIG-induced adverse effects was significantly lower in the premedicated group than in the non-premedicated group (18.4 VS 27.1%, $P = 0.04$). However, the results of a separate study indicated that the rate of immunoglobulin-induced immediate adverse events was not altered by premedication (29). With regards to thrombotic events, Huang et al. (119) implemented a protocol in which treatment with antiplatelets and anticoagulation before IVIG infusion eliminated IVIG-related thrombotic events. However, because their sample size was small, further studies are needed to determine the safety and efficacy of this protocol.

Prehydration with normal saline is also used to prevent immunoglobulin-induced adverse effects. Many studies have proposed that prehydration can be helpful for headache, thrombolysis, renal impairment, and hemolysis (63, 120, 121); however, the implementation protocol, the dose of saline (250 or 500 ml, etc.), and the duration of saline infusion remain unclear. All of these studies utilized a protocol that combined hydration and other measures; therefore, the efficacy of prehydration should be further evaluated in a well-designed study.

Switching From IVIG to SCIG or Other Immunoglobulin Preparations

Switching from IVIG to SCIG seems to be an effective strategy that attenuates immunoglobulin-induced adverse effects, especially for patients who have previously experienced severe adverse effects or are at high risk of developing adverse effects. An increasing number of well-designed studies show that SCIG can be used as a treatment for immunodeficiency diseases, multifocal motor neuropathy, chronic inflammatory demyelinating polyneuropathy, and myasthenia gravis (6, 122–136) (**Table 3**). The results of two randomized, crossover studies indicate that the rate of systematic adverse effects was lower following SCIG than following IVIG, and no severe adverse effects were reported in patients treated with SCIG (123, 135). However, the sample sizes of these two studies were small (30 and 20). Racosta et al. (137) performed a meta-analysis of reports that explored the efficacy and safety of SCIG VS IVIG and identified a total of 8 studies comprising 138 patients with inflammatory demyelinating polyneuropathies. Their results showed that the relative risk of moderate and/or systemic adverse effects was 28% lower in the SCIG group [95% confidence interval, 0.11–0.76]. Due to the small sample size of these studies, the efficiency of SCIG

TABLE 3 | Subcutaneous immunoglobulin (SCIG) treatment in a variety of diseases.

Reference	Sample	Diagnosis	Study design	SCIG dose	Rate of side effects	Severity
Misbah et al. (130)	8	Multifocal motor neuropathy	Prospective, open-label, multicenter study	271.8 ± 139.13 mg/kg (range, 100–488 mg/kg)	50% had 18 AEs 0.098 per infusion	Mild to moderate No discontinuations
Kanegane et al. (133)	25	Primary immunodeficiency	Prospective, multicenter, open-label, single-arm study	Not mentioned	96.0% had 269 AEs 0.461 per infusion	Mild to moderate No discontinuations
Empson et al. (131)	35	Primary immunodeficiency	Phase III, single-arm, open-label, multicenter study	Median 6.70 g/week (range, 3–13.5 g/week)	40% of patients 0.059 per infusion	Mild to moderate No discontinuations
Hoffmann et al. (128)	82	Primary and secondary antibody deficiencies	Prospective, observational, multicenter study	91 ± 31 mg/kg/week	2/82 patients had 2AEs	Local tissue reactions 1 patient discontinued
Thépot et al. (129)	65	Primary hypogammaglobulinemia	Monocentric, longitudinal trial	108 mg/kg (range, 62–174 mg/kg)	3/65 patients	Mild to moderate 3 patients switched to intravenous immunoglobulin
Berger et al. (126)	51	Primary immunodeficiency	Not mentioned	100–200 mg/kg/week	86.3% of patients 0.15 per infusion	1 severe adverse effect 2 patients withdrew
Spadaro et al. (134)	14	Hypogammaglobulinemia	Not mentioned	100 ± 4.4 mg/kg/week	Not mentioned	Not mentioned
Harbo et al. (127)	6	Multifocal motor neuropathy	Prospective, observational study	13–51 g per week	6/6 patients had local tissue reactions	Local tissue reactions 1 patient withdrew
Ochs et al. (124)	65	Primary immunodeficiency	Prospective, open-label, multicenter study	158 mg/kg (range, 155–165 mg/kg)	60/65 patients 0.52 per infusion	Mild to moderate 14 patients withdrew
Markvardsen et al. (132)	20	Chronic inflammatory demyelinating polyneuropathy	Randomized, single-blind, crossover study	0.4 g/kg	Not mentioned	Not mentioned
van Schaik et al. (136)	172	Chronic inflammatory demyelinating polyneuropathy	Randomized, multicenter, double-blind, placebo-controlled, parallel-group, phase III study	0.2 or 0.4 g/kg	30% in the low-dose group 34% in the high-dose group	Six (3%) patients had 11 serious adverse events
Beecher et al. (6)	23	Myasthenia gravis	Prospective, open-label, phase 3 trial	2 g/kg	Headache and injection site reactions were common	Mild to moderate No discontinuations
Markvardsen et al. (135)	30	Chronic inflammatory demyelinating polyneuropathy	Randomized, double-blind, placebo-controlled trial	4.8–48 g/week	6/15 patients	Mild to moderate No discontinuations
Gardulf et al. (122)	165	Primary immunodeficiency	Not mentioned	Not mentioned	17% of patients 0.03 per infusion	Mild to moderate No discontinuations
Eftimov et al. (125)	10	Multifocal motor neuropathy	Prospective, open-label, noncontrolled study	0.46 g/kg/month (range, 0.27–0.62)	9 patients developed local adverse events	Mild to moderate No discontinuations
Chapel et al. (123)	30	Primary immunodeficiency	Randomized, multicenter, open-label, crossover trial	Not mentioned	0.1 per infusion	Mild to moderate No discontinuations

should be further explored, and more randomized controlled trials with larger samples of patients with various diseases are needed.

It remains unclear how the dose should be adjusted when switching from IVIG to SCIG. Berger and colleagues found that using 137 and 153% of the IVIG dose when switching to SCIG produced the same effect in patients being treated for primary immunodeficiencies (138). Another study concluded that sustained serum IgG levels can be achieved after switching to SCIG despite the use of a reduced immunoglobulin dose in patients with primary hypogammaglobulinemia (129). Individualizing the dosage based on the disease state and the clinical response is preferable to using mean pharmacokinetic parameters when switching from IVIG to SCIG. In addition, more studies focused on pharmacokinetics in immune-mediated diseases are needed.

Detailed information regarding the immunoglobulin preparation should always be recorded, including the manufacturer, batch, and drug instructions. It is clear that the content, composition, and characteristics of each immunoglobulin preparation can adversely affect patients in different manners. Hence, if patients frequently develop adverse effects following administration with an IVIG preparation, switching to another immunoglobulin preparation may lead to fewer adverse effects (62).

Other Measures

Many patients develop immunoglobulin-associated adverse effects, and the majority of these effects are mild to moderate and resolve with appropriate treatment. The observed effects include immediate adverse effects, aseptic meningitis, hemolysis, neutropenia, and electrolyte disturbances. Some of these severe adverse effects should be treated according to the principle underlying the corresponding diseases, such as an effective antithrombotic therapy in patients with thrombosis or short-term renal replacement therapy in patients with severely damaged renal function.

FUTURE PROSPECTS

Immunoglobulin preparations have been widely used in a variety of diseases, but controlled studies have not been performed for many diseases, such as myasthenia gravis, some forms of lupus erythematosus, septic syndrome, and polymyositis. The improper usage of immunoglobulin increases the risk of adverse effects to some extent; therefore, further studies are needed to demonstrate the proper indications for the use of immunoglobulin.

The majority of adverse effects are associated with high doses of immunoglobulin; thus, determining individualized dosages to guarantee the efficacy of therapy and minimize adverse effects is an urgent focus. Ameratunga (139) suggested that the initial IVIG dose should be based on adjusted body weight in obese patients with primary immunodeficiency disorders. As this study was a single observation and focused on only obese patients, additional special populations, such as the elderly, should be studied to determine the parameters of individualized dosing for immunoglobulin therapy.

Many measures have been used to prevent or minimize immunoglobulin-related adverse effects, as summarized above. Given that these studies were case controlled or small sample size studies, the efficacy of these measures should be verified by randomized controlled studies or head-to-head studies with larger sample sizes. Simultaneously, the use of only one preventive measure may not prevent adverse effects, and a series of measures serving as a standard protocol may be effective for preventing serious adverse effects, such as combining prehydration with anti-thrombosis to minimize thrombotic events.

Currently, immunoglobulin may be given intravenously or subcutaneously to treat a variety of disorders. However, IVIG and SCIG preparations also result in adverse effects. It is possible that other routes of immunoglobulin administration may reduce the rate of adverse effects. In 1982, Barnes et al. (140) found that oral administration of immunoglobulin could be used for the prevention and treatment of rotavirus diarrhea in low-birth weight babies. Later, several meta-analysis studies concluded that oral administration of immunoglobulin could not prevent rotavirus diarrhea and necrotizing enterocolitis (141, 142). Although these studies have several limitations (small sample size and few well-designed studies), oral administration may be a promising preparation to attenuate the occurrence of adverse effects.

Many factors affect the rate of immunoglobulin-related adverse effects. Several characteristics of newer generation immunoglobulin products should be improved, including specific functions, purity, and biological safety. Thus, advanced separation and purification technologies should be developed.

AUTHOR CONTRIBUTIONS

YG and XT conceived the article and wrote the manuscript. XW and ZX reviewed and edited the manuscript. All authors read and approved the manuscript.

FUNDING

This study was supported by the medical research project of Chongqing Health and Family Planning Commission (2013-1-012) and the National Clinical Key Specialty Construction Foundation of China and the National Natural Science Foundation of China (Nos. 81471320, 8167051933, 81471319, 81671301). The authors have no other relevant affiliations or financial involvement with any organization or entity with a financial interest in or financial conflict with the subject matter or materials discussed in the manuscript apart from those disclosed.

REFERENCES

1. Barahona Afonso AF, Joao CM. The production processes and biological effects of intravenous immunoglobulin. *Biomolecules* (2016) 6(1):15. doi:10.3390/biom6010015
2. Pecoraro A, Crescenzi L, Granata F, Genovese A, Spadaro G. Immunoglobulin replacement therapy in primary and secondary antibody deficiency: the correct clinical approach. *Int Immunopharmacol* (2017) 52:136–42. doi:10.1016/j.intimp.2017.09.005
3. Qin YH, Zhou TB, Su LN, Lei FY, Zhao YJ, Huang WF. The efficacy of different dose intravenous immunoglobulin in treating acute idiopathic thrombocytopenic purpura: a meta-analysis of 13 randomized controlled trials. *Blood Coagul Fibrinolysis* (2010) 21(8):713–21. doi:10.1097/MBC.0b013e3283401490

4. Chen S, Dong Y, Yin Y, Krucoff MW. Intravenous immunoglobulin plus corticosteroid to prevent coronary artery abnormalities in Kawasaki disease: a meta-analysis. *Heart* (2013) 99(2):76–82. doi:10.1136/heartjnl-2012-302126
5. Oaklander AL, Lunn MP, Hughes RA, van Schaik IN, Frost C, Chalk CH. Treatments for chronic inflammatory demyelinating polyradiculoneuropathy (CIDP): an overview of systematic reviews. *Cochrane Database Syst Rev* (2017) 1:Cd010369. doi:10.1002/14651858.CD010369.pub2
6. Beecher G, Anderson D, Siddiqi ZA. Subcutaneous immunoglobulin in myasthenia gravis exacerbation: a prospective, open-label trial. *Neurology* (2017) 89(11):1135–41. doi:10.1212/WNL.0000000000004365
7. Olyaeemanesh A, Rahmani M, Goudarzi R, Rahimdel A. Safety and effectiveness assessment of intravenous immunoglobulin in the treatment of relapsing-remitting multiple sclerosis: a meta-analysis. *Med J Islam Repub Iran* (2016) 30:336.
8. Iro MA, Martin NG, Absoud M, Pollard AJ. Intravenous immunoglobulin for the treatment of childhood encephalitis. *Cochrane Database Syst Rev* (2017) 10:Cd011367. doi:10.1002/14651858.CD011367.pub2
9. Cherin P, Marie I, Michallet M, Pelus E, Dantal J, Crave JC, et al. Management of adverse events in the treatment of patients with immunoglobulin therapy: a review of evidence. *Autoimmun Rev* (2016) 15(1):71–81. doi:10.1016/j.autrev.2015.09.002
10. Raju TN. Emil Adolf von Behring and serum therapy for diphtheria. *Acta Paediatr* (2006) 95(3):258–9. doi:10.1111/j.1651-2227.2006.tb02222.x
11. Cohn EJ, Oncley JL, Strong LE, Hughes WL, Armstrong SH. Chemical, clinical, and immunological studies on the products of human plasma fractionation. I. The characterization of the protein fractions of human plasma. *J Clin Invest* (1944) 23(4):417–32. doi:10.1172/JCI101508
12. Bruton OC. Agammaglobulinemia. *Pediatrics* (1952) 9(6):722–8.
13. Eibl MM. History of immunoglobulin replacement. *Immunol Allergy Clin North Am* (2008) 28(4):737–64, viii. doi:10.1016/j.iac.2008.06.004
14. Imbach P, Barandun S, Baumgartner C, Hirt A, Hofer F, Wagner HP. High-dose intravenous gammaglobulin therapy of refractory, in particular idiopathic thrombocytopenia in childhood. *Helv Paediatr Acta* (1981) 36(1):81–6.
15. Matsumoto S, Kobayashi N, Gohya N. Clinical trials of sulfonated immunoglobulin preparation for intravenous administration. II. Adverse reactions. *Eur J Pediatr* (1981) 136(2):167–71. doi:10.1007/BF00441919
16. Seidling V, Hoffmann JH, Enk AH, Hadaschik EN. Analysis of high-dose intravenous immunoglobulin therapy in 16 patients with refractory autoimmune blistering skin disease: high efficacy and no serious adverse events. *Acta Derm Venereol* (2013) 93(3):346–9. doi:10.2340/00015555-1471
17. Manlhiot C, Tyrrell PN, Liang L, Atkinson AR, Lau W, Feldman BM. Safety of intravenous immunoglobulin in the treatment of juvenile dermatomyositis: adverse reactions are associated with immunoglobulin A content. *Pediatrics* (2008) 121(3):e626–30. doi:10.1542/peds.2007-1218
18. Friedman DF, Lukas MB, Larson PJ, Douglas SD, Manno CS. Clinical impact of anti-D in intravenous immunoglobulin. *Transfusion* (1997) 37(4):450–2. doi:10.1046/j.1537-2995.1997.37497265353.x
19. Thorpe SJ, Fox BJ, Dolman CD, Lawrence J, Thorpe R. Batches of intravenous immunoglobulin associated with adverse reactions in recipients contain atypically high anti-Rh D activity. *Vox Sang* (2003) 85(2):80–4. doi:10.1046/j.1423-0410.2003.00336.x
20. Lemm G. Composition and properties of IVIg preparations that affect tolerability and therapeutic efficacy. *Neurology* (2002) 59(12 Suppl 6):S28–32. doi:10.1212/WNL.59.12_suppl_6.S28
21. Sherer Y, Levy Y, Langevitz P, Rauova L, Fabrizzi F, Shoenfeld Y. Adverse effects of intravenous immunoglobulin therapy in 56 patients with autoimmune diseases. *Pharmacology* (2001) 62(3):133–7. doi:10.1159/000056085
22. Dashti-Khavidaki S, Aghamohammadi A, Farshadi F, Movahedi M, Parvaneh N, Pouladi N, et al. Adverse reactions of prophylactic intravenous immunoglobulin; a 13-year experience with 3004 infusions in Iranian patients with primary immunodeficiency diseases. *J Investig Allergol Clin Immunol* (2009) 19(2):139–45.
23. Aghamohammadi A, Farhoudi A, Nikzad M, Moin M, Pourpak Z, Rezaei N, et al. Adverse reactions of prophylactic intravenous immunoglobulin infusions in Iranian patients with primary immunodeficiency. *Ann Allergy Asthma Immunol* (2004) 92(1):60–4. doi:10.1016/S1081-1206(10)61711-5
24. Rachid R, Castells M, Cunningham-Rundles C, Bonilla FA. Association of anti-IgA antibodies with adverse reactions to gamma-globulin infusion. *J Allergy Clin Immunol* (2011) 128(1):228–30.e1. doi:10.1016/j.jaci.2011.01.061
25. Rachid R, Bonilla FA. The role of anti-IgA antibodies in causing adverse reactions to gamma globulin infusion in immunodeficient patients: a comprehensive review of the literature. *J Allergy Clin Immunol* (2012) 129(3):628–34. doi:10.1016/j.jaci.2011.06.047
26. Bichuetti-Silva DC, Furlan FP, Nobre FA, Pereira CT, Goncalves TR, Gouveia-Pereira M, et al. Immediate infusion-related adverse reactions to intravenous immunoglobulin in a prospective cohort of 1765 infusions. *Int Immunopharmacol* (2014) 23(2):442–6. doi:10.1016/j.intimp.2014.09.015
27. Nydegger UE, Sturzenegger M. Adverse effects of intravenous immunoglobulin therapy. *Drug Safety* (1999) 21(3):171–85. doi:10.2165/00002018-199921030-00003
28. Knezevic-Maramica I, Kruskall MS. Intravenous immune globulins: an update for clinicians. *Transfusion* (2003) 43(10):1460–80. doi:10.1046/j.1537-2995.2003.00519.x
29. Kaba S, Keskindemirci G, Aydogmus C, Siraneci R, Erol Cipe F. Immediate adverse reactions to intravenous immunoglobulin in children: a single center experience. *Eur Ann Allergy Clin Immunol* (2017) 49(1):11–4.
30. Sorensen PS, Wanscher B, Jensen CV, Schreiber K, Blinkenberg M, Ravnborg M, et al. Intravenous immunoglobulin G reduces MRI activity in relapsing multiple sclerosis. *Neurology* (1998) 50(5):1273–81. doi:10.1212/WNL.50.5.1273
31. Brannagan TH III. Intravenous gammaglobulin (IVIg) for treatment of CIDP and related immune-mediated neuropathies. *Neurology* (2002) 59(12 Suppl 6):S33–40. doi:10.1212/WNL.59.12_suppl_6.S33
32. Gerstenblith MR, Antony AK, Junkins-Hopkins JM, Abuav R. Pompholyx and eczematous reactions associated with intravenous immunoglobulin therapy. *J Am Acad Dermatol* (2012) 66(2):312–6. doi:10.1016/j.jaad.2010.12.034
33. Cohen Aubart F, Barete S, Amoura Z, Frances C, Lyon-Caen O, Lebrun-Vignes B. Intravenous immunoglobulins-induced eczematous eruption: a long-term follow-up study. *Eur J Intern Med* (2009) 20(1):70–3. doi:10.1016/j.ejim.2008.04.022
34. Savasan S, Tuzcu V, Warrier I, Karpawich P. Cardiac rhythm abnormalities during intravenous immunoglobulin G infusion for treatment of thrombocytopenia. *J Pediatr Hematol Oncol* (1997) 19(3):254–7. doi:10.1097/00043426-199705000-00015
35. Tufekci S, Coban A, Bor M, Yasa B, Nisli K, Ince Z. Cardiac rhythm abnormalities during intravenous immunoglobulin G(IVIG) infusion in two newborn infants: coincidence or association? *Clin Case Rep* (2015) 3(9):731–4. doi:10.1002/ccr3.329
36. Raheja H, Kumar V, Hollander G, Shani J, Greenberg Y. Intravenous immunoglobulin-induced profound bradycardia in a patient with idiopathic thrombocytopenic purpura. *Am J Ther* (2017):1–2. doi:10.1097/MJT.0000000000000654
37. Charhon N, Bonnet A, Schmitt Z, Charpiat B. A case of circulatory collapse during intravenous immunoglobulin therapy: a manageable adverse effect! *Anaesth Crit Care Pain Med* (2015) 34(2):113–4. doi:10.1016/j.accpm.2014.08.004
38. Rizk A, Gorson KC, Kenney L, Weinstein R. Transfusion-related acute lung injury after the infusion of IVIG. *Transfusion* (2001) 41(2):264–8. doi:10.1046/j.1537-2995.2001.41020264.x
39. Berger-Achituv S, Ellis MH, Curtis BR, Wolach B. Transfusion-related acute lung injury following intravenous anti-D administration in an adolescent. *Am J Hematol* (2008) 83(8):676–8. doi:10.1002/ajh.21185
40. Voulgari PV, Paschou S, Svarna E, Tsifetaki N, Drosos AA. Images in rheumatology. Transfusion-related acute lung injury during intravenous immunoglobulin treatment. *J Rheumatol* (2010) 37(1):190–1. doi:10.3899/jrheum.090725
41. Gupta V, Gupta P, Yadav TP. Transfusion related acute lung injury with intravenous immunoglobulin. *Indian Pediatr* (2011) 48(10):807–8.
42. Stoclin A, Delbos F, Dauriat G, Brugiere O, Boeri N, Metivier AC, et al. Transfusion-related acute lung injury after intravenous immunoglobulin treatment in a lung transplant recipient. *Vox Sang* (2013) 104(2):175–8. doi:10.1111/j.1423-0410.2012.01645.x
43. Quest GR, Gaal H, Clarke G, Nahirniak S. Transfusion-related acute lung injury after transfusion of pooled immune globulin: a case report. *Transfusion* (2014) 54(12):3088–91. doi:10.1111/trf.12731
44. Reddy DR, Guru PK, Blessing MM, Stubbs JR, Rabinstein AA, Wijdicks EF. Transfusion-related acute lung injury after IVIG for myasthenic crisis. *Neurocrit Care* (2015) 23(2):259–61. doi:10.1007/s12028-015-0115-z

45. Vlaar AP, Juffermans NP. Transfusion-related acute lung injury: a clinical review. *Lancet* (2013) 382(9896):984–94. doi:10.1016/S0140-6736(12)62197-7
46. Kumar R, Sedky MJ, Varghese SJ, Sharawy OE. Transfusion related acute lung injury (TRALI): a single institution experience of 15 years. *Indian J Hematol Blood Transfus* (2016) 32(3):320–7. doi:10.1007/s12288-015-0604-4
47. Woodruff RK, Grigg AP, Firkin FC, Smith IL. Fatal thrombotic events during treatment of autoimmune thrombocytopenia with intravenous immunoglobulin in elderly patients. *Lancet* (1986) 2(8500):217–8. doi:10.1016/S0140-6736(86)92511-0
48. Daniel GW, Menis M, Sridhar G, Scott D, Wallace AE, Ovanesov MV, et al. Immune globulins and thrombotic adverse events as recorded in a large administrative database in 2008 through 2010. *Transfusion* (2012) 52(10):2113–21. doi:10.1111/j.1537-2995.2012.03589.x
49. Ramírez E, Romero-Garrido JA, López-Granados E, Borobia AM, Pérez T, Medrano N, et al. Symptomatic thromboembolic events in patients treated with intravenous-immunoglobulins: results from a retrospective cohort study. *Thromb Res* (2014) 133(6):1045–51. doi:10.1016/j.thromres.2014.03.046
50. Funk MB, Gross N, Gross S, Hunfeld A, Lohmann A, Guenay S, et al. Thromboembolic events associated with immunoglobulin treatment. *Vox Sang* (2013) 105(1):54–64. doi:10.1111/vox.12025
51. Rajabally YA, Kearney DA. Thromboembolic complications of intravenous immunoglobulin therapy in patients with neuropathy: a two-year study. *J Neurol Sci* (2011) 308(1–2):124–7. doi:10.1016/j.jns.2011.05.035
52. Ho P, Khan S, Crompton D, Hayes L. Extensive cerebral venous sinus thrombosis after romiplostim treatment for immune thrombocytopenia (ITP) despite severe thrombocytopenia. *Intern Med J* (2015) 45(6):682–3. doi:10.1111/imj.12765
53. Moulis G, Audemard-Verger A, Arnaud L, Luxembourger C, Montastruc F, Gaman AM, et al. Risk of thrombosis in patients with primary immune thrombocytopenia and antiphospholipid antibodies: a systematic review and meta-analysis. *Autoimmun Rev* (2016) 15(3):203–9. doi:10.1016/j.autrev.2015.11.001
54. Severinsen MT, Engebjerg MC, Farkas DK, Jensen AO, Norgaard M, Zhao S, et al. Risk of venous thromboembolism in patients with primary chronic immune thrombocytopenia: a Danish population-based cohort study. *Br J Haematol* (2011) 152(3):360–2. doi:10.1111/j.1365-2141.2010.08418.x
55. Park KM, Yang EJ, Lim YT. Dural venous sinus thrombosis and pulmonary embolism following immunoglobulin treatment in pediatric patient with immune thrombocytopenic purpura. *J Pediatr Hematol Oncol* (2017) 39(8):e508–11. doi:10.1097/MPH.0000000000000841
56. Takemoto CM, Sohi S, Desai K, Bharaj R, Khanna A, McFarland S, et al. Hospital-associated venous thromboembolism in children: incidence and clinical characteristics. *J Pediatr* (2014) 164(2):332–8. doi:10.1016/j.jpeds.2013.10.025
57. Bentley P, Rosso M, Sadnicka A, Israeli-Korn S, Laffan M, Sharma P. Intravenous immunoglobulin increases plasma viscosity without parallel rise in blood pressure. *J Clin Pharm Ther* (2012) 37(3):286–90. doi:10.1111/j.1365-2710.2011.01287.x
58. Baba R, Shibata A, Tsurusawa M. Single high-dose intravenous immunoglobulin therapy for Kawasaki disease increases plasma viscosity. *Circ J* (2005) 69(8):962–4. doi:10.1253/circj.69.962
59. Fokkink W, Koch B, Ramakers C, van Doorn PA, van Gelder T, Jacobs BC. Pharmacokinetics and pharmacodynamics of intravenous immunoglobulin G maintenance therapy in chronic immune-mediated neuropathies. *Clin Pharmacol Ther* (2017) 102(4):709–16. doi:10.1002/cpt.693
60. Bonilla FA. Intravenous and subcutaneous immunoglobulin G replacement therapy. *Allergy Asthma Proc* (2016) 37(6):426–31. doi:10.2500/aap.2016.37.3987
61. Brannagan TH III, Nagle KJ, Lange DJ, Rowland LP. Complications of intravenous immune globulin treatment in neurologic disease. *Neurology* (1996) 47(3):674–7. doi:10.1212/WNL.47.3.674
62. Feldmeyer L, Benden C, Haile SR, Boehler A, Speich R, French LE, et al. Not all intravenous immunoglobulin preparations are equally well tolerated. *Acta Derm Venereol* (2010) 90(5):494–7. doi:10.2340/00015555-0900
63. Thornby KA, Henneman A, Brown DA. Evidence-based strategies to reduce intravenous immunoglobulin-induced headaches. *Ann Pharmacother* (2015) 49(6):715–26. doi:10.1177/1060028015576362
64. Kemmotsu Y, Nakayama T, Matsuura H, Saji T. Clinical characteristics of aseptic meningitis induced by intravenous immunoglobulin in patients with Kawasaki disease. *Pediatr Rheumatol Online J* (2011) 9:28. doi:10.1186/1546-0096-9-28
65. Bharath V, Eckert K, Kang M, Chin-Yee IH, Hsia CC. Incidence and natural history of intravenous immunoglobulin-induced aseptic meningitis: a retrospective review at a single tertiary care center. *Transfusion* (2015) 55(11):2597–605. doi:10.1111/trf.13200
66. Sekul EA, Cupler EJ, Dalakas MC. Aseptic meningitis associated with high-dose intravenous immunoglobulin therapy: frequency and risk factors. *Ann Intern Med* (1994) 121(4):259–62. doi:10.7326/0003-4819-121-4-199408150-00004
67. Jain RS, Kumar S, Aggarwal R, Kookna JC. Acute aseptic meningitis due to intravenous immunoglobulin therapy in Guillain-Barre syndrome. *Oxf Med Case Rep* (2014) 2014(7):132–4. doi:10.1093/omcr/omu051
68. Nakajima M. Posterior reversible encephalopathy complicating intravenous immunoglobulins in a patient with Miller-Fisher syndrome. *Eur Neurol* (2005) 54(1):58–60. doi:10.1159/000087720
69. Stetefeld HR, Lehmann HC, Fink GR, Burghaus L. Posterior reversible encephalopathy syndrome and stroke after intravenous immunoglobulin treatment in Miller-Fisher syndrome/Bickerstaff brain stem encephalitis overlap syndrome. *J Stroke Cerebrovasc Dis* (2014) 23(9):e423–5. doi:10.1016/j.jstrokecerebrovasdis.2014.05.034
70. Ribeiro BN, Salata TM, Borges RS, Marchiori E. Posterior reversible encephalopathy syndrome following immunoglobulin therapy in a patient with Miller-Fisher syndrome. *Radiol Bras* (2016) 49(1):58–9. doi:10.1590/0100-3984.2015.0129
71. Belmouaz S, Desport E, Leroy F, Teynie J, Hannequin J, Ayache RA, et al. Posterior reversible encephalopathy induced by intravenous immunoglobulin. *Nephrol Dial Transplant* (2008) 23(1):417–9. doi:10.1093/ndt/gfm594
72. Kao CD, Chen JT, Wu ZA, Shan DE, Liao KK. SIADH and seizure associated with immunoglobulin therapy. *Eur J Neurol* (2003) 10(6):748–9. doi:10.1046/j.1351-5101.2003.00695.x
73. Wright SE, Shaikh ZH, Castillo-Lugo JA, Tanriover B. Aseptic meningitis and abducens nerve palsy as a serious side effect of high dose intravenous immunoglobulin used in a patient with renal transplantation. *Transpl Infect Dis* (2008) 10(4):294–7. doi:10.1111/j.1399-3062.2007.00294.x
74. Rodriguez-Lozano A, Juarez-Echenique JC, Rivas-Larrauri F, Gamez-Gonzalez LB, Yamazaki-Nakashimada M. VI nerve palsy after intravenous immunoglobulin in Kawasaki disease. *Allergol Immunopathol (Madr)* (2014) 42(1):82–3. doi:10.1016/j.aller.2012.08.003
75. Emiroglu M, Alkan G, Kartal A, Cimen D. Abducens nerve palsy in a girl with incomplete Kawasaki disease. *Rheumatol Int* (2016) 36(8):1181–3. doi:10.1007/s00296-016-3515-2
76. Epstein JS, Zoon KC. Important drug warning: immune globulin intravenous (human) (IGIV) products. *Neonatal Netw* (2000) 19(2):60–2.
77. Pharmacovigilance A-CNd. *Enqête Officielle Immunoglobulines Humaines: Atteintes Rénales. Direction de l'Evaluation des Médicaments et des Produits Biologiques — Unité de Pharmacovigilance.* (2006).
78. Rault R, Piraino B, Johnston JR, Oral A. Pulmonary and renal toxicity of intravenous immunoglobulin. *Clin Nephrol* (1991) 36(2):83–6.
79. Hansen-Schmidt S, Silomon J, Keller F. Osmotic nephrosis due to high-dose immunoglobulin therapy containing sucrose (but not with glycine) in a patient with immunoglobulin A nephritis. *Am J Kidney Diseases* (1996) 28(3):451–3. doi:10.1016/S0272-6386(96)90505-3
80. Cayco AV, Perazella MA, Hayslett JP. Renal insufficiency after intravenous immune globulin therapy: a report of two cases and an analysis of the literature. *J Am Soc Nephrol* (1997) 8(11):1788–94.
81. Levine AA, Levine TD, Clarke K, Saperstein D. Renal and hematologic side effects of long-term intravenous immunoglobulin therapy in patients with neurologic disorders. *Muscle Nerve* (2017) 56(6):1173–6. doi:10.1002/mus.25693
82. Itkin YM, Trujillo TC. Intravenous immunoglobulin-associated acute renal failure: case series and literature review. *Pharmacotherapy* (2005) 25(6):886–92. doi:10.1592/phco.2005.25.6.886
83. Orbach H, Tishler M, Shoenfeld Y. Intravenous immunoglobulin and the kidney – a two-edged sword. *Semin Arthritis Rheum* (2004) 34(3):593–601. doi:10.1016/j.semarthrit.2004.06.003
84. Orbach H, Katz U, Sherer Y, Shoenfeld Y. Intravenous immunoglobulin: adverse effects and safe administration. *Clin Rev Allergy Immunol* (2005) 29(3):173–84. doi:10.1385/CRIAI:29:3:173
85. Levy JB, Pusey CD. Nephrotoxicity of intravenous immunoglobulin. *QJM* (2000) 93(11):751–5. doi:10.1093/qjmed/93.11.751

86. Bassilios N, Mercadal L, Deray G. Immunoglobulin as a risk factor for contrast media nephrotoxicity. *Nephrol Dial Transplant* (2001) 16(7):1513–4. doi:10.1093/ndt/16.7.1513
87. Kim AS, Broide DH. Acute renal dysfunction caused by nonsucrose intravenous immunoglobulin in common variable immunodeficiency. *Ann Allergy Asthma Immunol* (2017) 118(2):231–3. doi:10.1016/j.anai.2016.11.009
88. Daw Z, Padmore R, Neurath D, Cober N, Tokessy M, Desjardins D, et al. Hemolytic transfusion reactions after administration of intravenous immune (gamma) globulin: a case series analysis. *Transfusion* (2008) 48(8):1598–601. doi:10.1111/j.1537-2995.2008.01721.x
89. Desborough MJ, Miller J, Thorpe SJ, Murphy MF, Misbah SA. Intravenous immunoglobulin-induced haemolysis: a case report and review of the literature. *Transfus Med* (2014) 24(4):219–26. doi:10.1111/tme.12083
90. Bonilla FA. Adverse effects of immunoglobulin G therapy: thromboembolism and haemolysis. *Clin Exp Immunol* (2014) 178(Suppl 1):72–4. doi:10.1111/cei.12518
91. Chamouni P, Tamion F, Gueit I, Girault C, Lenain P, Varin R, et al. Adverse effect of polyvalent immunoglobulin in the treatment of Guillain-Barre syndrome. *Transfus Apher Sci* (2003) 28(2):117–24. doi:10.1016/S1473-0502(03)00012-0
92. Mohamed M, Bates G, Eastley B. Massive intravascular haemolysis after high dose intravenous immunoglobulin therapy. *Br J Haematol* (2013) 160(5):570. doi:10.1111/bjh.12182
93. Martinez C, Watson DJ, Shebl A, Wallenhorst C, Hubsch A, Simon TL. Impact of screening and exclusion of high anti-A titer donors on the risk of hemolytic anemia with intravenous immunoglobulin treatment – a hospital-based cohort study in the US. *Am J Hematol* (2017) 93(1):E17–20. doi:10.1002/ajh.24931
94. Markvardsen LH, Christiansen I, Harbo T, Jakobsen J. Hemolytic anemia following high dose intravenous immunoglobulin in patients with chronic neurological disorders. *Eur J Neurol* (2014) 21(1):147–52. doi:10.1111/ene.12287
95. Wilson JR, Bhoopalam H, Fisher M. Hemolytic anemia associated with intravenous immunoglobulin. *Muscle Nerve* (1997) 20(9):1142–5. doi:10.1002/(SICI)1097-4598(199709)20:9<1142::AID-MUS8>3.0.CO;2-8
96. Kim NY, Kim JH, Park JS, Kim SH, Cho YK, Cha DH, et al. A 2-month-old boy with hemolytic anemia and reticulocytopenia following intravenous immunoglobulin therapy for Kawasaki disease: a case report and literature review. *Korean J Pediatr* (2016) 59(Suppl 1):S60–3. doi:10.3345/kjp.2016.59.11.S60
97. Markvardsen LK, Jakobsen J. Relative leucopenia and hemolytic anemia following infusion of immunoglobulin. *Eur J Neurol* (2017) 24(12):e85. doi:10.1111/ene.13444
98. Majer RV, Green PJ. Neutropenia caused by intravenous immunoglobulin. *Br Med J* (1988) 296(6631):1262. doi:10.1136/bmj.296.6631.1262-a
99. Veys PA, Macey MG, Owens CM, Newland AC. Neutropenia following intravenous immunoglobulin. *Br Med J* (1988) 296(6639):1800. doi:10.1136/bmj.296.6639.1800-a
100. Matsuda M, Hosoda W, Sekijima Y, Hoshi K, Hashimoto T, Itoh S, et al. Neutropenia as a complication of high-dose intravenous immunoglobulin therapy in adult patients with neuroimmunologic disorders. *Clin Neuropharmacol* (2003) 26(6):306–11. doi:10.1097/00002826-200311000-00009
101. Bajaj NP, Henderson N, Bahl R, Stott K, Clifford-Jones RE. Call for guidelines for monitoring renal function and haematological variables during intravenous infusion of immunoglobulin in neurological patients. *J Neurol Neurosurg Psychiatry* (2001) 71(4):562–3. doi:10.1136/jnnp.71.4.562
102. Singh A, Arif F, Smith SD. Intravenous immunoglobulin-induced reversible neutropenia in a renal transplant patient. *Clin Nephrol* (2005) 64(3):246–8. doi:10.5414/CNP64246
103. Khan S, Dore PC, Sewell WA. Intravenous immunoglobulin-induced neutropenia. *Pediatr Allergy Immunol* (2010) 21(5):892–3. doi:10.1111/j.1399-3038.2009.00885.x
104. Koffman BM, Dalakas MC. Effect of high-dose intravenous immunoglobulin on serum chemistry, hematology, and lymphocyte subpopulations: assessments based on controlled treatment trials in patients with neurological diseases. *Muscle Nerve* (1997) 20(9):1102–7. doi:10.1002/(SICI)1097-4598(199709)20:9<1102::AID-MUS2>3.0.CO;2-C
105. Daphnis E, Stylianou K, Alexandrakis M, Xylouri I, Vardaki E, Stratigis S, et al. Acute renal failure, translocational hyponatremia and hyperkalemia following intravenous immunoglobulin therapy. *Nephron Clin Pract* (2007) 106(4):c143–8. doi:10.1159/000104424
106. From the Centers for Disease Control and Prevention. Outbreak of hepatitis C associated with intravenous immunoglobulin administration – United States, October 1993-June 1994. *JAMA* (1994) 272(6):424–5. doi:10.1001/jama.272.6.424
107. Centers for Disease Control and Prevention (CDC). Outbreak of hepatitis C associated with intravenous immunoglobulin administration – United States, October 1993-June 1994. *MMWR Morb Mortal Wkly Rep* (1994) 43(28):505–9.
108. Razvi S, Schneider L, Jonas MM, Cunningham-Rundles C. Outcome of intravenous immunoglobulin-transmitted hepatitis C virus infection in primary immunodeficiency. *Clin Immunol* (2001) 101(3):284–8. doi:10.1006/clim.2001.5132
109. Benwell N, Boan P, Raby E, McGettigan B. False positive hepatitis B virus core and surface antibodies due to intravenous immunoglobulin. *Intern Med J* (2017) 47(1):119–20. doi:10.1111/imj.13314
110. Parker S, Gil E, Hewitt P, Ward K, Reyal Y, Wilson S, et al. Case report: passive transfer of hepatitis B antibodies from intravenous immunoglobulin. *BMC Infect Dis* (2014) 14:99. doi:10.1186/1471-2334-14-99
111. Ramsay I, Gorton RL, Patel M, Workman S, Symes A, Haque T, et al. Transmission of hepatitis B core antibody and galactomannan enzyme immunoassay positivity via immunoglobulin products: a comprehensive analysis. *Clin Infect Dis* (2016) 63(1):57–63. doi:10.1093/cid/ciw222
112. Radomski KU, Lattner G, Schmidt T, Romisch J. Pathogen safety of a new intravenous immune globulin 10% liquid. *BioDrugs* (2017) 31(2):125–34. doi:10.1007/s40259-017-0212-y
113. Kocak ED, Wang BZ, Hall AJ. Bilateral uveitis following intravenous immunoglobulin administration. *Am J Ophthalmol Case Rep* (2017) 6:74–6. doi:10.1016/j.ajoc.2017.03.005
114. Uchida Y, Kato D, Adachi K, Toyoda T, Matsukawa N. Passively acquired thyroid autoantibodies from intravenous immunoglobulin in autoimmune encephalitis: two case reports. *J Neurol Sci* (2017) 383:116–7. doi:10.1016/j.jns.2017.11.002
115. Uygur Kucukseymen E, Yuksel B, Genc F, Ozaydin Goksu E, Yildiz S, Bicer Gomceli Y. Reversible splenial lesion syndrome after intravenous immunoglobulin treatment for Guillain-Barre syndrome. *Clin Neuropharmacol* (2017) 40(5):224–5. doi:10.1097/WNF.0000000000000236
116. Berger M. Principles of and advances in immunoglobulin replacement therapy for primary immunodeficiency. *Immunol Allergy Clin North Am* (2008) 28(2):413–37, x. doi:10.1016/j.iac.2008.01.008
117. Roberton DM, Hosking CS. Use of methylprednisolone as prophylaxis for immediate adverse infusion reactions in hypogammaglobulinaemic patients receiving intravenous immunoglobulin: a controlled trial. *Aust Paediatr J* (1988) 24(3):174–7.
118. Souayah N, Hasan A, Khan HM, Yacoub HA, Jafri M. The safety profile of home infusion of intravenous immunoglobulin in patients with neuroimmunologic disorders. *J Clin Neuromuscul Dis* (2011) 12(Suppl 4):S1–10. doi:10.1097/CND.0b013e3182212589
119. Huang L, Kanellis J, Mulley W. Slow and steady. Reducing thrombotic events in renal transplant recipients treated with IVIg for antibody-mediated rejection. *Nephrology* (2011) 16(2):239–42. doi:10.1111/j.1440-1797.2010.01399.x
120. Mignogna MD, Fortuna G, Leuci S, Ruoppo E, Adamo D, Fedele S. Analysis of thromboembolic risk related to high-dose intravenous immunoglobulin treatment: a preliminary clinical study of 10 patients with autoimmune mucocutaneous blistering diseases. *Clin Exp Dermatol* (2009) 34(2):145–50. doi:10.1111/j.1365-2230.2008.02809.x
121. Lasica M, Zantomio D. Severe intravenous immunoglobulin-induced hemolysis with pigment nephropathy managed with red cell exchange. *J Clin Apher* (2016) 31(5):464–6. doi:10.1002/jca.21416
122. Gardulf A, Andersen V, Bjorkander J, Ericson D, Froland SS, Gustafson R, et al. Subcutaneous immunoglobulin replacement in patients with primary antibody deficiencies: safety and costs. *Lancet* (1995) 345(8946):365–9. doi:10.1016/S0140-6736(95)90346-1
123. Chapel HM, Spickett GP, Ericson D, Engl W, Eibl MM, Bjorkander J. The comparison of the efficacy and safety of intravenous versus subcutaneous immunoglobulin replacement therapy. *J Clin Immunol* (2000) 20(2):94–100. doi:10.1023/A:1006678312925
124. Ochs HD, Gupta S, Kiessling P, Nicolay U, Berger M, Subcutaneous IgG Study Group. Safety and efficacy of self-administered subcutaneous immunoglobulin

in patients with primary immunodeficiency diseases. *J Clin Immunol* (2006) 26(3):265–73. doi:10.1007/s10875-006-9021-7
125. Eftimov F, Vermeulen M, de Haan RJ, van den Berg LH, van Schaik IN. Subcutaneous immunoglobulin therapy for multifocal motor neuropathy. *J Peripher Nerv Syst* (2009) 14(2):93–100. doi:10.1111/j.1529-8027.2009.00218.x
126. Berger M, Murphy E, Riley P, Bergman GE. Improved quality of life, immunoglobulin G levels, and infection rates in patients with primary immunodeficiency diseases during self-treatment with subcutaneous immunoglobulin G. *South Med J* (2010) 103(9):856–63. doi:10.1097/SMJ.0b013e3181eba6ea
127. Harbo T, Andersen H, Jakobsen J. Long-term therapy with high doses of subcutaneous immunoglobulin in multifocal motor neuropathy. *Neurology* (2010) 75(15):1377–80. doi:10.1212/WNL.0b013e3181f735ce
128. Hoffmann F, Grimbacher B, Thiel J, Peter HH, Belohradsky BH. Home-based subcutaneous immunoglobulin G replacement therapy under real-life conditions in children and adults with antibody deficiency. *Eur J Med Res* (2010) 15(6):238–45. doi:10.1186/2047-783X-15-6-238
129. Thepot S, Malphettes M, Gardeur A, Galicier L, Asli B, Karlin L, et al. Immunoglobulin dosage and switch from intravenous to subcutaneous immunoglobulin replacement therapy in patients with primary hypogammaglobulinemia: decreasing dosage does not alter serum IgG levels. *J Clin Immunol* (2010) 30(4):602–6. doi:10.1007/s10875-010-9417-2
130. Misbah SA, Baumann A, Fazio R, Dacci P, Schmidt DS, Burton J, et al. A smooth transition protocol for patients with multifocal motor neuropathy going from intravenous to subcutaneous immunoglobulin therapy: an open-label proof-of-concept study. *J Peripher Nerv Syst* (2011) 16(2):92–7. doi:10.1111/j.1529-8027.2011.00330.x
131. Empson MB, Tang ML, Pearce LK, Rozen L, Gold MS, Katelaris CH, et al. Efficacy, safety and pharmacokinetics of a novel subcutaneous immunoglobulin, Evogam(R), in primary immunodeficiency. *J Clin Immunol* (2012) 32(5):897–906. doi:10.1007/s10875-011-9641-4
132. Markvardsen LH, Debost JC, Harbo T, Sindrup SH, Andersen H, Christiansen I, et al. Subcutaneous immunoglobulin in responders to intravenous therapy with chronic inflammatory demyelinating polyradiculoneuropathy. *Eur J Neurol* (2013) 20(5):836–42. doi:10.1111/ene.12080
133. Kanegane H, Imai K, Yamada M, Takada H, Ariga T, Bexon M, et al. Efficacy and safety of IgPro20, a subcutaneous immunoglobulin, in Japanese patients with primary immunodeficiency diseases. *J Clin Immunol* (2014) 34(2):204–11. doi:10.1007/s10875-013-9985-z
134. Spadaro G, Pecoraro A, De Renzo A, Della Pepa R, Genovese A. Intravenous versus subcutaneous immunoglobulin replacement in secondary hypogammaglobulinemia. *Clin Immunol* (2016) 166-167:103–4. doi:10.1016/j.clim.2016.04.001
135. Markvardsen LH, Sindrup SH, Christiansen I, Olsen NK, Jakobsen J, Andersen H, et al. Subcutaneous immunoglobulin as first-line therapy in treatment-naive patients with chronic inflammatory demyelinating polyneuropathy: randomized controlled trial study. *Eur J Neurol* (2017) 24(2):412–8. doi:10.1111/ene.13218
136. van Schaik IN, Bril V, van Geloven N, Hartung H-P, Lewis RA, Sobue G, et al. Subcutaneous immunoglobulin for maintenance treatment in chronic inflammatory demyelinating polyneuropathy (PATH): a randomised, double-blind, placebo-controlled, phase 3 trial. *Lancet Neurol* (2018) 17(1):35–46. doi:10.1016/S1474-4422(17)30378-2
137. Racosta JM, Sposato LA, Kimpinski K. Subcutaneous versus intravenous immunoglobulin for chronic autoimmune neuropathies: a meta-analysis. *Muscle Nerve* (2017) 55(6):802–9. doi:10.1002/mus.25409
138. Berger M, Rojavin M, Kiessling P, Zenker O. Pharmacokinetics of subcutaneous immunoglobulin and their use in dosing of replacement therapy in patients with primary immunodeficiencies. *Clin Immunol* (2011) 139(2):133–41. doi:10.1016/j.clim.2011.01.006
139. Ameratunga R. Initial intravenous immunoglobulin doses should be based on adjusted body weight in obese patients with primary immunodeficiency disorders. *Allergy Asthma Clin Immunol* (2017) 13:47. doi:10.1186/s13223-017-0220-y
140. Barnes GL, Doyle LW, Hewson PH, Knoches AM, McLellan JA, Kitchen WH, et al. A randomised trial of oral gammaglobulin in low-birth-weight infants infected with rotavirus. *Lancet* (1982) 1(8286):1371–3. doi:10.1016/S0140-6736(82)92496-5
141. Foster JP, Seth R, Cole MJ. Oral immunoglobulin for preventing necrotizing enterocolitis in preterm and low birth weight neonates. *Cochrane Database Syst Rev* (2016) 4:CD001816. doi:10.1002/14651858.CD001816.pub3
142. Pammi M, Haque KN. Oral immunoglobulin for the prevention of rotavirus infection in low birth weight infants. *Cochrane Database Syst Rev* (2011) (11):Cd003740. doi:10.1002/14651858.CD003740.pub2

11

Reduced Luteinizing Hormone Induction Following Estrogen and Progesterone Priming in Female-to-Male Transsexuals

Toshiya Funabashi[1,2], Hideya Sakakibara[3,4], Fumiki Hirahara[3] and Fukuko Kimura[1,5]*

[1] Department of Physiology, Yokohama City University School of Medicine, Yokohama, Japan, [2] Department of Physiology, St. Marianna University School of Medicine, Kawasaki, Japan, [3] Department of Obstetrics and Gynecology, Yokohama City University School of Medicine, Yokohama, Japan, [4] Department of Gynecology, Yokohama City University Medical Center, Yokohama, Japan, [5] Tanaka Clinic Yokohama-Koen, Yokohama, Japan

***Correspondence:**
Toshiya Funabashi
t4-funabashi@marianna-u.ac.jp

Anatomical studies have suggested that one of the brain structures involved in gender identity is the bed nucleus of the stria terminalis, though this brain structure is probably not the only one to control gender identity. We hypothesized that, if this brain area also affected gonadotropin secretion in humans, transsexual individuals might produce different gonadotropin levels in response to exogenous stimulation. In the present study, we examined whether estrogen combined with progesterone might lead to a change in luteinizing hormone (LH) secretion in female-to-male (FTM) transsexual individuals. We studied female control subjects ($n = 9$), FTM transsexual subjects ($n = 12$), and male-to-female (MTF) transsexual subjects ($n = 8$). Ethinyl estradiol (50 μg/tablet) was administered orally, twice a day, for five consecutive days. After the first blood sampling, progesterone (12.5 mg) was injected intramuscularly. Plasma LH was measured with an immunoradiometric assay. The combination of estrogen and progesterone resulted in increased LH secretion in female control subjects and in MTF subjects, but this increase appeared to be attenuated in FTM transsexual subjects. In fact, the %LH response was significantly reduced in FTM subjects ($P < 0.05$), but not in MTF subjects ($P > 0.5$), compared to female control subjects. In addition, the peak time after progesterone injection was significantly delayed in FTM subjects ($P < 0.05$), but not in MTF subjects ($P > 0.5$), compared to female control subjects. We then compared subjects according to whether the combination of estrogen and progesterone had a positive (more than 200% increase) or negative (less than 200% increase) effect on LH secretion. A χ^2 analysis revealed significantly different ($P < 0.05$) effects on LH secretion between female controls (positive $n = 7$, negative $n = 2$) and FTM transsexual subjects (positive $n = 4$, negative $n = 8$), but not between female controls and MTF transsexual subjects (positive $n = 7$, negative $n = 1$). Thus, LH secretion in response to estrogen- and progesterone priming was attenuated in FTM subjects, but not in MTF subjects, compared to control females. This finding suggested that the brain area related to gender identity in morphological studies might also be involved in the LH secretory response in humans. Thus, altered brain morphology might be correlated to altered function in FTM transsexuals.

Keywords: transsexual, gender dysphoria, gender identity, estrogen, progesterone, luteinizing hormone, bed nucleus, human

INTRODUCTION

It is generally agreed that the rodent central nervous system is sexually differentiated. This includes the hypothalamus and the anterior pituitary, which control luteinizing hormone (LH) secretion. Female rodents, but not males, exhibit a surge of LH secretion that drives ovulation, which results from a "positive feedback" effect of estrogen (1). Androgen exposure during the neonatal period is thought to be critical for the development of sexual differentiation (2–5). Thus, the presence of a sex difference, or sexual dimorphism, is found in many brain structures, due to the organizational effects of sex steroids, which produce male- or female-like morphology.

The bed nucleus of the stria terminalis (BST) is one of several structures that show sexually dimorphic regions (6, 7). Moreover, neuronal fibers that project from the BST to various brain regions (8–10) are involved in many different types of motivational behaviors (11–13). In addition, the BST was shown to be involved in gonadotropin secretion (14–17). Indeed, estrogen-binding cells were found in the BST (18), where gonadal steroid receptors were expressed (19–21). The rat lateral subdivision of the BST is homologous to the human central BST (22, 23), which is thought be involved in gender identity in humans.

Gender identity disorder, or gender dysphoria (GD), is defined as a strong gender identification with the opposite sex; for example, female-to-male (FTM) transsexuals have a strong male gender identity, and thus, they want to reassign their physical sex (24–26). Although GD is a highly complex clinical situation, its etiology has been described by several environmental, genetic, and anatomical theories (27–30). Currently, there is morphological evidence that, in humans, the BST is related to gender identity (31–33). Studies have shown that the number of neurons in the BST (34) and the central BST size (35) in male-to-female (MTF) transsexual individuals corresponded to the respective norms for biological females. Conversely, FTM transsexual individuals exhibited a BST size that corresponded to the norm for biological males (35). It is unknown whether these structural features are causally related to sexual identity or whether they are indirectly correlated.

Taken together, findings from previous studies have led to the hypothesis that, if the same area of the central nervous system that controls LH secretions is also involved in gender identity, or conversely, if the causal factor(s) (as yet undetermined) that affects brain structure in GD can also account for LH secretion, then the LH secretory profile in subjects with GD might be different from the typical profile expected for a given sex. Gooren and colleagues studied this hypothesis in detail (36, 37) and concluded that the neuroendocrine regulation of LH secretion did not differ between transsexual and non-transsexual individuals, either males or females (24, 28). This result may be reasonable, since the neuroendocrine mechanism that regulates the cyclic release (surge) of LH in primates is not thought to be different between the sexes (5, 38). Indeed, estrogen was equally capable of inducing surge-like LH secretions in male rhesus monkeys (5, 38–40) and female monkeys (1). In humans, it was reported that a similar surge-like LH secretion could be induced by estrogen in gonadectomized men (41, 42).

However, androgen exposure during the neonatal period, which is essential for brain differentiation in rodents (2, 3, 38), may alter the LH secretory response later in life, even in female primates (39, 43–46). It was reported that, in estrogen-primed ovariectomized female rhesus monkeys, progesterone had a stimulatory effect on LH secretion (47, 48). Importantly, this stimulatory effect was unremarkable in orchidectomized male rhesus macaques pretreated with 17-β estradiol (49). Although one report suggested that a surge-like LH secretion could be induced in men with progesterone after estrogen priming (50), the response was not directly compared with responses in women subjects; thus, the amplitude of the effect was unclear. Therefore, we hypothesized that estrogen combined with progesterone might lead to a change in LH secretion in patients with GD.

SUBJECTS AND METHODS

Subjects

For the present study, we recruited healthy Japanese volunteers who had undergone either FTM or MTF transsexual procedures. All FTM subjects were diagnosed with GD by psychiatrists, independent of the present study. All MTF subjects self-reported that they were bilaterally orchidectomized. Although, ideally, MTF subjects should be compared to male control subjects with bilateral orchidectomies, we could not recruit these control subjects. Thus, we compared the MTF transsexual data to female control data. One month before the sampling experiment, MTF subjects were asked to stop their cross-gender hormone treatments. All subjects self-reported their sexual orientation.

Treatment

Ethinyl estradiol (50 μg) tablets were administered to all subjects orally twice per day (100 μg total per day) for five consecutive days (days 3 to 7). Day 1 of the experiment was the day that menstruation began in female and FTM subjects. In previous studies, this dose of estrogen alone did not induce LH secretion, but when combined with progesterone, it induced a surge-like LH secretion (51–53). The estrogen treatment period was chosen, based on previous reports (51–53) and on our previous experience with rats (54). Blood samples were drawn on day 7. After the blood sample was taken, progesterone (12.5 mg) was injected at the University Hospital, between 0830 and 0930 h. Then, sequential blood samples (1.0–1.5 ml each) were collected on the same day, at 1200, 1500, 1800, and 2100 h. The final blood sample was drawn at 0900 h the next day. All blood samples were drawn through a median cubital vein. Plasma was separated from the blood samples at 4°C and stored at −20°C.

Ethics

This study was conducted in accordance with the recommendations of the Ethical Guidelines for Medical and Health Research Involving Human Subjects, established by the Ministry of Education, Culture, Sports, Science, and Technology and the Ministry of Health, Labor and Welfare. We obtained written informed consent to participate in the study from all volunteers, in accordance with the Declaration of Helsinki. The protocol was approved by the institutional Ethics Committee of the Yokohama City University School of Medicine. Subjects were interviewed to obtain data on their general health condition, sexual orientation, and menstrual cycles.

Analytical Methods and Statistical Analyses

Plasma LH was measured with immunoradiometric assay kits (Daiichi Radioisotope Institute). The intra- and inter-assay coefficients of variation, estimated at the mean LH level of 7.6 mIU/ml, were 3.0 and 8.0%, respectively. We tested statistical significance, as appropriate, with the one-way ANOVA, followed by Fisher's Least Significant Differences (LSD) *post hoc* comparison; with the Kruskal–Wallis test, followed by Dunn's multiple comparison test; or with the χ^2 test. Significance was accepted at $P < 0.05$.

RESULTS

Subjects

A total of nine female control subjects, 12 FTM subjects, and 8 MTF subjects, aged 28.7 ± 2.7, 27.4 ± 1.5, and 39.3 ± 2.3 years, respectively, participated in blood sampling experiments. We found that the baseline LH levels (before injection) were higher in MTF subjects (**Figure 1**) than in the other subjects. This finding suggested that no negative feedback was present, consistent with the removal of the testes. All female control and 10 FTM subjects self-reported regular menstrual cycles (regular was defined as a menstrual cycle of 25–38 days). Sexual orientations were self-reported; all female control subjects were attracted to men. All FTM subjects were attracted to women. Among the MTF subjects, one was attracted to women, four were to men, and three were attracted to both.

Effects of Estrogen Combined With Progesterone on LH Secretion

The LH response to estrogen and progesterone was tentatively defined as positive, when LH levels were greater than 200% of the control level. This threshold was based on data from previous studies (55, 56). According to this criterion, 77.7% of control females and 33.3% of FTM subjects showed positive responses (**Table 1**, $P < 0.05$, χ^2 test). In addition, seven out of eight MTF subjects displayed positive responses, a similar proportion to that observed among control females ($P > 0.1$).

Representative changes in LH profiles over time are shown in **Figure 1**. The estrogen and progesterone treatment appeared to stimulate LH release in both female control and MTF subjects, but not in FTM subjects. The mean LH concentrations at each time point are shown in **Figure 2A**. We analyzed the %change in LH secretion. This analysis showed that the LH response in FTM subjects was significantly smaller than in female controls (**Figure 2B**, ANOVA $P < 0.05$, Fisher's LSD $P < 0.05$). On the other hand, the LH response in MTF subjects was not different from that observed in female controls (Fisher's LSD $P > 0.5$). The mean peak time of LH secretion in FTM subjects was significantly delayed compared to that observed in female controls (**Figure 2C**, Kruskal–Wallis $P < 0.01$, Dunn's multiple comparison $P < 0.05$). The mean peak time of LH secretion in MTF subjects was not different from that observed in female controls (Dunn's multiple comparison, no significant difference).

DISCUSSION

In the present study, FTM subjects were attracted to women, but the MTF subjects were attracted to women, men, or both sexes. This result was in good accord with previous reports (57–59). For example, Auer et al. (59) described an MTF group that comprised individuals attracted to women (gynephilic, 51%) or men (androphilic, 26%), and an FTM group that were attracted to women (gynephilic, 73%). These similarities to our data suggested that our sampling population was not biased.

By examining the LH response to estrogen combined with progesterone, we found that the neuroendocrine response was different between FTM subjects and female controls. We should consider the physiological meaning of this phenomenon. Progesterone is certainly an important factor for induction of the LH surge in the rodent (1, 60), the ewe (61), and the primate (47, 48). However, the physiological role of progesterone in the ovulation-induced LH surge has not been fully understood (62). For example, a primary question is, what is the source of progesterone? Progesterone in the follicular fluid in the ovary exhibits higher than in the blood of pregnant women and thus source of progesterone may be follicle cells (62). Progesterone may come from the central nervous system (63). Basically, in the menstrual cycle, a gonadotropin surge and follicular rupture occur, followed by the luteinization of granulosa cells. Granulosa cells then establish the corpus luteum and progesterone secretion increases. Thus, we speculated that, with the current understanding, it might be difficult to distinguish FTM subjects from control subjects, based solely on the LH response to estrogen, and suggest the importance of determining the LH controlling mechanism by means of progesterone treatment in transsexuals.

The majority of FTM subjects exhibited a regular menstrual cycle. Consequently, like female control subjects, they could reproduce the menstrual cycle, as shown by Gooren (24). We confirmed that some FTM subjects displayed a preovulatory LH surge (Funabashi and Kimura, unpublished observations), but we did not examine ovulation directly in this study. However, our previous studies suggested that there was a discrepancy in reproductive abilities; female rats exposed to a low dose of testosterone during the neonatal period displayed a surge-like LH secretion in response to the combination of estrogen and progesterone, but the number of gonadotropin-releasing hormone neurons that expressed Fos was attenuated (54). Since these rats exhibit a regular estrous cycle, these results are consistent with FTM in this study having a regular menstrual cycle, but exhibiting attenuated LH secretion in response to estrogen combined with progesterone. Thus, the discrepancy between the mechanism for controlling menstrual

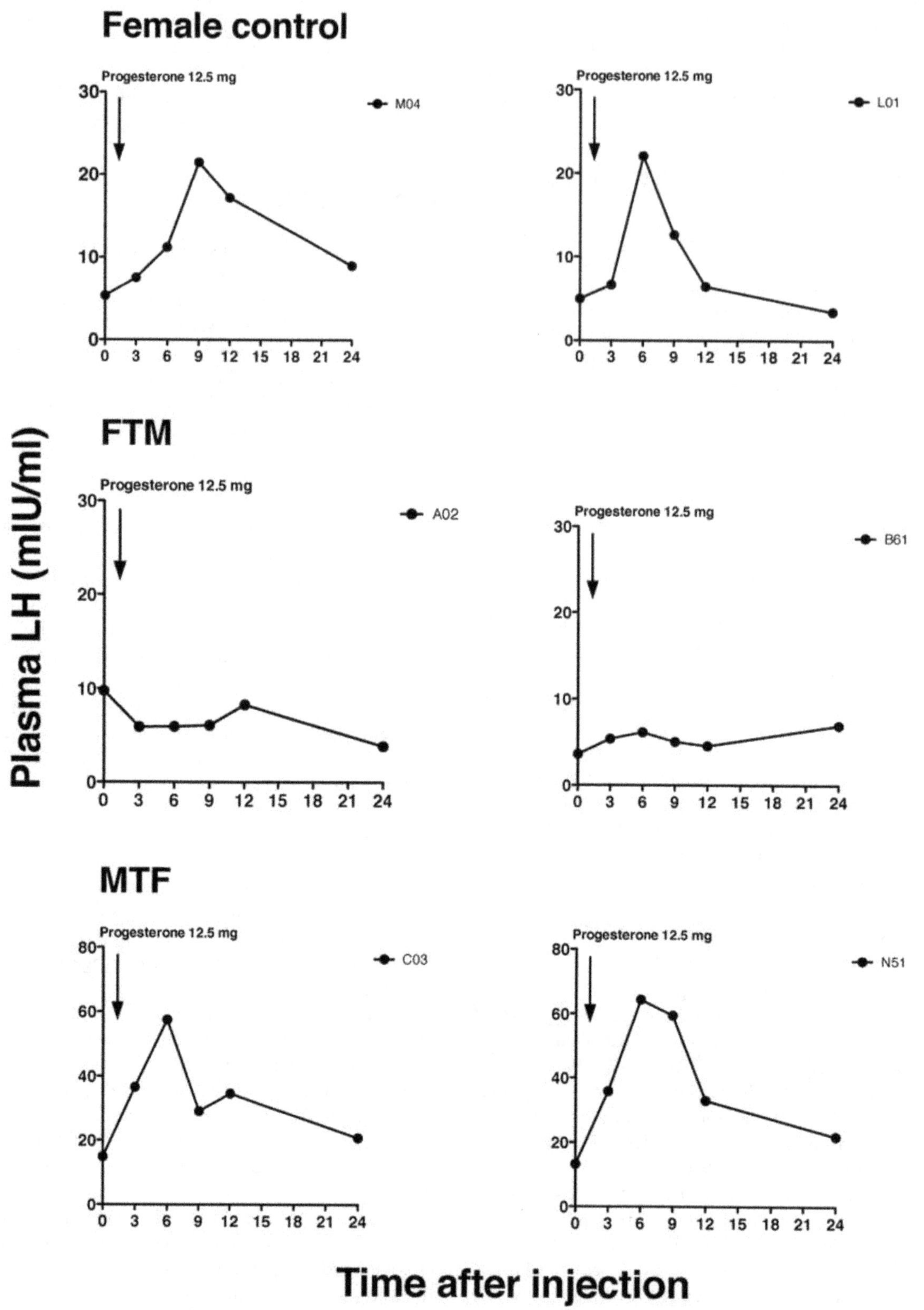

FIGURE 1 | Representative luteinizing hormone (LH) secretory patterns in transsexual individuals. Profiles of the LH secretory pattern in two female controls *(upper panels)*, two female-to-male transsexual (FTM) subjects *(middle panels)*, and two male-to-female transsexual (MTF) subjects *(lower panels)*, after estrogen priming (ethinyl estradiol, 100 μg for 5 days), and before (time 0) and after the progesterone injection. Each point indicates the plasma LH level. The arrow indicates the time of progesterone injection (12.5 mg).

TABLE 1 | Luteinizing hormone (LH) response to estrogen and progesterone stimulation, in control females and transsexual subjects.

Subjects	Number	LH response[a]		*P*-value
		Positive	Negative	
Control	9	7	2	
Female-to-Male	12	4	8	*
Male-to-Female	8	7	1	NS

[a]*The LH responses were classified as positive (more than 200% increase) or negative (less than 200% increase), compared to baseline. *P < 0.05 vs. female control subjects, based on the χ^2 test. NS = not significant.*

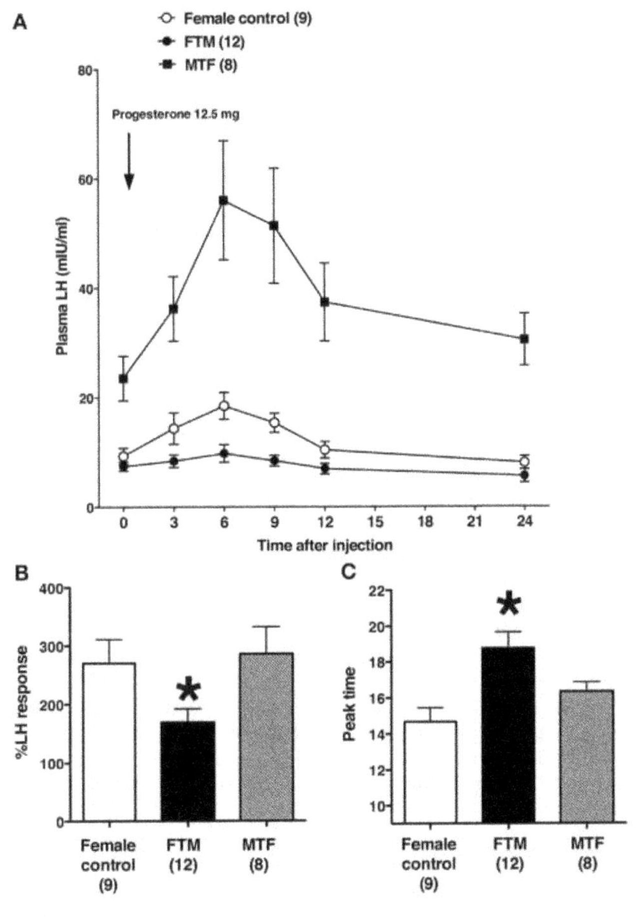

FIGURE 2 | Summary of the effects of estrogen and progesterone treatment on luteinizing hormone (LH) secretion in transsexuals. **(A)** Effects on LH secretion over time in female controls (open circles), female-to-male transsexual (FTM) subjects (closed circles), and male-to-female transsexual (MTF) subjects (closed squares). Each point and vertical line indicate the mean and SE, respectively. The LH level after 5 days of estrogen is shown at time 0. The arrow indicates the time of progesterone injection (12.5 mg). **(B)** The peak %changes in plasma LH are shown after estrogen and progesterone treatment, in female controls (*open bars*), FTM transsexual subjects (*filled bars*), and MTF transsexual subjects (*hatched bars*). **(C)** The time of peak plasma LH levels in subjects treated with estrogen and progesterone. Numbers in parentheses are the number of subjects in each group. Each bar and vertical line indicate the mean and SE, respectively; **P* < 0.05 vs. female control.

cycle and the steroid-induced LH surge may be reasonable but LH response by an exogenous stimulus is attenuated in FTM subjects.

We would like to discuss whether the LH controlling mechanism is different between the sexes in humans. A previous report found that this mechanism was not different between transsexual individuals and controls; therefore, they concluded that it was not sexually differentiated (24). In the present study, the majority of MTF subjects showed an increase in LH secretion in response to estrogen combined with progesterone, similar to female control subjects. This result suggested that the LH controlling mechanism was not sexually differentiated. This finding was supported by a previous report that suggested that a surge-like LH secretion could be induced in men by injecting progesterone after estrogen priming (50); however, that response was not compared with a response in women subjects in that report; therefore, sexual differentiation could not be ruled out. If it is reasonable to compare MTF subjects to FTM subjects, due to the opposite genetic backgrounds and sexual identities, different conclusions are drawn. Since LH responses in transsexuals were different, the alteration in sexual differentiation may be related to the GD etiology (25, 57). Thus, gender identity, sexual orientation, and reproduction might be sexually differentiated through different brain mechanisms. In previous studies, different brain areas were responsible for sexual orientation and gender identity; the suprachiasmatic nucleus and the bed nucleus of the stria terminalis, respectively (25, 28).

The main limitation of this study was the lack of a male control without testes, which prevented us from drawing conclusions. This study was also limited by the small number of GD subjects; thus, we lacked firm evidence to support our hypothesis. Consequently, our findings remain to be confirmed in future studies with larger numbers of subjects.

ETHICS STATEMENT

This study was conducted in accordance with the recommendations of the Ethical Guidelines for Medical and Health Research Involving Human Subjects, established by the Ministry of Education, Culture, Sports, Science, and Technology and the Ministry of Health, Labor and Welfare. We obtained written informed consent to participate in the study from all volunteers, in accordance with the Declaration of Helsinki. The protocol was approved by the institutional Ethics Committee of the Yokohama City University School of Medicine. Subjects were interviewed to obtain data on their general health condition, sexual orientation, and menstrual cycles.

AUTHOR CONTRIBUTIONS

TF and FK designed the study, analysis and interpretation of data, and assisted in the preparation of the manuscript. TF wrote the initial draft of the manuscript. All other authors have contributed to data collection. FK critically reviewed the manuscript. All authors approved the final version of the manuscript, and agreed to be accountable for all aspects of the work in ensuring that questions related to the accuracy or integrity of any part of the work are appropriately investigated and resolved.

ACKNOWLEDGMENTS

The present study was supported by JSPS KAKENHI, Grant Numbers 16659059 (to FK) and 17K08577 (to TF). The authors thank the Yokohama City University Hospital nursing staff for implementing the study protocol. The authors appreciate the support of A. K. for technical assistance.

FUNDING

The present study was supported by Grant-in-Aid for Exploratory Research (FK: 16659059) and Grant-in-Aid for Scientific Research (TF: 17K08577).

REFERENCES

1. Kalra SP, Kalra PS. Neural regulation of luteinizing hormone secretion in the rat. *Endocr Rev* (1983) 4(4):311–51. doi:10.1210/edrv-4-4-311
2. Gorski RA. Influence of age on the response to paranatal administration of a low dose of androgen. *Endocrinology* (1968) 82(5):1001–4. doi:10.1210/endo-82-5-1001
3. Arnold AP, Gorski RA. Gonadal steroid induction of structural sex differences in the central nervous system. *Annu Rev Neurosci* (1984) 7:413–42. doi:10.1146/annurev.ne.07.030184.002213
4. Gorski RA. Sexual dimorphisms of the brain. *J Anim Sci* (1985) 61(Suppl 3): 38–61. doi:10.1093/ansci/61.Supplement_3.38
5. Resko JA, Roselli CE. Prenatal hormones organize sex differences of the neuroendocrine reproductive system: observations on guinea pigs and nonhuman primates. *Cell Mol Neurobiol* (1997) 17(6):627–48. doi:10.1023/A:1022534019718
6. Segovia S, Guillamón A. Searching for sex differences in the vomeronasal pathway. *Horm Behav* (1996) 30:618–26. doi:10.1006/hbeh.1996.0065
7. Guillamón A, Segovia S. Sex differences in the vomeronasal system. *Brain Res Bull* (1997) 44:377–82. doi:10.1016/S0361-9230(97)00217-7
8. Moga MM, Saper CB, Gray TS. Bed nucleus of the stria terminalis: cytoarchitecture, immunohistochemistry, and projection to the parabrachial nucleus in the rat. *J Comp Neurol* (1989) 283:315–32. doi:10.1002/cne.902830302
9. Dong HW, Petrovich GD, Watts AG, Swanson LW. Basic organization of projections from the oval and fusiform nuclei of the bed nuclei of the stria terminalis in adult rat brain. *J Comp Neurol* (2001) 436:430–55. doi:10.1002/cne.1079
10. Dong HW, Swanson LW. Projections from the rhomboid nucleus of the bed nuclei of the stria terminalis: implications for cerebral hemisphere regulation of ingestive behaviors. *J Comp Neurol* (2003) 463:434–72. doi:10.1002/cne.10758
11. Toufexis D. Region- and sex-specific modulation of anxiety behaviours in the rat. *J. Neuroendocrinol* (2007) 19:461–73. doi:10.1111/j.1365-2826.2007.01552.x
12. de Vries GJ. Sex differences in vasopressin and oxytocin innervation of the brain. *Prog Brain Res* (2008) 170:17–27. doi:10.1016/S0079-6123(08)00402-0
13. Walker DL, Davis M. Role of the extended amygdala in short-duration versus sustained fear: a tribute to Dr. Lennart Heimer. *Brain Struct Funct* (2008) 213:29–42. doi:10.1007/s00429-008-0183-3
14. Kimura F, Kawakami M. Reanalysis of the preoptic afferents and efferents involved in the surge of LH, FSH and prolactin release in the proestrous rat. *Neuroendocrinology* (1978) 27(1–2):74–85. doi:10.1159/000122801
15. Beltramino C, Taleisnik S. Dual action of electrochemical stimulation of the bed nucleus of the stria terminalis on the release of LH. *Neuroendocrinology* (1980) 30(4):238–42. doi:10.1159/000123007
16. Pompolo S, Ischenko O, Pereira A, Iqbal J, Clarke IJ. Evidence that projections from the bed nucleus of the stria terminalis and from the lateral and medial regions of the preoptic area provide input to gonadotropin releasing hormone (GNRH) neurons in the female sheep brain. *Neuroscience* (2005) 132(2):421–36. doi:10.1016/j.neuroscience.2004.12.042
17. Yamada S, Uenoyama Y, Maeda KI, Tsukamura H. Role of noradrenergic receptors in the bed nucleus of the stria terminalis in regulating pulsatile luteinizing hormone secretion in female rats. *J Reprod Dev* (2006) 52(1):115–21. doi:10.1262/jrd.17071
18. Pfaff DW, Gerlach J, McEwen BS, Ferin M, Carmel P, Zimmerman EA. Autoradiographic localization of hormone-concentrating cells in the brain of the female rhesus monkey. *J Comp Neurol* (1976) 170(3):279–93. doi:10.1002/cne.901700302
19. Simerly RB, Chang C, Muramatsu M, Swanson LW. Distribution of androgen and estrogen receptor mRN-containing cells in the rat brain: an in situ Hybridization Study. *J Comp Neurol* (1990) 294:76–95. doi:10.1002/cne.902940107
20. Shughrue PJ, Merchenthaler I. Distribution of estrogen receptor β immunoreactivity in the rat central nervous system. *J Comp Neurol* (2001) 436:64–81. doi:10.1002/cne.1054
21. Mitra SW, Hoskin E, Yudkovitz J, Pear L, Wilkinson HA, Hayashi S, et al. Immunolocalization of estrogen receptor beta in the mouse brain: comparison with estrogen receptor alpha. *Endocrinology* (2003) 144(5):2055–67. doi:10.1210/en.2002-221069
22. Lesur A, Gaspar P, Alvarez C, Berger B. Chemoanatomic compartments in the human bed nucleus of the stria terminalis. *Neuroscience* (1989) 32:181–94. doi:10.1016/0306-4522(89)90117-6
23. Walter A, Mai J, Lanta L, Görcs T. Differential distribution of immunohistochemical markers in the bed nucleus of the stria terminalis in the human brain. *J Chem Neuroanat* (1991) 4(4):281–98. doi:10.1016/0891-0618(91)90019-9
24. Gooren L. The endocrinology of transsexualism: a review and commentary. *Psychoneuroendocrinology* (1990) 15(1):3–14. doi:10.1016/0306-4530(90)90041-7
25. Swaab DF, Chung WC, Kruijver FP, Hofman MA, Ishunina TA. Structural and functional sex differences in the human hypothalamus. *Horm Behav* (2001) 40(2):93–8. doi:10.1006/hbeh.2001.1682
26. Guillamón A, Junque C, Gomez-Gil E. A review of the status of brain structure research in transsexualism. *Arch Sex Behav* (2016) 45(7):1615–48. doi:10.1007/s10508-016-0768-5
27. Cohen-Kettenis PT, Gooren LJ. Transsexualism: a review of etiology, diagnosis and treatment. *J Psychosom Res* (1999) 46(4):315–33. doi:10.1016/S0022-3999(98)00085-3
28. Gooren L. The biology of human psychosexual differentiation. *Horm Behav* (2006) 50(4):589–601. doi:10.1016/j.yhbeh.2006.06.011
29. Castellanos-Cruz L, Bao A-M, Swaab DF. Sexual identity and sexual orientation. *Hormones, Brain and Behavior*. 3rd ed. Vol. 5 (2017). p. 279–90. doi:10.1016/B978-0-12-803592-4.00104-8
30. Roselli CE. Neurobiology of gender identity and sexual orientation. *J Neuroendocrinol* (2017). doi:10.1111/jne.12562
31. Chung WC, De Vries GJ, Swaab DF. Sexual differentiation of the bed nucleus of the stria terminalis in humans may extend into adulthood. *J Neurosci* (2002) 22(3):1027–33. doi:10.1523/JNEUROSCI.22-03-01027.2002
32. Swaab DF. Sexual differentiation of the brain and behavior. *Best Pract Res Clin Endocrinol Metab* (2007) 21(3):431–44. doi:10.1016/j.beem.2007.04.003
33. Garcia-Falgueras A, Swaab DF. Sexual hormones and the brain: an essential alliance for sexual identity and sexual orientation. *Endocr Dev* (2010) 17:22–35. doi:10.1159/000262525
34. Zhou JN, Hofman MA, Gooren LJ, Swaab DF. A sex difference in the human brain and its relation to transsexuality. *Nature* (1995) 378(6552):68–70. doi:10.1038/378068a0
35. Kruijver FP, Zhou JN, Pool CW, Hofman MA, Gooren LJ, Swaab DF. Male-to-female transsexuals have female neuron numbers in a limbic nucleus. *J Clin Endocrinol Metab* (2000) 85(5):2034–41. doi:10.1210/jcem.85.5.6564
36. Gooren LJ, Rao BR, van Kessel H, Harmsen-Louman W. Estrogen positive feedback on LH secretion in transsexuality. *Psychoneuroendocrinology* (1984) 9(3):249–59. doi:10.1016/0306-4530(84)90004-0
37. Gooren L. The neuroendocrine response of luteinizing hormone to estrogen administration in the human is not sex specific but dependent on the hormonal

environment. *J Clin Endocrinol Metab* (1986) 63(3):589–93. doi:10.1210/jcem-63-3-589
38. Karsch FJ, Dierschke DJ, Knobil E. Sexual differentiation of pituitary function: apparent difference bewteen primates and rodents. *Science* (1973) 179(72):484–6. doi:10.1126/science.179.4072.484
39. Steiner RA, Clifton DK, Spies HG, Resko JA. Sexual differentiation and feedback control of luteinizing hormone secretion in the rhesus monkey. *Biol Reprod* (1976) 15(2):206–12. doi:10.1095/biolreprod15.2.206
40. Hodges JK. Regulation of oestrogen-induced LH release in male and female marmoset monkeys (*Callithrix jacchus*). *J Reprod Fertil* (1980) 60(2):389–98. doi:10.1530/jrf.0.0600389
41. Kulin HE, Reiter EO. Gonadotropin and testosterone measurements after estrogen administration to adult men, prepubertal and pubertal boys, and men with hypogonadotropism: evidence for maturation of positive feedback in the male. *Pediatr Res* (1976) 10(1):46–51. doi:10.1203/00006450-197601000-00009
42. Barbarino A, De Marinis L. Estrogen induction of luteinizing hormone release in castrated adult human males. *J Clin Endocrinol Metab* (1980) 51(2):280–6. doi:10.1210/jcem-51-2-280
43. Barnes RB, Rosenfield RL, Ehrmann DA, Cara JF, Cuttler L, Levitsky LL, et al. Ovarian hyperandrogynism as a result of congenital adrenal virilizing disorders: evidence for perinatal masculinization of neuroendocrine function in women. *J Clin Endocrinol Metab* (1994) 79(5):1328–33. doi:10.1210/jcem.79.5.7962325
44. Dumesic DA, Abbott DH, Eisner JR, Goy RW. Prenatal exposure of female rhesus monkeys to testosterone propionate increases serum luteinizing hormone levels in adulthood. *Fertil Steril* (1997) 67(1):155–63. doi:10.1016/S0015-0282(97)81893-6
45. McCartney CR, Eagleson CA, Marshall JC. Regulation of gonadotropin secretion: implications for polycystic ovary syndrome. *Semin Reprod Med* (2002) 20(4):317–26. doi:10.1055/s-2002-36706
46. Abbott DH, Barnett DK, Levine JE, Padmanabhan V, Dumesic DA, Jacoris S, et al. Endocrine antecedents of polycystic ovary syndrome in fetal and infant prenatally androgenized female rhesus monkeys. *Biol Reprod* (2008) 79(1):154–63. doi:10.1095/biolreprod.108.067702
47. Clifton DK, Steiner RA, Resko JA, Spies HG. Estrogen-induced gonadotropin release in ovariectomized rhesus monkeys and its advancement by progesterone. *Biol Reprod* (1975) 13(2):190–4. doi:10.1095/biolreprod13.2.190
48. Terasawa E, Rodriguez-Sierra JF, Dierschke DJ, Bridson WE, Goy RW. Positive feedback effect of progesterone on luteinizing hormone (LH) release in cyclic female rhesus monkeys: LH response occurs in two phases. *J Clin Endocrinol Metab* (1980) 51(6):1245–50. doi:10.1210/jcem-51-6-1245
49. Resko JA, Horton LE. Effects of progesterone on estrogen-induced gonadotropin release in male rhesus macaques. *Endocrinology* (1983) 112(3):850–5. doi:10.1210/endo-112-3-850
50. Stearns EL, Winter JS, Faiman C. Positive feedback effect of progestin upon serum gonadotropins in estrogen-primed castrate men. *J Clin Endocrinol Metab* (1973) 37(4):635–8. doi:10.1210/jcem-37-4-635
51. Tsai CC, Yen SS. The effect of ethinyl estradiol administration during early follicular phase of the cycle on the gonadotropin levels and ovarian function. *J Clin Endocrinol Metab* (1971) 33(6):917–23. doi:10.1210/jcem-33-6-917
52. Cargille CM, Vaitukaitis JL, Bermudez JA, Ross GT. A differential effect of ethinyl estradiol upon plasma FSH and LH relating to time of administration in the menstrual cycle. *J Clin Endocrinol Metab* (1973) 36(1):87–94. doi:10.1210/jcem-36-1-87
53. Rakoff JS, Yen SS. Progesterone induced acute release of prolactin in estrogen primed ovariectomized women. *J Clin Endocrinol Metab* (1978) 47(4):918–21. doi:10.1210/jcem-47-4-918
54. Fukushima A, Furuta M, Kimura F, Akema T, Funabashi T. Testosterone exposure during the critical period decreases corticotropin-releasing hormone-immunoreactive neurons in the bed nucleus of the stria terminalis of female rats. *Neurosci Lett* (2013) 534:64–8. doi:10.1016/j.neulet.2012.11.065
55. Aono T, Minagawa J, Kinugasa T, Miyake A, Kurachi K. The diagnostic significance of LH-releasing hormone test in patients with amenorrhea. *Am J Obstet Gynecol* (1974) 119(6):740–8. doi:10.1016/0002-9378(74)90085-4
56. Miyake A, Tasaka K, Sakumoto T, Kawamura Y, Aono T. Estrogen induces the release of luteinizing hormone-releasing hormone in normal cyclic women. *J Clin Endocrinol Metab* (1983) 56(6):1100–2. doi:10.1210/jcem-56-6-1100
57. Okabe N, Sato T, Matsumoto Y, Ido Y, Terada S, Kuroda S. Clinical characteristics of patients with gender identity disorder at a Japanese gender identity disorder clinic. *Psychiatry Res* (2008) 157(1–3):315–8. doi:10.1016/j.psychres.2007.07.022
58. Nieder TO, Herff M, Cerwenka S, Preuss WF, Cohen-Kettenis PT, De Cuypere G, et al. Age of onset and sexual orientation in transsexual males and females. *J Sex Med* (2011) 8(3):783–91. doi:10.1111/j.1743-6109.2010.02142.x
59. Auer MK, Fuss J, Hohne N, Stalla GK, Sievers C. Transgender transitioning and change of self-reported sexual orientation. *PLoS One* (2014) 9(10):e110016. doi:10.1371/journal.pone.0110016
60. Everett JW, Sawyer CH. A neural timing factor in the mechanism by which progesterone advances ovulation in the cyclic rat. *Endocrinology* (1949) 45(6):581–95. doi:10.1210/endo-45-6-581
61. Caraty A, Skinner DC. Progesterone priming is essential for the full expression of the positive feedback effect of estradiol in inducing the preovulatory gonadotropin-releasing hormone surge in the ewe. *Endocrinology* (1999) 140:165–70. doi:10.1210/endo.140.1.6444
62. ZalaÂnyi S. Progesterone and ovulation. *Eur J Obstet Gynecol Reprod Biol* (2001) 98:152–9. doi:10.1016/S0301-2115(01)00361-X
63. Micevych P, Sinchak K. The neurosteroid progesterone underlies estrogen positive feedback of the LH surge. *Front Endocrinol* (2011) 2:90. doi:10.3389/fendo.2011.00090

12

Luteinizing Hormone Involvement in Aging Female Cognition: Not all is Estrogen Loss

Sabina Bhatta*[1]*, Jeffrey A. Blair*[1] *and Gemma Casadesus*[1,2]

[1] School of Biomedical Sciences, Kent State University, Kent, OH, United States, [2] Department of Biological Sciences, Kent State University, Kent, OH, United States

***Correspondence:**
Gemma Casadesus
gcasades@kent.edu

Pervasive age-related dysfunction in hypothalamic-pituitary-gonadal (HPG) axis is associated with cognitive impairments in aging as well as pathogenesis of age-related neurodegenerative diseases such as the Alzheimer's disease (AD). As a major regulator of the HPG axis, the steroid hormone estrogen has been widely studied for its role in regulation of memory. Although estrogen modulates both cognition as well as cognition associated morphological components in a healthy state, the benefits of estrogen replacement therapy on cognition and disease seem to diminish with advancing age. Emerging data suggests an important role for luteinizing hormone (LH) in CNS function, which is another component of the HPG axis that becomes dysregulated during aging, particularly in menopause. The goal of this review is to highlight the current existing literature on LH and provide new insights on possible mechanisms of its action.

Keywords: luteinizing hormone, luteinizing hormone receptor, cognition, menopause, estrogen, ovariectomy, inverse relationship

INTRODUCTION

Our ability to successfully treat midlife diseases has increased human longevity as well as the prevalence of age-associated neurodegenerative diseases such as the Alzheimer's disease (AD). While a small percentage of AD is precipitated by dominant mutations, the majority is sporadic and is highly associated with environmental/life-style choices as well as the physiological aging process. In fact, aging is the strongest risk factor for development for AD, the most common form of dementia (1–3). As baby boomers age, millions of people are at risk for AD and other cognitive diseases. This is especially relevant as the number of AD diagnosis is expected to rise from current 5.7 million to 14 million by 2050, and the cost of disease is projected to rise to 1.1 trillion dollars creating a broad economic and social impact. Therefore, identifying therapeutic targets to delay, modify, or cure the disease is of paramount importance.

Menopause, a hallmark of aging in women, is associated with dysfunctions in the hypothalamic-pituitary-gonadal (HPG) axis and is implicated in the pathogenesis of AD. Age-related declines in reproductive hormones lead to a disarray of the HPG axis as it is tightly regulated by positive and negative feedback loops involving gonadotropin releasing hormone (GnRH), gonadal steroids, and gonadotropins. The loss of any component leads to significant dysregulation of the system and any type of hormonal imbalance likely affects homeostasis resulting in functional decline throughout the body, including the brain (4–8). In fact, these declines in gonadal hormones, and associated increases in gonadotropins such as LH are implicated in cognitive dysfunction in aging as well as the pathogenesis of age-related disorders such as AD. This is particularly relevant for women as they have two-fold higher risk for development of AD after menopause compared to men.

HORMONE REPLACEMENT THERAPY (HRT) FOR COGNITION AND AD

Several studies attribute increased risk of AD to the menopausal loss of estrogen (9, 10) and considered estrogen replacement a promising therapeutic avenue to reduce the risk of AD (11–14). This was initially supported by early epidemiological studies identifying strong relationships between estrogen therapy in post-menopausal women and reductions in multiple types of memory decline, specifically, in menopausal women with and without AD (15, 16).

Clinically, estrogen replacement or HRT showed initial promise in smaller clinical retrospective (17–20) and prospective studies (21–23). However, a large scale, randomized, double-blind placebo-controlled trial, women's health initiative WIH found no overall cognitive benefits. While the use of estrogen immediately or after a smaller delay following onset of menopause was effective, HRT in women at least 15 years after onset of menopause slightly increased the risk of dementia instead (24–26). This discrepancy in actions of estrogen on memory and dementia risk lead several groups to hypothesize that a "critical period" may exist following onset of menopause where estrogen can confer benefits, beyond which it is ineffective and may instead exert harmful effects (27–31). These clinical observations were further supported by pre-clinical work in ovariectomized rodents (32) and primates (33) providing support for the existence of a critical window for the initiation of estrogen for optimal enhancement of cognitive function (34).

One mechanism purported to underlie the ineffectiveness of estrogen treatment beyond a critical period is the "*healthy cell bias*" wherein estrogen is beneficial to healthy cells, but detrimental to unhealthy ones (35, 36). This was further supported by the fact that critical plasticity and cognition related proteins such as BDNF (37) and the cholinergic system (38) differ in young and old rats. Based on the above theory, more recent clinical randomized trials addressed the potential benefit of estrogen therapy considering timing of replacement. Unfortunately, these studies have yielded little support for this hypothesis (39–42). Together, these data suggest that while estrogen is relevant and important for CNS function and structure during the reproductive periods, aspects beyond estrogen loss contribute to age-related menopausal dysfunction.

INVOLVEMENT OF LUTEINIZING HORMONE (LH) IN CNS FUNCTION AND AD

Accumulating evidence supports a role for LH in regulating cognition and AD-related parameters. LH, a gonadotropin hormone released from the anterior pituitary, functions to stimulate the production of sex steroids, which in turn negatively regulate hypothalamic GnRH release and further production of LH. In the absence of sex steroids providing negative feedback, LH levels drastically increase, as observed following menopause and andropause. Peripheral levels of LH increase three-fold in post-menopausal women (43) and two-fold in aging men (44). Importantly, these increases in peripheral LH levels correlate to cognitive deficits in aging men and women (45, 46) as well as AD patients (47–51). In fact, increased levels of peripheral LH in AD patients is associated with exacerbated pathology and cognitive deficits (50–52). Additionally, increased LH is correlated with increased plasma $A\beta_{1-40}$ and $A\beta_{1-42}$ levels in subjective memory complainers, suggesting LH may play a progressive role in early preclinical stages (51).

In rodents, earlier studies demonstrated that over-expression of LH in transgenic mice (53), or exogenous treatment with human LH (54) without any estrogen manipulations, impaired working memory. These studies are supported by work showing that chronic elevations in peripheral levels through exogenous application of the LH analog, human chorionic gonadotropin (hCG), results in similar attenuation of working memory as well as increases in total brain amyloid-β_{1-40} in a mouse model of AD (55, 56). Moreover, peripheral increase in hCG is capable of reversing estrogen associated benefits in spatial memory (55, 56).

Several studies involving pharmacological downregulation of peripheral LH after ovariectomy also support a role for LH in cognition and plasticity. To this end, work utilizing either GnRH super-agonist (57–60) or competitive antagonists (61–64) of the GnRH receptor reverse cognitive deficits (57–64) and neuronal plasticity loss (59, 60) in the absence of estrogen replacement. For example, several studies from our lab using GnRH super-agonist, leuprolide acetate, improved function in ovariectomized C57BL/6J mice (58, 60) as well as aged-ovariectomized 3xTg AD mice (59). Furthermore, these benefits were associated with activation of signaling cascades associated with long term potentiation (LTP), the cellular basis of learning and memory, Bryan et al. (58) in the absence of AD pathology (59), further supporting a direct role of LH-related mechanisms on cognition. More importantly, a key finding was that pharmacological reductions in peripheral levels of LH lead to cognitive improvements and rescue of dendritic spine density without any dependence on timing of treatment onset (60). This raises the exciting possibility that LH may provide an additional therapeutic target for rescuing cognitive and structural deficiencies associated with menopause, aging, and AD.

While there is no clinical data to support the benefits of peripheral downregulation of LH in menopausal women, clinical data in AD patients support its validity (65). A small, phase II, randomized, clinical trial, in female patients with moderate AD, showed that leuprolide acetate stabilized cognitive function in a subgroup treated with an acetylcholinesterase inhibitor, Aricept. Given Aricept is the primary treatment option for AD patients, these data are encouraging. However, while clinical and pre-clinical studies show promise for LH-related therapeutics, the mechanisms underlying these effects remain unknown to date. In the next sections, we highlight a potential mechanism of action of these therapies in relation to signaling and function of the LH receptor.

LH SIGNALING AND COGNITION

LH as well its receptor LHR are expressed in the CNS (66–69). Importantly, LHR is present in regions associated with learning and memory (68–70). Similarly, LHR is also expressed in the choroid plexus, ependymal cells of the third, fourth and lateral ventricles as well as the area postrema (68), which are areas involved in production and circulation of cerebrospinal fluid CSF as well as blood brain barrier transport, suggesting a potential modulatory role of LHR in BBB permeability.

The LHR is a G-protein-coupled receptor involved in production of sex steroids in the gonads through Gs cAMP/PKA, ERK and Gq PLC pathways. G_s signaling results in phosphorylation of MAPK and CREB, while G_q induces intracellular Ca^{2+} release and activation of several protein kinases such as PKA and CAMKII (71–74). LHR activated cAMP/PKA signaling cascades in the immortalized cultures of hippocampal and hypothalamic neurons *in vitro* (75, 76). Interestingly, these signaling cascades downstream of LHR are associated with gene expression and structural changes that are the hallmark of synaptic plasticity and memory formation in the CNS (77–80) and induction of LTP (81–84). Furthermore, active kinases trigger activation of transcriptional factors such as MAPK and CREB leading to gene expression and structural remodeling of the synapse. This ultimately leads to enhanced synaptic transmission and BDNF production, as well as plasticity of dendritic spines (79, 85–87). However, as previously discussed above, downregulation of peripheral LH in the OVX model lead to CAMKII autophosphorylation at Thr 286 and CAMKII dependent GluR1 Ser 831 phosphorylation (58), inhibition of GSK3β and upregulation of β-catenin in 3X Tg mouse model of AD (59), and improved cognitive function. Based on the known canonical signaling cascades ascribed to the LHR, these data, at least indirectly, suggest activation rather than inhibition of the LHR, thus, in conflict with the prevalent idea that LH signaling in the CNS is detrimental.

The idea that LH signaling in the CNS is detrimental stems from the supposition that LH crosses the blood-brain-barrier (BBB); however, LH is a large glycoprotein that is unlikely to penetrate the BBB without a transporter molecule. Furthermore, both human and animal studies show contradictory evidence on whether hCG or LH can cross the BBB. One study showed some permeability of hCG into CNS when administered at supra-physiological levels (88) while another did not (89). Moreover, studies show hCG is not BBB permeable in human choriocarcinomas models until a high threshold is reached (90, 91), especially in patients with normal levels of plasma LH (92). These data suggest that hCG and LH may not be permeable in normal or OVX conditions, thus, the supposition that the LHR is detrimental is difficult to reconcile.

BRAIN-SPECIFIC LH AS MECHANISM FOR LHR-MEDIATED CNS FUNCTION

Several earlier studies have demonstrated the expression of LH in the brain of various species (59, 66, 67), as well as its ability to modulate synaptic function (93–95), neurogenesis (96), and behavior (59, 88, 97, 98). *In vitro*, administration of the LH analog hCG, which binds and activates the LHR similarly to LH (99, 100), stimulates neurite outgrowth in rat neuronal culture and differentiation in PC12 cells through activation of the erk/MAPK pathway (99, 101). Erk/MAPK is a pathway that is critical for memory function and plasticity (78). Similarly, LHR activation *in vitro* also leads to stem cell differentiation (102), and protection against excitotoxicity in primary neurons (103).

LHR transcripts as well as functional receptors have been found in neurons and glial cells *in vitro* (94, 95). LHR was functional *in vitro* in neurons cultured at embryonic day 19. Similarly, hCG treatment of mixed glial cultures, from either P0 or P1 neonates, for 3 days lead to a dose-dependent increase in anti-inflammatory prostaglandin (PG), PGD2 and decrease in proinflammatory PGE2. These actions of LHR may be important for neonatal brain development and function as PGE2 inhibits the proliferation of glial cells, while PGD2 may do the exact opposite. Therefore, LHR signaling may be promoting controlled proliferation of glial cells during brain development (94).

While the above cited works cannot conclusively identify the source of LH in the brain, these studies demonstrate the presence of LH in cognition associated areas and its ability to mediate signaling and behavior. Furthermore, the highlighted *in vitro* work validates CNS LHR functionality and signaling consistent with cognition and neuroplasticity, both through neurons and glial cells. This said, how the LHR is involved in menopause and ovariectomy-induced cognitive and neuroplasticity loss remains unclear but may be explained through alterations in brain and peripheral levels of LH, as highlighted in the section below.

INVERSE RELATIONSHIP BETWEEN PERIPHERY AND THE BRAIN

Accumulating research shows that LH levels in the brain may have an inverse relationship to the periphery. For example, in studies of cycling adult female rats, hypothalamic LH decreased during proestrus, when a drastic 10-fold increase in LH occurs in the pituitary and periphery (104). Similarly, LH treatment into the median eminence (ME) of the hypothalamus in intact or castrated males and females significantly decreased both LH levels in the pituitary as well as the periphery (105). In a similar experiment, hCG treatment into the median eminence of hypothalamus in ovariectomized as well as intact mature female rats decreased peripheral LH (106).

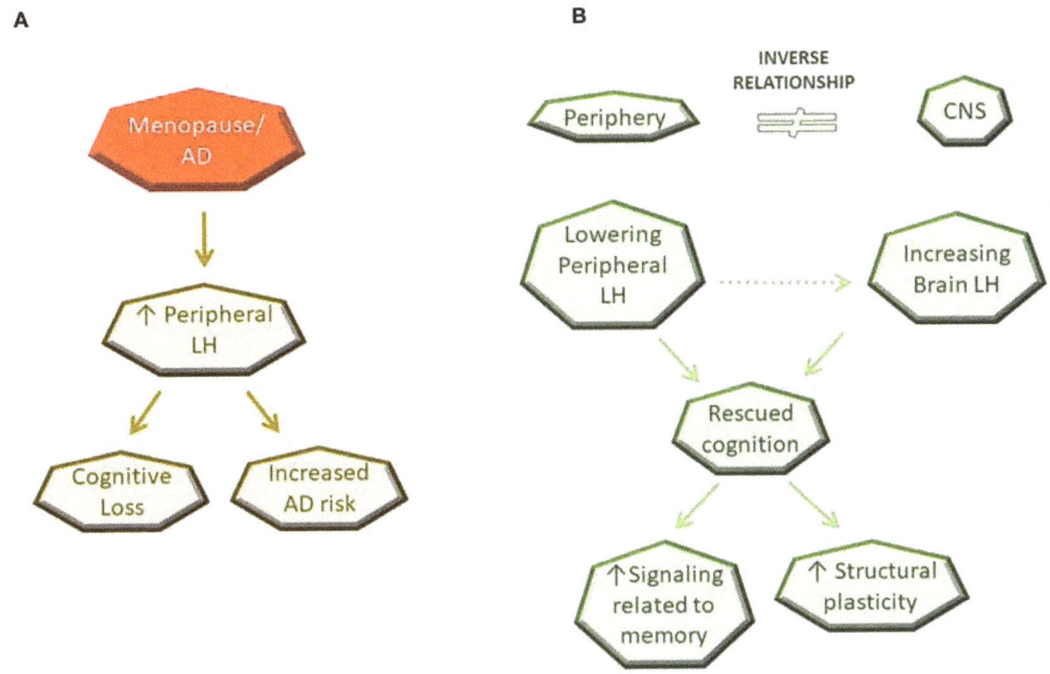

FIGURE 1 | Schematic diagram of current working model for LH action in the CNS. **(A)** Observation in the literature. **(B)** Potential mechanisms of LH action.

Additionally, LH mRNA levels are reduced in both the hippocampus and the cortex of human female AD brains (59), although they are increased in the periphery (47, 48). Interestingly, LH immunoreactivity is remarkably reversed when peripheral LH levels are downregulated and lead to improved cognition (59). These experiments, therefore, provide ample support to the idea of inverse relationship between peripheral LH and central LH, and further suggest that the LH and hCG in the periphery are capable of self-regulating their levels through short-loop feedback into the brain (105, 107, 108).

Interestingly, ovariectomized rats have no changes in hypothalamic LH, although the pituitary and serum LH levels are elevated eight-fold (104). Furthermore, the self-regulated decrease in peripheral LH in response to IV treatment of hCG and hLH seen in rabbits 2 weeks following castrations was absent 6 weeks following castrations, suggesting the sensitivity of the short-loop changes with time after castration (107). This begs the question of whether self-regulation of hypothalamic LH production is more pertinent than gonadal loss, and importantly, whether loss of this "short" feedback in menopause underlies the "critical period" sensitivity observed for estrogen. The fact that the LHR is rapidly internalized in the presence of its ligands (109–113) may provide a potential explanation for the loss of short-feedback loop, as impairments in LHR signaling due to ligand-induced internalization may reduce the ability to signal back to the hypothalamus. This may also explain the work postulating that activation of LHR is deleterious to cognition (52, 62, 88, 114) as the above studies used supraphysiological doses of exogenous hCG. In one of the studies above, deglycosylated hCG used as the LHR antagonist improved cognition; however, validation of the levels of LHR or verification of full deglycosylation of hCG was not performed (114). Therefore, further studies need to be carried out with careful consideration of LH dose and LHR internalization to clarify the role of LHR in the CNS.

An additional aspect that has confounded our ability to clearly dissect the function of the LHR in the CNS from that of loss of gonadal steroids is the fact that LHR has not been modulated in a brain-specific manner. For example, one article demonstrated that knocking out LHR in an AD mouse model attenuated the pathology and cognitive deficits (115). However, the LHR knockout model was global, not brain-specific, thus early developmental effects due to deficits in sex steroids, which are known in these animals, cannot be separated from the role of LHR loss.

CONCLUSIONS

Among a multitude of changes that occur with aging, menopause is a clear driver for development of AD in women. The role of steroid hormones in CNS function and structure, particularly during reproductive stages, is undisputed and here we provide evidence that LH and its receptor are important in CNS function as well as dysfunction as depicted in the working model of LH action in **Figure 1**. We also highlight a potential mechanism, specifically the inverse relationship of LH levels in the CNS vs. the periphery, to provide an explanation for the paradox observed between the ability of the LHR to activate cascades associated with learning, memory and neuroplasticity, and the findings demonstrating benefits of peripheral LH downregulation on these aspects. Further investigation is necessary to understand how the inverse relationship of LH between the periphery and the CNS is maintained as well as to identify the molecular mechanisms underlying LH-related memory and plasticity benefits in a CNS-specific manner. Genetic approaches targeting the LHR specifically within the brain are likely to be useful models to conclusively address the role of the LHR in CNS function and structure.

AUTHOR CONTRIBUTIONS

All authors listed have made a substantial, direct, and intellectual contribution to the work and approved it for publication.

FUNDING

Our works cited in this manuscript have been funded by the NIH grant, RF1 AG054654-01.

REFERENCES

1. Alzheimer's Association. 2018 Alzheimer's disease facts and figures. *Alzheimers Dement.* (2018) 14:367–429. doi: 10.1016/j.jalz.2018.02.001
2. Castellani RJ, Rolston RK, Smith M. Alzheimer disease. *Dis Mon.* (2011) 56:1–60. doi: 10.1016/j.disamonth.2010.06.001.Alzheimer
3. Maki PM, Henderson VW. Hormone therapy, dementia, and cognition: the Women's Health Initiative 10 years on. *Climacteric* (2012) 15:256–62. doi: 10.3109/13697137.2012.660613
4. McEwen BS, Alves SE, Bulloch K, Weiland NG. Clinically relevant basic science studies of gender differences and sex hormone effects. *Psychopharmacol Bull.* (1998) 34:251–9.
5. McEwen BS, Alves SE. Estrogen actions in the central nervous system. *Endocr Rev.* (1999) 20:279–307. doi: 10.1210/edrv.20.3.0365
6. Hojo Y, Hattori T-A, Enami T, Furukawa A, Suzuki K, Ishii H-T, et al. Adult male rat hippocampus synthesizes estradiol from pregnenolone by cytochromes P45017alpha and P450 aromatase localized in neurons. *Proc Natl Acad Sci USA.* (2004) 101:865–70. doi: 10.1073/pnas.2630225100
7. Gibbs RB. Estrogen therapy and cognition: a review of the cholinergic hypothesis. *Endocr Rev.* (2010) 31:224–53. doi: 10.1210/er.2009-0036
8. Bowen RL, Atwood CS. Living and dying for sex: a theory of aging based on the modulation of cell cycle signaling by reproductive hormones. *Gerontology* (2004) 50:265–90. doi: 10.1159/000079125
9. Launer LJ, Andersen K, Dewey ME, Letenneur L, Ott A, Amaducci LA, et al. Rates and risk factors for dementia and Alzheimer's disease. *Neurology* (1999) 52:78 LP–78.
10. Andersen K, Launer LJ, Dewey ME, Letenneur L, Ott A, Copeland JRM, et al. Gender differences in the incidence of AD and vascular dementia. *Neurology* (1999) 53:1992LP–1992.
11. Zandi PP, Carlson MC, Plassman BL, Welsh-Bohmer KA, Mayer LS, Steffens DC, et al. Hormone replacement therapy and incidence of Alzheimer disease in older women: the Cache County Study. *J Am Med Assoc.* (2002) 288:2123–9. doi: 10.1097/01.OGX.0000055761.75837.23
12. Kawas C, Resnick S, Morrison A, Brookmeyer R, Corrada M, Zonderman A, et al. A prospective study of estrogen replacement therapy and the risk of developing Alzheimer's disease: the Baltimore Longitudinal Study of Aging. *Neurology* (1997) 48:1517–21.
13. Hogervorst E, Williams J, Budge M, Riedel W, Jolles J. The nature of the effect of female gonadal hormone replacement therapy on cognitive function in post-menopausal women: a meta-analysis. *Neuroscience* (2000) 101:485–512. doi: 10.1016/S0306-4522(00)00410-3
14. Tang MX, Jacobs D, Stern Y, Marder K, Schofield P, Gurland B, et al. Effect of oestrogen during menopause on risk and age at onset of Alzheimer's disease. *Lancet* (1996) 348:429–32.
15. Hogervorst E, Yaffe K, Richards M, Huppert F. Hormone replacement therapy to maintain cognitive function in women with dementia. *Cochrane Database Syst. Rev.* (2009) 1:CD003799. doi: 10.1002/14651858.CD003799.pub2
16. Rocca WA, Grossardt BR, Shuster LT. Oophorectomy, estrogen, and dementia: a 2014 update. *Mol Cell Endocrinol.* (2014) 389:7–12. doi: 10.1016/j.mce.2014.01.020.Oophorectomy
17. Henderson VW, Paganini-Hill A, Emanuel CK, Dunn ME, Buckwalter JG. Estrogen replacement therapy in older women. Comparisons between Alzheimer's disease cases and nondemented control subjects. *Arch Neurol.* (1994) 51:896–900.
18. Kampen DL, Sherwin BB. Estrogen use and verbal memory in healthy postmenopausal women. *Obstet Gynecol.* (1994) 83:979–83.
19. Yaffe K, Sawaya G, Lieberburg I, Grady D. Estrogen therapy in postmenopausal women: effects on cognitive function and dementia. *J Am Med Assoc.* (1998) 279:688–95.
20. Yaffe K, Haan M, Byers A, Tangen C, Kuller L. Estrogen use, APOE, and cognitive decline: evidence of gene-environment interaction. *Neurology* (2000) 54:1949 LP–1954. doi: 10.1212/WNL.54.10.1949
21. Sherwin BB. Estrogen and/or androgen replacement therapy and cognitive functioning in surgically menopausal women. *Psychoneuroendocrinology* (1988) 13:345–57. doi: 10.1016/0306-4530(88)90060-1
22. Sherwin BB. Can estrogen keep you smart? Evidence from clinical studies. *J Psychiatry Neurosci.* (1999) 24:315–21.
23. Phillips SM, Sherwin BB. Effects of estrogen on memory function in surgically menopausal women. *Psychoneuroendocrinology* (1992) 17:485–95.
24. Shumaker SA, Legault C, Rapp SR, Thal L, Wallace RB, Ockene JK, et al. Estrogen plus progestin and the incidence of dementia and mild cognitive impairment in postmenopausal women: the women's health initiative memory study: a randomized controlled trial. *JAMA* (2003) 289:2651–62. doi: 10.1001/jama.289.20.2651
25. Shumaker SA, Legault C, Rapp SR, Thal L, Lane DS, Fillit H, et al. Conjugated equine estrogens and incidence of probable dementia and mild cognitive impairment in postmenopausal women Women' s Health Initiative Memory Study. *JAMA* (2004) 291:2947–58. doi: 10.1001/jama.291.24.2947
26. Espeland MA, Rapp SR, Shumaker SA, Brunner R, Manson JE, Sherwin BB, et al. Conjugated equine estrogens and global cognitive function in postmenopausal women Women' s Health Initiative Memory Study. *JAMA* (2004) 291:2959–68. doi: 10.1001/jama.291.24.2959
27. Resnick SM, Henderson VW. Hormone therapy and risk of Alzheimer disease: a critical time. *J Am Med Assoc.* (2002) 288:2170–2. doi: 10.1001/jama.288.17.2170
28. Henderson VW. Hormone therapy and Alzheimer's disease: benefit or harm? *Expert Opin Pharmacother.* (2004) 5:389–406. doi: 10.1517/14656566.5.2.389
29. Sherwin BB. Estrogen and cognitive functioning in women: lessons we have learned. *Behav Neurosci.* (2012) 126:123–7. doi: 10.1037/a0025539
30. Shao H, Breitner JCS, Whitmer RA, Wang J, Hayden K, Wengreen H, et al. Hormone therapy and Alzheimer disease dementia: new findings from the cache county study. *Neurology* (2012) 79:1846–52. doi: 10.1212/WNL.0b013e318271f823
31. Singh M, Simpkins JW, Bimonte-Nelson HA, Brinton RD. Window of opportunity for estrogen and progestin intervention in brain aging and Alzheimer's disease. *Brain Res.* (2013) 1514:1–2. doi: 10.1016/j.brainres.2013.04.044
32. Gibbs R. Long-term treatment with estrogen and progesterone enhances acqui- sition of a spatialmemory task by ovariectomized aged rats. *Neurobiol Aging* (2000) 21:107–16. doi: 10.1016/S0197-4580(00)00103-2
33. Lacreuse A, Wilson ME, Herndon JG. Estradiol, but not raloxifene, improves aspects of spatial working memory in aged ovariectomized rhesus monkeys. *Neurobiol Aging* (2002) 23:589–600. doi: 10.1016/S0197-4580(02)00002-7

34. Gibbs RB, Gabor R. Estrogen and cognition: applying preclinical findings to clinical perspectives. *J Neurosci Res.* (2003) 74:637–43. doi: 10.1002/jnr.10811
35. Zhao L, Chen S, Ming Wang J, Brinton RD. 17beta-estradiol induces Ca2+ influx, dendritic and nuclear Ca2+ rise and subsequent cyclic AMP response element-binding protein activation in hippocampal neurons: a potential initiation mechanism for estrogen neurotrophism. *Neuroscience* (2005) 132, 299–311. doi: 10.1016/j.neuroscience.2004.11.054
36. Brinton RD. The healthy cell bias of estrogen action: mitochondrial bioenergetics and neurological implications. *Trends Neurosci.* (2008) 31:529–37. doi: 10.1016/j.tins.2008.07.003
37. Jezierski MK, Sohrabji F. Neurotrophin expression in the reproductively senescent forebrain is refractory to estrogen stimulation. *Neurobiol Aging* (2001) 22:311–21. doi: 10.1016/S0197-4580(00)00230-X
38. Markowska AL, Savonenko AV. Effectiveness of estrogen replacement in restoration of cognitive function after long-term estrogen withdrawal in aging rats. *J. Neurosci.* (2002) 22:10985–95. doi: 10.1523/JNEUROSCI.22-24-10985.2002
39. Espeland MA, Shumaker SA, Leng I, Manson JE, Brown CM, LeBlanc ES, et al. Long-term effects on cognitive function of postmenopausal hormone therapy prescribed to women aged 50 to 55 years. *JAMA Intern Med.* (2013) 173:1429–36. doi: 10.1001/jamainternmed.2013.7727
40. Gleason CE, Dowling NM, Wharton W, Manson JAE, Miller VM, Atwood CS, et al. Effects of hormone therapy on cognition and mood in recently postmenopausal women: findings from the randomized, controlled KEEPS-cognitive and affective study. *PLoS Med.* (2015) 12:e1833. doi: 10.1371/journal.pmed.1001833
41. Henderson VW, St John JA, Hodis HN, McCleary CA, Stanczyk FZ, Shoupe D, et al. Cognitive effects of estradiol after menopause. *Neurology* (2016) 87:699–708. doi: 10.1212/WNL.0000000000002980
42. Imtiaz B, Tuppurainen M, Rikkonen T, Kivipelto M, Soininen H, Kröger H, et al. Postmenopausal hormone therapy and Alzheimer disease. *Neurology* (2017) 88:1062–8. doi: 10.1212/WNL.0000000000003696
43. Chakravarti S, Collins WP, Forecast JD, Newton TR, Oram DH, Studd JWW. Hormonal profiles after the menopause. *Br Med J.* (1976) 2:784–7. doi: 10.1136/bmj.2.6039.784
44. Neaves WB, Johnson L, Porter JC, Parker CRJ, Petty CS. Leydig cell numbers, daily sperm production, and serum gonadotropin levels in aging men. *J Clin Endocrinol Metab.* (1984) 59:756–63. doi: 10.1210/jcem-59-4-756
45. Hyde Z, Flicker L, Almeida OP, McCaul KA, Jamrozik K, Hankey GJ, et al. Higher luteinizing hormone is associated with poor memory recall: the health in men study. *J Alzheimers Dis.* (2010) 19:943–51. doi: 10.3233/JAD-2010-1342
46. Rodrigues MA, Verdile G, Foster JK, Hogervorst E, Joesbury K, Devine A, et al. Gonadotropins and cognition in older women. *J Alzheimers Dis.* (2008) 13:267–74. doi: 10.3233/JAD-2008-13304
47. Short RA, Bowen RL, O'Brien PC, Graff-Radford NR. Elevated gonadotropin levels in patients with Alzheimer disease. *Mayo Clin Proc.* (2001) 76:906–9. doi: 10.4065/76.9.906
48. Butchart C, Ismailoglu F, Myint PK, Musonda P, Lunt CJ, Pai Y, et al. Identification of possible determinants of inpatient mortality using Classification and Regression Tree (CART) analysis in hospitalized oldest old patients. *Arch Gerontol Geriatr.* (2013) 56:188–91.doi: 10.1016/j.archger.2012.07.005
49. Hogervorst E, Bandelow S, Combrinck M, Smith AD. Low free testosterone is an independent risk factor for Alzheimer's disease. *Exp. Gerontol.* (2004) 39:1633–9. doi: 10.1016/j.exger.2004.06.019
50. Verdile G, Yeap BB, Clarnette RM, Dhaliwal S, Burkhardt MS, Chubb SAP, et al. Luteinizing hormone levels are positively correlated with plasma amyloid-beta protein levels in elderly men. *J Alzheimers Dis.* (2008) 14:201–8. doi: 10.3233/JAD-2008-14208
51. Verdile G, Laws SM, Henley D, Ames D, Bush AI, Ellis KA, et al. Associations between gonadotropins, testosterone and beta amyloid in men at risk of Alzheimer's disease. *Mol Psychiatry* (2014) 19:69–75. doi: 10.1038/mp.2012.147
52. Verdile G, Asih PR, Barron AM, Wahjoepramono EJ, Ittner LM, Martins RN. The impact of luteinizing hormone and testosterone on beta amyloid (Aβ) accumulation: animal and human clinical studies. *Horm Behav.* (2015) 76:81–90. doi: 10.1016/j.yhbeh.2015.05.020
53. Casadesus G, Milliken EL, Webber KM, Bowen RL, Lei Z, Rao CV, et al. Increases in luteinizing hormone are associated with declines in cognitive performance. *Mol Cell Endocrinol.* (2007) 269:107–11. doi: 10.1016/j.mce.2006.06.013
54. Wahjoepramono EJ, Wijaya LK, Taddei K, Bates KA, Howard M, Martins G, et al. Direct exposure of guinea pig CNS to human luteinizing hormone increases cerebrospinal fluid and cerebral beta amyloid levels. *Neuroendocrinology* (2011) 94:313–22. doi: 10.1159/000330812
55. Berry AS, Tomidokoro Y, Ghiso J, Thornton J. Human chorionic gonadotropin (a luteinizing hormone homologue) decreases spatial memory and increases brain amyloid-beta levels in female rats. *Horm Behav.* (2008) 54:143–52. doi: 10.1016/j.yhbeh.2008.02.006
56. Barron AM, Verdile G, Taddei K, Bates KA, Martins RN. Effect of chronic hCG administration on Alzheimer's-related cognition and A beta accumulation in PS1KI mice. *Endocrinology* (2010) 151:5380–8. doi: 10.1210/en.2009-1168
57. Casadesus G, Webber KM, Atwood CS, Pappolla M, Perry G, Bowen RL, et al. Luteinizing hormone modulates cognition and amyloid-beta deposition in Alzheimer APP transgenic mice. *Biochim Biophys Acta* (2006) 1762:447–52. doi: 10.1016/j.bbadis.2006.01.008
58. Bryan KJ, Mudd JC, Richardson SL, Chang J, Lee HG, Zhu X, et al. Down-regulation of serum gonadotropins is as effective as estrogen replacement at improving menopause-associated cognitive deficits. *J Neurochem.* (2010) 112:870–81. doi: 10.1111/j.1471-4159.2009.06502.x
59. Palm R, Chang J, Blair J, Garcia-Mesa Y, Lee H, Castellani RJ, et al. Down-regulation of serum gonadotropins but not estrogen replacement improves cognition in aged-ovariectomized 3xTg AD female mice. *J Neurochem.* (2014) 130:115–25. doi: 10.1111/jnc.12706
60. Blair JA, Palm R, Chang J, McGee H, Zhu X, Wang X, et al. Luteinizing hormone downregulation but not estrogen replacement improves ovariectomy-associated cognition and spine density loss independently of treatment onset timing. *Horm Behav.* (2016) 78:60–6. doi: 10.1016/j.yhbeh.2015.10.013
61. McConnell SE, Alla J, Wheat E, Romeo RD, McEwen B, Thornton JE. The role of testicular hormones and luteinizing hormone in spatial memory in adult male rats. *Horm Behav.* (2012) 61:479–86. doi: 10.1016/j.yhbeh.2012.01.003
62. Ziegler SG, Thornton JE. Low luteinizing hormone enhances spatial memory and has protective effects on memory loss in rats. *Horm Behav.* (2010) 58:705–13. doi: 10.1016/j.yhbeh.2010.07.002
63. Telegdy G, Adamik A, Tanaka M, Schally AV. Effects of the LHRH antagonist Cetrorelix on affective and cognitive functions in rats. *Regul Pept.* (2010) 159:142–7. doi: 10.1016/j.regpep.2009.08.005
64. Telegdy G, Tanaka M, Schally AV. Effects of the LHRH antagonist Cetrorelix on the brain function in mice. *Neuropeptides* (2009) 43:229–34. doi: 10.1016/j.npep.2009.03.001
65. Bowen RL, Perry G, Xiong C, Smith MA, Atwood CS. A clinical study of lupron depot in the treatment of women with AD: preservation of cognitive function in patients taking an acetylcholinesterase inhibitor and treated with high dose lupron over 48 weeks. *J Alzheimer's Dis.* (2015) 34:549–60. doi: 10.3233/JAD-141626
66. Emanuele NV, Anderson J, Andersen E, Connick E, Baker G, Kirsteins L, et al. Extrahypothalamic brain luteinizing hormone: characterization by radioimmunoassay, chromatography, radioligand assay and bioassay. *Neuroendocrinology* (1983) 36, 254–260.
67. Glass JD, McClusky ME. Immunoreactive luteinizing hormone-containing neurons in the brain of the white-footed mouse, Peromyscus leucopus. *Experientia* (1987) 43:188–90.
68. Lei ZM, Rao CV, Kornyei JL, Licht P, Hiatt ES. Novel expression of human chorionic gonadotropin/luteinizing hormone receptor gene in brain. *Endocrinology* (1993) 132:2262–70.
69. Apaja PM, Harju KT, Aatsinki JT, Petäjä-Repo UE, Rajaniemi HJ. Identification and structural characterization of the neuronal luteinizing hormone receptor associated with sensory systems. *J Biol Chem.* (2004) 279:1899–906. doi: 10.1074/jbc.M311395200
70. Hämäläinen T, Poutanen M, Huhtaniemi I. Age- and sex-specific promoter function of a 2-kilobase 5′-flanking sequence of themurine luteinizing

hormone receptor gene in transgenic mice. *Endocrinology* (1999) 140:5322–9.
71. Ascoli M, Fanelli F, Segaloff DL. The lutropin/choriogonadotropin receptor, A 2002 perspective. *Endocr Rev.* (2002) 23:141–74. doi: 10.1210/edrv.23.2.0462
72. Herrlich A, Kühn B, Grosse R, Schmid A, Schultz G, Gudermann T. Involvement of Gs and Gi proteins in dual coupling of the luteinizing hormone receptor to adenylyl cyclase and phospholipase C. *J Biol Chem.* (1996) 271:16764–72.
73. Gudermann T, Nichols C, Levy FO, Birnbaumer M, Birnbaumer L. Ca2+ mobilization by the LH receptor expressed in Xenopus oocytes independent of 3',5'-cyclic adenosine monophosphate formation: evidence for parallel activation of two signaling pathways. *Mol Endocrinol.* (1992) 6:272–8.
74. Gudermann T, Birnbaumer M, Birnbaumer L. Evidence for dual coupling of the murine luteinizing hormone receptor to adenylyl cyclase and phosphoinositide breakdown and Ca2+ mobilization. *J Biol Chem.* (1992) 267:4479–88.
75. Lei ZM, Rao CV. Novel presence of luteinizing hormone/human chorionic gonadotropin (hCG) receptors and the down-regulating action of hCG on gonadotropin- releasing hormone gene expression in immortalized hypothalamic GT1-7 neurons. *Mol Endocrinol.* (1994) 8:1111–21. doi: 10.1210/mend.8.8.7997235
76. Zhang W, Lei ZM, Rao CV. Immortalized hippocampal cells contain functional luteinizing hormone/human chorionic gonadotropin receptors. *Life Sci.* (1999) 65:2083–98. doi: 10.1016/S0024-3205(99)00474-9
77. Atkins CM, Selcher JC, Petraitis JJ, Trzaskos JM, Sweatt JD. The MAPK cascade is required for mammalian associative learning. *Nat Neurosci.* (1998) 1:602–9.
78. English JD, Sweatt JD. A requirement for the mitogen-activated protein kinase cascade in hippocampal long term potentiation. *J Biol Chem.* (1997) 272:19103–6.
79. Matsuzaki M, Honkura N, Ellis-Davies GC, Kasai H. Structural basis of long-term potentiation in single dendritic spines. *Nature* (2004) 429:761–6. doi: 10.1038/nature02617
80. Kasai H, Matsuzaki M, Noguchi J, Yasumatsu N, Nakahara H. Structure-stability-function relationships of dendritic spines. *Trends Neurosci.* (2003) 26:360–8.doi: 10.1016/S0166-2236(03)00162-0
81. Roche KW, O'Brien RJ, Mammen AL, Bernhardt J, Huganir RL. Characterization of multiple phosphorylation sites on the AMPA receptor GluR1 subunit. *Neuron* (1996) 16:1179–88.
82. Barria A, Muller D, Derkach V, Griffith LC, Soderling TR. Regulatory phosphorylation of AMPA-type glutamate receptors by CaMKII during long-term potentiation. *Science* (1997) 276:2042–5.
83. Mammen AL, Kameyama K, Roche KW, Huganir RL. Phosphorylation of the alpha-amino-3-hydroxy-5-methylisoxazole-4-propionic acid receptor GluR1 subunit by calcium/calmodulin-dependent kinase II. *J Biol Chem.* (1997) 272:32528–33.
84. Lee HK, Barbarosie M, Kameyama K, Bear MF, Huganir RL. Regulation of distinct AMPA receptor phosphorylation sites during bidirectional synaptic plasticity. *Nature* (2000) 405:955–9. doi: 10.1038/350 16089
85. Nusser Z, Lujan R, Laube G, Roberts JD, Molnar E, Somogyi P. Cell type and pathway dependence of synaptic AMPA receptor number and variability in the hippocampus. *Neuron* (1998) 21:545–59.
86. Matsuzaki M, Ellis-Davies GC, Nemoto T, Miyashita Y, Iino M, Kasai H. Dendritic spine geometry is critical for AMPA receptor expression in hippocampal CA1 pyramidal neurons. *Nat Neurosci.* (2001) 4:1086–92. doi: 10.1038/nn736
87. Jezierski MK, Sohrabji F. Estrogen enhances retrograde transport of brain-derived neurotrophic factor in the rodent forebrain. *Endocrinology* (2003) 144:5022–9. doi: 10.1210/en.2003-0724
88. Lukacs H, Hiatt ES, Lei ZM, Rao CV. Peripheral and intracerebroventricular administration of human chorionic gonadotropin alters several hippocampus-associated behaviors in cycling female rats. *Horm Behav.* (1995) 29:42–58.
89. Ondo JG, Mical RS, Porter JC. Passage of Radioactive Substances from CSF to Hypophysial Portal Blood1. *Endocrinology* (1972) 91:1239–46.
90. McCormick JB. Gonadotrophin in urine and spinal fluid; quantitative studies for chorionic moles and choriocarcinomas. *Obstet Gynecol.* (1954) 3:58–66.
91. Tashima CK, Timberger R, Burdick R, Leavy M, Rawson RW. Cerebrospinal fluid titer of chorionic gonadotropin in patients with intracranial metastatic choriocarcinoma. *J Clin Endocrinol Metab.* (1965) 25:1493–5. doi: 10.1210/jcem-25-11-1493
92. Bagshawe KD, Orr AHH, Rushworth AGJ. Relationship between concentrations of human chorionic gonadotropin in plasma and cerebrospinal fluid. *Nature* (1968) 217:950–1.
93. Gallo RV, Johnson JH, Kalra SP, Whitmoyer DI, Sawyer CH. Effects of luteinizing hormone on multiple-unit activity in the rat hippocampus. *Neuroendocrinology* (1972) 9:149–57. doi: 10.1159/000122046
94. AL-Hader AA, Lei ZM, Rao CV. Novel expression of functional luteinizing hormone/chorionic gonadotropin receptors in cultured glial cells from neonatal rat brains. *Biol Reprod.* (1997) 56:501–7. doi: 10.1095/biolreprod56.2.501
95. AL-Hader AA, Lei ZM, Rao CV. Neurons from fetal rat brains contain functional luteinizing hormone/chorionic gonadotropin receptors. *Biol Reprod.* (1997) 56:1071–6. doi: 10.1095/biolreprod,56.5.1071
96. Mak GK, Enwere EK, Gregg C, Pakarainen T, Poutanen M, Huhtaniemi I, et al. Male pheromone-stimulated neurogenesis in the adult female brain: possible role in mating behavior. *Nat Neurosci.* (2007) 10:1003–11. doi: 10.1038/nn1928
97. Zhao C, Deng W, Gage FH. Mechanisms and Functional Implications of Adult Neurogenesis. *Cell* (2008) 132:645–60. doi: 10.1016/j.cell.2008.01.033
98. Yang E-J, Nasipak BT, Kelley DB. Direct action of gonadotropin in brain integrates behavioral and reproductive functions. *Proc Natl Acad Sci USA.* (2007) 104:2477–82. doi: 10.1073/pnas.0608391104
99. Menon KMJ, Menon B. Structure, function and regulation of gonadotropin receptors - A perspective. *Mol Cell Endocrinol.* (2012) 356:88–97. doi: 10.1016/j.mce.2012.01.021
100. McFarland KC, Sprengel R, Phillips HS, Kohler M, Rosemblit N, Nikolics K, et al. Lutropin-choriogonadotropin receptor: an unusual member of the G protein-coupled receptor family. *Science* (1989) 245:494–9. doi: 10.1126/science.2502842
101. Meng XL, Rennert OM, Chan WY. Human chorionic gonadotropin induces neuronal differentiation of PC12 cells through activation of stably expressed lutropin/choriogonadotropin receptor. *Endocrinology* (2007) 148:5865–73. doi: 10.1210/en.2007-0941
102. Gallego MJ, Porayette P, Kaltcheva MM, Bowen RL, Vadakkadath Meethal S, Atwood CS. The pregnancy hormones human chorionic gonadotropin and progesterone induce human embryonic stem cell proliferation and differentiation into neuroectodermal rosettes. *Stem Cell Res Ther.* (2010) 1:28. doi: 10.1186/scrt28
103. Movsas TZ, Weiner RL, Greenberg MB, Holtzman DM, Galindo R. Pretreatment with human chorionic gonadotropin protects the neonatal brain against the effects of hypoxic-ischemic injury. *Front Pediatr.* (2017) 5:232. doi: 10.3389/fped.2017.00232
104. Emanuele N, Oslapas R, Connick E, Kirsteins L, Lawrence AM. Hypothalamic LH may play a role in control of pituitary LH release. *Neuroendocrinology* (1981) 33:12–7. doi: 10.1111/j.1752-1688.2007.00005.x
105. David MA, Fraschini F, Martini L. Control of LH secretion: role of a "Short" feedback mechanism1. *Endocrinology* (1966) 78:55–60. doi: 10.1210/endo-78-1-55
106. Hirono M, Igarashi M, Matsumoto S. The direct effect of HCG upon pituitary gonadotrophin secretion. *Endocrinology* (1972) 90:1214–9. doi: 10.1210/endo-90-5-1214
107. Molitch M, Edmonds M, Jones EE, Odell WD. Short-loop feedback control of luteinizing hormone in the rabbit. *Am J Physiol.* (1976) 230:907–10.
108. Patritti-laborde N, Wolfsen ADAR, Heber D, Odell WD. Luteinizing hormone in the rabbit. *J Clin Invest.* (1979) 64:1066–9.
109. Hu Z. Hormonal regulation of LH receptor mRNA and expression in the rat ovary. *FEBS Lett.* (1990) 274:181–4. doi: 10.1016/0014-5793(90)81359-V
110. Segaloff DL, Sprengel R, Nikolics K, Ascoli M. Structure of the lutropin/choriogonadotropin receptor. *Recent Prog Horm Res.* (1990) 46:261–3.
111. Peegel H, Randolph JJ, Midgley AR, Menon KM. *In situ* hybridization of luteinizing hormone/human chorionic gonadotropin receptor messenger

ribonucleic acid during hormone-induced down-regulation and the subsequent recovery in rat corpus luteum. *Endocrinology* (1994) 135:1044–51. doi: 10.1210/endo.135.3.8070346

112. Min KS, Liu X, Fabritz J, Jaquette J, Abell AN, Ascoli M. Mutations that induce constitutive activation and mutations that impair signal transduction modulate the basal and/or agonist-stimulated internalization of the lutropin/choriogonadotropin receptor. *J Biol Chem.* (1998) 273:34911–9. doi: 10.1074/jbc.273.52.34911
113. Kishi M, Liu X, Hirakawa T, Reczek D, Bretscher A, Ascoli M. Identification of two distinct structural motifs that, when added to the C-terminal tail of the rat LH receptor, redirect the internalized hormone-receptor complex from a degradation to a recycling pathway. *Mol Endocrinol.* (2001) 15:1624–35. doi: 10.1210/me.15.9.1624
114. Burnham V, Sundby C, Laman-Maharg A, Thornton J. Luteinizing hormone acts at the hippocampus to dampen spatial memory. *Horm Behav.* (2017) 89:55–63. doi: 10.1016/j.yhbeh.2016.11.007
115. Lin J, Li X, Yuan F, Lin L, Cook CL, Rao CV, et al. Genetic ablation of luteinizing hormone receptor improves the amyloid pathology in a mouse model of alzheimer disease. *J Neuropathol Exp Neurol.* (2010) 69:253–61. doi: 10.1097/NEN.0b013e3181d072cf

13

Estrogen Protects Neurotransmission Transcriptome During Status Epilepticus

Dumitru A. Iacobas [1,2*], ***Sanda Iacobas*** [1,3], ***Nino Nebieridze*** [4†], ***Libor Velíšek*** [4,5,6] ***and Jana Velíšková*** [4,6,7]

[1] Center for Computational Systems Biology, Prairie View A&M University, Prairie View, TX, United States, [2] DP Purpura Department of Neuroscience, Albert Einstein College of Medicine, New York, NY, United States, [3] Department of Pathology, New York Medical College, Valhalla, NY, United States, [4] Department of Cell Biology & Anatomy, New York Medical College, Valhalla, NY, United States, [5] Department of Pediatrics, New York Medical College, Valhalla, NY, United States, [6] Department of Neurology, New York Medical College, Valhalla, NY, United States, [7] Department of Obstetrics & Gynecology, New York Medical College, Valhalla, NY, United States

****Correspondence:***
Dumitru A. Iacobas
daiacobas@pvamu.edu

Women with epilepsy commonly have premature onset of menopause. The decrease in estrogen levels is associated with increased occurrence of neurodegenerative processes and cognitive decline. Previously, we found that estradiol (E2) replacement in ovariectomized (OVX) female rats significantly reduced the seizure-related damage in the sensitive hilar region of hippocampal dentate gyrus (DG). However, the complex mechanisms by which E2 empowers the genomic fabrics of neurotransmission to resist damaging effects of status epilepticus (SE) are still unclear. We determined the protective effects of the estradiol replacement against kainic acid-induced SE-associated transcriptomic alterations in the DG of OVX rats. Without E2 replacement, SE altered expression of 44% of the DG genes. SE affected all major functional pathways, including apoptosis (61%), Alzheimer's disease (47%), cell cycle (59%), long-term potentiation (62%), and depression (55%), as well as synaptic vesicle cycle (62%), glutamatergic (53%), GABAergic (49%), cholinergic (52%), dopaminergic (55%), and serotonergic (49%) neurotransmission. However, in rats with E2 replacement the percentage of significantly affected genes after SE was reduced to the average 11% (from 8% for apoptosis to 32% for GABAergic synapse). Interestingly, while SE down-regulated most of the synaptic receptor genes in oil-injected females it had little effect on these receptors after E2-replacement. Our novel Pathway Protection analysis indicated that the E2-replacement prevented SE-related damage from 50% for GABA to 75% for dopaminergic transmission. The 15% synergistic expression between genes involved in estrogen signaling (ESG) and neurotransmission explains why low E2 levels result in down-regulation of neurotransmission. Interestingly, in animals with E2-replacement, SE switched 131 synergistically expressed ESG-neurotransmission gene pairs into antagonistically expressed gene pairs. Thus, the ESG pathway acts like a buffer against SE-induced alteration of neurotransmission that may contribute to the E2-mediated maintenance of brain function after the SE injury in postmenopausal women. We also show that the long-term potentiation is lost in OVX rats following SE but not in those with E2 replacement. The electrophysiological findings in OVX female rats with SE are corroborated by the high percentage of long-term potentiation regulated genes (62%) in oil-injected while only 13% of genes were regulated following SE in E2-replaced rats.

Keywords: beta-estradiol, cholinergic synapse, dentate gyrus, dopaminergic synapse, GABAergic synapse, glutamatergic synapse, jun oncogene, serotonergic synapse

INTRODUCTION

Special considerations are necessary for women with epilepsy. Irregularities in ovarian function (reflected in menstrual cycles), may affect the likelihood of seizures (Harden et al., 1999; Herzog et al., 2004; Velíšková and DeSantis, 2013). Especially women with seizures originating in temporal lobe (temporal lobe epilepsy, TLE) often have premature ovarian failure/early menopause (late thirties-early forties), which may affect seizure rate (Klein et al., 2001; Isojarvi, 2003; Pennell, 2009) and further contribute to cognitive decline, dementia, and vulnerability to neuronal dysfunction (Shuster et al., 2010; Rocca et al., 2011). The female sex hormones (especially β-estradiol, E2) have neuroprotective effects including attenuation of seizure-induced hippocampal damage and cognitive decline. The E2 effects involve complex transcriptomic mechanisms that are still poorly understood. Therefore, estrogen effects on seizures and their consequences need to be further investigated to determine beneficial effects of hormone therapy in women with epilepsy.

In this report, we analyze alterations in neurotransmission transcriptome of the hippocampal dentate gyrus (DG) induced by status epilepticus (SE) in ovariectomized (OVX) female rats and compare to changes in OVX rats with E2 replacement. In addition to the standard analyses based on our genomic fabric paradigm approach (Iacobas et al., 2012, 2017; Iacobas, 2016), we used also novel quantifiers termed Weighted Pathway Regulation (WPR) and Pathway Protection (PPR). The new quantifiers are not affected by the arbitrarily introduced cut-offs for the absolute fold-change and *p*-value to consider a gene as significantly regulated. We focused on the interplay between the estrogen signaling (ES) pathway and five types of neurotransmission: glutamatergic (GLU), GABAergic (GABA), dopaminergic (DA), cholinergic (ACH), and serotonergic (5HT). Since estrogen acts through estrogen receptors, which are ligand-induced transcription factors, we wanted to determine the extent of its effects on gene transcription under condition of SE-induced hippocampal damage.

Abbreviations: 5HT, Serotonergic synapse pathway; ACH, cholinergic synapse pathway; ALZ, Alzheimer's disease pathway; APO, apoptosis pathway; CC, cell cycle pathway; CG, common genes; CUT, absolute fold-change cut-off to consider a gene as regulated; DA, dopaminergic synapse pathway; DG, dentate gyrus; E2, β-estradiol; ESG, estrogen signaling pathway; FC, fold-change; GABA, GABAergic synapse pathway; GLU, glutamatergic synapse pathway; KA, kainic acid; LTD, long-term depression pathway; LTP, long-term potentiation pathway; OVX, ovariectomized; PPR, Pathway Protection; SE, status epilepticus; SVC, synaptic vesicle cycle pathway; TBS, theta burst stimulation; TLE, temporal lobe epilepsy; TPR, Transcriptomic Protection; WPR, Weighted Pathway Regulation

In order to understand the magnitude of the SE-related damage and the protection provided by the E2 we have included also data on several other pathways: apoptosis (APO), cell cycle (CC), synaptic vesicle cycle (SVC), long-term potentiation (LTP), long-term depression (LTD), and Alzheimer's disease (ALZ).

Because estrogen signaling ESG and neurotransmission have several genes in common, we considered these common genes as the main vehicles through which ESG regulates the synaptic connection and as such, the brain circuitry. The common genes were identified using the Kyoto Encyclopedia of Genes and Genomes developed by Kanehisa Laboratories (Kanehisa et al., 2017). These genes are: adenylcyclases (*Adcy2, Adcy3, Adcy5, Adcy6, Adcy7, Adcy8, Adcy9*), oncogenes (*Akt1, Ak3, Fos, Hras, Kras, raf1, Src*), transcription factors (*Atf4, Atf6b*), calmodulins (*Calm1, Calm2, Calm3*), membrane receptors (*Gabbr1, Gabbr2, Grm1, Itpr1, Itpr2*), binding proteins (*Creb1, Creb3l1, Gnai1, Gnai2, Gnai3, Gnao1, Gnaq*), ion channels (*Kcnj3, Kcnj5, Kcnj9*), and kinases (*Map2k1, Mapk1, Mapk3, Pik3ca, Pik3cb*).

In addition, we show the complex transcriptomic regulation of the hippocampal DG neurotransmission by E2 replacement that is functionally important to preserve neuronal plasticity following SE. Results bring essential insights into E2-neurotransmission interactions, which are interesting beyond the seizures for understanding sex-specific and hormonal modulated depression/anxiety, stress processing, memory, and cognition.

MATERIALS AND METHODS

Animals

Experiments were carried out according to the Revised Guide for the Care and Use of Laboratory Animals and approved by the New York Medical College Animal Care and Use Committee. We used 8–9 week old female Sprague-Dawley rats (Taconic Farms) kept on a 12-h light/dark cycle (lights on at 07:00 a.m.) with food and water *ad libitum*. Rats were OVX (=castrated) under ketamine/xylazine (70/10 mg/kg intraperitoneally) anesthesia and, 1 week later, injected subcutaneously with either 17β-estradiol benzoate (2 μg/0.1 ml/day; Sigma-Aldrich, St. Louis, MO) or sterile peanut oil (0.1 ml; controls) daily at 10:00 for 4 consecutive days (Velíšková and Velíšek, 2007), a treatment producing E2 levels within a physiological range (Neal-Perry et al., 2005). Measurements of vaginal impedance confirmed the successful OVX as well as E2-replacement.

SE was induced by injection of kainic acid (12.5 mg/kg intraperitoneally) 24 h following the last oil/E2 injection.

Animals were observed for seizure occurrence and only animals with at least2 h of continuous forelimb clonus seizures were included for further experiments. There were no differences in seizure severity or duration between the treatment groups as described previously (Velíšková and Velíšek, 2007). SE was terminated by diazepam (10 mg/kg i.p.) injection. Control animals received saline as well as diazepam injections. Tissue from all groups was collected 24 h after SE. As illustrated in **Figure 1A**, studies were performed on four groups of OVX female rats: CON (castrated, oil-injected, no SE), CEN (castrated, E2-replaced, no SE), COS (castrated, oil-injected, SE), and CES (castrated, E2-replaced, SE). CON and CEN animals were obtained as previously described (Velíšková et al., 2015). All rats were decapitated under light isoflurane anesthesia. Separate groups of identically treated female rats were used for *in vitro* electrophysiology experiments.

Electrophysiology *in Vitro*

After decapitation, the brains were removed. Transverse combined entorhinal cortex-hippocampal slices (400 μm thick) were cut with a vibratome (Leica model DTK-1000) in ice-cold artificial cerebrospinal fluid (aCSF; in mM: NaCl 126, KCl 5, NaH_2PO_4 1.25, $MgCl_2$ 2, $CaCl_2$ 2, $NaHCO_3$ 26, and glucose 10; pH 7.36). Recordings started following 1 h pre-incubation in an interface chamber in a pre-warmed (34–35°C) and oxygenated (5% CO_2/95% O_2) aCSF. Field excitatory postsynaptic potentials (fEPSPs) were recorded with a glass microelectrode (2 M NaCl; 2–5 MΩ) placed in the middle third of the DG molecular layer as described previously (Nebieridze et al., 2012). Medial perforant path axons were stimulated once each 30 s with a bipolar stainless-steel stimulating electrode (FHC Inc.; Bowdoinham, ME). Baseline fEPSPs were recorded using a stimulus intensity that produced ~30% of maximal fEPSP slope.

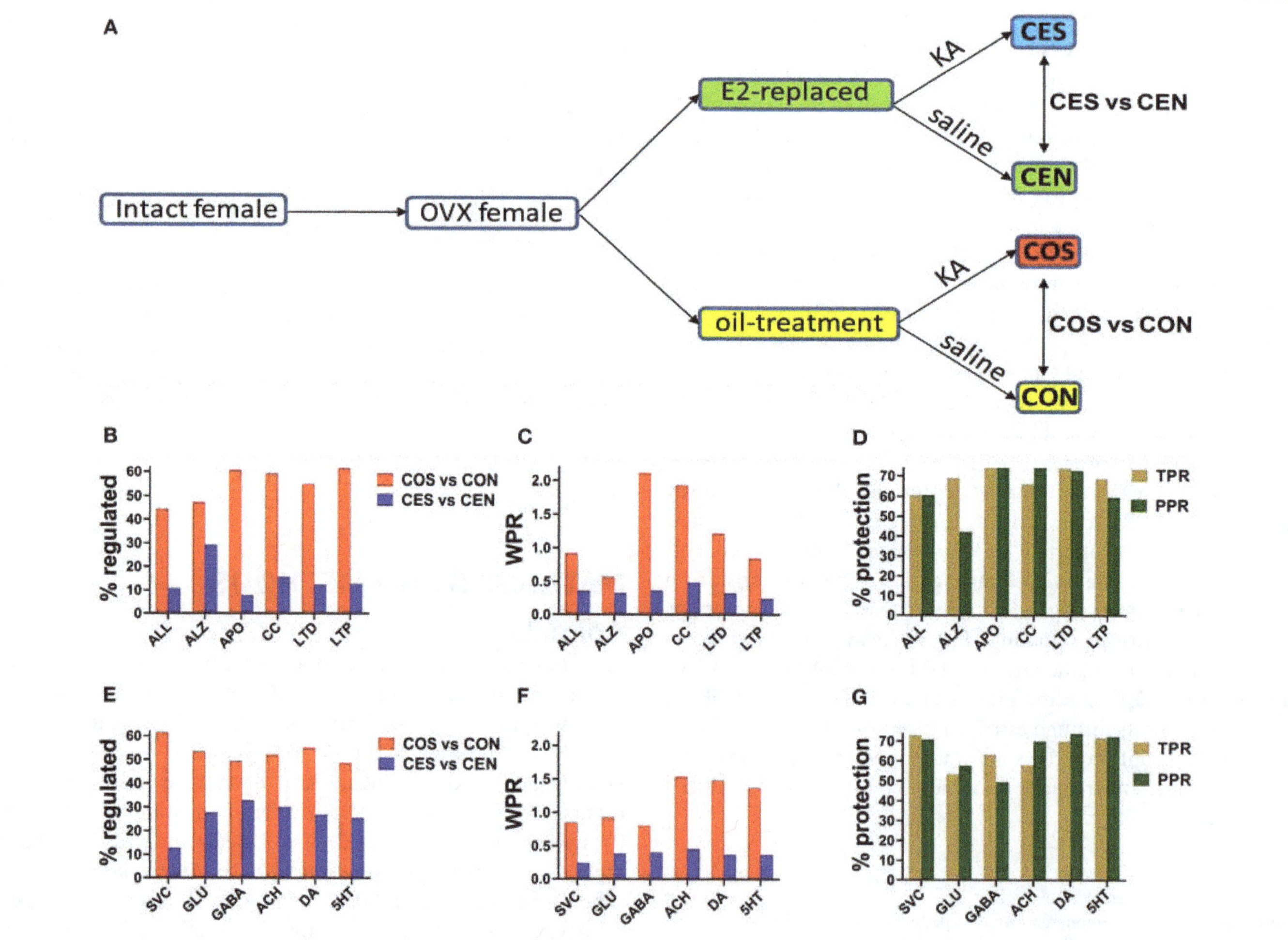

FIGURE 1 | (A) Experimental design. OVX, ovariectomy; KA, kainic acid; saline, KA vehicle. Animals were injected with oil or 2 μg of β-estradiol benzoate for 4 days subcutaneously. **(B,E)** Percentage of the regulated genes within the entire transcriptome (ALL) and included in the analyzed pathways in CES and COS groups with respect to CEN, respectively CON groups. ALZ, Alzheimer's disease, APO, apoptosis, CC, cell cycle, LTD, long-term depression, LTP, long-term potentiation, SVC, synaptic vesicle cycle, GLU, glutamatergic synapse, GABA, GABAergic synapse, ACH, cholinergic synapse, DA, dopaminergic synapse, 5HT, serotonergic synapse. Note the massive effect of SE on the gene expression. **(C,F)** WPR scores for selected pathways. In **(B,C,E,F)** lower is better (less damaging). **(D,G)** Protection against transcriptomic regulation in E2-replaced animals quantified by both TPR (percent reduction of the number of significantly regulated genes) and PPR (percent reduction of WPR). Note that DA had the largest (better) protection as quantified by PPR.

A

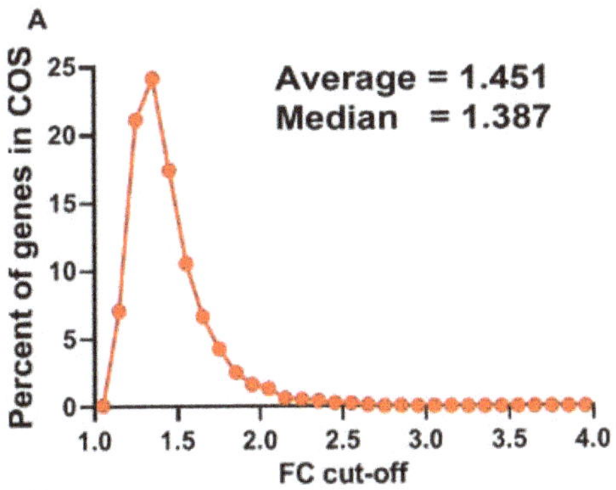

B

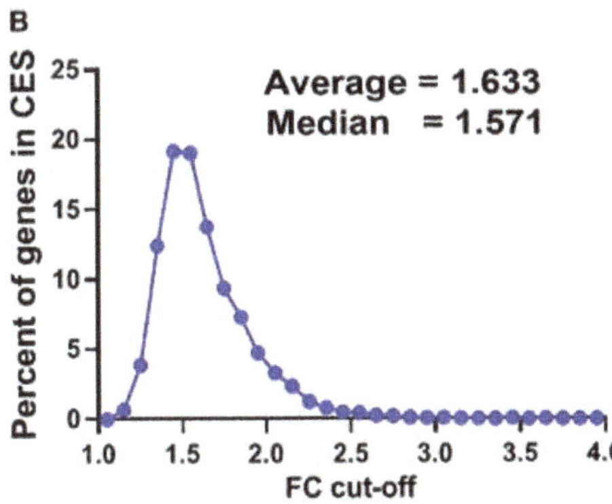

C

GENE	DESCRIPTION	COS	P-VAL	CUT	CES	P-VAL	CUT
Abl1	C-abl oncogene 1, receptor tyrosine kinase	1.417	0.0135	1.298	1.209	0.2329	1.404
Adcy2	Adenylate cyclase 2 (brain)	-1.242	0.0403	1.240	-1.601	0.1721	1.633
Akt1	V-akt murine thymoma viral oncogene homolog 1	-1.258	0.2300	1.390	2.037	0.0282	1.851
Anapc10	Anaphase promoting complex subunit 10	1.399	0.0069	1.217	-1.042	0.7288	1.324
App	Amyloid beta (A4) precursor protein	-1.312	0.1315	1.440	1.471	0.0282	1.405
Atf6	cyclic AMP-dependent transcription factor ATF-6 alpha	1.307	0.0399	1.286	1.430	0.2531	1.869
Atp5c1	ATP synthase, H+ transporting, mitochondrial F1 complex, gamma polypeptide 1	-1.274	0.0706	1.249	1.465	0.0300	1.405
Atp5f1	ATP synthase, H+ transporting, mitochondrial F0 complex, subunit B1	-1.372	0.0103	1.227	-1.153	0.5587	1.618
Atp5g3	ATP synthase lipid-binding protein, mitochondrial	-1.407	0.0235	1.331	-1.244	0.3088	1.575
Atp5h	ATP synthase, H+ transporting, mitochondrial F0 complex, subunit d	1.352	0.0189	1.262	1.337	0.0210	1.267
Atp6v0d1	ATPase, H+ transporting, lysosomal 38kDa, V0 subunit d1	-1.496	0.0147	1.319	-1.106	0.7187	1.763
Atp6v0e1	ATPase, H+ transporting, lysosomal 9kDa, V0 subunit e1	1.487	0.0322	1.423	1.317	0.2341	1.618
Bace2	Beta-site APP-cleaving enzyme 2	1.244	0.0201	1.167	-1.200	0.3373	1.435
Bbc3	Bcl-2 binding component 3	1.308	0.0039	1.169	1.354	0.0929	1.452
Cacna1c	Calcium channel, voltage-dependent, L type, alpha 1C subunit	-1.463	0.0003	1.150	-1.214	0.3446	1.520
Ccnd3	Cyclin D3	1.457	0.0375	1.406	1.691	0.0964	1.851
Ccne1	Cyclin E1	1.289	0.0338	1.228	1.043	0.7747	1.401
Ccnh	Cyclin H	1.236	0.0093	1.183	1.413	0.0719	1.448
Cdc16	Cell division cycle 16 homolog (S. cerevisiae)	1.237	0.0012	1.104	1.180	0.0349	1.154
Cdc25b	Cell division cycle 25 homolog B (S. pombe)	-1.432	0.0224	1.280	-1.092	0.6493	1.503
Cdk5	Cyclin-dependent kinase 5	-1.417	0.0062	1.242	1.665	0.0802	1.769
Cdk7	Cell division protein kinase 7	1.372	0.0075	1.233	-1.261	0.1020	1.295
Chrna7	nicotinic receptor alpha 7 subunit	2.226	0.0473	2.297	1.986	0.0370	1.873
Cox7a2	Cytochrome c oxidase subunit VIIa polypeptide 2	1.381	0.0286	1.332	1.554	0.0017	1.250
Cyp2d4	Cytochrome P450 2D18	-1.439	0.0067	1.264	-1.213	0.4188	1.609
Dab2ip	DAB2 interacting protein	-1.490	0.0181	1.240	-1.073	0.5871	1.345
Gabarap	GABA(A) receptor-associated protein	1.387	0.0078	1.214	-1.047	0.7416	1.358
Grid2	Glutamate receptor, ionotropic, delta 2	1.333	0.0402	1.294	1.400	0.0519	1.411
Grin2a	Glutamate receptor, ionotropic, N-methyl D-aspartate 2A	-3.135	0.0165	1.434	1.466	0.0377	1.421
Hras	Harvey rat sarcoma virus oncogene	-1.371	0.0235	1.201	-1.055	0.7105	1.374
Htr2c	5-hydroxytryptamine (serotonin) receptor 2C	-1.880	0.0441	2.309	1.481	0.0356	1.357
Htr7	5-hydroxytryptamine receptor 7	-1.496	0.0231	1.362	5.885	0.0308	1.627
Ide	Insulin degrading enzyme	1.300	0.0112	1.184	1.246	0.1405	1.370
Igf1	Insulin-like growth factor 1	1.380	0.0286	1.305	1.247	0.1595	1.382
Kcnj4	Potassium inwardly-rectifying channel, subfamily J, member 4	-1.442	0.0446	1.266	-1.268	0.2939	1.559
Lmnb2	Lamin B2	1.438	0.0103	1.261	-1.152	0.5359	1.592
Ncstn	Nicastrin	2.498	0.0003	1.422	1.377	0.0072	1.236
Ndufa12	NADH dehydrogenase (ubiquinone) 1 alpha subcomplex, 12	-1.448	0.0118	1.310	1.091	0.4688	1.320
Ndufa8	NADH dehydrogenase (ubiquinone) 1 alpha subcomplex, 8	-1.353	0.0059	1.174	-1.728	0.1440	1.743
Ndufb3	NADH dehydrogenase (ubiquinone) 1 beta subcomplex 3	-1.482	0.0032	1.246	1.249	0.4350	1.696
Ndufs3	NADH dehydrogenase (ubiquinone) Fe-S protein 3	-1.441	0.0031	1.147	1.171	0.1607	1.282
Ndufs7	NADH dehydrogenase (ubiquinone) Fe-S protein 7	-1.381	0.0009	1.140	-1.093	0.5711	1.410
Ndufs8	NADH dehydrogenase (ubiquinone) Fe-S protein 8	-1.298	0.0070	1.169	1.652	0.0687	1.437
Ndufv2	NADH dehydrogenase (ubiquinone) flavoprotein 2	-1.253	0.0140	1.189	-2.107	0.0485	1.636
Ngf	Beta-nerve growth factor	1.482	0.0434	1.422	1.009	0.9628	1.546
Nsf	N-ethylmaleimide-sensitive factor	-1.795	0.0334	1.393	1.382	0.0383	1.360
Orc3l	Origin recognition complex, subunit 3-like (yeast)	1.811	0.0130	1.400	1.352	0.0391	1.338
Orc4l	Origin recognition complex, subunit 4-like (yeast)	1.439	0.0287	1.367	-3.314	0.0616	2.072
Parp2	Poly (ADP-ribose) polymerase 2	1.349	0.0065	1.212	1.303	0.3259	1.743
Pik3r2	Phosphoinositide-3-kinase, regulatory subunit 2 (beta)	-2.094	0.0112	1.342	1.251	0.0179	1.200
Plcb4	Phospholipase C, beta 4	-1.406	0.0474	1.254	1.129	0.6187	1.665
Plcl1	Phospholipase C-like 1	1.230	0.0332	1.186	-1.052	0.6377	1.289
Prkcb	Protein kinase C, beta	-1.380	0.0051	1.217	1.984	0.0581	1.997
Psenen	Presenilin enhancer 2 homolog (C. elegans)	-1.413	0.0182	1.227	1.179	0.0940	1.197
Raf1	V-raf-leukemia viral oncogene 1	1.363	0.0410	1.344	3.783	0.3266	2.821
Sdhd	Succinate dehydrogenase complex, subunit D, integral membrane protein	1.288	0.0008	1.117	1.003	0.9819	1.341
Shank1	SH3 and multiple ankyrin repeat domains 1	1.365	0.0048	1.208	1.032	0.0208	1.695
Slc1a3	Solute carrier family 1 (glial high affinity glutamate transporter), member 3	-1.270	0.0322	1.251	1.522	0.2295	1.993
Slc6a1	Solute carrier family 6 (neurotransmitter transporter, GABA), member 1	-1.444	0.0050	1.228	-1.583	0.0814	1.425
Stx1b	Syntaxin-1B	-1.464	0.0470	1.349	1.599	0.1610	1.940
Tgfb3	Transforming growth factor, beta 3	1.325	0.0061	1.170	-1.350	0.3318	1.682
Ywhag	Tyrosine 3-monooxygenase/tryptophan 5-monooxygenase activation protein, gamma polypeptide	-1.345	0.4417	1.832	1.251	0.0156	1.194
Ywhaz	Tyrosine 3-monooxygenase/tryptophan 5-monooxygenase activation protein, zeta polypeptide	1.249	0.6008	2.211	1.449	0.0278	1.357

FIGURE 2 | Power of the flexible fold-change cut-off. **(A)** Distribution of the fold-change cut-offs for the COS vs. CON comparison. COS, expression ratio in the comparison COS vs. CON, CES, expression ratio in the comparison CES vs. CEN. When all 12,710 quantified unigenes are considered, CUT values range from 1.055 for *Pcyt1a* to 4.062 for *Scgb1c1*, with the average 1.451. **(B)** Distribution of the fold-change cut-offs for the CES vs. CEN comparison. When all 12,710 quantified unigenes are considered, CUT values range from 1.109 for *Mapk1ip1l* to 3.877 for *Ttr*, with the average 1.633. **(C)** "False negatives" and "false positive" regulation hits from the analyzed functional pathways. Note that expression ratio 2.226 was not enough for *Chrna7* to be considered as up-regulated in COS vs. CON comparison (CUT = 2.297) but 1.986 was enough in CES vs. CEN (CUT = 1.873).

LTP was induced by theta burst stimulation (TBS; 10 bursts delivered at interburst interval 200 ms; each burst consisted of 10 stimuli at 100 Hz). The stimulus intensity has not been changed during the TBS. Picrotoxin (50 μM; Abcam, Cambridge, MA, USA) was bath applied during the experiment to enhance the LTP.

Microarray

Two hours after the onset of continuous seizures, under light isoflurane anesthesia the rats were decapitated, brains were removed and hippocampal DG were isolated. Four animals were used from each of the four groups of OVX female rats (CON, CEN, COS, and CES). Previously described experimental protocol (Kravchick et al., 2016) was used for RNA extraction, purification, fluorescent labeling and reverse transcription, and hybridization with Agilent Rat GE 4 × 44k v3 microarrays in the "multiple yellow" design (Iacobas et al., 2006). In this design, differently labeled biological replicates are co-hybridized with each microarray. A non-control microarray spot is valid if the foreground fluorescence is at least twice its background. We normalize the background-subtracted fluorescence of each valid spot to the median of all same-label valid spots in the array, and compute the average for all spots probing the same transcript (thus eliminating the array redundancy). Same label average values for each transcript are then compared across experimental conditions and results averaged for the two colors. An in-house developed iterative algorithm renormalizes all data sets across the fluorescent labels and experimental conditions until the average change of expression ratios between successive iterations falls below 5%.

Functional Pathways

We used Kyoto Encyclopedia of Genes and Genomes (KEGG) maps developed by Kanehisa Laboratories (Kanehisa et al., 2017) to select the genes responsible for estrogen signaling pathway (map04915) and for cholinergic (map04725), glutamatergic (map04724), GABAergic (map04727), dopaminergic (map04728), and serotonergic (map04726) transmissions. KEGG maps were also used for apoptosis (map04210), cell cycle (map04110), synaptic vesicle cycle (map04721), long-term potentiation (map04720), long-term depression (map04730), and Alzheimer's disease (map05010) pathways. Although KEGG designed map04730 for the cerebellar long-term depression the basic molecular mechanisms are likely to occur also in the DG.

Data Analysis

According to our laboratory standard (Lee et al., 2017), a gene was considered as regulated (here by SE in oil-injected/E2-replaced females with respect to the corresponding non-SE animals) if the absolute fold-change (FC) exceeded the combined contributions of the technical noise and biological variability (CUT, cut-off). The regulation was considered significant if the *p*-value of the heteroscedastic *t*-test of the equality of the average expression levels in the compared conditions with the Bonferroni-type correction for redundant spots probing the same gene (Iacobas et al., 2005) was below 0.05. This FC cut-off

TABLE 1 | Genes turned on/off by E2 replacement alone (in non-SE rats) and genes turned on by SE (in COS animals) but prevented by E2 replacement (CES rats).

Gene	Symbol
Genes turned on by estradiol replacement alone	
Chemokine (C-C motif) receptor 10	Ccr10
Fibronectin type III domain containing 5	Fndc5
G protein-coupled receptor 39	Gpr39
Short coiled-coil protein	Scoc
Unc-5 homolog C (*C. elegans*)	Unc5c
Genes turned off by estradiol replacement alone	
Leukocyte cell derived chemotaxin 1	Lect1
Genes whose turned on by se was prevented by estradiol replacement	
ARP1 actin-related protein 1 homolog B (yeast)	Actr1b
A disintegrin and metalloprotease domain 4	Adam4
ArfGAP with GTPase domain, ankyrin repeat, and PH domain 1	Agap1
Adenosylhomocysteinase-like 1	Ahcyl1
Aldehyde dehydrogenase family 1, subfamily A7	Aldh1a7
Amyotrophic lateral sclerosis 2 (juvenile) homolog (human)	Als2
ATPase, H+ transporting, lysosomal V0 subunit A2	Atp6v0a2
Dopamine receptor D2	Drd2
Family with sequence similarity 53, member B	Fam53b
Forkhead box C2	Foxc2
Gonadotropin-releasing hormone 1 (luteinizing-releasing hormone)	Gnrh1
HECT, C2 and WW domain containing E3 ubiquitin protein ligase 2	Hecw2
Helicase, lymphoid specific	Hells
Hepatocyte growth factor	Hgf
Minichromosome maintenance complex component 4	Mcm4
Myelin gene regulatory factor	Mrf
Myosin, heavy chain 10, non-muscle	Myh10
Nuclear transcription factor-Y alpha	Nfya
Patatin-like phospholipase domain containing 3	Pnpla3
Surfactant protein C	Sftpc
Sarcoglycan zeta	Sgcz
Seven in absentia 1A	Siah1a
SLAM family member 8	Slamf8
Solute carrier family 39 (zinc transporter), member 14	Slc39a14
Syntaxin 2	Stx2
SMT3 suppressor of mif two 3 homolog 3 (*S. cerevisiae*)	Sumo3
Transcription factor AP-2 beta	Tcfap2b
Tetratricopeptide repeat domain 33	Ttc33
Ubiquitin-associated protein 2	Ubap2
Unc-5 homolog D (*C. elegans*)	Unc5d
Zinc finger, C4H2 domain containing	Zc4h2
Zinc metallopeptidase, STE24 homolog (*S. cerevisiae*)	Zmpste24
Zinc finger, MYM-type 4	Zmym4
Zinc finger protein 286A	Znf286a

computed for every single gene includes in the regulated list the "false negatives" of the traditionally uniform 1.5 × (very stably expressed genes across biological replicates that are probed by very clean spots with 1.5 > FC > CUT). In addition, it eliminates most of the "false positives" from the variably expressed genes that are also probed by not so clean spots (1.5 < FC < CUT).

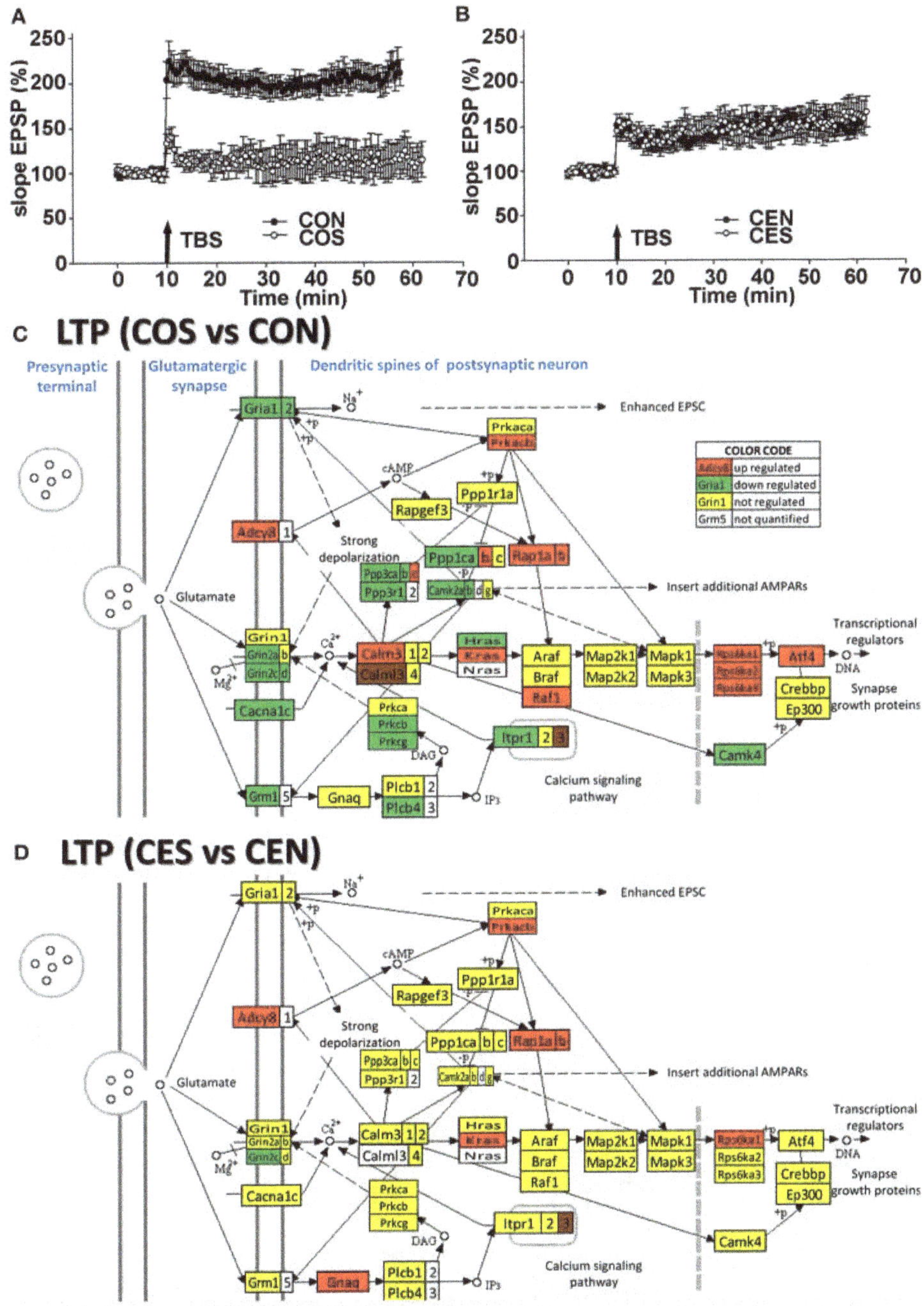

FIGURE 3 | Electrophysiology and transcriptomics of the long-term potentiation (LTP). **(A,B)** Medial perforant path LTP in the DG in OVX rats is lost following SE but preserved in E2-replaced animals. LTP induced by TBS following SE (filled circles) compared to rats with no seizures (open circles). An arrow marks a moment when the TBS was administered. In slices from oil-injected rats exposed to SE (COS; $n = 5$), TBS-induced LTP was severely reduced compared to LTP from rats with no SE (CON; $n = 10$). In contrast, the magnitude of TBS-induced LTP in slices from E2-replaced OVX rats following SE (CES; $n = 5$) was not different from LTP in slices from rats with no seizure experience (CEN; $n = 10$). **(C,D)** Dramatic regulation of LTP associated genes by SE in OVX rats compared to their non-SE counterparts (COS vs. CON) is in contrast to protection against the transcriptomic regulation of LTP associated genes in E2 replaced animals (CES vs. CEN). As specified in the "COLOR CODE" inset table, red/green/yellow background of the gene symbol indicates up-/down-/no regulation, while the white background indicates that expression of that gene was not quantified. Note the significantly lower number of regulated genes in rats with E2 replacement.

In addition to the percentages of up-/down-regulated genes, we have also computed the Weighted Pathway Regulation (WPR) and Pathway Protection (PPR, similar to Pathway Restoration Efficiency) that we have recently introduced (Iacobas et al., 2017). WPR and PPR are free of the arbitrary FC and p-value cut-offs to consider a gene as significantly regulated and take also into account the magnitude and significance of each gene regulation. Thus, a gene with 2 × fold-change at p-val = 0.01 contributes to WPR more than twice than a gene with 1.5 × fold-change at p-val = 0.05. This approach is different from the percentage of regulated genes that not only depends on the arbitrarily introduced cut-offs but treats all

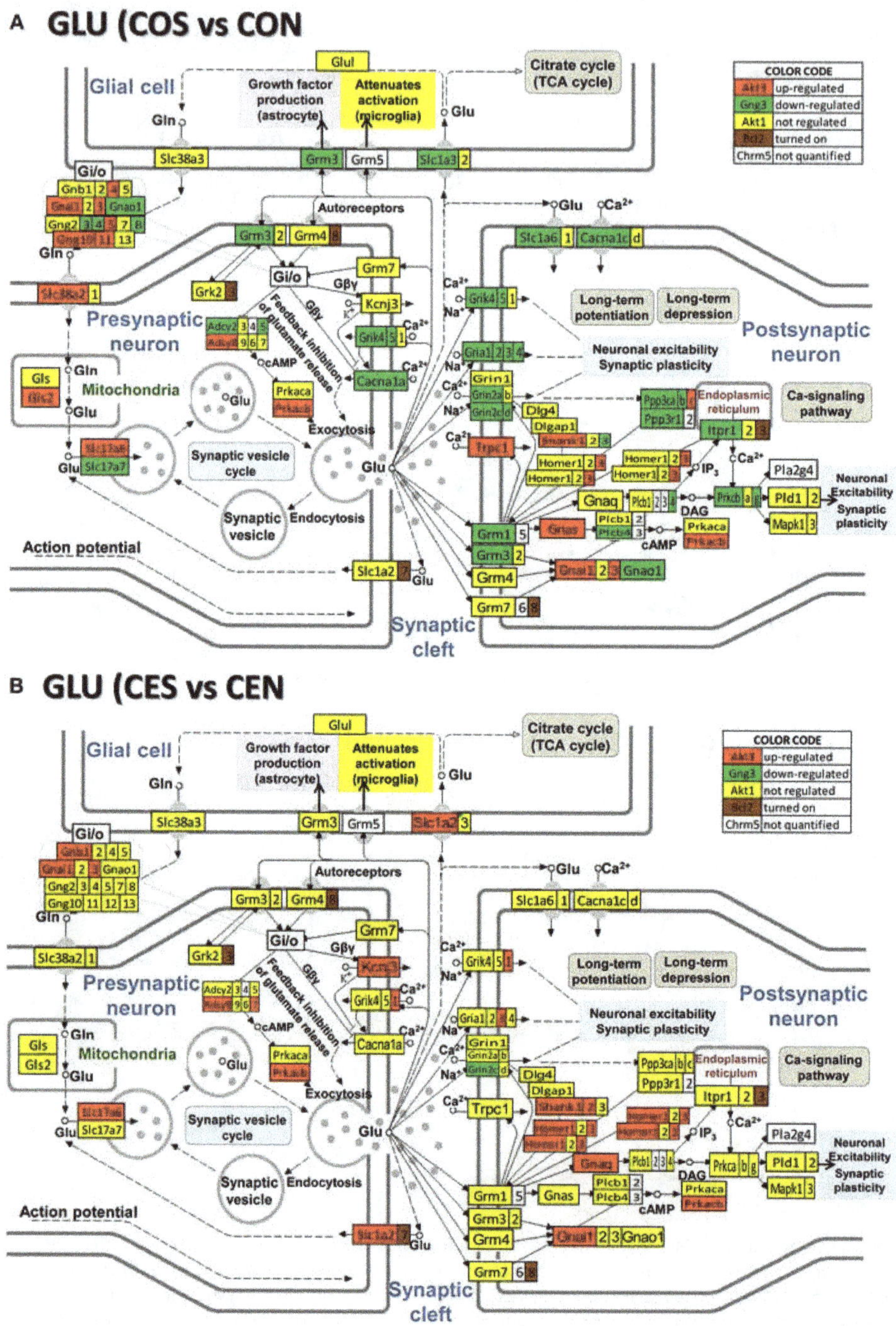

FIGURE 4 | Regulation of the glutamatergic synapse pathway by SE in OVX rats with (CES)/without (COS) E2-replacement with respect to their non-SE counterparts (CEN and CON). Note the large number of down-regulated genes by SE in oil injected rats [e.g., metabotropic glutamate receptor 3, *Grm3* in **(A)**] whose expression was not affected by SE in rats with E2 replacement **(B)**.

regulated genes as equal contributors. We have used also the Transcriptomic Protection (TPR), similar to the Transcriptomic Recovery Efficacy (Lachtermacher et al., 2011; Soares et al., 2011), representing the reduction of the percentage of regulated genes while considering also the side effects (i.e., the percentage of the regulated genes by the E2-replacement alone).

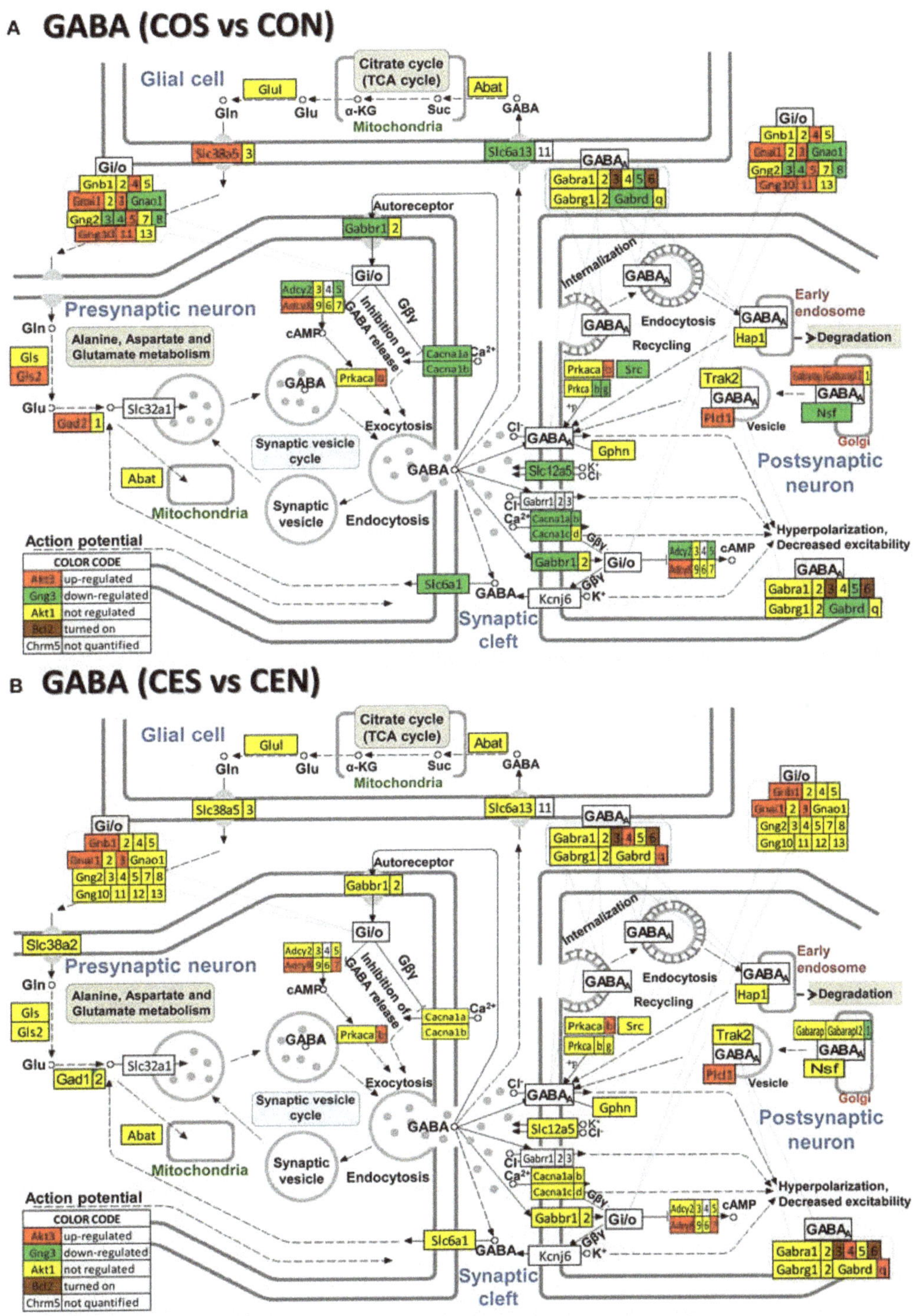

FIGURE 5 | Regulation of the GABAergic synapse pathway by SE in OVX rats with (CES)/without (COS) E2-replacement with respect to their non-SE counterparts (CEN and CON). Note large number of genes down-regulated by SE in oil-injected animals [e.g., GABA B receptor 1, *Gabbr1* in **(A)**] whose expression was not affected by SE in rats with E2 replacement **(B)**.

Transcriptomic Networks

For each condition (CON, COS, CEN, CES) we determined how much expression of each gene is coordinated with expression of each other gene by computing Pearson correlation coefficient between the expression levels of the two genes among biological replicates. Expression coordination of two genes may result from several molecular mechanisms that may include (but it is not restricted to) the regulation of the expressions of both genes by a common transcription factor. We used coordination analysis (Iacobas et al., 2007a; Iacobas and Iacobas, 2010) to determine the transcriptomic networks by which genes in the estrogen signaling pathway controls the genes involved in all

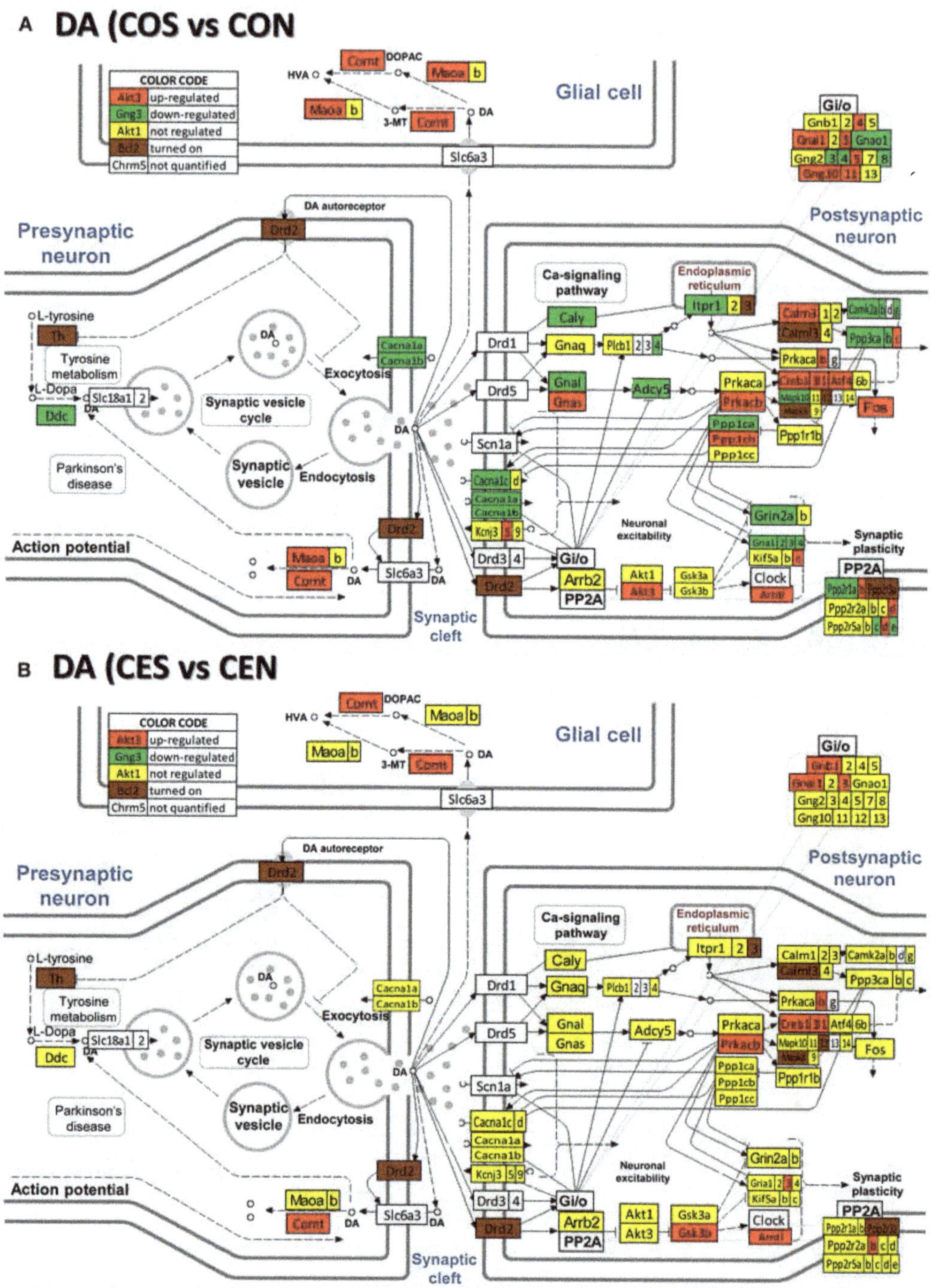

FIGURE 6 | Regulation of the dopaminergic synapse pathway by SE in OVX rats with (CES)/without (COS) E2-replacement with respect to their non-SE counterparts (CEN and CON). Note the number of genes down-regulated by SE in oil-injected animals [e.g., DOPA decarboxylase, *Ddc* in **(A)**] whose expression was not affected by SE in rats with E2 replacement **(B)**.

types of neurotransmission in the female DG. The analysis is based on our principle of "transcriptomic stoichiometry" (Iacobas et al., 2007b; Iacobas, 2016) stating that genes whose encoded proteins are working together in functional pathways should be coordinately expressed to produce the pathway players in the right proportions. In a previous paper (Iacobas et al., 2007c), we have shown that the transcriptomic networks do not stop at the cellular border. Instead, they may cross it to link pathways from (phenotypically similar or distinct) neighboring cells via intercellular signaling (Iacobas et al., 2006d).

RESULTS

We quantified expressions of 12,710 distinct genes in all 16 samples and computed 80,765,695 Pearson correlation coefficients among these genes for each of the four conditions. Detailed experimental procedure and raw and normalized gene

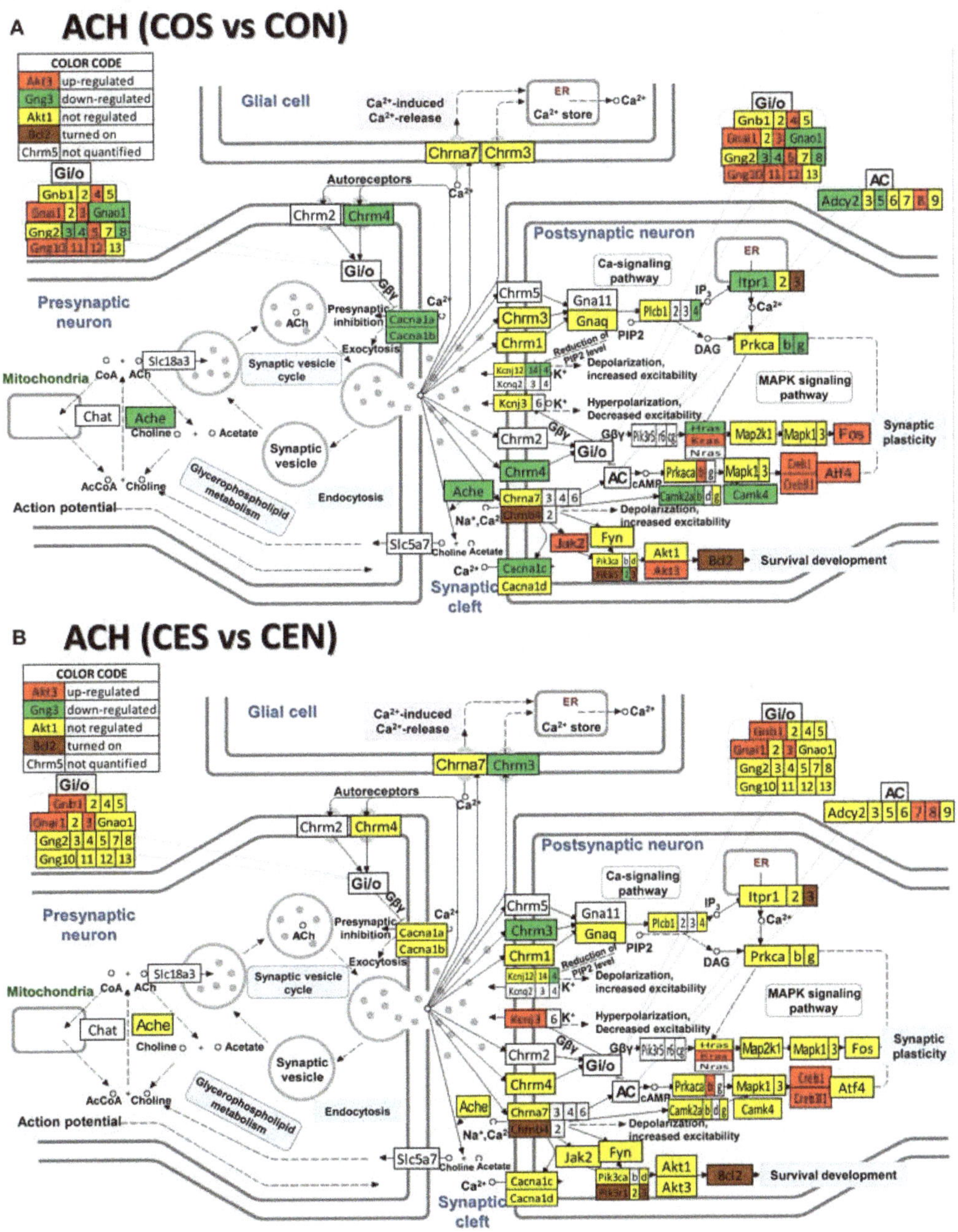

FIGURE 7 | Regulation of the cholinergic synapse pathway by SE in OVX rats with (CES)/without (COS) E2-replacement with respect to their non-SE counterparts (CEN and CON). Again, note the large number of genes down-regulated by SE in oil-injected animals [e.g., acetylcholinesterase, *Ache* in **(A)**] whose expression was not affected by SE in rats with E2 replacement **(B)**.

expression data are publically available at http://www.ncbi.nlm.nih.gov/geo as GSE60013 and GSE107725.

Gene Expression Regulation by SE and Protection by E2 Replacement

Figures 1B,E present the percentage of the SE-related regulated genes from all analyzed pathways in COS and CES groups with respect to their corresponding controls (CON and CEN groups). Of note is the substantial reduction of the percentage of regulated genes in OVX rats with EB replacement compared to the animals that received only oil. Note that larger percentages of genes were altered synaptic pathways than the overall alteration percentage in the entire transcriptome. **Figures 1C,F** present the WPR scores for selected pathways, confirming the

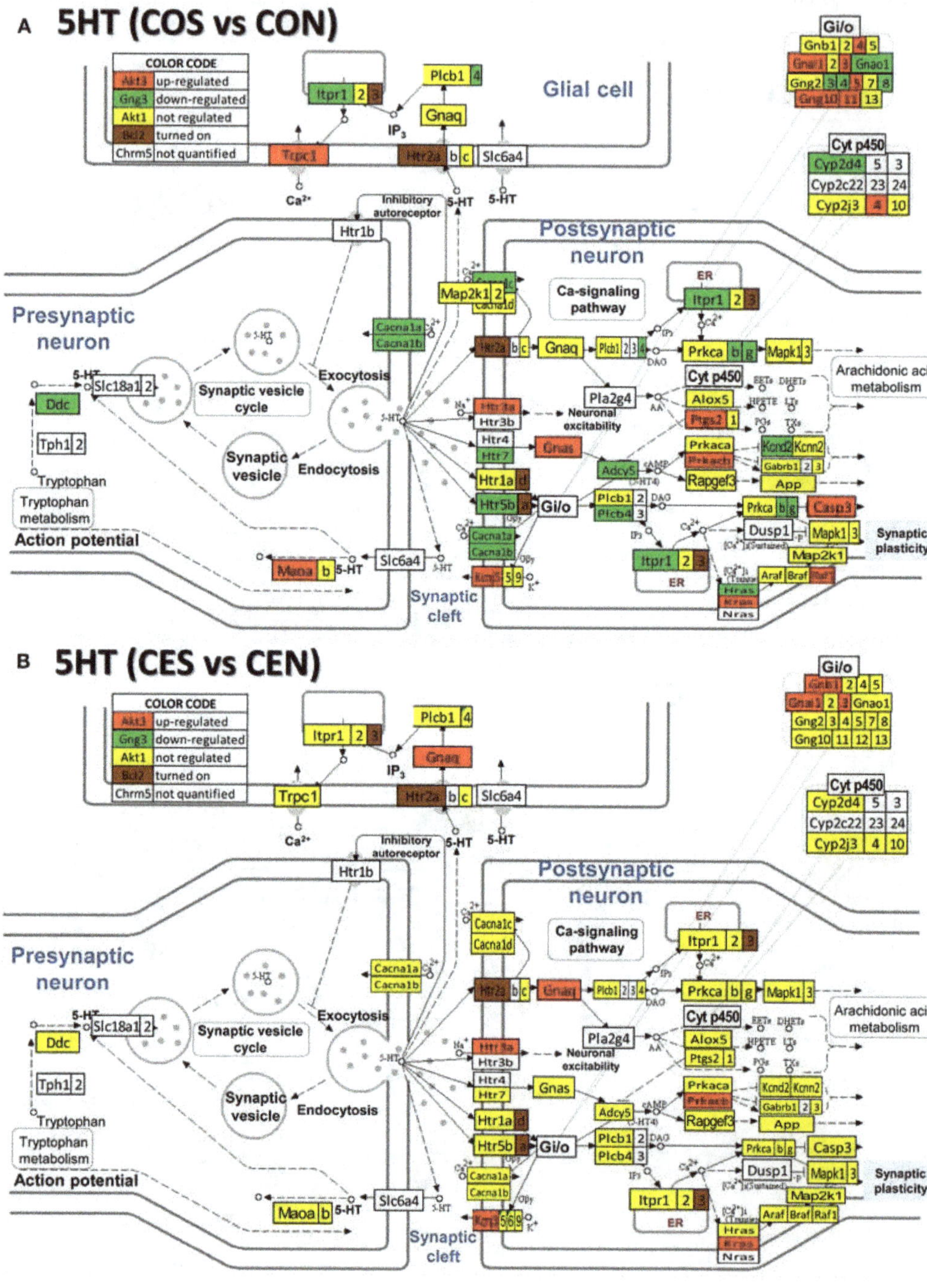

FIGURE 8 | Regulation of the serotonergic synapse pathway by SE in OVX with (CES)/without (COS) E2-replacement with respect to their non-SE counterparts (CEN and CON). Note the number of down-regulated genes by SE in oil-injected animals [e.g. serotonin receptor 5B, *Htr5b* in **(A)**] whose expression was not affected by SE in rats with E2 replacement **(B)**.

substantially lower alteration of these pathways in rats with E2 replacement. **Figures 1D,G** present the protection against SE alteration in E2 replaced animals as quantified by both TPR and PPR.

The expression ratios (x, negative for down-regulation), the absolute fold-change cut-offs (CUT) and the *p*-values for all regulated genes in the analyzed pathways are listed in the **Supplementary Table S1**. In order to illustrate how our method of flexible FC cut-off works, we present in **Figure 2** the distributions of the FC cut-offs and the list of "false negatives" (e.g., *Abl1* with 1.5 > COS = 1.477 > CUT = 1.298) and "false positives" (e.g., *Chrna7* with 1.5 < COS = 2.226 < CUT = 2.297) selected from the **Supplementary Table S1**. Of note from **Figure 1C** is that the FC ranges from 1.104 (for the "false negative" *Cdc16* in COS) to 2.821 (for *Raf1* in CES).

In addition to regulate the expression of thousands genes, both SE and E2 replacement separately or together turned ON/OFF many other genes. **Table 1** lists the turned on/off genes by E2 replacement alone in non-SE rats and the genes whose turning on by SE was prevented by E2 replacement.

Effects of SE on the LTP in the Hippocampal DG of OVX Oil-Injected and E2 Replaced Female Rats

To confirm the functional protection provided by the E2 replacement against SE, we compared the TBS-induced LTP in the hippocampal DG of animals with no SE experience to LTP from animals following kainic acid-induced SE. In oil-injected OVX females (no E2 replacement), we found that the TBS-induced LTP was lost following SE (**Figure 3A**) while in OVX

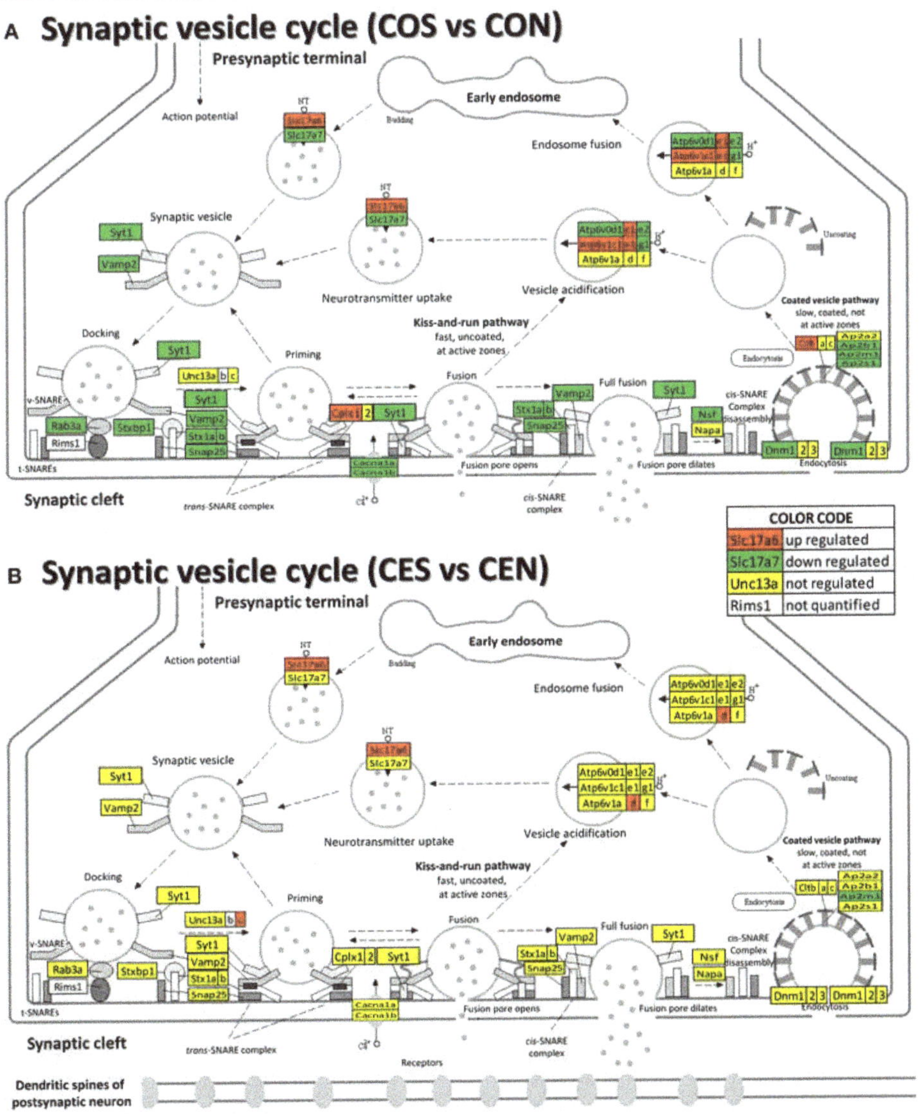

FIGURE 9 | Regulation of the synaptic vesicle cycle pathway by SE in OVX with (CES)/without (COS) E2-replacement with respect to their non-SE counterparts (CEN and CON). Note that in oil-injected animals **(A)** the vesicle cycle was altered by SE in all phases but only few genes were affected in animals with E2 replacement **(B)**.

rats with E2 replacement, the magnitude of the TBS-induced LTP in the DG was not affected by SE (**Figure 3B**). These data are in accord with the transcriptomic findings (**Figures 3C,D**). Thus, the LTP data clearly demonstrate that the DG plasticity was functionally severely compromised and associated with dramatic gene regulation in the LTP pathway following SE in OVX animals. In contrast, the SE did not disturb the LTP in animals with E2 replacement.

Regulation of Neurotransmission Pathways by SE w/o E2 Replacement

Figures 4–8 present the regulation of GLU, GABA, DA, ACH, and 5HT pathways by SE in OVX rats w/o E2-replaced with respect to their non-SE counterparts. Of note is the large number (58!) of down-regulated genes in oil-injected animals whose expression was preserved in E2-replaced rats. The protected genes include: adenylate cyclases (*Adcy2, Adcy5*), calcium (*Cacna1a, Cacna1b, Cacna1c*), potassium (*Kcnd2, Kcnj14*), and solute carrier (*Slc12a5, Slc17a7, Slc1a3, Slc1a6, Slc6a1, Slc6a13*) channels and kinases (*Camk2a, Camk2b, Camk4, Mapk10, Pik33r2, Prkcb, Prkcg*). E2 replacement preserved also expression of several receptor genes: *Chrm4, Gabr1, Gabr5, Gabrd, Gnal, Gnao1, Gng3, Gng4, Gria1, Gria2, Gria4, Grik4, Grik5, Grin2a, Grin2d, Grm1, Grm3, Htr5b, Htr7, Itpr1*). Moreover, the down-regulation of *Gria3* in oil-treated animals was switched to up-regulation in E2-replaced. E2 replacement also protected some binding proteins (*Gnb4, Gng10, Gng11, Gng12, Gng5*) and oncogenes (*Akt3, Fos, Jun, Raf1*) against the SE-related upregulation. However, other genes, not affected by SE in oil-injected animals were regulated in E2-replaced ones (*Adcy7, Chrm3, Gabarapl1, Gabra4, Gabrq, Gnb1, Grik1, Gsk3b, Homer1, Kcnj3, Ppp2r2b, Shank2, Slc1a2, Sos2*). The protection against SE-related down-regulation of *Itpr1* and calcium channels is particularly important for the role these genes play in the intercellular calcium signaling (Iacobas et al., 2006d).

Our data show (**Figure 9**) that also the synaptic vesicle cycle (SVC) was massively altered by SE in oil-injected females and on much smaller scale in rats with E2 replacement.

SE Remodels the Transcriptomic Networks by Which the ESG Pathway Controls Neurotransmission

We found that SE not only regulates the ESG pathway (**Figure 10**) but also profoundly remodeled the transcriptomic networks by which ESG regulates neurotransmission. Interestingly, in animals with E2 replacement, SE turned

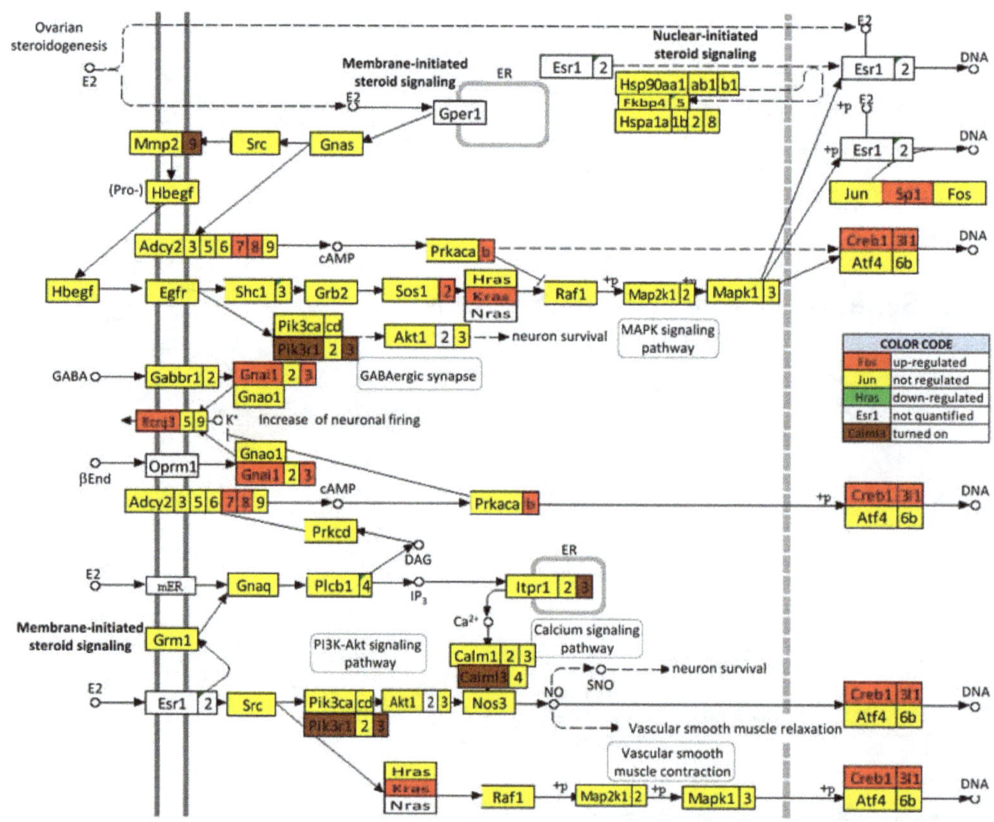

FIGURE 10 | Regulation of the estrogen signaling pathway by SE in OVX females with E2 replacement. Note that, in addition to up-regulating *Adcy7, Adcy8, Creb1, Creb3l1, Gnai1, Gnai3, Kcnj3, Kras, Prkacb,* and *Sp1*, SE turned on *Calml3, Itpr3, Mmp9, Pik3r1,* and *Pik3r3*. No gene of this pathway was found as down-regulated or turned off by SE.

on the very important *Pik3r1* and *Pik3r3* [phosphoinositide-3-kinase regulatory subunits 1 (alpha) and 3 (gamma)] that control numerous major pathways via the PI3K-AKT signaling.

Figures 11A and **12A** present the transcriptomic networks that interlink ESG pathway genes with glutamatergic and cholinergic transmission via common genes in OVX animals with E2 replacement. **Figures 11B**, **12B** show how SE altered these networks. The analysis revealed high degree (15%) of synergistic expression between genes involved in ESG pathway and all types of neurotransmission. This synergism means that when the ESG diminishes, the expression of neurotransmission genes decreases as well. This may explain why decline in E2 levels is associated with increased incidence of neurodegenerative diseases.

We also noticed that in animals with E2 replacement the synergistic expression of 131 ESG-neurotransmission gene pairs was switched by SE into antagonistic expression (albeit 25 pairs were switched from antagonistically to synergistically expressed). Thus, when expression of the ESG gene partner decreases, the expression of the paired neurotransmission gene goes up, likely compensating for the decrease of other synapse molecular factors. **Figure 13** presents the ESG-neurotransmission gene pairs that switched their expression coordination from synergistic to antagonistic or *vice versa* in E2-replaced animals following SE. For instance, the transcription factor *Jun*, known for its role in synaptic plasticity and term memory formation (Alberini, 2009) had 13 synergistic-to-antagonistic switch(with: *Arrb2, Ddc, Dlg4, Gabra1, Gabra2, Gabr4, Gabrg2, Gng2, Gria2, Gria3, Grik5,*

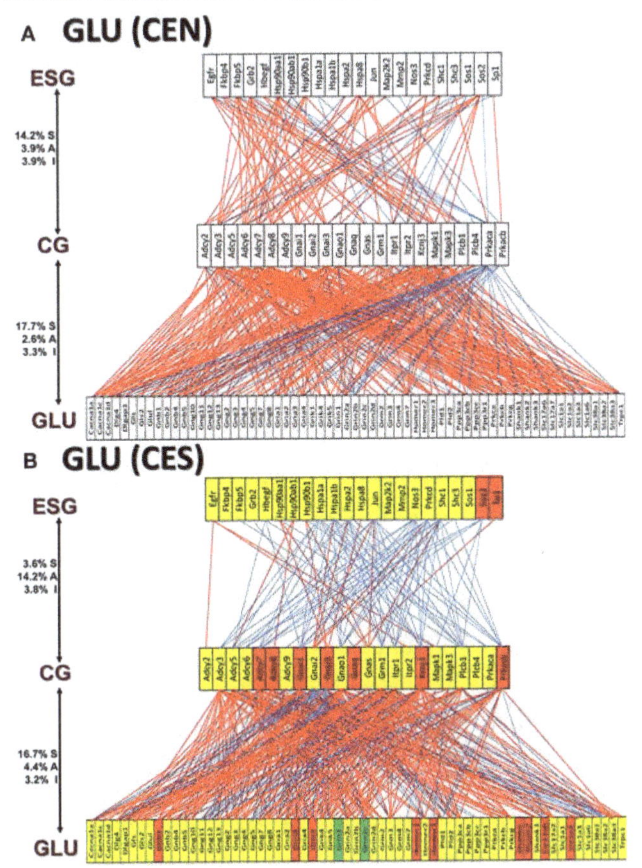

FIGURE 11 | The transcriptomic networks by which the estrogen-signaling (ESG) pathway genes regulate the glutamatergic synapse (GLU) genes through expression coordination with the common genes (CG) between the two pathways in OVX rats with E2-replacement. **(A)** Networks in the DG of non-SE animals. A red/blue line indicates that the linked genes are significantly (p-value < 0.05) synergistically/antagonistically expressed, respectively. Numbers on the left side represent the percentages of the synergistically (S)/antagonistically (A)/independently (I) expressed pairs that can be formed between the two groups of genes. **(B)** Networks in the DG of SE animals. Red/green/yellow background of the gene symbol indicates that that gene was up-/down-/not regulated by SE. Note that there is a substantial shift from synergistic to antagonistic expression between ESG and CG groups in SE animals.

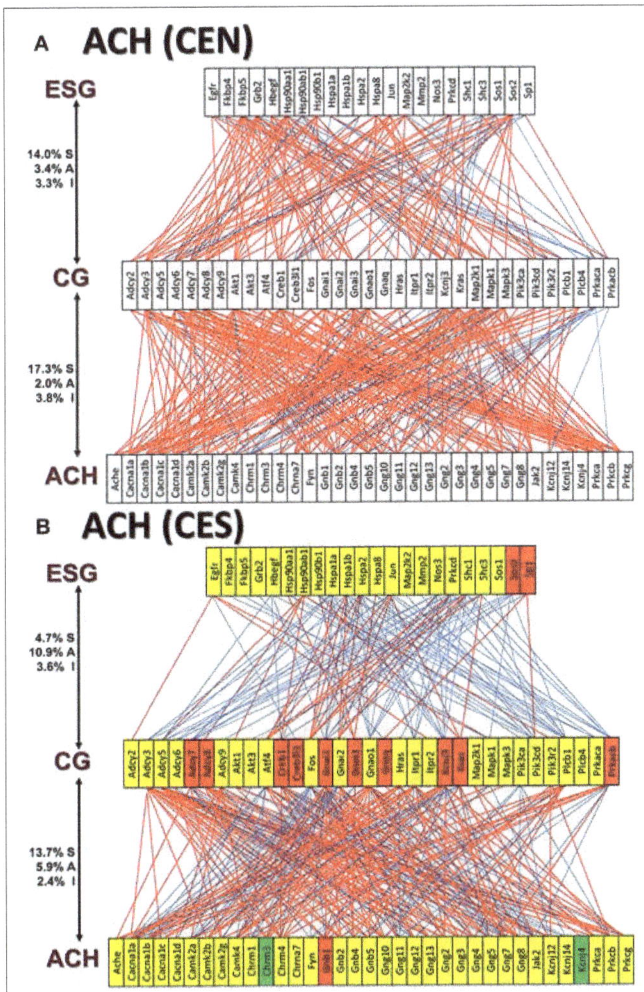

FIGURE 12 | The transcriptomic networks by which the estrogen-signaling (ESG) pathway genes regulate the cholinergic synapse (ACH) genes through expression coordination with the common genes (CG) between the two pathways in OVX rats with E2-replacement. **(A)** Networks in the DG of non-SE animals. **(B)** Networks in the DG of SE animals. Note the substantial shift from synergistic to antagonistic expression between ESG and CG groups in SE animals.

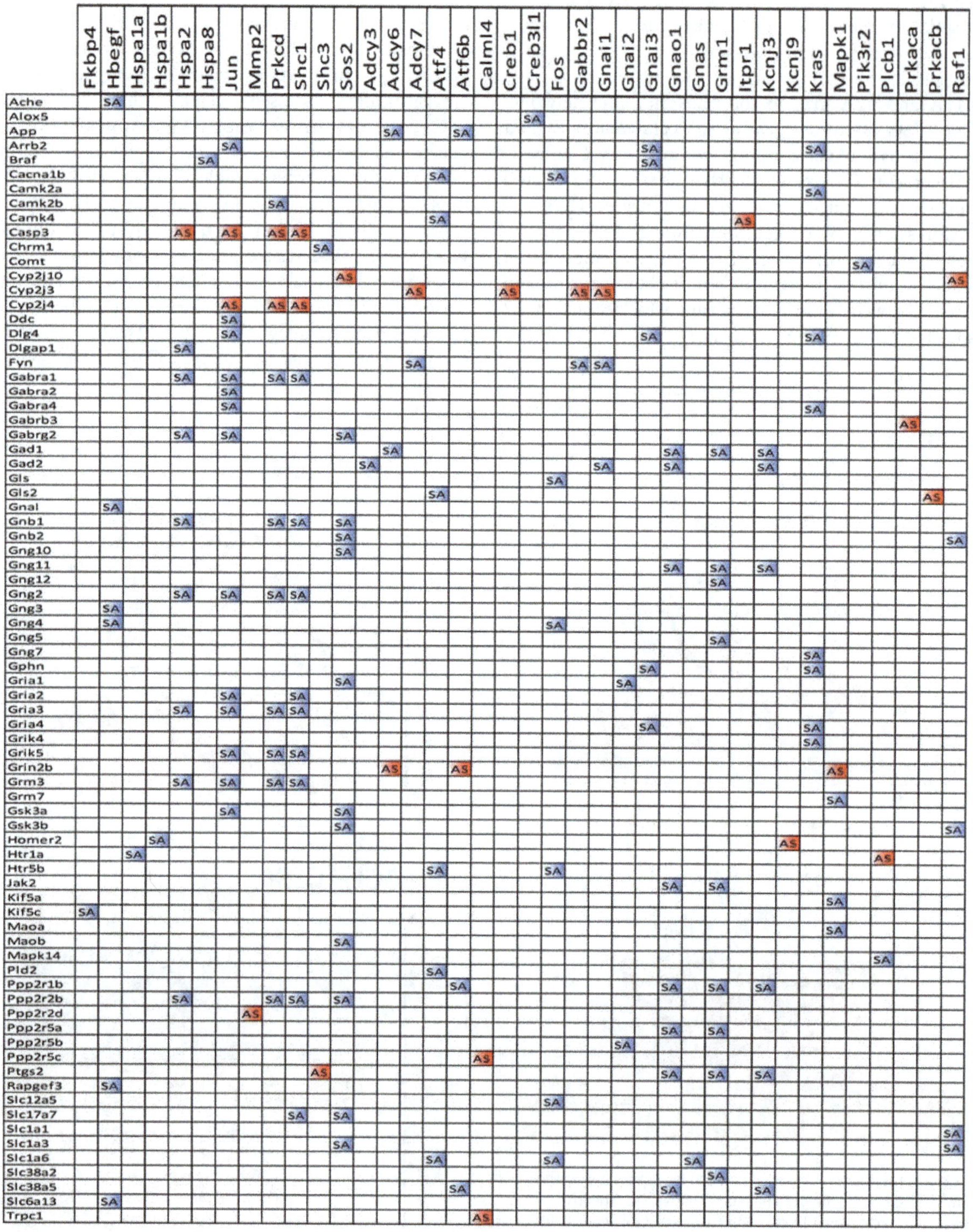

FIGURE 13 | ES-neurotransmission gene pairs that switched their expression coordination from synergistic to antagonistic (white to blue bullets) or from antagonistic to synergistic (white to red bullets) following SE.

Grm3, Gsk3a) and 2 antagonistic-to synergistic ones (*Casp3, Cyp2j3*).

It is interesting how the expression coordination of *Jun* with major synapse membrane receptors depends on the E2 presence and changes following SE. As illustrated in **Figure 14**, the E2-replacement doubled the number of synergistically expressed partners for *Jun* among the synaptic receptors and turned *Gabra1* from an independently to a synergistically expressed

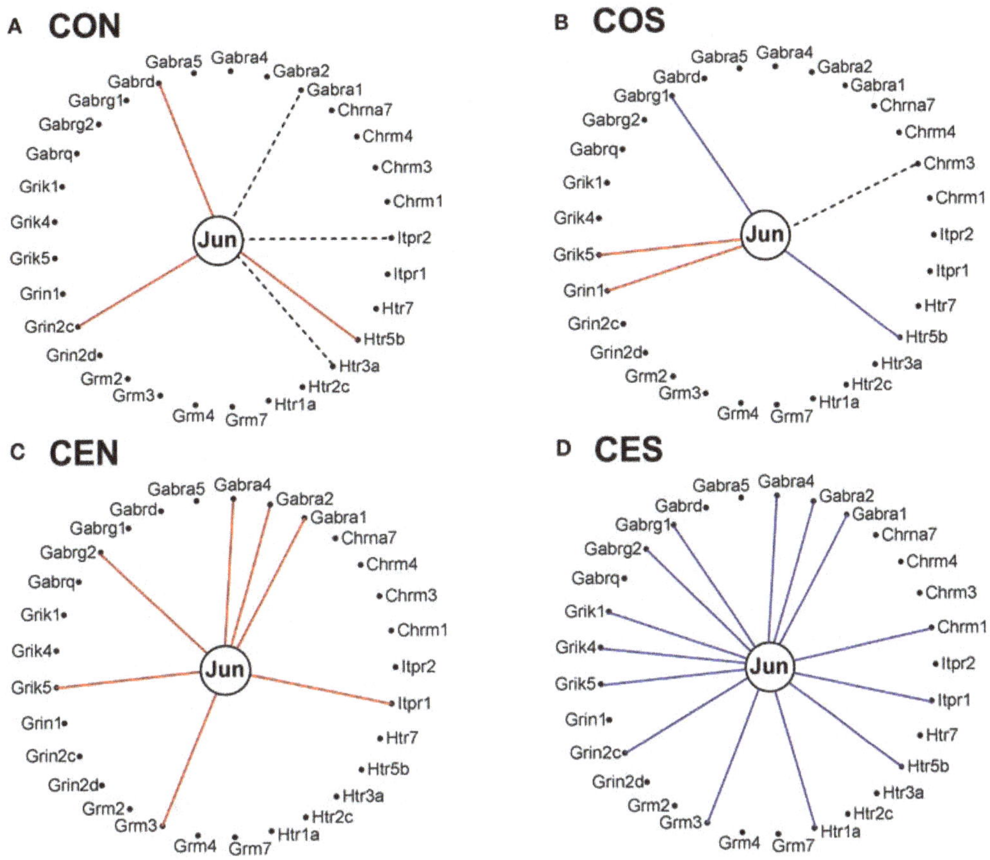

FIGURE 14 | Expression correlation of Jun oncogene with some synapse membrane receptors in the DG of OVX rat female rats. **(A)** Oil-injected, non-SE rats; **(B)** Oil-injected SE rats; **(C)** E2-replaced, non-SE rats; **(D)** E2-replaced, SE rats. A continuous red/blue line indicates significant (P-value < 0.05) expression synergism/antagonism of *Jun* with the linked gene, an interrupted black line indicates significant (p-value < 0.05) expression independence, while missing lines mean that we have not enough evidence to categorize the expression coordination of *Jun* with that gene.

gene. In both oil-injected and E2-replaced animals, SE induced antagonistic expression of *Jun* with several synaptic receptors.

DISCUSSION

We show that the well-known neuroprotective effects of E2, in this case against SE-induced hippocampal damage, involve complex, multifactorial changes including alteration of neurotransmission pathways. Our study stresses the importance of considering global genomic changes when studying effects of steroid hormones. The neuroprotective effects of E2 against SE-induced damage involve widespread regulation of neurotransmitter systems. Our data further shows that loss of estrogen leads to a state of transcriptomic instability, which may significantly contribute to neuronal vulnerability and, consequently, may render the system more susceptible to neurodegenerative processes. We identified a large number of down-regulated genes in the neurotransmission pathways induced by SE in oil-injected females and interpreted this finding as the major culprit for most of SE features. Indeed, E2 replacement led to restoration of the expression of many of these genes and we consider this as a good indication of the E2 protective role of brain circuitry.

The overall technical noise of the arrays hybridized with samples from oil-injected animals is practically equal to that of the samples from E2-replaced animals as indicated by comparing the control spots. Hence, the lower average (and median) of the FC distribution in the COS vs CON results from the reduction of expression variability in the compared conditions. This result is consistent with our robust finding in hundreds of transcriptomic experiments that the expression variability is larger in tissues of animals closer to their normal condition than in disease conditions. As presented in a previous publication (Iacobas, 2016) CES and CEN are closer to the conditions of intact females with/without SE than are COS and CEN.

The coordination analysis of the over 80 mil gene pairs in each condition, sorted in numerous interplays among the genomic fabrics of functional pathways provides an enormous amount of information. Complete presentation of this information is not possible to cover in a single report. Therefore, we have selected some results that may enhance our understanding of the complex molecular mechanisms triggered by the SE and the neuroprotective role of E2 replacement on brain circuitry.

Studies in patients with epilepsy suggest that particularly in the DG, seizure-induced hippocampal damage (sclerosis) is associated with memory deficits (Helmstaedter et al., 1997; Grunwald et al., 1999a,b). Recordings from resected human hippocampal specimens indicate that in patients with temporal lobe epilepsy (TLE) that was associated with hippocampal sclerosis, TBS-induced LTP in the DG is lost (Beck et al., 2000). Our present data show that following kainic acid-induced SE, a model of seizures originating in the temporal lobe (Velíšková et al., 2000; Velíšková and Velíšek, 2007), TBS-induced LTP is severely impaired in slices from oil-injected, but not E2-replaced OVX rats. Interestingly, an MRI study has demonstrated that young women are less likely to develop TLE-associated hippocampal damage suggesting possible protective effects of female ovarian hormones (Briellmann et al., 2000). Indeed, our previous studies showed that kainic-acid-induced SE was associated with severe neuronal loss in the vulnerable hilar region of the DG in OVX rats but the neuronal damage was significantly ameliorated in E2-replaced animals (Velíšková et al., 2000; Velíšková and Velíšek, 2007). We would like to emphasize that in OVX rats, the dose of E2 used in our studies produces circulating levels of E2 within the physiological range (Neal-Perry et al., 2005). This E2 dose is not only neuroprotective against the SE-induced hippocampal damage but it also has a mild anticonvulsant effect (Velíšková et al., 2000; Velíšková and Velíšek, 2007). Others have used various doses of E2 and showed consistent neuroprotective effects against seizure-induced hippocampal neuronal damage regardless the E2 dose but the supraphysiological E2 levels were associated with a proconvulsant effect (see Velíšková and DeSantis, 2013 for detailed review).

Very important findings of this study concern Jun oncogene (*Jun*) expression regulation and coordination with neurotransmission genes. As part of the activator protein-1 (AP-1), *Jun* is involved in major cellular processes including differentiation, proliferation and cell survival, frequently leading to cancerous processes, (Papoudou-Bai et al., 2017; Shrihari, 2017; Tewari et al., 2017). Significant up-regulation of *Jun* by SE in oil-injected rats (2.9x) can explain vast occurrence of SE-related brain damage through activation of pro-apoptotic genes (Kravchick et al., 2016). Importantly, expression of *Jun* was not altered by SE in E2-replaced animals, proving again the important protection E2 provides to the brain likely through its interference with apoptotic process here represented by *Jun*.

In a recent study (Iacobas et al., 2018) on a rat model of infantile spasms, we have analyzed how the epileptic spasms alter the neurotransmission in the hypothalamic arcuate nucleus and how the ACTH or PMX53 (a potent complement C5ar1 antagonist) treatment recovers most of these alterations. Thus, the question exists whether initiation of the E2 replacement in adult OVX females following the SE would also rescue the deteriorating effects of SE.

AUTHOR CONTRIBUTIONS

DI designed the microarray experiment, developed the analytical methods, and analyzed the data. SI performed the microarray experiment and the primary analysis. NN performed most of the animal work and analyzed the electrophysiology LTP data. LV contributed the biological interpretation of the experimental results. JV designed and supervised the entire project. All authors contributed to the manuscript writing.

ACKNOWLEDGMENTS

The studies were supported by the NIH grants NS-072966 (LV) and JV was partially supported by NS092786.

SUPPLEMENTARY MATERIAL

Supplementary Table S1 | Significantly regulated genes in the analyzed pathways. COS/CON, CES/CEN = expression ratios (negative for down-regulation) in the respective comparisons, CUT = fold-change cut-off computed for each gene in each comparison to be considered as regulated. Red/green background of the expression ratio indicates significant up/down regulation while yellow background indicates not significant regulation.

REFERENCES

1. Alberini, C. M. (2009). Transcription factors in long-term memory and synaptic plasticity. *Physiol. Rev.* 89, 121–145. doi: 10.1152/physrev.00017.2008
2. Beck, H., Goussakov, I. V., Lie, A., Helmstaedter, C., and Elger, C. E. (2000). Synaptic plasticity in the human dentate gyrus. *J. Neurosci.* 20, 7080–7086. doi: 10.1523/JNEUROSCI.20-18-07080.2000
3. Briellmann, R. S., Berkovic, S. F., and Jackson, G. D. (2000). Men may be more vulnerable to seizure-associated brain damage. *Neurology* 55, 1479–1485. doi: 10.1212/WNL.55.10.1479
4. Grunwald, T., Beck, H., Lehnertz, K., Blumcke, I., Pezer, N., Kurthen, M., et al. (1999b). Evidence relating human verbal memory to hippocampal N- methyl-D-aspartate receptors. *Proc. Natl. Acad. Sci. U.S.A.* 96, 12085–12089. doi: 10.1073/pnas.96.21.12085
5. Grunwald, T., Beck, H., Lehnertz, K., Blumcke, I., Pezer, N., Kutas, M., et al. (1999a). Limbic P300s in temporal lobe epilepsy with and without Ammon's horn sclerosis. *Eur. J. Neurosci.* 11, 1899–1906. doi: 10.1046/j.1460-9568.1999.00613.x
6. Harden, C. L., Pulver, M. C., Ravdin, L., and Jacobs, A. R. (1999). The effect of menopause and perimenopause on the course of epilepsy. *Epilepsia* 40, 1402–1407. doi: 10.1111/j.1528-1157.1999.tb02012.x
7. Helmstaedter, C., Gleissner, U., Di Perna, M., and Elger, C. E. (1997). Relational verbal memory processing in patients with temporal lobe epilepsy. *Cortex* 33, 667–678. doi: 10.1016/S0010-9452(08)70724-X
8. Herzog, A. G., Harden, C. L., Liporace, J., Pennell, P., Schomer, D. L., Sperling, M., et al. (2004). Frequency of catamenial seizure exacerbation in women with localization-related epilepsy. *Ann. Neurol.* 56, 431–434. doi: 10.1002/ana.20214
Iacobas, D. A. (2016). The genomic fabric perspective on the transcriptome between universal quantifiers and personalized genomic medicine. *Biol. Theor.* 11, 123–137. doi: 10.1007/s13752-016-0245-3
9. Iacobas, D. A., Chachua, T., Iacobas, S., Benson, M. J., Borges, K., Veliskova, J., et al. (2018). ACTH and PMX53 recover the normal synaptic transcriptome in a rat model of infantile spasms. *Sci. Rep.* 8:5722. doi: 10.1038/s41598-018-24013-x
10. Iacobas, D. A., Fan, C., Iacobas, S., Spray, D. C., and Haddad, G. G. (2006). Transcriptomic changes in developing kidney exposed to chronic hypoxia. *Biochem. Biophys. Res. Comm.* 349, 329–338. doi: 10.1016/j.bbrc.2006.08.056

11. Iacobas, D. A., Iacobas, S., and Spray, D. C. (2007b). Connexin43 and the brain transcriptome of the newborn mice. *Genomics* 89, 113–123. doi: 10.1016/j.ygeno.2006.09.007
12. Iacobas, D. A., Iacobas, S., and Spray, D. C. (2007c). Connexin-dependent transcellular transcriptomic networks in mouse brain. *Prog. Biophys. Mol. Biol.* 94, 168–184. doi: 10.1016/j.pbiomolbio.2007.03.015
13. Iacobas, D. A., Iacobas, S., Tanowitz, H. B., deCarvalho, A. C., and Spray, D. C. (2017). Functional genomic fabrics are remodeled in a mouse model of Chagasic cardiomyopathy and restored following cell therapy. *Microbes Infect.* 20, 185–195. doi: 10.1016/j.micinf.2017.11.003
14. Iacobas, D. A., Iacobas, S., Urban-Maldonado, M., and Spray, D. C. (2005). Sensitivity of the brain transcriptome to connexin ablation. *Biochim. Biophys. Acta* 1711, 183–196. doi: 10.1016/j.bbamem.2004.12.002
15. Iacobas, D. A., Iacobas, S., Werner, P., Scemes, E., and Spray, D. C. (2007a). Alteration of transcriptomic networks in adoptive-transfer experimental autoimmune encephalomyelitis. *Front. Integr. Neurosci.* 1:10. doi: 10.3389/neuro.07.010.2007
16. Iacobas, D. A., Suadicani, S. O., Spray, D. C., and Scemes, E. (2006d). A stochastic 2D model of intercellular Ca2+ wave spread in glia. *Biophys. J.* 90, 24–41. doi: 10.1529/biophysj.105.064378
17. Iacobas, S., and Iacobas, D. A. (2010). Astrocyte proximity modulates the myelination gene fabric of oligodendrocytes. *Neuron Glia Biol.* 6, 157–169. doi: 10.1017/S1740925X10000220
18. Iacobas, S., Thomas, N. M., and Iacobas, D. A. (2012). Plasticity of the myelination genomic fabric. *Mol. Gen. Genom.* 287, 237–246. doi: 10.1007/s00438-012-0673-0
19. Isojarvi, J. I. (2003). Reproductive dysfunction in women with epilepsy. *Neurology* 61(6Suppl. 2), S27–34. doi: 10.1212/WNL.61.6_suppl_2.S27
20. Kanehisa, M., Furumichi, M., Tanabe, M., Sato, Y., and Morishima, K. (2017). KEGG: new perspectives on genomes, pathways, diseases and drugs. *Nucleic Acids Res.* 45, D353–D361. doi: 10.1093/nar/gkw1092
21. Klein, P., Serje, A., and Pezzullo, J. C. (2001). Premature ovarian failure in women with epilepsy. *Epilepsia* 42, 1584–1589. doi: 10.1046/j.1528-1157.2001.13701r.x
22. Kravchick, D. O., Hrdinka, M., Iacobas, S., Iacobas, D. A., Kreutz, M. R., and Jordan, B. A. (2016). Synaptonuclear messenger PRR7 inhibits c-Jun ubiquitination and regulates NMDA mediated excitotoxicity. *EMBO J.* 35, 1923–1934. doi: 10.15252/embj.201593070
23. Lachtermacher, S., Esporcatte, B. L. B., Fortes, F. S. A., Rocha, N. N., Montalvo, F., Costa, P., et al. (2011). Functional and transcriptomic recovery of infarcted mouse myocardium treated with bone marrow mononuclear cells. *Stem Cell Rev.* 8, 251–261. doi: 10.1007/s12015-011-9282-2
24. Lee, P. R., Cohen, J. E., Iacobas, D. A., Iacobas, S., and Fields, R. D. (2017). Gene-regulatory networks activated by pattern-specific generation of action potentials in dorsal root ganglia neurons. *Sci. Rep.* 7:43765. doi: 10.1038/srep43765
25. Neal-Perry, G. S., Zeevalk, G. D., Santoro, N. F., and Etgen, A. M. (2005). Attenuation of preoptic area glutamate release correlates with reduced luteinizing hormone secretion in middle-aged female rats. *Endocrinology* 146, 4331–4339. doi: 10.1210/en.2005-0575
26. Nebieridze, N., Zhang, X. L., Chachua, T., Velíšek, L., Stanton, P. K., and Velíšková, J. (2012). β-Estradiol unmasks mGluR-mediated metaplasticity in the female dentate gyrus. *Psychoneuroendocrinology* 37, 1845–1854. doi: 10.1016/j.psyneuen.2012.03.023
27. Papoudou-Bai, A., Hatzimichael, E., Barbouti, A., and Kanavaros, P. (2017). Expression patterns of the activator protein-1 (AP-1) family members in lymphoid neoplasms. *Clin. Exp. Med.* 17, 291–304. doi: 10.1007/s10238-016-0436-z
28. Pennell, P. B. (2009). Hormonal aspects of epilepsy. *Neurol. Clin.* 27, 941–965. doi: 10.1016/j.ncl.2009.08.005
29. Rocca, W. A., Grossardt, B. R., and Shuster, L. T. (2011). Oophorectomy, menopause, estrogen treatment, and cognitive aging: clinical evidence for a window of opportunity. *Brain Res.* 1379, 188–198. doi: 10.1016/j.brainres.2010.10.031
30. Shrihari, T. G. (2017). Dual role of inflammatory mediators in cancer. *Ecancermedicalscience* 11:721. doi: 10.3332/ecancer.2017.721
31. Shuster, L. T., Rhodes, D. J., Gostout, B. S., Grossardt, B. R., and Rocca, W. A. (2010). Premature menopause or early menopause: long-term health consequences. *Maturitas* 65, 161–166. doi: 10.1016/j.maturitas.2009.08.003
32. Soares, M. B., Lima, R. S., Souza, B. S. F., Vasconcelos, J. F., Rocha, L. L., dos Santos, R. R., et al. (2011). Reversion of gene expression alterations in hearts of mice with chronic chagasic cardiomyopathy after transplantation of bone marrow cells. *Cell Cycle* 10, 1448–1455. doi: 10.4161/cc.10.9.15487
33. Tewari, D., Nabavi, S. F., Nabavi, S. M., Sureda, A., Farooqi, A. A., Atanasov, A. G., et al. (2017). Targeting activator protein 1 signaling pathway by bioactive natural agents: possible therapeutic strategy for cancer prevention and intervention. *Pharmacol. Res.* 128, 366–375. doi: 10.1016/j.phrs.2017.09.014
34. Velíšková, J., and DeSantis, K. A. (2013). Sex and hormonal influences on seizures and epilepsy. *Horm. Behav.* 63, 267–277. doi: 10.1016/j.yhbeh.2012.03.018
35. Velíšková, J., and Velíšek, L. (2007). β-estradiol increases dentate gyrus inhibition in female rats via augmentation of hilar neuropeptide, Y. *J. Neurosci.* 27, 6054–6063. doi: 10.1523/JNEUROSCI.0366-07.2007
36. Velíšková, J., Iacobas, D. A., Iacobas, S., Sidyelyeva, G., Chachua, T., and Velíšek, L. (2015). Estradiol regulates neuropeptide Y release and the gene coupling with GABAergic and glutamatergic synapse in adult female rat dentate gyrus. *J. Neuroendocrinol.* 27, 911–920. doi: 10.1111/jne.12332
37. Velíšková, J., Velíšek, L., Galanopoulou, A. S., and Sperber, E. F. (2000). Neuroprotective effects of estrogens on hippocampal cells in adult female rats after status epilepticus. *Epilepsia* 41, S30–S35. doi: 10.1111/j.1528-1157.2000.tb01553.x

14

The Role of Estrogen Receptor β in the Dorsal Raphe Nucleus on the Expression of Female Sexual Behavior in C57BL/6J Mice

Kazuhiro Sano[1†], Chihiro Morimoto[1†], Mariko Nataka[1], Sergei Musatov[2‡], Mumeko C. Tsuda[1], Naoko Yamaguchi[3], Toshiro Sakamoto[4] and Sonoko Ogawa[1]*

[1] Laboratory of Behavioral Neuroendocrinology, University of Tsukuba, Tsukuba, Japan, [2] Laboratory of Molecular Neurosurgery, Department of Neurological Surgery, Weill Cornell Medical College, New York, NY, United States, [3] Department of Medicine, Aichi Medical University, Nagakute, Japan, [4] Department of Health Sciences, Kyoto Tachibana University, Kyoto, Japan

***Correspondence:**
Sonoko Ogawa
ogawa@kansei.tsukuba.ac.jp

†These authors have contributed equally to this work.

‡Deceased.

17β-Estradiol (E_2) regulates the expression of female sexual behavior by acting through estrogen receptor (ER) α and β. Previously, we have shown that ERβ knockout female mice maintain high level of lordosis expression on the day after behavioral estrus when wild-type mice show a clear decline of the behavior, suggesting ERβ may be involved in inhibitory regulation of lordosis. However, it is not identified yet in which brain region(s) ERβ may mediate an inhibitory action of E_2. In this study, we have focused on the dorsal raphe nucleus (DRN) that expresses ERβ in higher density than ERα. We site specifically knocked down ERβ in the DRN in ovariectomized mice with virally mediated RNA interference method. All mice were tested weekly for a total of 3 weeks for their lordosis expression against a stud male in two consecutive days: day 1 with the hormonal condition mimicking the day of behavioral estrus, and day 2 under the hormonal condition mimicking the day after behavioral estrus. We found that the level of lordosis expression in ERβ knockdown (βERKD) mice was not different from that of control mice on day 1. However, βERKD mice continuously showed elevated levels of lordosis behavior on day 2 tests, whereas control mice showed a clear decline of the behavior on day 2. These results suggest that the expression of ERβ in the DRN may be involved in the inhibitory regulation of sexual behavior on the day after behavioral estrus in cycling female mice.

Keywords: adeno-associated virus-mediated RNA interference, estrogen receptor β, estrogen receptor α, lordosis, dorsal raphe nucleus, estrogen, progesterone, serotonin

INTRODUCTION

The expression of female sexual behavior undergoes cyclic change during an estrus cycle. An ovarian hormone, 17β-estradiol (E_2) plays an essential role in this cyclic regulation of the behavior. In rodents, lordosis, a stereotypical female sexual behavior is expressed at high levels only during the time around ovulation, the period called as "behavioral estrus" occurring subsequently to the exponential elevation of circulating E_2. E_2 is known to act through at least two receptor subtypes, estrogen receptor (ER) α and β. Studies using knockout mouse models have shown that the level of sexual behavioral expression is greatly reduced in ERα knockout (αERKO) females (1–3) whereas in the ERβ knockouts (βERKO), such alteration is not observed (4, 5). It has also been reported that the selective ERα agonist, propyl-pyrazole triol facilitates female sexual behavior in ovariectomized female rat whereas the selective ERβ agonist, diarylpropionitrile (DPN) is unable to do so (6). Furthermore, Musatov et al. (7) demonstrated that the site-specific knockdown of ERα in the ventromedial nucleus of the hypothalamus (VMN) leads to a complete disappearance of female sexual behavior in mice. These studies collectively suggest that E_2 action through ERα, particularly in the VMN, is necessary for normal display of female sexual behavior whereas ERβ may not be involved in facilitatory regulation of female sexual behavior by E_2. However, close observation of gonadally intact βERKO mice has revealed an intriguing behavioral phenotype that the period of behavioral estrus may be extended in βERKO females (4). In these mice, the level of sexual receptivity was reported to stay high until the day after behavioral estrus when their respective wild-type (WT) mice show a clear decline of the behavior. In addition, except the day of behavioral estrus and the day after, βERKO females express very little receptive behavior similar to WT females (4). To replicate this finding in more hormonally controlled setting, we performed a preliminary experiment in ovariectomized βERKO females treated with exogenous ovarian steroids. We found that these females continuously showed elevated levels of lordosis expression 72 h after estradiol benzoate (EB) and 24 h after progesterone administration that mimic typical hormonal condition of the day after behavioral estrus (unpublished data). These findings collectively suggest that E_2 is not only promoting sexual behavior in females during the behavioral estrus with ERα dependent mechanisms but also involved in active inhibition of lordosis expression on the day after behavioral estrus by acting through ERβ. To further test this hypothesis and elucidate possible neural mechanisms of ERβ-mediated inhibitory regulation of lordosis, we aimed to identify the responsible brain site(s) in this study.

The dorsal raphe nucleus (DRN) is one of the brain areas that possibly act inhibitory on the expression of female sexual behavior. Lesions of this area are reported to increase lordosis expression in both EB-treated ovariectomized female rat and EB-treated castrated male rat (8–11) whereas the electrical stimulation of the DRN can lead to marked and immediate suppression of lordosis in ovariectomized female rat hormonally primed with EB and progesterone (12). In addition to its possible inhibitory role in the regulation of female sexual behavior, the DRN is also known for high levels of ERβ expression that is about two-fold of that of ERα within the nucleus (13, 14). Thus, it is reasonable to hypothesize that the DRN may be the brain site responsible for ERβ-mediated inhibitory action of E_2 in female sexual behavior. To test this hypothesis, we employed a virally mediated RNA interference method and examined the effects of site-specific knockdown of ERβ in the DRN on the expression of lordosis behavior.

MATERIALS AND METHODS

Subjects

Adult C57BL/6J female mice originally purchased from a commercial breeder (CLEA, Japan) and maintained in a breeding colony at the University of Tsukuba. All mice were housed under standard conditions (23 ± 2°C) with a 12:12-h light/dark cycle (lights off at 12:00). Food and water were provided *ad libitum*. All procedures were approved by the Animal Care and Use Committee and the Recombinant DNA Use Committee at the University of Tsukuba and conducted strictly in accordance with the National Institutes of Health guidelines. All efforts were made to minimize the number of animals and their suffering.

Design of Small Hairpin (sh) RNA for ER β Silencing

Adeno-associated virus (AAV) vectors expressing an shRNA against either the sequence specific for the ERβ gene (AAV-shERβ: 5′-GATCCCCGCCACGAATCAGTGTACCATCTTCCTGTCAATGGTACACTGATTCGTGGCTTTTTGGAAT-3′ and 5′-CTAGATTCCAAAAAGCCACGAATCAGTGTACCATTGACAGGAAGATGGTACACTGATTCGTGGCGGG-3′) or the sequence specific for luciferase (LUC) as control (AAV-shLUC: 5′-GATCCCCCCGCTGGAGAGCAACTGCATCTTCCTGTCAATGCAGTTGCTCTCCAGCGGTTTTTGGAAT-3′ and 5′-CTAGATTCCAAAAACCGCTGGAGAGCAACTGCATTGACAGGAAGATGCAGTTGCTCTCCAGCGGGGG-3′) were used. The nucleotides specific for ERβ or LUC are underlined. These vectors also express enhanced green fluorescent protein (GFP) as a reporter to visually detect transduced neurons.

Stereotaxic Surgery

Adult female mice (11.4 ± 2.2 weeks old) were assigned to either vector treatment (i) AAV-shERβ [ERβ knockdown (βERKD)] or (ii) AAV-shLUC (Control). They were anesthetized with sodium pentobarbital (60 mg/kg) and placed in a stereotaxic frame. A 5 μl Hamilton syringe inclined at 25° was aimed at the DRN [anteroposterior, −4.96 mm, mediolateral, 0.00 mm; dorsoventral, −3.40 mm] that was determined based on The Mouse Brain Stereotaxic Coordinates (15). Each mouse was injected with 0.5 μl of either AAV-shERβ or AAV-shLUC (10^{12} packaged genomic particles) using a micropump injector (World Precision Instruments Inc., USA). The injection lasted 5 min, and the needle was left in place for an additional 10 min following the end of infusion. Mice were then group housed with their littermates (4–5 mice/cage) until they were used for behavioral studies.

Ovariectomy and Hormone Treatment

Two weeks after stereotaxic surgery, all mice were ovariectomized (OVX) under isoflurane inhalation anesthesia. Mice were then individually housed in plastic cages (19 cm × 29 cm × 19 cm). All female mice were hormonally treated with weekly subcutaneous injections of EB (5 μg/0.1 ml sesame oil) followed by progesterone (P; 250 μg/0.1 ml sesame oil) at 44–46 h later, to mimic hormonal conditions in cycling females.

Sexual Behavior Test

Starting 1 week after OVX, all mice were weekly tested for sexual behavior against a sexually experienced male (gonadally intact ICR/Jcl) mouse in the males' home cages on two consecutive days, for a total of six trials during 3 weeks. For each week, mice were first tested 4–5 h after P injection which mimic the day of behavioral estrous (day 1), then tested again 24 h later (day 2)

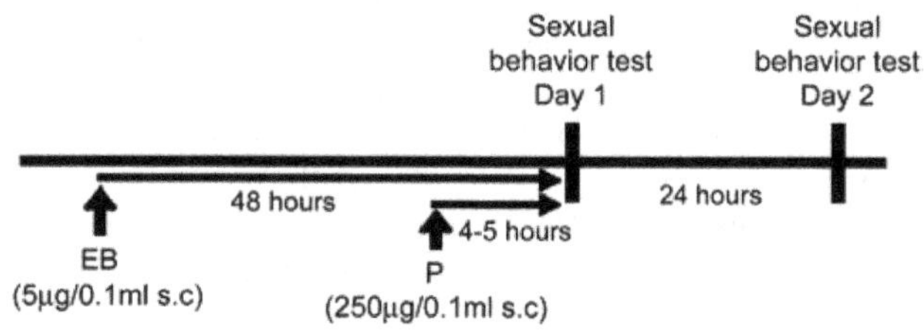

FIGURE 1 | Experimental paradigm.

(**Figure 1**). Each test was performed during the dark phase (starting 2–3 h after lights off) of the light/dark cycle under red light illumination. Each test lasted until females received 15 mounts or intromissions. Male intromissions were terminated (after about 8 thrusts) by the experimenter after female's behavioral responses were scored. Lordosis quotient (LQ) was calculated by dividing the number of lordosis responses by 15, the number of mounts or intromissions. In addition, each lordosis posture was given a score of 1–3 depending on the degree of dorsiflexion of the vertebral column and behaviors. For calculation of Lordosis Quality Scores, only lordosis responses that were given a score between 1 and 3 were included and averaged in each mouse. Mice with no lordosis response were excluded from the analysis in each test.

Tissue Preparation for Immunohistochemistry

Two weeks after the completion of behavioral testing, all mice were given subcutaneous injection of EB (5 µg/0.1 ml sesame oil). Forty-eight hours later, the time point matching the hormonal condition of day 1 tests, they were deeply anesthetized with a solution of 1:1 mixture of sodium pentobarbital (60 mg/kg) and heparin (1,000 U/kg) and transcardially perfused with 0.1 M phosphate-buffered saline (PBS; pH 7.2) followed by 4% paraformaldehyde (PFA) in 0.1 M phosphate buffer (PB; pH 7.2). Brains were removed and post-fixed overnight at 4°C in 4% PFA in 0.1 M PB. They were then rinsed with 0.1 M PB and cryoprotected in 0.1 M PB containing 30% sucrose.

Immunohistochemistry

Free-floating coronal sections (35 µm thickness) prepared on freezing microtome were split into four series (140 µm apart). One series of sections from each mouse was incubated in a rinse buffer, PBS-X (PBS and 0.2% Triton X-100), containing 1% hydrogen peroxide for 20 min to inhibit endogenous peroxidase activity, and then blocked in an incubation buffer (3% skim milk and 3% bovine serum albumin in PBS-X) for 2 h at room temperature. After the blocking process, they were incubated in a goat polyclonal anti-GFP antiserum (1:5,000; ab6673, Abcam) dissolved in the incubation buffer overnight at 4°C. Sections were then treated with a 1:250 dilution of biotinylated rabbit anti-goat secondary antibody (Vector Laboratories) in the incubation buffer for 2 h at room temperature, followed by 1 h incubation with avidin-biotin complex (Vectastain ABC Elite kit, Vector Laboratories) in TBS. After the completion of antiserum reaction procedures, sections were visualized with 0.02% diaminobenzidine and 0.003% hydrogen peroxide in TBS. A few sections from each group were also processed for immunohistochemical staining for ERβ. They were incubated in a rinse buffer, PBS-X, containing 1% hydrogen peroxide for 20 min, and then blocked in an incubation buffer (5% bovine serum albumin in PBS-X) for 2 h at room temperature. After the blocking process, they were incubated in a goat polyclonal anti-ERβ antiserum (1:1,000; Z8P, lot 10766190, Zymed Laboratories) dissolved in the incubation buffer for three days at 4°C. Sections were then treated with a1:250 dilution of biotinylated goat anti-rabbit secondary antibody (Vector Laboratories) in the incubation buffer for 4 h at room temperature, followed by 1 h incubation with avidin-biotin complex (Vectastain ABC Elite kit, Vector Laboratories) in TBS. After the completion of antiserum reaction procedures, sections were visualized with 0.03% diaminobenzidine, 0.15% $NiNH_4SO_4$, and 0.003% hydrogen peroxide in TBS.

All sections were mounted in gelatin-coated slides, air-dried and dehydrated through ascending alcohol series, which were cleared with xylene, and cover slipped with Permount (Fisher Scientific, USA). To verify the specificity of the immunohistochemical procedures, we included negative controls in which the primary antiserums were omitted from the staining procedure. In these conditions, neither cells nor fibers were stained.

The seven sections containing the DRN [Bregma −4.24 to −5.20 mm (15)] were obtained and photographed at 40× magnification with a digital camera mounted on an Olympus microscope (DP21, Olympus, Japan). To verify successful infusion of shRNA in the DRN, the distribution of GFP immunoreactive cells was evaluated on these seven sections.

Statistics

Lordosis quotients in the Control and βERKD groups were analyzed by a three-way analysis of variance (ANOVA) for repeated measurements for the main effects of vector treatment, day, week, and their interactions. LQs in the missed βERKD group were analyzed by a two-way ANOVA for repeated measurement for the main effect of day and week, and their interactions. ANOVAs were followed by Bonferroni *post hoc* test when it was appropriate. Lordosis Quality Scores were analyzed and compared by Mann–Whitney *U* test between day 1 and day 2 in each week in each vector treatment group. All data were presented as mean ± SEM. Statistically significant differences were considered at $p < 0.05$ (two-tailed). LQs were analyzed using SPSS 21.0 (SPSS Inc., Chicago, IL, USA) statistical package, and Lordosis Quality Scores were analyzed using StatView 5.0.1 (SAS Institute Inc., Cary, NC, USA).

RESULTS

Verification of Transfection

Similar to previous reports in the medial amygdala and medial preoptic area (16), the efficacy of the vector in silencing the expression of ERβ site-specifically in the DRN was confirmed as shown in **Figure 2**.

Successful infusion of shRNA in the DRN was confirmed in 12 females injected with AAV-shLUC (Control) and 10 females with AAV-shERβ (βERKD) (**Figure 3**). In addition to these mice in

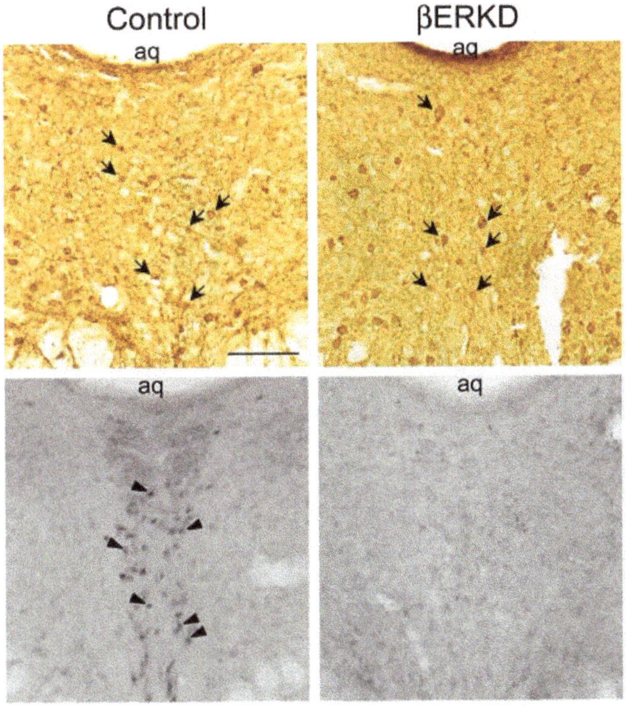

FIGURE 2 | Representative photomicrographs of immunohistochemically labeled cells for green fluorescent protein (GFP) in brain sections of control and ERβ knockdown (βERKD) groups (top panels), and those for estrogen receptor (ER) β in the adjacent sections (bottom panels). GFP and ERβ immunoreactive cells were detected by the methods described in the present and previous studies (16). The scale bar in the panel represents 100 μm. Arrows in the top panels indicate GFP stained cells, and arrow heads in the bottom panel indicate ERβ stained cells.

which AAV-shERβ was successfully infused into the entire DRN, there were five females in which AAV-shERβ was not spread in the mediodorsal area of dorsal part of the nucleus (**Figure 4**). These animals were classified as a missed βERKD group, and their behavioral data were analyzed separately. The mediodorsal area of dorsal part of the DRN was defined as the area within a 0.2 mm diameter circle placed on right below the bottom edge of the aqueduct and ranging from Bregma −4.48 to −4.84 mm (15) (**Figure 4**).

Effect of ERβ Knockdown in the DRN on the LQ

Knocking down of ERβ in the DRN dramatically affected LQ in day 2, but not in day 1. As shown in **Figure 5**, Control and βERKD showed similar levels of LQ on day 1 test in each week. In the Control group, the LQs were greatly decreased on day 2 compared with day 1 in all three weekly tests, whereas βERKD showed similar levels of LQ on day 2 as those on day 1 in all three tests. Three-way repeated measures ANOVA revealed significant effects of Day [$F(1, 20) = 22.247$, $P < 0.0001$], Treatment [$F(1, 20) = 4.881$, $P < 0.05$], and Week [$F(2, 40) = 37.487$, $P < 0.0001$]. There were significant interactions between Treatment and Day [$F(1, 20) = 5.518$, $P < 0.05$], Treatment and Week [$F(2, 40) = 3.876$, $P < 0.05$]. There were no statistically significant interactions between Day and Week [$F(2, 40) = 0.390$, ns] or Treatment, Day, and Week [$F(2, 40) = 0.381$, ns]. *Post hoc* analysis revealed that LQ on day 2 was lower than day 1 in the Control group alone (the day 1 vs. the day 2 in each test, $P < 0.01$, for control) in each test. However, there was no significant difference between day 1 and day 2 in LQ of βERKD in each test.

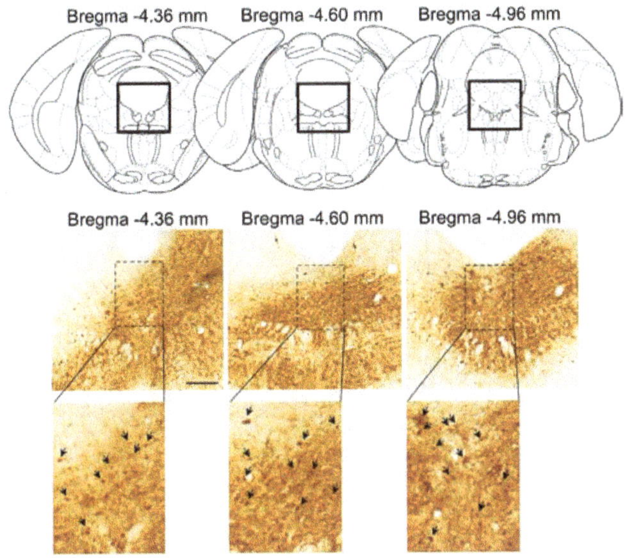

FIGURE 3 | Representative distribution pattern of adeno-associated virus within the dorsal raphe nucleus determined based on green fluorescent protein immunohistochemistry. The scale bar represents 200 μm.

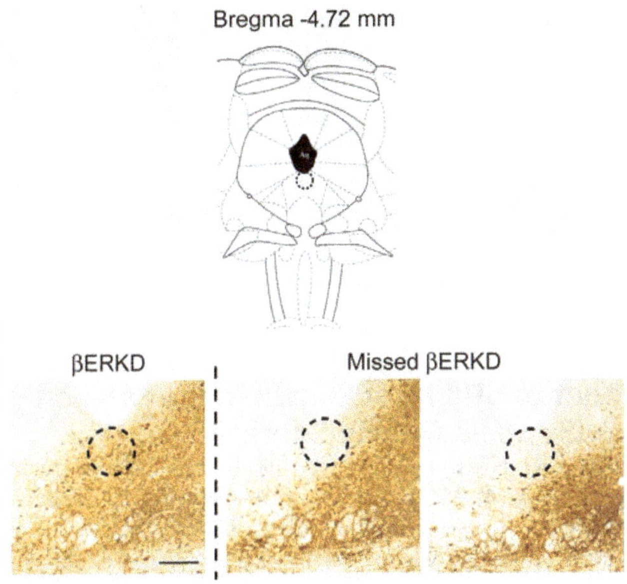

FIGURE 4 | Comparison of distribution pattern of adeno-associated virus within the mediodorsal area of dorsal part of the dorsal raphe nucleus (Bregma −4.72 mm) determined by green fluorescent protein immunohistochemistry in successful ERβ knockdown (βERKD) (left) and missed βERKD (middle and right) mice. The scale bar represents 200 μm.

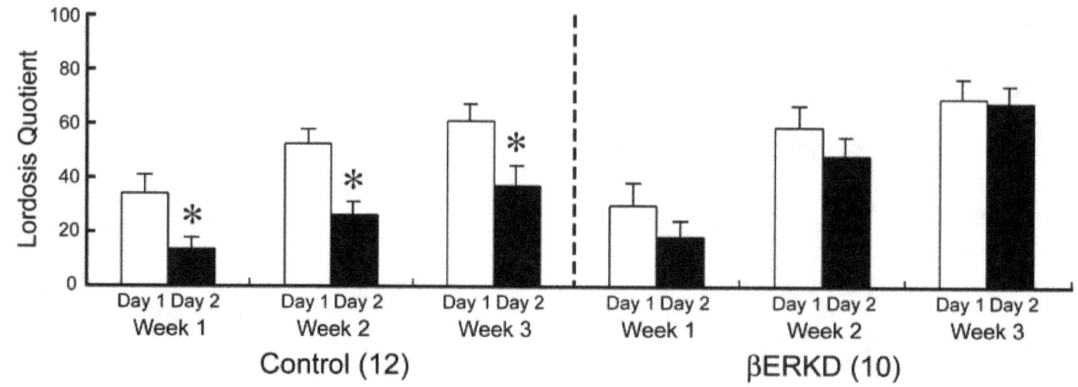

FIGURE 5 | Effect of estrogen receptor (ER) β knockdown in the dorsal raphe nucleus on Lordosis quotient (LQ). LQ of control (left) and ERβ knockdown (βERKD) (right) in each test. *$P < 0.05$ vs. day 1. Data presented as mean ± SEM.

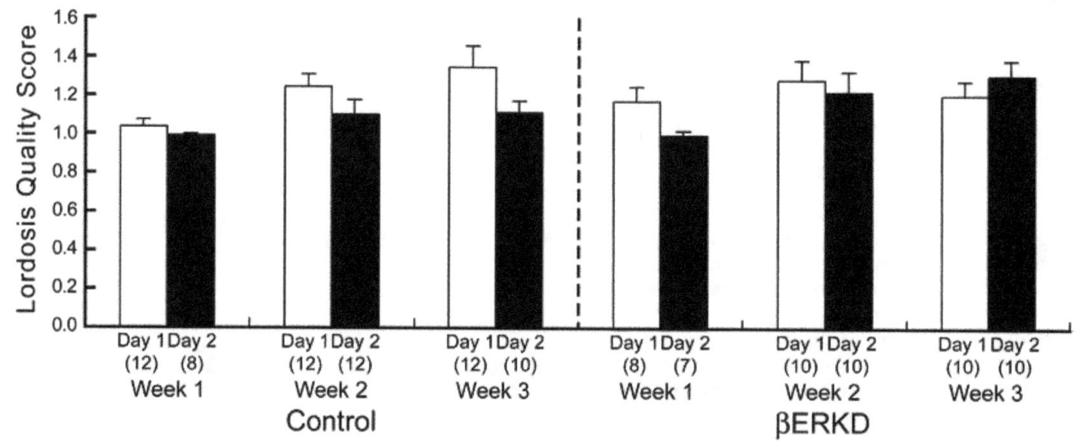

FIGURE 6 | Lordosis Quality Score of control (left) and ERβ knockouts (right) mice in each test. There was no difference between day 1 and day 2 in each week regardless of treatment group. The number in parentheses showed the number of mice which expressed lordosis (i.e., lordosis score of higher than 1) in each test.

Effect of ERβ Knockdown in the DRN on the Lordosis Quality Score

Estrogen receptor β knockdown did not affect the Lordosis Quality Score (**Figure 6**). Mann–Whitney U test revealed that there was no difference between day 1 and day 2 of Lordosis Quality Score in each week regardless of treatment group (Control: Week 1; $U = 44.000$, Week 2; $U = 40.500$, Week 3; $U = 33.500$, βERKD: Week 1; $U = 16.000$, Week 2; $U = 43.000$, Week 3; $U = 33.000$, all ns).

LQ of Missed βERKD Group

Behavioral data shown above included only mice in which the range of vector infusion covered the entire targeted area, but not elsewhere. These βERKD mice maintained the LQ that was equivalent to day 1 in day 2. On the other hand, such effect was absent if the virus did not spread into the mediodorsal area of dorsal part in the DRN. Two-way repeated measures ANOVA revealed significant effects of Day [$F(1, 4) = 21.574$, $P < 0.05$] and Week [$F(2, 8) = 7.704$, $P < 0.05$]. There were no statistically significant interactions between Day and Week [$F(2, 8) = 0.141$, ns].

DISCUSSION

In this study, we demonstrated that knocking down of ERβ in the DRN altered female sexual behavior on the day after behavioral estrus without affecting the behavior on the day of behavioral estrus. Our results showed that LQ between βERKD and Control mice was at a similar level on day 1 test performed at 44–46 h after EB and 4–6 h after progesterone injection that mimicked hormonal states of the day of behavioral estrus. By contrast, on day 2 test which corresponds to the day after behavioral estrus, βERKD mice still showed similar levels of LQ in comparison with their LQ on day 1 in each of three test. Control mice showed greatly decreased levels of LQ on day 2 compared with day 1 (**Figure 5**). These findings are consistent with previous studies using βERKO mice in which both gonadally intact and hormonally manipulated ovariectomized βERKO females continuously showed elevated levels of receptivity on the day after behavioral estrus [(4); unpublished data]. Thus, our finding suggests that the DRN is one of the brain sites responsible for the ERβ-mediated inhibitory regulation of female sexual behavioral expression on the day after behavioral estrus. On the other hand, Lordosis

Quality Score that indicates the quality of each lordosis was not different between day 1 and day 2 in both βERKD and Control groups (**Figure 6**). The brain sites responsible for the qualitative aspect of lordosis posture and possible involvement of gonadal steroids are not known. Our data indicate that ERβ expressed in the DRN may not be involved in the qualitative regulation of lordosis responses.

Furthermore, the knockdown effect was absent if the virus did not spread into the mediodorsal area within the dorsal part of the DRN even though the infusion was successful elsewhere within the nucleus (**Figures 4** and **7**). This finding may indicate that even within the DRN, the mediodorsal area of dorsal part is the most critical area for the ERβ-mediated inhibition of female sexual behavior on the day after behavioral estrus.

The exact mechanism of this ERβ-mediated inhibitory regulation of female sexual behavior has yet to be elucidated. However, it is possible to hypothesize that ERβ in the DRN may be involved in inhibition of female sexual behavior by intervening the serotonergic systems. Serotonin is known to act inhibitory on the expression of female sexual behavior through its binding to 5HT-1A receptors (17). The DRN is the largest serotonin synthesizing nucleus whose projections directly innervate the VMN and MPOA where 5HT-1A receptors are highly abundant (18–20). Selective lesions of serotonergic neurons projecting from the DRN to the VMN have been reported to facilitate lordosis (21). On the other hand, site-specific activation of 5HT-1A receptors either in the VMN or MPOA by local infusion of selective agonist, 8-hydroxy-2-(di-*n*-propylamino) tetralin (8-OH-DPAT) reduces the expression of lordosis in hormonally primed ovariectomized and gonadally intact proestrus female rats (22–24). Within the DRN, more than 95% of ERβ expressing neurons are serotonergic (14), and the majority of serotonergic neurons that project into the MPOA express ERβ (25). Furthermore, the administration of 17β-estradiol or ERβ-specific agonists, DPN to ovariectomized female rats are reported to enhance mRNA expression of tryptophan hydroxylase 2 (TPH 2), the rate-limiting enzyme for serotonin synthesis (26). In addition, the TPH 2 mRNA expression is greatly reduced in the DRN of βERKO female mice (14). Thus, ERβ in the DRN is possibly mediating the inhibition of female sexual behavior by upregulating the activity of the serotonergic system within the DRN that further activates 5HT-1A receptors expressed in hypothalamic regions such as the VMN and MPOA. The expression of 5HT-1A receptors in these regions seems to be also upregulated by estrogen (20, 27). Interestingly, a recent study by Spiteri et al. (28) reported that the site-specific knockdown of ERα in the MPOA, the region also known for its inhibitory role on the expression of female sexual behavior, increase the lordosis expression in response to a low dose EB treatment that generally fails to stimulate lordosis in ovariectomized females. Thus, the inhibitory action of the MPOA on the female sexual behavior seems to be ERα mediate although the crucial role of ERα in the VMN in the facilitation of the behavior is well known (7).

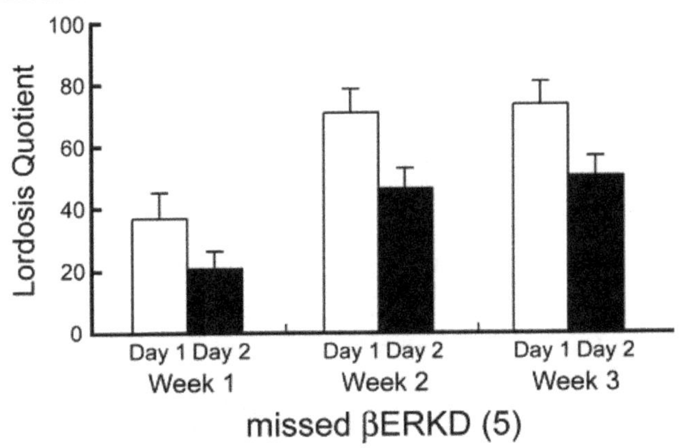

FIGURE 7 | Lordosis quotient of missed ERβ knockdown (βERKD) mice. Data presented as mean ± SEM.

Collectively with these studies, our present findings provide a significant piece to lay out the possible mechanism underling the cyclic regulation of female sexual behavior. Thus, on the day of behavioral estrus, high levels of circulating estradiol simultaneously (1) facilitate behavioral expression *via* ERα-mediated genomic action in the VMN, (2) upregulate 5HT-1A receptor expression *via* ERα in the hypothalamic areas such as the VMN and MPOA, while (3) upregulate TPH 2, the rate-limiting enzyme for serotonin synthesis in the DRN *via* ERβ. On the day after behavioral estrus, serotonin release by serotonergic neurons in the DRN may activate 5HT-1A receptors in the VMN and/or the MPOA and inhibit lordosis expression.

In addition to serotonin, progesterone is also known to inhibit the expression of female sexual behavior in its long-term effect while its short-term effect is facilitatory. Progesterone acts through progesterone receptor (PR), and the expression of the receptor is highly dependent on estrogen action. In female mice, the expression of PR in the VMN is known to be upregulated by estrogen *via* ERα (7). Whereas in the DRN, it seems to be ERβ dependent since EB administration still upregulate PR expression in the DRN of ovariectomized αERKO female mice (29). Moreover, estrogen-induced PR expression in the DRN found in αERKO female is suspected to be on the serotonergic neuron since the majority of PR immunoreactive cells coexpressed TPH immunoreactivity in these females (29). Therefore, it is reasonable to hypothesize that PR upregulation by E_2 in the DRN is mediated ERβ by and this progesterone–PR signaling pathway, in turn, may contribute the activation of serotonergic system that inhibits the expression of female sexual behavior on the day after behavioral estrus.

In this study, we focused on lordosis that reflects more of consummatory aspects. However, we cannot exclude the possible effect of ERβ knockdown in the DRN on behavioral components other than lordosis itself. Ogawa et al. (4) reported that gonadally intact βERKO female mice exhibited slightly higher levels of proceptivity throughout the estrous cycle compared with WT mice. Thus, in future experiments, it will be important to investigate the site-specific involvement of ERβ in the DRN in the appetitive aspects of female sexual behavior. It is also important to directly monitor or manipulate neuronal activity of ERβ- and/or PR-expressing cells and the serotonergic system within the DRN during both estrus and non-estrus phase to further elucidate neuronal and intracellular mechanisms of ERβ-mediated inhibitory regulation of female sexual behavior. Moreover, it is our great interest to investigate site-specific involvement of ERβ in brain regions other than the DRN such as the MPOA, the region also involved in the inhibitory regulation of female sexual behavior and known to highly express ERβ.

CONCLUSION

The main aim for this study was to elucidate site-specific involvement of ERβ expressed in the DRN in the inhibitory regulation of sexual behavior in female mice. This study demonstrated that βERKD mice continuously showed elevated levels of receptivity even on the day after behavioral estrus, whereas control mice showed greatly reduced receptivity on the day after behavioral estrus compared with the day of estrus. Therefore, the findings in this study suggest that ERβ in the DRN may be involved in the inhibition of female sexual behavior on the day after behavioral estrus. This is the first study to demonstrate the site-specific involvement of ERβ in the inhibitory regulation of female sexual behavior.

ETHICS STATEMENT

All procedures were approved by the Animal Care and Use Committee and the Recombinant DNA Use Committee at the University of Tsukuba and conducted strictly in accordance with the National Institutes of Health guidelines. All efforts were made to minimize the number of animals and their suffering.

AUTHOR CONTRIBUTIONS

KS, CM, and SO designed research and wrote the paper. KS, CM, MN, SM, MT, NY, and TS performed research and analyzed data. SM and SO contributed new reagents/analytic tools; KS and CM equally contributed to the study. SM designed and prepared the viral vectors expressing shRNAs used in this study.

FUNDING

This work was supported by Grant-in-Aid for Scientific Research 15H05724 to SO.

REFERENCES

1. Rissman EF, Early AH, Taylor JA, Korach KS, Lubahn DB. Estrogen receptors are essential for female sexual receptivity. *Endocrinology* (1997) 138:507–10. doi:10.1210/endo.138.1.4985
2. Ogawa S, Gordan JD, Taylor J, Lubahn D, Korach K, Pfaff DW. Reproductive functions illustrating direct and indirect effects of genes on behavior. *Horm Behav* (1996) 30:487–94. doi:10.1006/hbeh.1996.0052
3. Ogawa S, Eng V, Taylor J, Lubahn DB, Korach KS, Pfaff DW. Roles of estrogen receptor-alpha gene expression in reproduction-related behaviors in female mice. *Endocrinology* (1998) 139:5070–81. doi:10.1210/endo.139.12.6357
4. Ogawa S, Chan J, Chester AE, Gustafsson JÅ, Korach KS, Pfaff DW. Survival of reproductive behaviors in estrogen receptor beta gene-deficient (betaERKO) male and female mice. *Proc Natl Acad Sci U S A* (1999) 96:12887–92. doi:10.1073/pnas.96.22.12887
5. Kudwa AE, Rissman EF. Double oestrogen receptor alpha and beta knockout mice reveal differences in neural oestrogen-mediated progestin receptor induction and female sexual behaviour. *J Neuroendocrinol* (2003) 15:978–83. doi:10.1046/j.1365-2826.2003.01089.x
6. Mazzucco CA, Walker HA, Pawluski JL, Lieblich SE, Galea LAM. ERalpha, but not ERbeta, mediates the expression of sexual behavior in the female rat. *Behav Brain Res* (2008) 191:111–7. doi:10.1016/j.bbr.2008.03.016
7. Musatov S, Chen W, Pfaff DW, Kaplitt MG, Ogawa S. RNAi-mediated silencing of estrogen receptor {alpha} in the ventromedial nucleus of hypothalamus abolishes female sexual behaviors. *Proc Natl Acad Sci U S A* (2006) 103:10456–60. doi:10.1073/pnas.0603045103
8. Kakeyama M, Negishi M, Yamanouchi K. Facilitatory effect of ventral cut of dorsal raphe nucleus on lordosis in female rats. *Endocr J* (1997) 44:589–93. doi:10.1507/endocrj.44.589
9. Kakeyama M, Yamanouchi K. Lordosis in male rats: the facilitatory effect of mesencephalic dorsal raphe nucleus lesion. *Physiol Behav* (1992) 51:181–4. doi:10.1016/0031-9384(92)90221-M
10. Kakeyama M, Yamanouchi K. Inhibitory effect of baclofen on lordosis in female and male rats with dorsal raphe nucleus lesion or septal cut. *Neuroendocrinology* (1996) 63:290–6. doi:10.1159/000126968
11. Kakeyama M, Yamanouchi K. Lordosis in male rats: effect of dorsal raphe nucleus cuts. *Horm Behav* (1997) 32:60–7. doi:10.1006/hbeh.1997.1409
12. Arendash GW, Gorski RA. Suppression of lordotic responsiveness in the female rat during mesencephalic electrical stimulation. *Pharmacol Biochem Behav* (1983) 19:351–7. doi:10.1016/0091-3057(83)90064-3
13. Mitra SW, Hoskin E, Yudkovitz J, Pear L, Wilkinson HA, Hayashi S, et al. Immunolocalization of estrogen receptor beta in the mouse brain: comparison with estrogen receptor alpha. *Endocrinology* (2003) 144:2055–67. doi:10.1210/en.2002-221069
14. Nomura M, Akama KT, Alves SE, Korach KS, Gustafsson JÅ, Pfaff DW, et al. Differential distribution of estrogen receptor (ER)-alpha and ER-beta in the midbrain raphe nuclei and periaqueductal gray in male mouse: predominant role of ER-beta in midbrain serotonergic systems. *Neuroscience* (2005) 130:445–56. doi:10.1016/j.neuroscience.2004.09.028
15. Paxinos G, Franklin KBJ. *The Mouse Brain in Stereotaxic Coordinates*. 2nd ed. San Diego: Academic Press (2001).
16. Nakata M, Sano K, Musatov S, Yamaguchi N, Sakamoto T, Ogawa S. Effects of prepubertal or adult site-specific knockdown of estrogen receptor beta in the medial preoptic area and medial amygdala on social behaviors in male mice. *eNeuro* (2016) 3:1–14. doi:10.1523/ENEURO.0155-15.2016
17. Snoeren EMS, Veening JG, Olivier B, Oosting RS. Serotonin 1A receptors and sexual behavior in male rats: a review. *Pharmacol Biochem Behav* (2014) 121:102–14. doi:10.1016/j.pbb.2013.11.007
18. Azmitia EC, Segal M. An autoradiographic analysis of the differential ascending projections of the dorsal and median raphe nuclei in the rat. *J Comp Neurol* (1978) 179:641–67. doi:10.1002/cne.901790311
19. Ishimura K, Takeuchi Y, Fujiwara K, Tominaga M, Yoshioka H, Sawada T. Quantitative analysis of the distribution of serotonin-immunoreactive cell bodies in the mouse brain. *Neurosci Lett* (1988) 91:265–70. doi:10.1016/0304-3940(88)90691-X
20. Flügge G, Pfender D, Rudolph S, Jarry H, Fuchs E. 5HT1A-receptor binding in the brain of cyclic and ovariectomized female rats. *J Neuroendocrinol* (1999) 11:243–9. doi:10.1046/j.1365-2826.1999.00317.x
21. Moreines J, Kelton M, Luine VN, Pfaff DW, McEwen BS. Hypothalamic serotonin lesions unmask hormone responsiveness of lordosis behavior in adult male rats. *Neuroendocrinology* (1988) 47:453–8. doi:10.1159/000124949
22. Uphouse L, Caldarola-Pastuszka M. Female sexual behavior following intracerebral infusion of the 5-HT1A agonist, 8-OH-DPAT, into the medial preoptic area. *Brain Res* (1993) 601:203–8. doi:10.1016/0006-8993(93)91711-Z
23. Jackson A, Uphouse L. Dose-dependent effects of estradiol benzoate on 5-HT1A receptor agonist action. *Brain Res* (1998) 796:299–302. doi:10.1016/S0006-8993(98)00238-8
24. Uphouse L, White S, Harrison L, Hiegel C, Majumdar D, Guptarak J, et al. Restraint accentuates the effects of 5-HT2 receptor antagonists and a 5-HT1A receptor agonist on lordosis behavior. *Pharmacol Biochem Behav* (2003) 76:63–73. doi:10.1016/S0091-3057(03)00194-1
25. Lu H, Ozawa H, Nishi M, Ito T, Kawata M. Serotonergic neurones in the dorsal raphe nucleus that project into the medial preoptic area

contain oestrogen receptor beta. *J Neuroendocrinol* (2001) 13:839–45. doi:10.1046/j.1365-2826.2001.00695.x

26. Donner N, Handa RJ. Estrogen receptor beta regulates the expression of tryptophan-hydroxylase 2 mRNA within serotonergic neurons of the rat dorsal raphe nuclei. *Neuroscience* (2009) 163:705–18. doi:10.1016/j.neuroscience.2009.06.046
27. King TS, Steger RW, Morgan WW. Effect of ovarian steroids to stimulate region-specific hypothalamic 5-hydroxytryptamine synthesis in ovariectomized rats. *Neuroendocrinology* (1986) 42:344–50. doi:10.1159/000124461
28. Spiteri T, Ogawa S, Musatov S, Pfaff DW, Ågmo A. The role of the estrogen receptor alpha in the medial preoptic area in sexual incentive motivation, proceptivity and receptivity, anxiety, and wheel running in female rats. *Behav Brain Res* (2012) 230:11–20. doi:10.1016/j.bbr.2012.01.048
29. Alves SE, McEwen BS, Hayashi S, Korach KS, Pfaff DW, Ogawa S. Estrogen-regulated progestin receptors are found in the midbrain raphe but not hippocampus of estrogen receptor alpha (ERalpha) gene-disrupted mice. *J Comp Neurol* (2000) 427:185–95. doi:10.1002/1096-9861(20001113)427:2<185:AID-CNE2>3.0.CO;2-G

15

Brain Aromatase Modulates Serotonergic Neuron by Regulating Serotonin Levels in Zebrafish Embryos and Larvae

Zulvikar Syambani Ulhaq and Mitsuyo Kishida*

Graduate School of Science and Technology, Kumamoto University, Kumamoto, Japan

***Correspondence:**
Mitsuyo Kishida
mkishida@gpo.kumamoto-u.ac.jp

Teleost fish are known to express two isoforms of P450 aromatase, a key enzyme for estrogen synthesis. One of the isoforms, brain aromatase (AroB), *cyp19a1b*, is highly expressed during early development of zebrafish, thereby suggesting its role in brain development. On the other hand, early development of serotonergic neuron, one of the major monoamine neurons, is considered to play an important role in neurogenesis. Therefore, in this study, we investigated the role of AroB in development of serotonergic neuron by testing the effects of (1) estradiol (E_2) exposure and (2) morpholino (MO)-mediated AroB knockdown. When embryos were exposed to E_2, the effects were biphasic. The low dose of E_2 (0.005 μM) significantly increased serotonin (5-HT) positive area at 48 hour post-fertilization (hpf) detected by immunohistochemistry and relative mRNA levels of tryptophan hydroxylase isoforms (*tph1a*, *tph1b*, and *tph2*) at 96 hpf measured by semi-quantitative PCR. To test the effects on serotonin transmission, heart rate and thigmotaxis, an indicator of anxiety, were analyzed. The low dose also significantly increased heart rate at 48 hpf and decreased thigmotaxis. The high dose of E_2 (1 μM) exhibited opposite effects in all parameters. The effects of both low and high doses were reversed by addition of estrogen receptor (ER) blocker, ICI 182,780, thereby suggesting that the effects were mediated through ER. When AroB MO was injected to fertilized eggs, 5-HT-positive area was significantly decreased, while the significant decrease in relative *tph* mRNA levels was found only with *tph2* but not with two other isoforms. AroB MO also decreased heart rate and increased thigmotaxis. All the effects were rescued by co-injection with AroB mRNA and by exposure to E_2. Taken together, this study demonstrates the role of brain aromatase in development of serotonergic neuron in zebrafish embryos and larvae, implying that brain-formed estrogen is an important factor to sustain early development of serotonergic neuron.

Keywords: estradiol, brain aromatase, biphasic manner, serotonergic neuron, zebrafish, early development

INTRODUCTION

Biosynthesis of estrogen is catalyzed by the action of cytochrome P450 aromatase, a product of *cyp19a1* gene (1, 2). Contrary to mammals, zebrafish and many other teleosts have two isoforms of aromatase gene, *cyp19a1a* and *cyp19a1b*, encoding ovarian and brain aromatase, respectively (3, 4), and their predominant expression in respective tissues indicates differential regulation and functions. Fish brain is characterized by having much higher aromatase expression in brain compared to mammals (5). At the same time, fish brain has been reported to exhibit elevated neuroregenerative capacity compared to mammals (6–8). Widespread proliferation zones are detected in zebrafish brain (6, 9), while only limited areas such as subependymal and subgranular zones exhibit proliferation in mammals (7). Such high neurogenic activity in teleost fish may be attributed to increased synthesis of estrogen due to the elevated expression of brain aromatase. Indeed, expression of brain aromatase is localized in radial glial cells (RGCs), which differentiate into neurons and other glial cells contributing to adult neurogenesis as well as developmental neurogenesis (10–12). Developmental studies in zebrafish show that expression of brain aromatase in embryos increases rapidly after 12 hour post-fertilization (hpf), and is regulated by positive feedback loop through its own product, estrogen, acting on estrogen response element of *cyp19a1b* (3, 13, 14). Therefore, the zebrafish model expressing elevated levels of brain aromatase in early development is suitable to investigate the functional significance of aromatase and neural estrogen in developing brain.

Serotonin (5-HT), a neurotransmitter produced by multiple enzymatic steps including a rate-limiting action of tryptophan hydroxylase (TPH), plays a major role in a number of physiological processes and pathological conditions, such as depression (15, 16), stress (15, 17), cardiac function (18), reward seeking behavior (19), and anxiety (15, 20). In addition, serotonergic neuron is known to be involved in neurogenic activities (21). It has been reported that 5-HT is critically involved in the brain plasticity, neural trafficking, synapse formation, and network construction during development (22, 23). Serotonergic neurons in raphe nuclei extend their axons to the forebrain possibly modulating the differentiation of neuronal progenitors (24). Early ontogeny of serotonergic system may further suggest its role in brain development (25). Raphe 5-HT populations in human brain are considered as the earliest to be identified (24, 26).

Serotonergic neurons in mammalian brain are localized mainly in raphe nuclei of brain stem, which project into accumbens, hypothalamus, substantia nigra, and periaqueductal gray (22, 23). On the other hand, 5-HT-positive cell bodies are detected mainly in three populations in adult fish brain: pretectal area, posterior tuberculum/hypothalamus, and raphe (27, 28). Interestingly, distributions of serotonergic populations and their fibers overlap with highly proliferative areas of fish brain, which may indicate serotonergic regulation in adult neurogenesis in fish (27). In adult zebrafish, serotonin has been shown to promote regeneration of motor neurons by acting on progenitor cells (29).

It is well documented that serotonergic neuron is one of the targets of estrogen in mammals (30, 31). In macaques, estrogen increases gene expression and protein contents for TPH (32), and decreases gene expression of the serotonin reuptake transporter and the 5HT1A autoreceptor (33, 34). In mammals, both ERα and ERβ are expressed in 5-HT neurons with differential distributions depending on species and sex (35–37). ERβ has been shown to regulate *tph2* expression in serotonergic neurons (38, 39). Similarly in teleost fish, effects of ovarian steroids on serotonin system have been reported in some species. In tilapia, the response of 5-HT content in brain to E_2 treatment was dependent on developmental stages. Treatment between days 7 and 10 posthatching decreased 5-HT content, while the treatment at later stages increased it (40). Similar result was obtained in Japanese sea bass, which shows a significant decrease in brain 5-HT content in fingerlings after E_2 treatment, while the content increased in juvenile group (41). Indeed, overlapping distributions of ER with raphe 5-HT innervation in telencephalon and diencephalon of adult zebrafish brain implies close association of ER and serotonergic neurons (27, 42). It has been reported that ERβ exhibits broad distribution along the brain ventricles of telencephalon and diencephalon in adult zebrafish (43), though co-localization of ER in serotonergic neurons has yet to be documented in fish.

Therefore, in this study, we tested the hypothesis that brain aromatase modulates serotonergic neuron in early development of zebrafish. In order to elucidate a possible role of brain-formed estrogen, we first examined the effects of exogenous E_2 and then MO-mediated knockdown of brain aromatase on parameters such as 5-HT contents, relative *tph* expression levels, heart rate, and thigmotaxis in zebrafish embryos and larvae.

MATERIALS AND METHODS

Fish Maintenance and Embryo Culture

Adult zebrafish (*Danio rerio*) were obtained from the local pet shop and reared in a 60-L tank. Water temperature was maintained at 26–30°C, and the light regime was 14 h of light starting at 10:00 followed by 10 h of dark. Fish were fed with TetraMin (Tetra Japan Inc.) twice a day. Fertilized eggs were collected within 15 min after fertilization and washed in embryo medium (EM) (0.004% $CaCl_2$, 0.163% $MgSO_4$, 0.1% NaCl, and 0.003% KCl) to remove debris. Embryos were transferred to a 6-well plastic plate (30 embryos in 8 mL of EM per well), and incubated at 28 ± 0.5°C. The medium was changed daily. All experimental procedures and maintenance of fish were conducted in accordance with the Guide for Care and Use of Laboratory Animals published by the US National Institutes of Health.

Exposure Experiments

Stock solutions of 17β-estradiol (E_2) (Sigma-Aldrich) at 10 mM, ICI 182,780 (ICI) (Tocris Bioscience) at 10 mM, and dexamethasone (DEX) (Wako) at 100 mM were prepared in dimethyl sulfoxide (DMSO), and diluted with EM to the final concentrations indicated in the experiments. Quipazine maleate salt (Q) (Sigma-Aldrich) and fluoxetine hydrochloride (FLX) (Wako) were dissolved in ethanol at 100 and 10 mM, respectively, which were further diluted with EM to the final concentrations used in the experiments. Control embryos were cultured in 0.1% DMSO or ethanol. Exposure started at 2 hpf and continued till embryos and larvae were subjected to the assays. The media were changed daily.

Morpholino (MO) Microinjection

Morpholino antisense oligos were purchased from Gene Tool. MO sequences are shown in **Table 1**. MOs were dissolved in distilled water to 50 mg/mL and stored at −20°C. Before injection,

MO solution was heated at 65°C for 5 min and further diluted to the working concentrations (2.5 and 5 ng/nL) with deionized H_2O containing rhodamine B (Wako). The final concentration of rhodamine B was 0.08%. MO was injected into embryos at one to four cell stages using a glass microcapillary injection needle attached to the automatic nanoliter injector (Drummond Scientific). Injection volume was set at 2.3 nL per embryo. After the injection, embryos were observed under the fluorescence microscope (Leica M165 FC), and embryos that did not exhibit red fluorescence were discarded. To examine the effect of MO-mediated AroB knockdown, AroB MO designed to block translation was injected (2.5 and 5 ng/nL). Uninjected embryos (C), embryos injected with 5 ng/nL of standard control MO (Std MO), and inverted AroB MO (InvB MO) served as control groups. MO to block translation of *cyp19a1a*, ovarian aromatase (AroA MO) was also tested for 5-HT immunohistochemistry. As it has been reported that MO injection will cause off-target effect such as apoptosis through activation of *p53* gene (44, 45), MO to block translation of p53 (p53 MO) at 2 ng/nL was co-injected with AroB MO at 5 ng/nL.

For rescue experiments, the AroB mRNA (30 pg/nL) was co-injected with AroB MO (5 ng/nL). The full length AroB cDNA was obtained by One Step PrimeScript RT-PCR Kit (Takara) using total RNA from 7-dpf zebrafish larvae and AroB primers (**Table 2**). Amplified products were purified with NucleoSpin Gel and PCR Clean-up (Machery-Nagel) and subcloned into pGEM-T Easy Vector (Promega). Nucleotide sequences and orientation of the inserts were verified by DNA sequencing analysis carried out using BigDye Terminator v3.1 Cycle Sequencing Kit (Applied Biosystems) and ABI 3130 xl genetic analyzer (Applied Biosystems). Plasmid DNA was linearized with *SalI* and the full length AroB mRNA was transcribed *in vitro* by MAXIscript T7 Kit (Ambion).

TABLE 1 | Morpholino (MO) sequences.

Name	Sequence	Reference
AroA MO (ovarian aromatase MO) Genebank Acc. No.: AF226620	GGAGCAGATCACCTGCCATAAGAAC	This paper
InvA MO (inverted ovarian aromatase MO)	CAAGAATACCGTCCACTAGACGAGG	This paper
AroB MO (brain aromatase MO) Genebank Acc. No.: AF226619	ATCCTTTACCACATGCTCCATCATC	This paper
InvB MO (inverted brain aromatase MO)	CTACTACCTCGTACACCATTTCCTA	This paper
Std MO (standard control MO)	CCTCTTACCTCAGTTACAATTTATA	Gene tools
p53 MO Genebank Acc. No.: NM 131327	GCGCCATTGCTTTGCAAGAATTG	(44, 45)

Western Blot and Dot Blot Analysis

The antiserum to brain aromatase was produced in a rabbit against the synthetic peptide, CNSNGETADNRTSKE of zebrafish AroB (Sigma-Genosys). This peptide sequence has been used to raise the specific antibody as previously described (47). To confirm the specificity of the antiserum, Western blot of brain extract was conducted. Adult female zebrafish were exposed to E_2 (5 and 25 ng/L) or vehicle alone (0.00025% DMSO) for 24 h (three fish per group). Brains were pooled and homogenized in HBST buffer (100 mM NaCl, 10 mM HEPES, 0.5% Triton-X 100, 0.01% TPCK, and 0.01% TLCK). After centrifugation at 10,000 *g* for 10 min, protein concentrations in supernatant were measured using BCA protein assay kit (Thermo Scientific). Extracts (30 μg protein/sample) were separated on 12.5% SDS-PAGE and transferred to a PVDF membrane. Precision Plus Protein Unstained Standards (Bio-Rad) were used for size reference. After blocking by 1% skim milk in PBS for 1 h, the membrane was incubated with the AroB antiserum (1:500) for 2 h, and then with the secondary antibody

TABLE 2 | PCR primers and conditions.

Gene	Primer sequence (5′ → 3′)	Size of PCR product (bp)	Amplification profile
tph1a	F: TTCAAGGACAATGTCTATCG R: GGGAGTCGCAGTGTTTGATG Genebank Acc. No.: AF548566 (46)	214	94°C—30 s 55°C—30 s 72°C—60 s (35 cycles)
tph1b	F: TACCTGCAGAACCTGCCTCT R: AGAGAAGACCAGCCCCGTAT Genebank Acc. No.: BC154120 (46)	430	94°C—30 s 55°C—30 s 72°C—60 s (35 cycles)
tph2	F: GTGTGAACTCCAAAGCAGCA R: TGGTATTCCTTCCCCATCTG Genebank Acc. No.: AB125219 (46)	684	94°C—30 s 55°C—30 s 72°C—60 s (35 cycles)
cyp19a1b (AroB)	F: TTAAAGAGGTGTGTCTGTATGTGAGGTG R: GGAATTTACTCTGTGCGCCTTTAAATGT Genebank Acc. No: BC076104	1,435	42°C—10 min 94°C—30 s 60°C—15 s 72°C—90 s (40 cycles)
β-Actin	F: GGTATGGGACAGAAAGACAG R: AGAGTCCATCACGATACCAG Genebank Acc. No: AF025305 (3)	330	94°C—30 s 58°C—30 s 72°C—60 s (34 cycles)

conjugated with alkaline phosphatase (AP) (Abcam) (1:1,000) for 1 h. After washing, the membrane was incubated in AP buffer (0.1 M Tris–HCl, pH 9.5, 0.1 M NaCl, 1 M MgCl) for 1 min. Signals were developed for 2–3 min in BCIP/NBT substrate (Roche) diluted at 1:50 in AP buffer, and the reaction was stopped by 0.5 M EDTA. All the incubation steps were done at RT. The antiserum to ovarian aromatase was raised in a rabbit using a synthetic peptide, CKPDVYFRLDWLHKKHKRD of zebrafish AroA (Sigma-Genosys). Similarly, Western blot with the antiserum (1:500) was performed using the ovarian extract prepared with HBST buffer from three adult fish (30 μg/lane).

To examine the effect of MO-mediated AroB knockdown, dot blot analysis using 120 larvae at 6 dpf collected from 4 separate MO injection experiments were pooled and extracted similarly as described for the brain extract. Extracts containing 40 μg protein (3 μL) were spotted onto nitrocellulose membrane (GVS Life Science). The membrane was treated similarly as in Western blot except for the concentration of the secondary antibody at 1:2,000. Density of the blots were analyzed with NIH ImageJ software. Blots of embryo extracts treated with the pre-immunized rabbit serum were used as a negative control to subtract from the density obtained with the AroB antiserum. No changes were observed among controls (uninjected, standard control MO, and inverted AroB MO) (data not shown). The effect of MO-mediated AroA knockdown was also examined by dot blot analysis. Briefly, pooled 120 embryos at 2 dpf collected from 5 separate embryo cohorts were extracted. Extracts containing 30 μg protein (3 μL) were spotted onto nitrocellulose membrane and subjected to immunostaining using AroA antiserum at 1:500. No changes were observed among controls including inverted AroA MO (data not shown).

5-HT Immunohistochemistry

Whole-mount immunohistochemistry for 5-HT was carried out according to the previous studies (48, 49). 2-dpf embryos were fixed in 4% paraformaldehyde in PBS overnight at 4°C. Fixed embryos were rinsed in PBS, bleached in 3% H_2O_2 for 30 min and stored in methanol at −20°C until use. For immunostaining, embryos were washed in PBS containing 0.1% Tween-20 and 0.5% Triton X-100 (PBSTX), and then permeabilization was achieved by incubation in deionized H_2O for 60 min at RT followed by 100% acetone for 8 min at −20°C. Non-specific binding was blocked by incubation in 10% normal goat serum (NGS) and 3% BSA for 3 h at RT. After several washes with PBSTX, embryos were incubated in rabbit polyclonal anti 5-HT (ImmunoStar) diluted at 1:500 in 10% NGS/PBS containing 0.3% Triton-X 100 for 2 days at 4°C. After rinsing in PBSTX for 4 h, embryos were incubated in the goat anti-rabbit IgG Alexa Fluor 488 (Molecular Probes Invitrogen Detection Technologies) diluted at 1:100 in 10% NGS/PBS overnight at 4°C. After thorough washing in PBSTX, embryos were mounted in 0.5% agarose and observed under the fluorescence microscope (Leica M165 FC). Negative controls processed by omitting incubation with the primary antibody or by replacing the primary antibody with normal rabbit serum showed no positive signals. For measurement of 5-HT-positive area, focus was adjusted on the field with the largest positive area, and NIH ImageJ software was used to quantify manually outlined areas. Immunostaining was performed using five to eight embryos per group, and the experiments were done in triplicate.

RT-PCR

Total RNA was extracted from larvae at 4 and 7 dpf (25 larvae/group) using ISOGEN II (Nippon Gene) and treated with DNase free (Ambion). cDNA was synthesized from 1 μg total RNA using Reverse Transcription System (Promega). A total reaction volume of 25 μL containing 2× GoTaq Green Master Mix (Promega), 10 μM of each primer, and 1 μL cDNA was subjected to PCR using Program Temp Control System PC708 (Astec). β-Actin was used as an internal control. Amplification conditions and primer sequences are listed in **Table 2**. The amplified products were separated on a 2% agarose gel. Levels of mRNAs expression were analyzed by NIH ImageJ software and normalized by the expression level in the control group at each developmental time. Experiments were done in triplicate.

Heart Rate Measurement

Embryos at 2 dpf were individually placed in a well of a 12-well culture plate containing 500 μL of corresponding experimental medium and kept for 15 min to allow heartbeats to resume a steady rate. Heart beats were counted manually for 15 s under a stereo microscope (Leica 58APO). Ten embryos were used for each group. Experiments were repeated three times with eggs collected from different spawns.

Thigmotaxis Assay

Assay was performed according to the protocols described previously (49, 50). Briefly, zebrafish larvae at 6 dpf were transferred into a 6-well tissue culture plate with one fish per well containing 4 mL EM. The bottom of each well was divided into two portions designated as inner and outer zones. After habituation at 28°C for 2 h followed by acclimation under the video camera for 5 min, swimming activity was recorded for 5 min. For each group, 12 larvae were used. Data from 36 larvae from three different spawns were pooled and analyzed to express % of time a fish spent in the outer zone.

Statistical Analysis

Data are presented as mean ± SEM. Statistical differences between groups were evaluated by one-way ANOVA followed by Tukey's or least significant difference *post hoc* test using IBM SPSS statistics version 19. Unpaired Student's *t*-test was used for the dot blot analysis. Kruskal-Wallis test and Mann–Whitney *U* test were used for thigmotaxis assays, as the data did not meet the assumptions required for parametric testing. Significant differences were accepted when $p < 0.05$.

RESULTS

Effect of E_2 Exposure on Serotonergic Neuron

5-HT-positive neurons were detected in the embryos at 2 dpf by whole-mount fluorescent immunohistochemistry (**Figure 1A**). Positively stained neurons were located in pretectal and thalamic

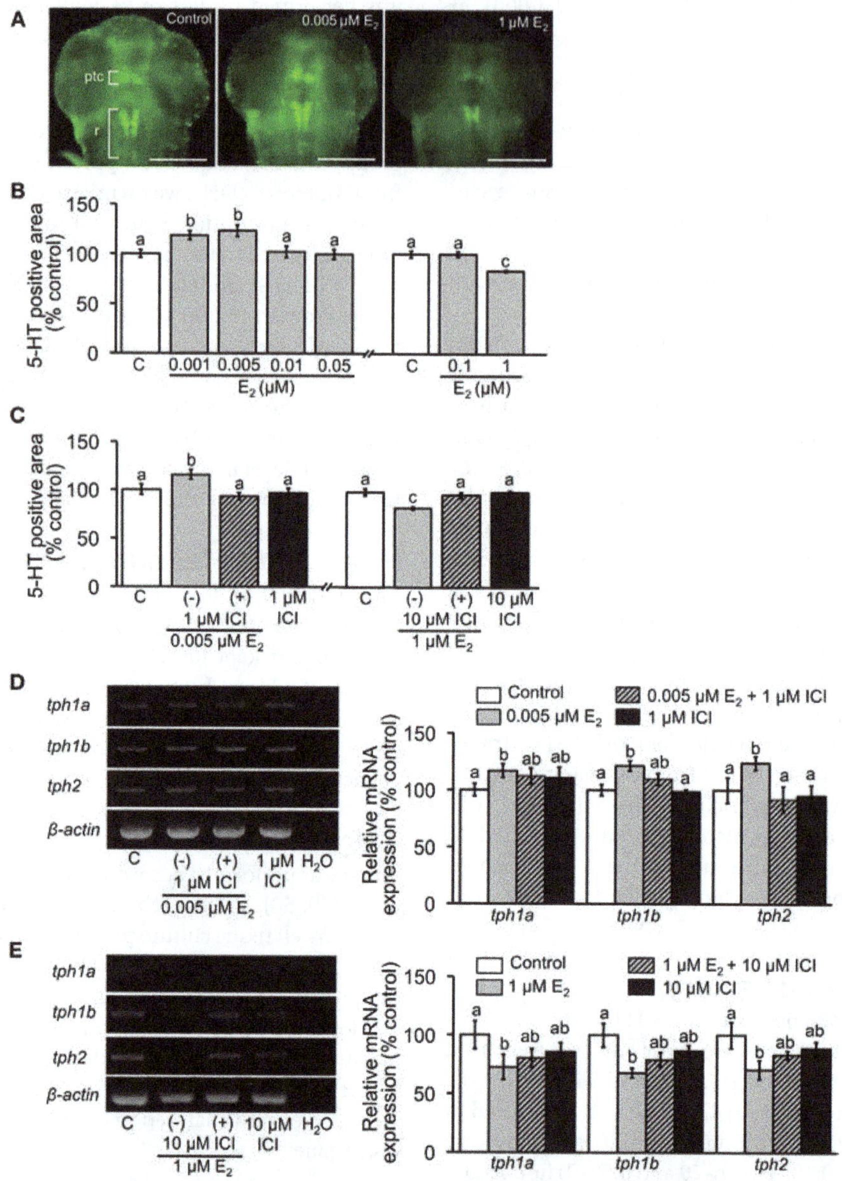

FIGURE 1 | Effect of E_2 on 5-HT-positive area and relative expression of *tph* isoforms. **(A)** Representative images of ventral view of head region showing 5-HT-positive cells in pretectal and thalamic complex (ptc) and raphe (r) at 2 dpf. Scale bar: 200 μm. **(B,C)** Measurements of the area of 5-HT-positive neurons in the experiment of E_2 exposure and co-incubation of E_2 and ICI, respectively. **(D,E)** Semi-quantitative PCR for expression of *tph* isoforms in 4 dpf larvae in the experiments of exposure to low and high doses of E_2 and co-incubation with ICI, respectively. Data are presented as a mean ± SEM. Different letters in each graph indicate significant differences ($p < 0.05$).

complex and raphe as reported previously (48, 51–54). 5-HT-positive areas were significantly increased when exposed to low doses E_2 (0.001 and 0.005 μM) but decreased in high dose (1 μM) exposure (**Figure 1B**). Effects of both low and high doses E_2 were significantly reversed by addition of 1 or 10 μM ICI, respectively (**Figure 1C**).

Relative expression levels of *tph* isoforms at 4 dpf were analyzed by semi-quantitative PCR. Significant increase in expression was detected in all *tph* isoforms when embryos were exposed to low-dose E_2 (0.005 μM). Addition of 1 μM ICI completely reversed the decreased expression of *tph2*, while expressions of *tph1a* and *tph1b* were reversed partially (**Figure 1D**). Conversely, high-dose E_2 exposure significantly decreased expression levels of all isoforms, which was partially reversed by addition of 10 μM ICI (**Figure 1E**).

When the embryos were exposed to E_2, the heart rate at 2 dpf was significantly increased in the 0.005 μM group, while significant decrease was found in the 0.1 and 1 μM groups (**Figure 2A**). Addition of 1 and 10 μM ICI significantly reversed the effects caused by low or high dose of E_2, respectively (**Figure 2A**). To verify the role of serotonergic signaling in regulation of heart rate, effects of Q (5-HT agonist) and FLX (5-HT selective re-uptake

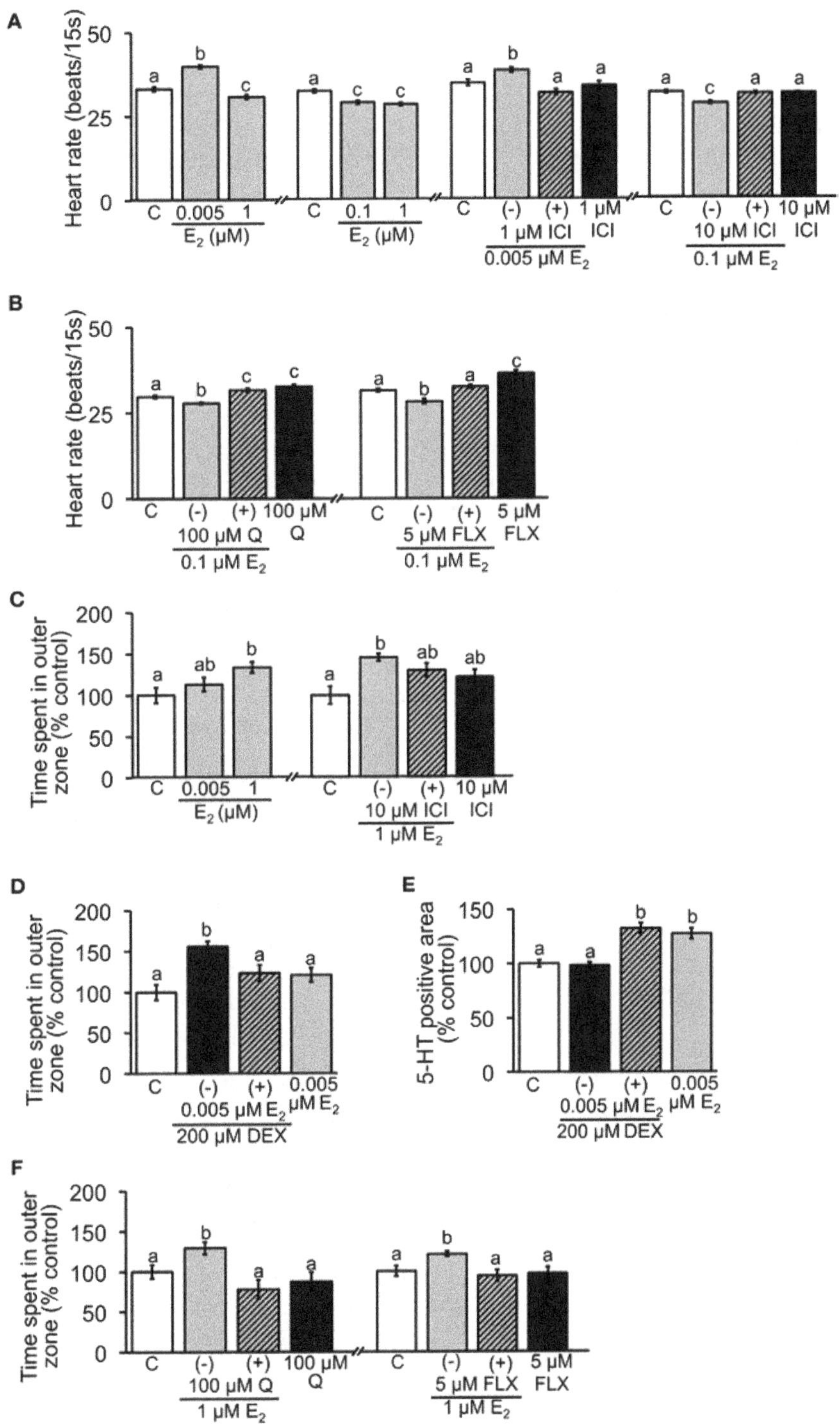

FIGURE 2 | Effect of E_2 on heart rate and thigmotaxis. Heart rate was measured in 2-dpf embryos; **(A)** exposure to low and high doses of E_2 and co-incubation with ICI; **(B)** co-incubation of E_2 and Q or FLX to examine involvement of serotonin signaling. Thigmotaxis assay was performed to evaluate anxiety level in 6-dpf larvae; **(C)** exposure to low and high doses of E_2 and co-incubation with ICI; **(D)** anxiolytic effect of low dose of E_2 when larvae were exposed to 200 μM DEX. **(E)** Measurements of 5-HT-positive neuron area in 2-dpf embryos exposed to DEX and low dose of E_2. **(F)** Effects of co-incubation of E_2 and Q or FLX on thigmotaxis to examine involvement of serotonin signaling. Data are presented as a mean ± SEM. Different letters in each graph indicate significant differences ($p < 0.05$).

inhibitor) were tested. Co-incubation with 0.1 μM E_2 significantly reversed the decreased heart rate caused by E_2. Heart rate was significantly increased when exposed to Q or FLX alone (**Figure 2B**).

Thigmotaxis assay was performed using 6-dpf larvae. Exposure to 1 μM E_2 increased the time fish spent in outer zone, suggesting that anxiety was increased, but no significant difference was observed in 0.005 μM E_2 group (**Figure 2C**). Addition of 10 μM ICI partially reversed the increase caused by 1 μM E_2 (**Figure 2C**). To further examine the effect of low-dose E_2, embryos were exposed to 200 μM DEX and subjected to the assay. DEX alone increased the time, but co-incubation with 0.005 μM E_2 significantly reduced the increase (**Figure 2D**). Immunostaining for 5-HT showed that co-incubation of low-dose E_2 and DEX increased the positive staining, although DEX alone had no effect (**Figure 2E**). To verify the role of serotonergic signaling in thigmotaxis assay, effects of Q and FLX were tested. Both Q and FLX significantly decreased the time fish spent in outer zone caused by 1 μM E_2 exposure (**Figure 2F**).

Validation of MO-Mediated Knockdown Using the Specific Antisera

Specificity of the antisera to AroB and AroA was examined by Western blot. The anti-AroB revealed a single band at the expected size of 50 kDa in brain extract from the fish exposed to E_2 at 25 ng/L (47) (**Figure 3A**). The anti-AroA detected a single band at the expected size of 75 kDa in the ovarian extract (**Figure 3A**), which is in agreement with the previous study (55). In addition, immunohistochemistry of the ovary showed similar localization of AroA as previously described (56) (data not shown).

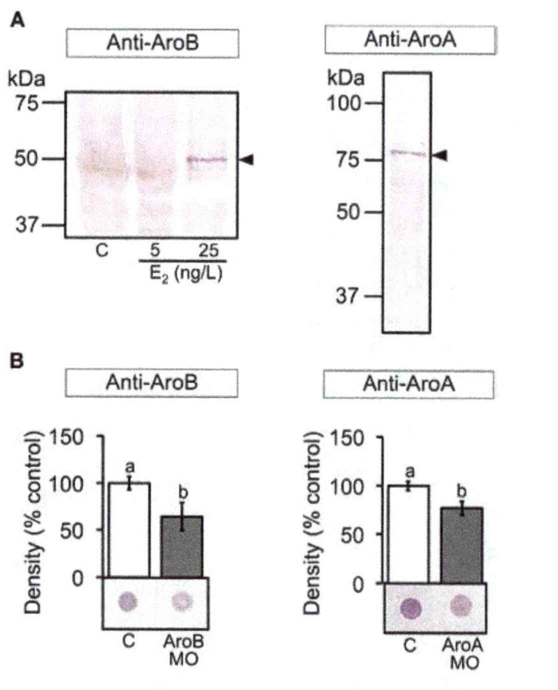

FIGURE 3 | Validation of MO-mediated knockdown on translation. **(A)** Western blots of brain extracts from control and E_2 exposed fish and ovarian extract from untreated fish were stained with the antiserum to AroB and AroA, respectively, showing a positive band at the expected size for each aromatase as indicated by arrowheads. **(B)** Dot blots of 6 and 2 dpf larval extracts using the antiserum to AroB and AroA, respectively, were analyzed. Representative blots are shown in each graph. Data are presented as a mean ± SEM. Different letters in each graph indicate significant differences ($p < 0.05$).

The dot blot analysis of the larval extracts showed that both AroB and AroA MO injections significantly decreased immunoreactivity compared to the uninjected control, indicating decreased translation of AroB and AroA, respectively (**Figure 3B**). Std MO, InvB, or InvA MO did not show any significant difference compared to the uninjected control (data not shown).

Effect of MO-Mediated Knockdown of AroB on Serotonergic Neuron

When AroB MO was injected, 5-HT-positive area was significantly decreased in the 5 ng/L group and partially decreased in the 2.5 ng/nL group compared to the uninjected control (**Figure 4A**). Injections of Std MO and InvB MO did not show any significant difference in 5-HT-positive areas compared to the uninjected control (**Figure 4A**). Moreover, the injection of AroA did not show any changes (**Figure 4A**). The decrease in 5-HT-positive area caused by AroB was completely rescued by co-injection of 30 pg/nL AroB mRNA (**Figure 4B**) and partially rescued by E_2 exposure at 0.1 μM (**Figure 4C**). When p53 MO was co-injected with AroB MO to examine off-target effect, no significant difference in 5-HT-positive area was observed, suggesting that decrease in 5-HT-positive area caused by AroB MO is not due to apoptosis caused by *p53* activation (**Figure 4D**).

The effect of AroB MO injection on relative expression of *tph* isoforms was evaluated by semi-quantitative PCR using 7-dpf larvae. While expression levels of *tph1a* and *tph1b* showed no significant changes, expression of *tph2* isoform was significantly decreased and partially rescued by E_2 exposure at 0.1 μM (**Figure 4E**).

Heart rate of AroB MO injected embryos was significantly decreased compared to the uninjected or Std MO and InvB MO injected controls (**Figure 5A**). The decrease caused by AroB MO was rescued either by co-injection of AroB mRNA or by exposure to 0.1 μM E_2 (**Figures 5B,C**). Exposure to 100 μM Q as well as to 5 μM FLX (**Figure 5D**) reversed the decrease to the control level.

In thigmotaxis assay, AroB MO injection caused significant increase in time fish spent in outer zone compared to the uninjected, Std MO injected, and InvB MO injected controls (**Figure 5E**). This effect of AroB MO was rescued either by co-injection of AroB mRNA or by exposure to 0.1 μM E_2 (**Figures 5F,G**). Exposure to 100 μM Q as well as to 5 μM FLX reversed the time fish spent in outer zone increased by AroB MO injection (**Figure 5H**).

DISCUSSION

The aim of this study is to elucidate the role of estradiol and brain aromatase in modulation of serotonergic neurons in early development of zebrafish, as the early ontogeny of serotonergic system may be one of the important factors for neuronal growth and brain development. We demonstrated that exogenous administration of E_2 biphasically affected parameters such as 5-HT-positive areas, relative expression of *tph* isoforms, heart rate and thigmotactic behavior with stimulation and suppression of serotonin system at the low dose and the high dose,

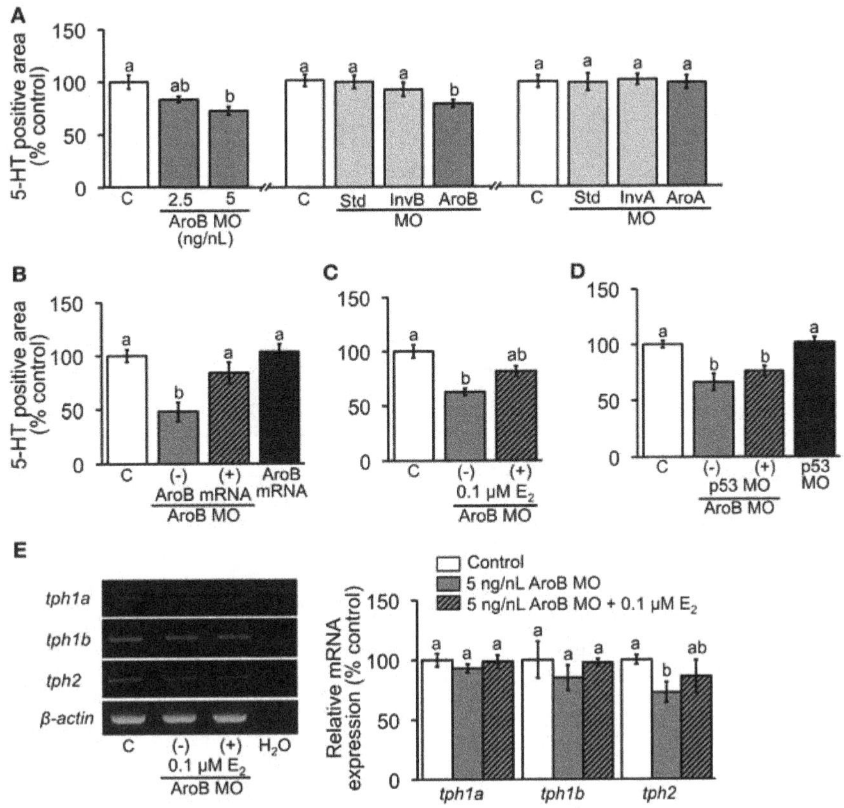

FIGURE 4 | AroB MO-mediated effect on serotonergic neuron. 5-HT-positive neuron area was measured in 2-dpf embryos; **(A)** injection of AroB MO and control MOs (Std MO, InvB MO and AroA MO); **(B,C)** co-injection of AroB mRNA and exposure to E_2, respectively, to rescue the effect of AroB MO; **(D)** co-injection of p53 MO to test off-target effect of AroB MO. **(E)** Semi-quantitative PCR measurement of expression of *tph* isoforms in 6-dpf larvae injected with AroB MO with and without exposure to E_2. Data are presented as a mean ± SEM. Different letters in each graph indicate significant differences ($p < 0.05$).

respectively, through acting on ER. On the other hand, activities of serotonergic neurons were suppressed by AroB MO-mediated knockdown, suggesting that brain-formed E_2 in early development stimulates serotonergic neurons, which is in accordance with the results of the low-dose E_2. Recent study shows that MO-mediated brain aromatase knockdown results in a significant decrease in E_2 concentration in 48 hpf embryos (57), which supports that our MO experiments reflect the reduction of estrogen production.

Non-monotonic dose responses of hormones and endocrine-disrupting chemicals have been widely documented (58). Estrogen among other hormones is known to exhibit biphasic dose-dependent effects in various physiological processes (59–66). However, only limited information is available in regards to serotonin system. There is one study in fish showing that low dose of E_2 stimulated monoamine oxidase activity and decreased 5-HT content in hypothalamus in ovariectomized catfish, while the result was opposite for high dose (67). Our study demonstrates that biphasic dose-dependent effects of E_2 on serotonergic neuron in fish, and shows that the effects or both low and high doses are mediated through ER, indicating physiological relevance. The effect of the low dose of E_2, stimulating serotonergic neuron, is likely to reflect the role of endogenous E_2 in embryos, as AroB MO-mediated effects demonstrate that brain-formed estrogen is necessary to maintain activity of serotonergic neuron in embryos. Mechanisms of biphasic responses are complex, but may be in part controlled by downregulation and desensitization of receptors (57, 68). Thus, effects of high doses of E_2 on serotonergic neuron in this study may be due to downregulation/desensitization of ERs. Sequence analysis of the promoter region of zebrafish *tph* isoforms shows the presence of 1/2 ERE in the upstream of transcription start site in all isoforms, suggesting possible nuclear action of estrogen, though their functional analysis is yet to be reported. In human serotonergic cell line, binding of E_2 and ERβ has been shown to directly interact with 1/2 ERE of *tph2* promoter to elicit gene expression (39). In addition to the classical action of E_2 on nuclear receptors membrane ERs plays an important role in brain (69, 70). Interaction between membrane ERs and the metabolic glutamate receptor in the brain provides a rapid and transient E_2 action (71, 72). Membrane bound G-protein-coupled ER, GPER/GPR30, also known to be involved in modulating rapid non-genomic action of E_2, plays a role in several brain areas (73). Estrogen action through GPR30 has been suggested in regulation of serotonergic neuron in mammals (74). Further studies are required to elucidate the mechanisms by which estrogen regulates serotonergic neuron in zebrafish.

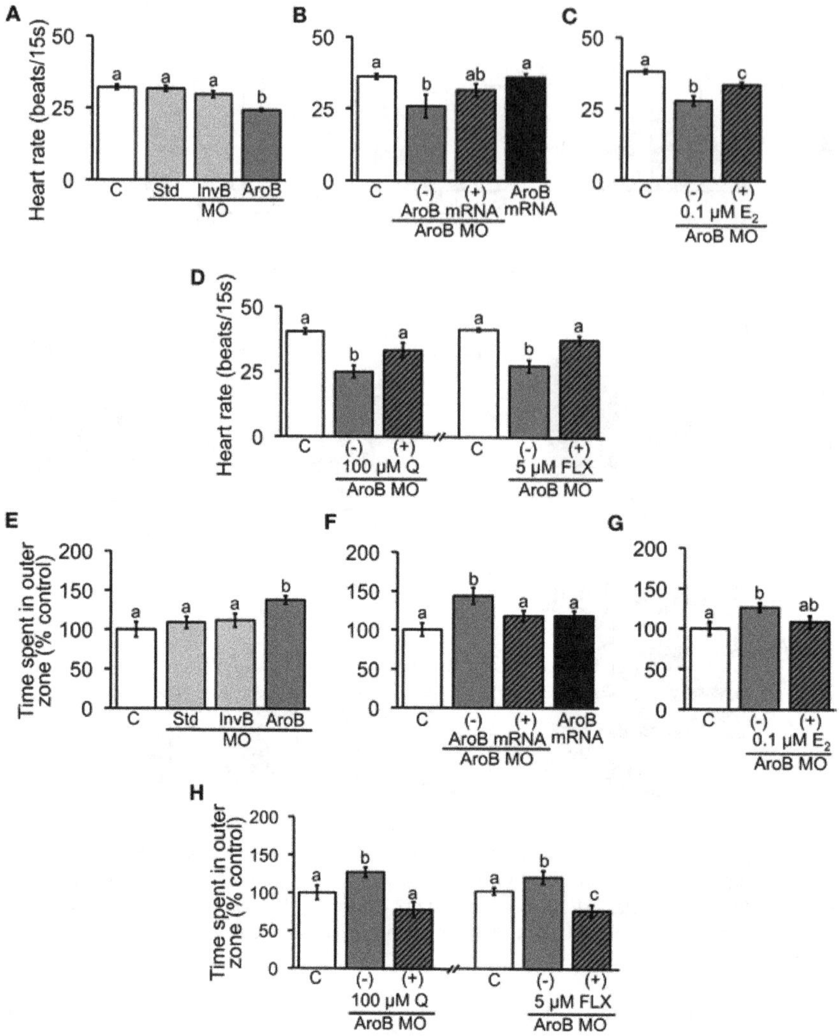

FIGURE 5 | AroB MO-mediated effect on heart rate and thigmotaxis. Heart rate was measured in 2-dpf embryos; **(A)** injection of AroB MO and control MOs; **(B,C)** co-injection of AroB mRNA and exposure to E_2, respectively, to rescue the effect of AroB MO; **(D)** injection of AroB MO with and without exposure to Q and FLX to examine involvement of serotonin signaling. Thigmotaxis assay was conducted using 6-dpf larvae; **(E)** injection of AroB MO and control MOs; **(F,G)** co-injection of AroB mRNA and exposure to E_2, respectively, to rescue the effect of AroB MO; **(H)** injection of AroB MO with and without exposure to Q and FLX to examine involvement of serotonin signaling. Data are presented as a mean ± SEM. Different letters in each graph indicate significant differences ($p < 0.05$).

Attenuation of serotonergic neuron by AroB MO-mediated knockdown clearly demonstrated that brain-formed estrogen is necessary to maintain the serotonin system to control heart rate and anxiety behavior in early development of zebrafish. Validity of AroB knockdown was supported by several lines of evidence. Immunoreactivity to the antiserum specific to AroB was decreased in AroB MO injected embryos. In addition to no significant effects found in the controls including standard MO, inverted AroB MO and AroA MO-injected embryos, AroB MO-mediated effects were rescued by co-injection of AroB mRNA and exposure to E_2. Off-target effect of MO injection was also examined by knockdown of *p53*, showing that the decreased 5-HT-positive area caused by AroB MO is not through activation of *p53*. The decrease in 5-HT-positive area by AroB MO injection indicates that brain-formed estrogen stimulates 5-HT synthesis, which is in accordance with the stimulatory effect of low-dose E_2. When the relative expressions of *tph* isoforms were examined in AroB MO injected embryos, only *tph2* expression was significantly decreased by AroB MO, which is well supported by the previous studies showing *tph2* but not *tph1* is expressed in raphe 5-HT neurons (54, 75, 76). Expression of *tph2* in 5-HT neurons in pretectal and hypothalamic complex starts to appear at 60 hpf (76). On the other hand, whereas in the exposure experiments, expressions of all isoforms were affected by E_2; increased by low dose and decreased by high dose. The results support the previous studies reporting that *tph2* expressed in brain is responsible for 5-HT synthesis in the zebrafish (27, 28, 54). Thus, we provide the evidence that brain-formed estrogen stimulates *tph2* expression to maintain 5-HT content in the serotonin neuron. The effects of E_2 exposure on *tph* isoforms indicate E_2 also modulates serotonin biosynthesis in tissues outside the brain. 5-HT has been reported to be produced in various organs including intestine which is the major source of 5-HT in the body and TPH1 is responsible for its synthesis (54, 77). Investigation of estrogen regulation of serotonin production in intestine during development would be a future research interest.

The parameters of physiological functions of serotonin system, heart rate, and thigmotactic behavior were measure to verify the activity of serotonergic neuron. The results were in accordance to the changes in 5-HT levels in the neurons; the increased 5-HT levels are accompanied by the increased heart rate and decreased thigmotactic behavior, while the contrary was true for the decreased 5-HT levels. Serotonin is known to be involved in cardiovascular function, and the effect of central serotonergic neuron is mediated through autonomic nervous system in mammals (18). Our result of the low-dose (0.005 μM) E_2 which increased heart rate corroborates the effect of MO-mediated AroB knockdown, indicating that nanomolar level of brain-formed estrogen, or even lower level in the tissue, stimulates serotonergic neuron to increase the heart rate. Exposure to quipazine (serotonin agonist), or fluoxetine (selective serotonin reuptake inhibitor, SSRI) completely reversed the decreased heart rate caused by the high dose (0.1 μM) E_2, or AroB MO injection confirming that heart rate is under the control of serotonin signaling. Taken together with a recent study showing that GPER in the pituitary of zebrafish embryo regulates heart rate through thyroid hormone (78), estrogen in brain centrally regulates heart rate through various mechanisms. On the other hand, cardiac functions are directly regulated by estrogen (79) and aromatase has been detected in the heart tissues such as myocardium in mice (80–82). Therefore, it is possible that AroB MO injection may affect aromatase expression in the heart and locally produced estrogen modulates heart rate. In some teleost fish, both ovarian and brain aromatases are expressed in the heart (83–85), but in ricefield eel only brain aromatase is detected (86), while only ovarian aromatase is present in spotted scat (87). These difference may be due to technical difference as well as differences in species and developmental and physiological status. Our preliminary analysis indicated the expression of ovarian aromatase but not the brain form in adult zebrafish heart (data not shown), suggesting that our result of MO injection is likely to be mediated through knockdown of brain aromatase expressed in the brain not in the heart. However, expression of aromatase in the heart during development needs to be verified.

Thigmotaxis is an evolutionally conserved behavior associated with fear and has been shown to be affected by anxiolytic and anxiogenic compounds (88); thus, it has been used to measure anxiety levels in animals including fish (89–92). Our present study shows the high dose E_2 (1 μM), which decreased the 5-HT level, significantly increased anxiety (increased time spent in outer zone), and this increase was abolished by addition of 5-HT agonist (Q) or SSRI (FLX), indicating the effect of high dose E_2 is mediated through serotonin signaling. Similarly, increased anxiety by AroB MO was also abolished by Q or FLX, which supports our hypothesis that brain-formed estrogen modulates serotonergic neuron. Despite our expectation, the low-dose E_2 (0.005 μM), which increased the 5-HT level, did not cause reduction of anxiety. Therefore, we further examined to see if the low-dose E_2 exerts anxiolytic effect in the larvae exposed to DEX to induce stress, and indeed, low-dose E_2 decreased the anxiety level. Thus, our data demonstrate a negative correlation between anxiety behavior and 5-HT level, which is in accordance with previous studies. In mammals, depletion of 5-HT level in rat brain induces anxiety (93) and acute reduction of tryptophan increases the anxiety level in patients of a social anxiety disorder (94). The role of 5-HT in anxiety is also reported in zebrafish (20, 95). Buspirone, partial agonist for 5-HT1A receptor, exerts anxiolytic-like effect in zebrafish (96). The phenotype of zebrafish leopard strain, which is characterized by increased anxiety-like behavior, is rescued by acute treatment with FLX (97). Taken together, we provide the evidence that brain-formed E_2 has an important role in modulating anxiety through serotonergic transmission.

In contrast to mammalian brain, where aromatase is expressed in both neuron and glia (98, 99), it is well documented that brain aromatase in fish is exclusively expressed in RGCs along the ventricles of forebrain, midbrain, and hindbrain serving as neural progenitors (10, 11, 47). While most RGCs are transformed into astrocytes by the time of adulthood in mammalian brain (100), presence of RGCs persists throughout the lifespan of zebrafish, which is considered to be one of the contributing factors for high capacity of neuronal proliferation (101). On the other hand, serotonin is known to play a role in neurogenesis (102). In adult zebrafish, it has been reported that projection of 5-HT neurons in raphe to ventricular surface of the brain, where highly proliferative cells are found. In addition, expression of 5-HT receptors are localized in ventricular surface in larval and adult zebrafish (27, 103). Thus, it may be possible that RGCs in ventricular surface are innervated by 5-HT neurons in raphe and modulated for neurogenesis. Interestingly, it has been reported that AroB-positive RGCs in PVO area in adult zebrafish has an ability to differentiate into serotonergic neuron (104). Taken together with our present study providing the evidence that brain-formed estrogen is necessary to maintain the levels of 5-HT in neurons in raphe, we can hypothesize that differentiation of AroB-expressing RGCs in serotonin neurons is regulated by serotonin neuron in raphe, whose activity is modulated by estrogen produced by AroB. It has been shown that placenta aromatase activity and expression are stimulated by serotonergic 5-HT2A receptor signaling (105). In goldfish, AroB expression in RGCs *in vitro* is upregulated by dopamine with modulation by E_2 (106). Nonetheless, estrogen biosynthesis and homeostasis in CNS are regulated and fine-tuned by multiple factors like neurotransmitters and hormones, so that diverse functions of estrogen can be coordinated.

In conclusion, this study demonstrates that estradiol exhibits a biphasic effect on serotonergic neuron, and that brain aromatase, thus brain-formed estrogen plays a significant role in modulating serotonin levels to sustain appropriate development and functions of serotonergic neurons which regulate heart rate and anxiety behavior in zebrafish embryos and larvae. Considering the role of serotonergic neurons in neural development and neurogenesis, it is possible to postulate that one of the mechanisms of brain aromatase and brain-formed estrogen to regulate neurogenesis in teleost brain may be through modulation of serotonergic system, which awaits future investigation.

ETHICS STATEMENT

All experimental procedures and maintenance of fish were conducted in accordance with the Guide for Care and Use of Laboratory Animals published by the US National Institutes of Health.

AUTHOR CONTRIBUTIONS

ZU and MK designed the experiments. ZU performed the experiments and analyzed the data. ZU and MK wrote the paper.

ACKNOWLEDGMENTS

ZU was supported by MEXT (Ministry of Education, Culture, Sports, Science and Technology, Japan) scholarship. We would like to thank Prof. Akiyoshi Takahashi and Assoc. Prof. Kanta Mizusawa for helping ZU to generate AroB mRNA, and Prof. Kazufumi Takamune for his support with western blot experiments.

REFERENCES

1. Simpson ER, Davis SR. Minireview: aromatase and the regulation of estrogen biosynthesis-some new perspectives. *Endocrinology* (2001) 142(11): 4589–94. doi:10.1210/endo.142.11.8547
2. Cui J, Shen Y, Li R. Estrogen synthesis and signaling pathways during ageing: from periphery to brain. *Trends Mol Med* (2013) 19(3):197–209. doi:10.1016/j.molmed.2012.12.007
3. Kishida M, Callard GV. Distinct cytochrome P450 aromatase isoforms in zebrafish (*Danio rerio*) brain and ovary are differentially programmed and estrogen regulated during early development. *Endocrinology* (2001) 142(2):740–50. doi:10.1210/endo.142.2.7928
4. Callard GV, Greytak SR, Novillo A, Cotter CA, Mayer RK. Brain aromatase in fish: perspective and comparative approaches. In: Balthazart J, Ball G, editors. *Brain Aromatase, Estrogen, and Behavior*. New York: Oxford University Press (2013). p. 13–42.
5. Pasmanik M, Callard GV. Changes in brain aromatase and 5 alpha-reductase activities correlate significantly with seasonal reproductive cycles in goldfish (*Carassius auratus*). *Endocrinology* (1988) 122(4):1349–56. doi:10.1210/endo-122-4-1349
6. Zupanc GKH. Adult neurogenesis and neuronal regeneration in the brain of teleost fish. *J Physiol Paris* (2008) 102(4–6):357–73. doi:10.1016/j.jphysparis.2008.10.007
7. Adolf B, Chapouton P, Lam CS, Topp S, Tannhäuser B, Strähle U, et al. Conserved and acquired features of adult neurogenesis in the zebrafish telencephalon. *Dev Biol* (2006) 295(1):278–93. doi:10.1016/j.ydbio.2006.03.023
8. Grandel H, Kaslin J, Ganz J, Wenzel I, Brand M. Neural stem cells and neurogenesis in the adult zebrafish brain: origin, proliferation dynamics, migration and cell fate. *Dev Biol* (2006) 295(1):263–77. doi:10.1016/j.ydbio.2006.03.040
9. Schmidt R, Strähle U, Scholpp S. Neurogenesis in zebrafish – from embryo to adult. *Neural Dev* (2013) 8:3. doi:10.1186/1749-8104-8-3
10. Forlano PM, Deitcher DL, Myers DA, Bass AH. Anatomical distribution and cellular basis for high levels of aromatase activity in the brain of teleost fish: aromatase enzyme and mRNA expression identify glia as source. *J Neurosci* (2001) 21(22):8943–55. doi:10.1523/JNEUROSCI.21-22-08943.2001
11. Tong SK, Mouriec K, Kuo MW, Pellegrini E, Gueguen MM, Brion F, et al. A cyp19a1b-gfp (aromatase B) transgenic zebrafish line that expresses GFP in radial glial cells. *Genesis* (2009) 47:67–73. doi:10.1002/dvg.20459
12. Radakovits R, Barros CS, Belvindrah R, Patton B, Müller U. Regulation of radial glial survival by signals from the meninges. *J Neurosci* (2009) 29(24):7694–705. doi:10.1523/JNEUROSCI.5537-08.2009
13. Sawyer SJ, Gerstner KA, Callard GV. Real-time PCR analysis of cytochrome P450 aromatase expression in zebrafish: gene specific tissue distribution, sex differences, developmental programming, and estrogen regulation. *Gen Comp Endocrinol* (2006) 147(2):108–17. doi:10.1016/j.ygcen.2005.12.010
14. Diotel N, Vaillant C, Gabbero C, Mironov S, Fostier A, Gueguen MM, et al. Effects of estradiol in adult neurogenesis and brain repair in zebrafish. *Horm Behav* (2013) 63(2):193–207. doi:10.1016/j.yhbeh.2012.04.003
15. Graeff FG, Guimarães FS, De Andrade TGCS, Deakin JFW. Role of 5-HT in stress, anxiety and depression. *Pharmacol Biochem Behav* (1996) 54(1): 129–41. doi:10.1016/0091-3057(95)02135-3
16. Michelsen KA, Schmitz C, Steinbusch HWM. The dorsal raphe nucleus-from silver stainings to a role in depression. *Brain Res Rev* (2007) 55(2):329–42. doi:10.1016/j.brainresrev.2007.01.002
17. Bravo JA, Dinan TG, Cryan JF. Early-life stress induces persistent alterations in 5-HT1A receptor and serotonin transporter mRNA expression in the adult rat brain. *Front Mol Neurosci* (2014) 7(24):1–9. doi:10.3389/fnmol.2014.00024
18. Côté F, Fligny C, Fromes Y, Mallet J, Vodjdani G. Recent advances in understanding serotonin regulation of cardiovascular function. *Trends Mol Med* (2004) 10(5):232–8. doi:10.1016/j.molmed.2004.03.007
19. Nakamura K. The role of the dorsal raphé nucleus in reward-seeking behavior. *Front Integr Neurosci* (2013) 7(60):1–18. doi:10.3389/fnint.2013.00060
20. Herculano AM, Maximino C. Serotonergic modulation of zebrafish behavior: towards a paradox. *Prog Neuropsychopharmacol Biol Psychiatry* (2014) 55:50–66. doi:10.1016/j.pnpbp.2014.03.008
21. Berg DA, Belnoue L, Song H, Simon A. Neurotransmitter mediated control of neurogenesis in the adult vertebrate brain. *Development* (2013) 140(2):2548–61. doi:10.1242/dev.088005
22. Charnay Y, Léger L. Brain serotonergic circuitries. *Dialogues Clin Neurosci* (2010) 12(4):471–87.
23. Lesch KP, Waider J. Serotonin in the modulation of neural plasticity and networks: implications for neurodevelopmental disorders. *Neuron* (2012) 76(1):175–91. doi:10.1016/j.neuron.2012.09.013
24. Herlenius E, Lagercrantz H. Neurotransmitters and neuromodulators during early human development. *Early Hum Dev* (2001) 65(1):21–37. doi:10.1016/S0378-3782(01)00189-X
25. Sodhi MS, Sanders-Bush E. Serotonin and brain development. *Int Rev Neurobiol* (2004) 59:111–74. doi:10.1016/S0074-7742(04)59006-2
26. Sundström E, Kolare S, Souverbie F, Samuelsson EB, Pschera H, Lunell NO, et al. Neurochemical differentiation of human bulbospinal monoaminergic neurons during the first trimester. *Brain Res Dev Brain Res* (1993) 75(1):1–12. doi:10.1016/0165-3806(93)90059-J
27. Lillesaar C. The serotonergic system in fish. *J Chem Neuroanat* (2011) 41(4):294–308. doi:10.1016/j.jchemneu.2011.05.009
28. Gaspar P, Lillesaar C. Probing the diversity of serotonin neurons. *Philos Trans R Soc Lond B Biol Sci* (2012) 367(1601):2382–94. doi:10.1098/rstb.2011.0378
29. Barreiro-Iglesias A, Mysiak KS, Scott AL, Reimer MM, Yang Y, Becker CG, et al. Serotonin promotes development and regeneration of spinal motor neurons in zebrafish. *Cell Rep* (2015) 13(5):924–32. doi:10.1016/j.celrep.2015.09.050
30. McEwen BS, Elves SE. Estrogen actions in the central nervous system. *Endocr Rev* (1999) 20(3):279–307. doi:10.1210/edrv.20.3.0365
31. Bethea CL, Lu NZ, Gundlah C, Streicher JM. Diverse actions of ovarian steroids in the serotonin neural system. *Front Neuroendocrinol* (2002) 23(1):41–100. doi:10.1006/frne.2001.0225
32. Pecins-Thompson M, Brown NA, Kohama SG, Bethea CL. Ovarian steroid regulation of tryptophan hydroxylase mRNA expression in rhesus macaque. *J Neurosci* (1996) 16(21):7021–9. doi:10.1523/JNEUROSCI.16-21-07021.1996
33. Pecins-Thompson M, Brown NA, Bethea CL. Regulation of serotonin re-uptake transporter mRNA expression by ovarian steroids in rhesus macaques.

Brain Res Mol Brain Res (1998) 53(1–2):120–9. doi:10.1016/S0169-328X(97)00286-6

34. Pecins-Thompson M, Bethea CL. Ovarian steroid regulation of serotonin-1A autoreceptor messenger RNA expression in the dorsal raphe of rhesus macaques. *Neuroscience* (1999) 89(1):267–77. doi:10.1016/S0306-4522(98)00326-1
35. Gundlah C, Lu NZ, Mirkes SJ, Bethea CL. Estrogen receptor beta (ERβ) mRNA and protein in serotonin neurons of macaques. *Mol Brain Res* (2001) 91:14–22. doi:10.1016/S0169-328X(01)00108-5
36. Sheng Z, Kawano J, Yanai A, Fujinaga R, Tanaka M, Watanabe Y, et al. Expression of estrogen receptors (α, β) and androgen receptor in serotonin neurons of the rat and mouse dorsal raphe nuclei; sex and species differences. *Neurosci Res* (2004) 49:185–96. doi:10.1016/j.neures.2004.02.011
37. Bethea CL, Phu K, Belikova Y, Bethea SC. Localization and regulation of reproductive steroid receptors in the raphe serotonin system of male macaques. *J Chem Neuroanat* (2015) 6(6–67):19–27. doi:10.1016/j.jchemneu.2015.04.001
38. Donner N, Handa RJ. Estrogen receptor beta regulates the expression of tryptophanhydroxylase 2 mRNA within serotonergic neurons of the rat dorsal raphe nuclei. *Neuroscience* (2009) 163(2):705–18. doi:10.1016/j.neuroscience.2009.06.046
39. Hiroi R, Handa RJ. Estrogen receptor-β regulates human tryptophan hydroxylase-2 through an estrogen response element in the 5' untranslated region. *J Neurochem* (2013) 127(4):487–95. doi:10.1111/jnc.12401
40. Tsai CL, Wang LH, Chang CF, Kao CC. Effects of gonadal steroids on brain serotonergic and aromatase activity during the critical period of sexual differentiation in tilapia, *Oreochromis mossambicus*. *J Neuroendocrinol* (2000) 12(9):894–8. doi:10.1046/j.1365-2826.2000.00536.x
41. Thilagam H, Gopalakrishnan S, Bo J, Wang KJ. Comparative study of 17β-estradiol on endocrine disruption and biotransformation in fingerlings and juveniles of Japanese sea bass *Lateolabrax japonicas*. *Mar Pollut Bull* (2014) 85:332–7. doi:10.1016/j.marpolbul.2014.05.024
42. Diotel N, Do Rego JL, Anglade I, Vaillant C, Pellegrini E, Vaudry H, et al. The brain of teleost fish, a source, and a target of sexual steroids. *Front Neurosci* (2011) 5:137. doi:10.3389/fnins.2011.00137
43. Coumailleau P, Pellegrini E, Adrio F, Diotel N, Nicolau JC, Nasri A, et al. Aromatase, estrogen receptors and brain development in fish and amphibians. *Biochim Biophys Acta* (2015) 1849(2):152–62. doi:10.1016/j.bbagrm.2014.07.002
44. Langheinrich U, Hennen E, Stott G, Vacun G. Zebrafish as a model organism for the identification and characterization of drugs and genes affecting p53 signaling. *Curr Biol* (2002) 12(23):2023–8. doi:10.1016/S0960-9822(02)01319-2
45. Robu ME, Larson JD, Nasevicius A, Beiraghi S, Brenner C, Farber SA, et al. p53 activation by knockdown technologies. *PLoS Genet* (2007) 3(5):e78. doi:10.1371/journal.pgen.0030078
46. Bashammakh S. *The Developmental Role of the Serotonin System [Dissertation Thesis]*. Berlin: Freie Universität Berlin (2007). Available from: http://edocs.fu-berlin.de/diss/receive/FUDISS_thesis_000000003162
47. Menuet A, Pellegrini E, Brion F, Gueguen MM, Anglade I, Pakdel F, et al. Expression and estrogen-dependent regulation of the zebrafish brain aromatase gene. *J Comp Neurol* (2005) 485(4):304–20. doi:10.1002/cne.20497
48. Aihart MJ, Lee DH, Wilson TD, Miller BE, Miller MN, Skalko RG, et al. Adverse effects of serotonin depletion in developing zebrafish. *Neurotoxicol Teratol* (2012) 34(1):152–60. doi:10.1016/j.ntt.2011.08.008
49. Jannat M, Sugiyono, Kishida M. Nitrite (NO_2^-) perturbs the activitu of serotonergic neuron during early development of zebrafish. *Int J Eng Res Sci Tech* (2014) 3(4):1–11.
50. Norton WHJ. Measuring larval zebrafish behavior: locomotion, thigmotaxis, and startle. In: Kalueff AV, Stewart AM, editors. *Zebrafish Protocols for Neurobehavioral Research*. Totowa, NJ: Humana Press (2012). p. 3–19.
51. Brustein E, Chong M, Holmqvist B, Drapeau P. Serotonin patterns locomotor network activity in the developing zebrafish by modulating quiescent periods. *J Neurobiol* (2003) 57(3):303–22. doi:10.1002/neu.10292
52. Holzschuh J, Gimeno AB, Ettl AK, Dürr K, Knapik EW, Driever W. Noradrenergic neurons in the zebrafish hindbrain are induced by retinoic acid and require tfap2a for expression of the neurotransmitter phenotype. *Development* (2003) 130(23):5741–54. doi:10.1242/dev.00816
53. Wang Y, Takai R, Yoshioka H, Shirabe K. Characterization and expression of serotonin transporter genes in zebrafish. *Tohoku J Exp Med* (2006) 208(3):267–74. doi:10.1620/tjem.208.267
54. Bashammakh S, Wurtele M, Kotnik K, Seyfried SA, Bader M. Serotonin is required for pharyngeal arch morphogenesis in zebrafish. *ScienceOpen Res* (2015):1–9. doi:10.14293/S2199-1006.1.SOR-LIFE.AWPDLZ.v1
55. Liu W, Chen C, Chen L, Wang L, Li J, Chen Y, et al. Sex-dependent effects of microcystin-LR on hypothalamic-pituitary-gonad axis and gametogenesis of adult zebrafish. *Sci Rep* (2016) 6:22819. doi:10.1038/srep22819
56. Caulier M, Brion F, Chadili E, Turies C, Piccini B, Porcher JM, et al. Localization of steroidogenic enzymes and Foxl2a in the gonads of mature zebrafish (*Danio rerio*). *Comp Biochem Physiol A Mol Integr Physiol* (2015) 188:96–106. doi:10.1016/j.cbpa.2015.06.016
57. Alharthy KM, Albaqami FF, Thornton C, Corrales J, Willett KL. Mechanistic evaluation of benzo[a]pyrene's developmental toxicities mediated by reduced cyp19a1b activity. *Toxicol Sci* (2017) 155(1):135–47. doi:10.1093/toxsci/kfw182
58. Vandenberg LN, Colborn T, Heyes TB, Heindel JJ, Jacobs DR, Lee D, et al. Hormones and endocrine-disrupting chemicals: low-dose effects and non-monotonic dose responses. *Endocr Rev* (2012) 33(3):378–455. doi:10.1210/er.2011-1050
59. Voss AK, Fortune JE. Estradiol-17-β has a biphasic effect on oxytocin secretion by bovine granulosa cells. *Biol Reprod* (1993) 48:1404–9. doi:10.1095/biolreprod48.6.1404
60. Sobel MI, Winkel CA, Macy LB, Liao P, Bjornsson TD. The regulation of plasminogen activators and plasminogen activator inhibitor type 1 in endothelial cells by sex hormones. *Am J Obstet Gynecol* (1995) 173:801–8. doi:10.1016/0002-9378(95)90344-5
61. Banerjee SK, Campbell DR, Weston AP, Banerjee DK. Biphasic estrogen response on bovine adrenal medulla capillary endothelial cell adhesion, proliferation and tube formation. *Mol Cell Biochem* (1997) 177:97–105. doi:10.1023/A:100688802
62. Weiss-Messer E, Ber R, Barkey RJ. Prolactin and MA-10 Leydig cell steroidogenesis: biphasic effects of prolactin and signal transduction. *Endocrinology* (1996) 137:5509–18. doi:10.1210/endo.137.12.8940378
63. Yokoyama K, Hayashi M, Mogi C, Sasakawa Y, Watanabe G, Taya K, et al. Dose-dependent effects of a glucocorticoid on protein production. *Endocr J* (2008) 55(2):405–14. doi:10.1507/endocrj.K07E-063
64. Mazziotti G, Giustina A. Glucocorticoids and the regulation of growth hormone secretion. *Nat Rev Endocrinol* (2013) 9:265–76. doi:10.1038/nrendo.2013.5
65. Zhang L, Yulong M, Qin P, Deng Y, Zhang Z, Hou Y, et al. The effects of various estrogen doses on the proliferation and differentiation of cultured neural stem cells. *J Cell Sci Ther* (2016) 7:247. doi:10.4172/2157-7013.1000247
66. Houshmand F, Faghihi M, Imani A, Kheiri S. Effect of different doses of oxytocin on cardiac electrophysiology and arrhythmias induced by ischemia. *J Adv Pharm Technol Res* (2017) 8(4):131–7. doi:10.4103/japtr.JAPTR_178_16
67. Senthilkumaran B, Joy KP. Effects of ovariectomy and oestradiol replacement on hypothalamic serotonergic and monoamine oxidase activity in the catfish, *Heteropneustes fossilis*: a study correlating plasma oestradiol and gonadotrophin levels. *J Endocrinol* (1994) 142(2):193–203. doi:10.1677/joe.0.1420193
68. Oliveira CA, Mehecha GAB, Carnes K, Prins GS, Saunders PTK, França L, et al. Differential hormonal regulation of estrogen receptors ERα and ERβ and androgen receptor expression in rat efferent ductules. *Reproduction* (2004) 128(1):73–86. doi:10.1530/rep.1.00136
69. McCarthy MM. Estradiol and the developing brain. *Physiol Rev* (2008) 88(1):91–134. doi:10.1152/physrev.00010.2007
70. Micevych PE, Mermelstein PG, Sinchak K. Estradiol membrane-initiated signaling in the brain mediates reproduction. *Trends Neurosci* (2017) 40(11):654–66. doi:10.1016/j.tins.2017.09.001
71. Boulware MI, Mermelstein PG. Membrane estrogen receptors activate metabotropic glutamate receptors to influence nervous system physiology. *Steroids* (2009) 74(7):608–13. doi:10.1016/j.steroids.2008.11.013
72. Cover KK, Maeng LY, Lebrón-Milad K, Milad MR. Mechanisms of estradiol in fear circuitry: implications for sex differences in psychopathology. *Transl Psychiatry* (2014) 5(4):e422. doi:10.1038/tp.2014.67
73. Micevych PE, Kelly MJ. Membrane estrogen receptor regulation of hypothalamic function. *Neuroendocrinology* (2012) 96(2):103–10. doi:10.1159/000338400
74. Xu H, Qin S, Carassco GA, Dai Y, Filardo EJ, Prossnitz ER, et al. Extra-nuclear estrogen receptor GPR30 regulates serotonin function in rat hypo-

thalamus. *Neuroscience* (2009) 158(4):1599–607. doi:10.1016/j.neuroscience.2008.11.028

75. Teraoka H, Russell C, Regan J, Chandrasekhar A, Concha ML, Yokoyama R, et al. Hedgehog and Fgf signaling pathways regulate the development of tphR-expressing serotonergic raphe neurons in zebrafish embryos. *J Neurobiol* (2004) 60(3):275–88. doi:10.1002/neu.20023
76. Lillesaar C, Tannhäuser B, Stigloher C, Kremmer E, Bally-Cuif L. The serotonergic phenotype is acquired by converging genetic mechanisms within the zebrafish central nervous system. *Dev Dyn* (2007) 236(4):1072–84. doi:10.1002/dvdy.21095
77. Côté F, Thévenot E, Fligny C, Fromes Y, Darmon M, Ripoche MA, et al. Disruption of the nonneuronal tph1 gene demonstrates the importance of peripheral serotonin in cardiac function. *Proc Natl Acad Sci U S A* (2003) 100(23):13525–30. doi:10.1073/pnas.2233056100
78. Romano SN, Edwards HE, Sounder JP, Ryan KJ, Cui X, Gorelick DA. G protein-coupled estrogen receptor regulates embryonic heart rate in zebrafish. *PLoS Genet* (2017) 13(10):e1007069. doi:10.1371/journal.pgen.1007069
79. Babiker FA, De Windt LJ, van Eickels M, Grohe C, Meyer R, Doevendans PA. Estrogenic hormone action in the heart: regulatory network and function. *Cardiovasc Res* (2002) 53(3):709–19. doi:10.1016/S0008-6363(01)00526-0
80. Bell JR, Mellor KM, Wollermann AC, Ip WT, Reichelt ME, Meachem SJ, et al. Aromatase deficiency confers paradoxical postischemic cardioprotection. *Endocrinology* (2011) 152(12):4937–47. doi:10.1210/en.2011-1212
81. Jazbutyte V, Stumpner J, Redel A, Lorenzen JM, Roewer N, Thum T, et al. Aromatase inhibition attenuates desflurane-induced preconditioning against acute myocardial infarction in male mouse heart in vivo. *PLoS One* (2012) 7(8):e42032. doi:10.1371/journal.pone.0042032
82. Connernet JJ, Spratt DI. Aromatase blockade is associated with increased mortality in acute illness in male mice. *J Endocr Soc* (2017) 1(9):1113–9. doi:10.1210/js.2017-00128
83. Chang X, Kobayashi T, Senthilkumaran B, Kobayashi-Kajura H, Sudhakumari CC, Nagahama Y. Two types of aromatase with different encoding genes, tissue distribution and developmental expression in Nile tilapia (*Oreochromis niloticus*). *Gen Comp Endocrinol* (2005) 141(2):101–15. doi:10.1016/j.ygcen.2004.11.020
84. Choi JY, Park JG, Jeong HB, Lee YD, Takemura A, Kim SJ. Molecular cloning of cytochrome P450 aromatases in the protogynous wrasse, *Halichoeres tenuispinis*. *Comp Biochem Physiol B Biochem Mol Biol* (2005) 141(1):49–59. doi:10.1016/j.cbpc.2005.01.009
85. Matsuoka MP, van Nes S, Andersen Ø, Benfey TJ, Reith M. Real-time PCR analysis of ovary- and brain-type aromatase gene expression during Atlantic halibut (*Hippoglossus hippoglossus*) development. *Comp Biochem Physiol B Biochem Mol Biol* (2006) 144(1):128–35. doi:10.1016/j.cbpb.2006.02.008
86. Zhang Y, Zhang W, Yang H, Zhou W, Hu C, Zhang L. Two cytochrome P450 aromatase genes in the hermaphrodite ricefield eel *Monopterus albus*: mRNA expression during ovarian development and sex change. *J Endocrinol* (2008) 199(2):317–31. doi:10.1677/JOE-08-0303
87. Liu H, Mu X, Gui L, Su M, Li H, Zhang G, et al. Characterization and gonadal expression of FOXL2 relative to Cyp19a genes in spotted scat *Scatophagus argus*. *Gene* (2015) 561(1):6–14. doi:10.1016/j.gene.2014.12.060
88. Walz N, Mühlberger A, Pauli P. A human open field test reveals thigmotaxis related to agoraphobic fear. *Biol Psychiatry* (2016) 80(5):390–7. doi:10.1016/j.biopsych.2015.12.016
89. Treit D, Fundytus M. Thigmotaxis as a test for anxiolytic activity in rats. *Pharmacol Biochem Behav* (1988) 31:959–62. doi:10.1016/0091-3057(88)90413-3
90. Prut L, Belzung C. The open field as a paradigm to measure the effects of drugs on anxiety-like behaviors: a review. *Eur J Pharmacol* (2003) 463:3–33. doi:10.1016/S0014-2999(03)01272-X
91. Schönrr SJ, Steenbergen PJ, Richardson MK, Champagne DL. Measuring thigmotaxis in larval zebrafish. *Behav Brain Res* (2012) 228(2):367–74. doi:10.1016/j.bbr.2011.12.016
92. Champagne DL, Hoefnagels CC, de Kloet RE, Richardson MK. Translating rodent behavioral repertoire to zebrafish (*Danio rerio*): relevance for stress research. *Behav Brain Res* (2010) 214(2):332–42. doi:10.1016/j.bbr.2010.06.001
93. Gurtman CG, Morley KC, Li KM, Hunt GE, McGregor IS. Increased anxiety in rats after 3,4-methylenedioxymethamphetamine: association with serotonin depletion. *Eur J Pharmacol* (2002) 446(1–3):89–96. doi:10.1016/S0014-2999(02)01820-4
94. Argyropoulos SV, Hood SD, Adrover M, Bell CJ, Rich AS, Nash JR, et al. Tryptophan depletion reverses the therapeutic effect of selective serotonin reuptake inhibitors in social anxiety disorder. *Biol Psychiatry* (2004) 56(7):503–9. doi:10.1016/j.biopsych.2004.07.006
95. Jia M, Pittman J. Deficits in striatal dopamine and hippocampal serotonin following induction of anxiety/depressive-like behaviors by bisphenol A. *Arch Neurosci* (2014) 2(1):e18555. doi:10.5812/archneurosci.18555
96. Gebauer DL, Pagnussat N, Piato AL, Schaefer IC, Bonan CD, Lara DR. Effects of anxiolytics in zebrafish: similarities and differences between benzodiazepines, buspirone and ethanol. *Pharmacol Biochem Behav* (2011) 99(3):480–6. doi:10.1016/j.pbb.2011.04.021
97. Maximino C, Puty B, Matos Oliveira KR, Herculano AM. Behavioral and neurochemical changes in the zebrafish leopard strain. *Genes Brain Behav* (2013) 12(5):576–82. doi:10.1111/gbb.12047
98. Martínez-Cerdeño V, Noctor SC, Kriegstein AR. Estradiol stimulates progenitor cell division in the ventricular and subventricular zones of the embryonic neocortex. *Eur J Neurosci* (2006) 24(12):3475–88. doi:10.1111/j.1460-9568.2006.05239.x
99. Yague JG, Muñoz A, de Monasterio-Schrader P, Defelipe J, Garcia-Segura LM, Azcoitia I. Aromatase expression in the human temporal cortex. *Neuroscience* (2006) 138(2):389–401. doi:10.1016/j.neuroscience.2005.11.054
100. Liu X, Bolteus AJ, Balkin DM, Henschel O, Bordey A. GFAP-expressing cells in the postnatal subventricular zone display a unique glial phenotype intermediate between radial glia and astrocytes. *Glia* (2006) 54(5):394–410. doi:10.1002/glia.20392
101. Pellegrini E, Mouriec K, Anglade I, Menuet A, Le Page Y, Guegeun MM, et al. Identification of aromatase-positive radial glial cells as progenitor cells in the ventricular layer of the forebrain in zebrafish. *J Comp Neurol* (2007) 501(1):150–67. doi:10.1002/cne.21222
102. Djavadian RL. Serotonin and neurogenesis in the hippocampal dentate gyrus of adult mammals. *Acta Neurobiol Exp (Wars)* (2004) 64(2):189–200.
103. Norton WH, Folchert A, Bally-Cuif L. Comparative analysis of serotonin receptor (HTR1A/HTR1B families) and transporter (slc6a4a/b) gene expression in the zebrafish brain. *J Comp Neurol* (2008) 511(4):521–42. doi:10.1002/cne.21831
104. Pérez MR, Pellegrini E, Nicolau JC, Gueguen MM, LeGuillou DM, Merot Y, et al. Relationships between radial glial progenitors and 5-HT neurons in the paraventricular organ of adult zebrafish-potential effects of serotonin on adult neurogenesis. *Eur J Neurosci* (2013) 38(9):3292–301. doi:10.1111/ejn.12348
105. Klempan T, Hudon-Thibeault AA, Oufkir T, Vaillancourt C, Sanderson JT. Stimulation of serotonergic 5-HT2A receptor signaling increases placental aromatase (CYP19) activity and expression in BeWo and JEG-3 human choriocarcinoma cells. *Placenta* (2011) 32(9):651–6. doi:10.1016/j.placenta.2011.06.003
106. Xing L, Esau C, Trudeau VL. Direct regulation of aromatase b expression by 17β-estradiol and dopamine D1 receptor agonist in adult radial glial cells. *Front Neurosci* (2016) 9:504. doi:10.3389/fnins.2015.00504

16

The Different Clinical Features Between Autoimmune and Infectious Status Epilepticus

Chih-Hsiang Lin [1], Yan-Ting Lu [1], Chen-Jui Ho [1], Fu-Yuan Shih [2] and Meng-Han Tsai [1]*

[1] Department of Neurology, Kaohsiung Chang Gung Memorial Hospital, College of Medicine, Chang Gung University, Kaohsiung, Taiwan, [2] Department of Neurosurgery, Kaohsiung Chang Gung Memorial Hospital, College of Medicine, Chang Gung University, Kaohsiung, Taiwan

***Correspondence:**
Meng-Han Tsai
menghan@cgmh.org.tw

Objective: The prognosis of status epilepticus (SE) is highly related to the underlying etiology. Inflammation of the central nervous system (CNS), including infection and autoimmune encephalitis, is one of the treatable conditions causing SE. The initial presentation of infectious and autoimmune CNS disorders can be quite similar, which may be difficult to differentiate at the beginning. However, treatment for these entities can be quite different. In this study, we aim to identify the differences in clinical features among patients with infectious and autoimmune SE, which could help the clinicians to select initial investigation and ensuing therapies that may improve overall outcomes.

Methods: This was a retrospective study that included 501 patients with SE within a period of 10.5-years. Patients with inflammatory etiology were collected and separated into infectious and autoimmune SE. The symptoms at onset, SE semiology, status epilepticus severity score, and END-IT score at admission, treatment for SE, and outcome (modified Rankin Scale) on discharge and last follow-up were recorded. Data on the first cerebrospinal fluid, electroencephalography, and magnetic resonance imaging were also collected.

Results: Forty-six (9.2%) of the 501 patients had SE with inflammatory etiology. Twenty-five (5%) patients were autoimmune SE and 21 (4.2%) were infectious SE. Patients with autoimmune SE have younger age and female predominance. As for clinical presentations, psychosis, non-convulsive SE, and super refractory SE were more common in patients with autoimmune SE. Nevertheless, the prognosis showed no difference between the two groups.

Conclusion: The different initial clinical presentations and patient characteristics may provide some clues about the underlying etiology of SE. When inflammatory etiology is suspected in patients with SE, younger age, female sex, psychosis, non-convulsive SE, and super refractory SE are clinical features that suggest an autoimmune etiology.

Keywords: status epilepticus, inflammatory, autoimmune, infection, autoantibody

INTRODUCTION

Status epilepticus (SE) is a neurological emergency associated with significant morbidity and mortality that usually requires admission to an intensive care unit (1–3). The goal when treating SE is to terminate the clinical and electrographic seizure activities as soon as possible (4). Even though antiepileptic drugs (AEDs) can be used to control seizures (5), the prognosis of SE is highly related to age and the underlying etiology (6–8). To further improve outcomes, targeted management of the underlying causes may be required (4, 9).

Brain inflammation can also cause SE (10, 11), including central nervous system (CNS) infections and autoimmune encephalitis (12). These conditions can be treated and may result in significantly different outcomes (13–15). Altered mental status is the most common initial presentation of inflammatory SE (12). However, it is an ambiguous sign that provides little information on the underlying etiology. Currently available investigations could help in initial differential diagnosis but have some limitations. Laboratory tests such as bacterial or viral culture, polymerase chain reaction (PCR) for specific pathogens, or autoantibody testing may not be immediately available (13, 16) and the results may take a few days or weeks to return. Cerebrospinal fluid (CSF) studies are useful to confirm the diagnose of bacterial infections, but are less effective in distinguishing between viral infections and autoimmune processes (13, 17). Magnetic resonance imaging (MRI) can provide evidence of CNS inflammation, but not the underlying cause of the inflammation (18). Electroencephalography (EEG) may sometimes show patterns that suggest a specific diagnosis, such as extreme delta brush in patients with anti-N-methyl-D-aspartate (NMDA) receptor encephalitis, but the findings are mostly non-specific (19).

Only two studies have specifically addressed the differences between infectious and autoimmune etiology. Spatola et al. were the first to report that patients with an infectious etiology were older in age and had a more severe clinical presentation at first encounter (20). Subsequently, Shin et al. found that patients with an autoimmune etiology were younger (11). Herein, we retrospectively reviewed our patients with SE and an inflammatory etiology over a 10.5-year period. We aimed to identify the presenting factors that may assist clinicians in differentiating the two entities earlier, which may lead to faster targeted treatment and better patient outcomes.

MATERIALS AND METHODS

Study Design

We retrospectively reviewed the medical records of all patients with SE admitted to the Neurological Intensive Care Unit at Kaohsiung Chang Gung Memorial Hospital between January 2006 and July 2016. This study was approved by the Chang Gung Medical Foundation Institutional Review Board.

Definitions and Criteria

SE was defined as 5 min or more of continuous clinical and/or electrographic seizure activity or recurrent seizure activity without recovery (returning to baseline) between seizures (21). Refractory SE was defined as SE not responded to first-line therapy (benzodiazepine) or second-line therapy and requiring general anesthesia (22). Super refractory SE was defined as SE continues 24 h or more after the onset of anesthesia, including those cases in which the SE recurs on the reduction or withdrawal of anesthesia (22). The semiology and etiology of SE were classified according to the International League Against Epilepsy Task Force report (23).

Inflammatory SE was defined as SE due to acute inflammation of the brain parenchyma, with or without the involvement of the meninges (12), and further divided into SE due to CNS infection and autoimmune SE. Autoimmune SE included autoimmune encephalitis and systemic autoimmune disorders causing SE (23). Patients with an identified etiology for SE such as cerebrovascular disease, intracranial tumor, head trauma, metabolic disturbance, alcohol-related, AED withdrawal, neurodegenerative disease, mitochondrial disease, and medically refractory epilepsy were excluded. Patients with an unknown etiology and those without CSF data were also excluded from this study.

Autoimmune SE was defined as suggested by previous experts' consensus (16):

1. Subacute onset (rapid progression of fewer than 3 months) of working memory deficits (short-term memory loss), altered mental status, or psychiatric symptoms.
2. At least one of the followings:
    - New focal CNS findings
    - Seizures not explained by a previously known seizure disorder
    - CSF pleocytosis (white blood cell count of more than five cells per mm3)
    - MRI features suggestive of encephalitis
3. Reasonable exclusion of alternative causes

SE patients who had positive neuronal surface auto-antibodies testing (EUROIMMUN, Autoimmune Encephalitis Mosaic 6 assay, Germany) in serum or CSF were also considered as autoimmune SE.

Infectious SE was diagnosed if microbiologic studies demonstrated an infectious agent. Those without evidence of microbiologic studies would have to fulfill one of the underlying criteria (20): (1) fever>38.5°C, (2) increased white blood cell count or C-reactive protein, (3) findings highly suggestive of a bacterial infection, such as turbid CSF, neutrophilic pleocytosis, or low CSF to serum glucose ratio (<0.5), or (4) clinical picture suggestive of a viral origin plus lymphocytic pleocytosis on CSF study with positive PCR result or serology test shows a 4-fold increase of viral antibodies 3 weeks after the onset of illness (24).

Clinical information was recorded using a standardized evaluation form, including the symptoms at onset, SE semiology and classification, status epilepticus severity score (STESS) (25) and the END-IT score (26) at admission, treatment for SE, and outcome at discharge and last follow-up. A STESS score ≥3 (25) or an END-IT score ≥3 (26) suggested a poor outcome. Data on the first acquired CSF, EEG, and MRI studies were collected. The EEG was described according to

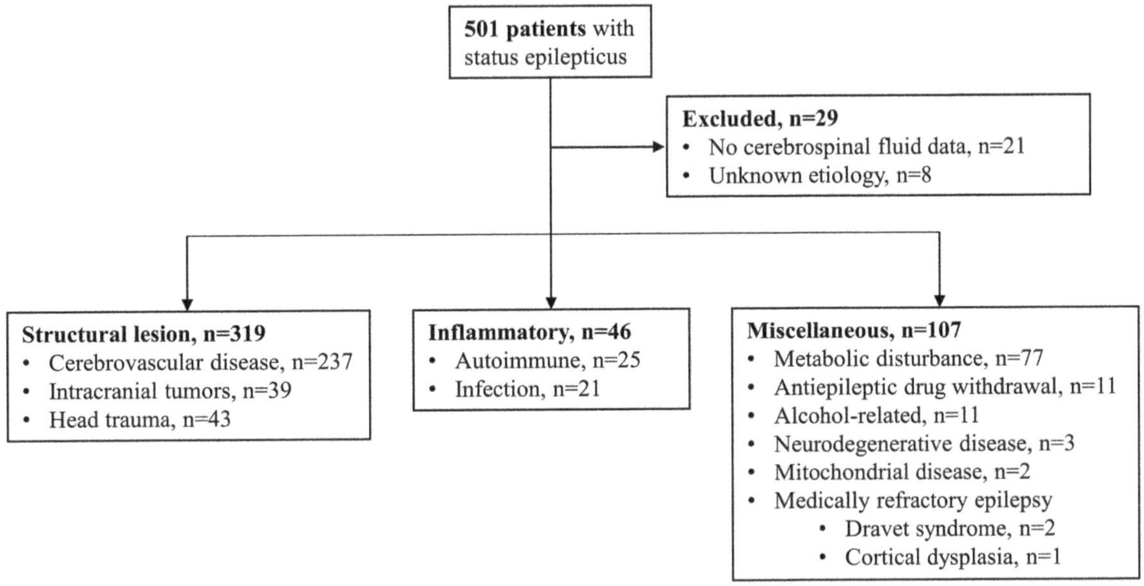

FIGURE 1 | Study population and etiologies of status epilepticus.

the 2012 American Clinical Neurophysiology Society's (ACNS) Standardized Critical Care EEG Terminology (27), which we categorized into background slowing activity, sporadic epileptiform discharge, periodic discharge, and electrographic seizures (11). MRI findings including the location and symmetry of signal changes on fluid-attenuated inversion recovery (FLAIR) and diffusion-weighted imaging (DWI) were recorded (10). Clinical outcomes at discharge and the last follow-up were graded using the modified Rankin Scale (mRS). A good outcome was defined as an mRS score <3 and a poor outcome was defined as an mRS score ≧3.

Statistical Analysis

Statistical analyses were performed using the IBM SPSS Statistics for Windows (version 22; IBM Corp., Armonk, NY, United States). To compare demographic data between infectious and autoimmune groups, categorical variables were assessed using Chi-square or Fisher exact tests, and continuous variables were compared using the Mann-Whitney U-test. $p < 0.05$ was considered as statistically significant.

RESULTS

During the 10.5-year study period (January 2006–June 2016), 501 patients with SE were reviewed, of whom 46 (9.2%) had an inflammatory etiology, including 25 females (54.3%) and 21 males (45.7%). Of the excluded patients, 237 had cerebrovascular disease, 77 had metabolic disturbances, 43 had head trauma, 39 had intracranial tumors, 11 had AED withdrawal, 11 had alcohol-related SE, three had neurodegenerative diseases, two had mitochondrial diseases, and three had medically refractory epilepsy. Of the three patients with medically refractory epilepsy, two had Dravet syndrome and one had focal cortical dysplasia. Patients without CSF data ($n = 21$) and those with an unknown etiology ($n = 8$) were also excluded (**Figure 1**).

The clinical characteristics of the 46 patients with inflammatory SE are presented in **Table 1**. Among the 46 patients, 25 (54.3%) had autoimmune SE, and 21 (45.7%) had infectious SE. In the patients with autoimmune SE, five were related to anti-NMDA receptor encephalitis, four were related to Hashimoto encephalopathy, one was related to CNS lupus, one was related to anti-collapsin response mediator protein 5 encephalitis, and 14 were diagnosed according to the criteria of autoimmune encephalitis (16). Of these 14 patients, five had received cell-based anti-neuronal antibody assays with negative results. The remaining nine patients did not receive anti-neuronal auto-antibody tests as the test was not available at the time of diagnosis. With regards to the patients with infectious SE, six had bacterial infections, 12 had viral infections, two had cryptococcal meningitis, and one had Creutzfeldt-Jakob disease.

The clinical features of infectious and autoimmune SE are compared in **Table 2**. The median age at onset of the patients with autoimmune SE was younger than that of the patients with infectious SE (32 vs. 56, $p = 0.015$), and more of the patients with autoimmune SE were female compared to those with infectious SE (68.0 vs. 38.1%, $p = 0.043$). The initial presentation of both groups was similar, including the STESS and END-IT score at admission, onset symptoms, and latency of seizures after the initial symptoms. Psychosis was the presenting symptom only in the autoimmune SE group (24.0 vs. 0.0%, $p = 0.025$) and non-convulsive SE was more prevalent among the patients with autoimmune SE compared to those with infectious SE (32.0 vs. 4.8%, $p = 0.027$). Refractory SE occurred more commonly in the autoimmune SE than in the infectious SE group, but the difference was not statistically significant (88.0 vs. 66.7%, $p = 0.081$). Super refractory SE was more common in the autoimmune SE group than in the infectious SE group (41.3 vs. 19.0%, $p = 0.007$). The number of AEDs used was similar between both groups, but the use of general anesthesia was more common in the autoimmune SE group than in the infectious SE group (64.0 vs. 23.8%, $p = 0.006$). However, the duration of admission or ICU stay, mRS score at discharge, and mortality rate during admission were similar between the two groups. The sensitivity and specificity for STESS to predict the outcome at discharge were 70.6 and 44.8%, respectively, compared to 68.8 and 45.5% at last follow-up. The sensitivity and specificity for the END-IT score to predict the outcome at discharge were 9.4 and 100.0%, respectively, compared to 21.4 and 100.0% at last follow-up.

The results of CSF and EEG are presented in **Table 3** and the MRI findings are summarized in **Table 4**. Patients with infectious SE had a higher median CSF protein level (93.0 mg/dL vs. 34.8 mg/dL, $p = 0.014$), higher median white blood cell count (20 vs. 3 cell/mm^3, $p = 0.011$), higher percentage of neutrophilic predominance (52.9 vs. 15.4%, $p = 0.034$), and higher percentage of low CSF/blood glucose ratio (56.3 vs. 24.0%, $p = 0.036$) compared to the patients with autoimmune SE, who had a higher percentage of lymphocytic predominance (84.6 vs. 47.1%, $p = 0.034$). There was no significant difference in IgG index between the two groups. The autoimmune SE group tended to have a higher rate of background slowing activity in the first EEG, but the difference between autoimmune and infection was not statistically different (56.0 vs. 28.6%, $p = 0.081$). The presence of sporadic epileptiform discharge, periodic discharge, or electrographic seizure was similar among the two groups in the first EEG study. With regards to the first MRI findings, an abnormal FLAIR signal was observed in 11 patients with autoimmune SE and eight patients with infectious SE. A restricted diffusion signal on DWI was found in 14 patients with autoimmune SE and 10 patients with infectious SE. However, there were no significant differences in abnormalities in the FLAIR and DWI signals between the two groups. Detailed descriptions of the locations of the abnormal signals on FLAIR and DWI are presented in **Table 4**.

TABLE 1 | Demographic data of inflammatory SE patients.

	Patients (n = 46)
Onset age (years)	45 (28–60)
Female	25 (54.3)
Onset symptom	
Fever	24 (52.2)
Decreased consciousness	17 (37.0)
Seizure	10 (21.7)
Upper respiratory tract infection	8 (17.4)
Headache	6 (13.0)
Psychosis	6 (13.0)
Fatigue	3 (6.5)
Cognitive decline	1 (2.2)
Latency of seizure after onset symptoms (days)	3 (0–7)
STESS ≥3 at admission	18 (39.1)
END-IT score ≥3 at admission	**43 (93.5)**
SE with prominent motor symptoms	37 (80.4)
Generalized convulsive SE	25 (54.3)
Epilepsia partialis continua	6 (13.0)
Focal onset evolving into bilateral convulsive SE	4 (8.7)
Myoclonic SE with coma	1 (2.2)
Hyperkinetic SE	1 (2.2)
Non-convulsive SE	9 (19.6)
Non-convulsive SE with coma	6 (13.0)
Myoclonic absence status	1 (2.2)
Non-convulsive SE without impairment of consciousness	1 (2.2)
Aphasic status	1 (2.2)
Number of AEDs used	**3 (2-3)**
Refractory SE	**36 (78.3)**
Super refractory SE	**19 (41.3)**
Required general anesthesia for SE control	21 (45.7)
Death during admission	13 (28.3)
Days of admission	39 (26-79)
Days in ICU	33.5 (11-60)
More than two AEDs at discharge	17 (36.9)
Good outcome at discharge (mRS<3)	17 (36.9)
Good outcome at last follow up (mRS<3)	16 (34.8)

Continuous variables were presented as median (interquartile range)
Categorical variables were presented as n (%).
AED, antiepileptic drug; ICU, intensive care unit; mRS, modified Rankin Scale; SE, status epilepticus; STESS, status epilepticus severity score.

DISCUSSION

Inflammatory SE is a previously under-recognized subgroup of SE. In the current study, 9.2% of all cases of SE were related to an inflammatory etiology, which is in accordance with previous studies (range from 6 to 12.8%) (11, 20). Inflammatory SE has two main etiologies, infectious, and autoimmune SE, which is at times difficult to differentiate at the initial presentation. We found that younger age, female sex, the presence of psychosis, non-convulsive SE, lymphocytic predominance in CSF were more commonly observed in the patients with autoimmune SE, while a high CSF total protein level, pleocytosis, and reduced glucose ratio were more common in those with infectious SE. EEG and MRI are important tools to confirm the diagnosis of SE and exclude structural lesions (19, 28), but were not particularly helpful in the current study.

Among all patients with SE, infection accounted for 4.2% and autoimmune accounted for 5%. This suggests that autoimmune SE is as common as infectious SE (20, 29), and therefore clinical features that can distinguish the two entities are important for intensive care physicians who care for patients with SE. We observed some differences in the presenting features of those with autoimmune and infectious SE. The age at onset was younger in the patients with autoimmune SE, which has also been reported in two previous studies (11, 20). Female predominance was also observed in the autoimmune SE group in this study, which is in accordance with previous reports that reported females predominance in autoimmune encephalitis and systemic autoimmune disorders (14, 30, 31).

TABLE 2 | Comparison of the clinical features of autoimmune and infectious SE.

	Autoimmune SE (n = 25)	Infectious SE (n = 21)	p-value	OR (95% CI)
Onset age (years)	32 (23–49.5)	56 (36.5–68.5)	0.015	
Female	17 (68.0)	8 (38.1)	0.043	0.29 (0.09–0.98)
Onset symptom				
Fever	13 (52.0)	11 (52.4)	0.979	0.99 (0.31–3.15)
Decrease consciousness	9 (36.0)	8 (38.1)	0.883	0.91 (0.28–3.04)
Seizure	6 (24.0)	4 (19.0)	0.685	1.34 (0.32–5.58)
Upper respiratory tract infection	5 (20.0)	3 (14.3)	0.611	1.50 (0.31–7.19)
Headache	2 (8.0)	4 (19.0)	0.268	0.37 (0.06–2.26)
Psychosis	6 (24.0)	0 (0.0)	0.025	
Fatigue	1 (4.0)	2 (9.5)	0.450	0.4 (0.03–4.70)
Cognitive decline	0 (0.0)	1 (4.8)	0.806	0.41 (0.01–11.68)
Latency of seizure after onset symptoms (days)	3 (0–7)	2 (0–8.5)	0.892	
STESS ≥3 at admission	11 (44.0)	7 (33.3)	0.460	1.57 (0.47–5.23)
END-IT score ≥3 at admission	**23 (92.0)**	**20 (95.2)**	**1.000**	**1.74 (0.15–20.65)**
SE with prominent motor symptoms	17 (68.0)	20 (95.2)	0.027	0.11 (0.01–0.94)
Generalized convulsive SE	11	14		
Epilepsia partialis continua	3	3		
Focal onset evolving into bilateral convulsive SE	2	2		
Myoclonic SE with coma	0	1		
Hyperkinetic SE	1	0		
Non-convulsive SE	8 (32.0)	1 (4.8)	0.027	9.41 (1.07–83.01)
Non-convulsive SE with coma	5	1		
Myoclonic absence status	1	0		
Non-convulsive SE without impairment of consciousness	1	0		
Aphasic status	1	0		
Number of AED used	**3 (2–3)**	**3 (1–3)**	**0.159**	
Refractory SE	**22 (88.0)**	**14 (66.7)**	**0.081**	**3.67(0.81–16.59)**
Super refractory SE	**15 (41.3)**	**4 (19.0)**	**0.007**	**6.38 (1.65–24.63)**
Required general anesthesia for SE control	16 (64.0)	5 (23.8)	0.006	5.69 (1.56–20.76)
Death during admission	5 (20.0)	8 (38.1)	0.175	0.41 (0.11–1.52)
Days of admission	40 (21–91)	33 (26–77.5)	0.817	
Days in ICU	34 (10.5-63.5)	33 (15–57)	0.869	
More than two AEDs at discharge	11 (44.0)	6 (28.6)	0.280	1.96 (0.57–6.74)
Good prognosis at discharge (mRS<3)	11 (44.0)	6 (28.6)	0.280	1.96 (0.57–6.74)
Good prognosis at last follow up (mRS<3)	10 (66.7)	6 (50.0)	0.381	2.00 (0.42–9.52)

Continuous variables were presented as median (interquartile range).
Categorical variables were presented as n (%).
AED, antiepileptic drug; CI, confidence interval; ICU, intensive care unit; mRS, modified Rankin Scale; OR, odds ratio; SE, status epilepticus; STESS, status epilepticus severity score.

The onset symptoms of autoimmune SE can be various. Alteration in mental status is the cardinal symptom (12), but provides little information about the underlying etiology. In our patients, the presenting symptoms of inflammatory SE included fever, decreased consciousness, seizure, upper respiratory tract infection, headache, psychosis, fatigue, and cognitive decline. Of note, psychosis was present only in those with autoimmune SE and not in those with infectious SE. Other studies have also reported that psychosis is the dominant presenting symptom among patients with autoimmune encephalitis (14, 29, 32, 33). In addition, we found that more of the patients with autoimmune SE had non-convulsive SE compared to those with infectious SE, which was not reported in the two previous studies (11, 20). This may be due to the difficulty in recognizing non-convulsive SE clinically without EEG monitoring or because it was not specifically looked for. Super refractory SE was also more prevalent in the autoimmune SE group, which may be due to the difficulty in making a diagnosis and the ineffectiveness of traditional SE treatment to control seizure activity without immunotherapy (34). When non-convulsive SE or psychosis followed by SE occurs in patients with a young age and female sex, autoimmune SE should be considered.

CSF studies are an important tool to identify the cause of SE, however, such studies can be challenging clinically. Neutrophilic predominant pleocytosis usually points toward a bacterial infection or the early stage of viral encephalitis, especially in the first 24 to 48 hours (24). Lymphocytic predominant pleocytosis was associated with autoimmune SE in our study,

TABLE 3 | The findings of the first cerebrospinal fluid (CSF) and electroencephalography (EEG) studies.

	Autoimmune SE (n = 25)	Infectious SE (n = 21)	p-value	OR (95% CI)
The first CSF findings				
CSF protein (mg/dL)	34.8 (23.5–110.9)	93.0 (38.1–260.9)	0.014	
CSF WBC count (cell/mm^3)	3 (0–18)	20 (2.5–536)	0.011	
Neutrophilic predominance	2 (15.4)	9 (52.9)	0.034	0.162 (0.03–0.96)
Lymphocytic predominance	11 (84.6)	8 (47.1)	0.034	6.19 (1.04–36.78)
[a]CSF/Blood glucose ratio <0.5	6 (24.0)	9 (56.3)	0.036	0.25 (0.06–0.95)
[b]IgG index >0.6	11 (55.0)	4 (66.7)	0.612	0.61 (0.09–4.14)
The first EEG finding				
Normal	1 (4.0)	3 (14.3)	0.318	0.25 (0.02–2.61)
Background slowing activity	14 (56.0)	6 (28.6)	0.081	0.51 (0.24–1.09)
Sporadic epileptiform discharge	2 (8.0)	4 (19.0)	0.239	2.38 (0.48–11.74)
Periodic discharge	3 (12.0)	3 (14.3)	0.769	1.19 (0.27–5.29)
Electrographic seizure	5 (20.0)	5 (23.8)	0.688	1.19 (0.4–3.56)

Continuous variables were presented as median (interquartile range).
Categorical variables were presented as n (%).
CI, confidence interval; OR, odds ratio; SE, status epilepticus; WBC, white blood cell.
a The CSF/blood glucose ratio was available in 16 patients with infectious and all patients with autoimmune etiology.
b The IgG index was available in six patients with infectious and 20 patients with autoimmune etiology.

but it was also often seen in cases of viral encephalitis-related SE (17, 24). Intensive care physicians often face a dilemma over whether to use antiviral therapy or immunotherapy when the diagnosis is unclear. Other parameters of the CSF can aid in the differential diagnosis, as our data suggested that the patients with an infectious etiology usually had a higher CSF protein level, although prolonged SE itself may result in a milder elevation of lactate and/or total protein levels. This was also reported by Oyanguren et al. who found similar white blood cell count between patients with viral infections and autoimmune processes, but that the protein level was higher in those with a CNS viral infection (35). Therefore, a high protein level in patients with lymphocytic predominance pleocytosis may suggest a viral etiology.

MRI can aid in the search for the etiology of SE, but with limitations. Limbic encephalitis may present as an increased FLAIR/T2 signal or abnormal DWI in the medial temporal lobes (36–38), and it can be used in helping to make the diagnosis of autoimmune encephalitis (16). Prolonged SE itself can also cause similar changes to some viral infectious in MRI signal with DWI abnormalities in the hippocampus and pulvinar (39), particularly herpes simplex encephalitis (18). Furthermore, these MRI patterns may not be present in all types of autoimmune SE and one study reported that 60% of the MRI findings in patients with anti-NMDA encephalitis may have been normal (14). Our data showed that no specific MRI findings could differentiate autoimmune and infectious SE.

EEG is routinely used to evaluate patients with seizures or disturbed consciousness. Slow background activity was more dominant in autoimmune patients compared with other etiologies of seizure (40), although we found no statistical difference in EEG findings between the two groups. Our study showed that at an early stage of inflammatory SE, it remains difficult to differentiate the two entities using currently available para-clinical investigations. The early use of auto-antibody assays may be needed when autoimmune SE is suspected clinically.

We found that general anesthesia was more commonly used in the patients with autoimmune SE. This is in accordance with previous studies in which patients with autoimmune SE were less responsive to AEDs (11, 20, 30, 41). The reason why AEDs are less effective for autoimmune SE remains to be clarified, although it is well-known that the treatment of autoimmune SE requires prompt immunotherapy (14, 15), which may then reduce the use of general anesthesia.

The functional outcomes were similar in both infectious and autoimmune groups with a similar mRS score at discharge and similar mortality rate during admission. However, most of our patients had a poor outcome at discharge or last follow-up (63.0 and 65.2%, respectively). Our study showed that the predictive values of STESS and END-IT scores were not in the same direction. That is, STESS was more sensitive but END-IT was more specific in terms of predicting the outcomes at discharge. More studies may be needed to compare the use of these two scores. In addition to functional impairments, a recent study reported that patients also had substantial impairments in their quality of life after SE (42). Our patients with autoimmune SE had a mortality rate of 20%, which is similar to other studies ranging from 10 to 23% (20, 30, 43). A recent population-based study conducted in Germany reported a hospital mortality rate for all types of SE of 14.8% with a higher rate in those with refractory SE and super refractory SE (15.0 and 39.9%, respectively) (44). The higher mortality rate in patients with autoimmune etiology compared to those with all-cause SE may be related to the high percentage of super refractory SE among patients with an autoimmune etiology. This higher mortality rate compared to all-cause SE emphasize the need for rapid recognition of the condition and prompt treatment toward the underlying causes in addition to standard SE care.

TABLE 4 | The findings of magnetic resonance imaging study.

	Autoimmune SE (n = 25)	Infectious SE (n = 21)	p-value	OR (95% CI)
FLAIR and T2 abnormalities	11 (44)	8 (38.1)	0.685	1.28 (0.39–4.17)
Lateralization				
Unilateral	5 (20.0)	3 (14.3)	0.729	0.72 (0.11–4.62)
Bilateral	6 (24.0)	5 (23.8)		
Location				
Temporal lobe	9 (36)	5 (23.8)		
Mesial temporal lobe	7 (28)	4 (19)		
Lateral temporal lobe	2 (8)	1 (4.8)		
Frontal lobe	6 (24)	3 (14.3)		
Parietal lobe	7 (28)	2 (9.5)		
Occipital lobe	7 (28)	4 (19)		
Basal ganglion	0 (0)	2 (9.5)		
Multiple lobes	7 (28)	3 (14.3)	0.367	2.10 (0.41–10.66)
DWI abnormalities	14 (56)	10 (50)	0.688	1.27 (0.39–4.14)
Lateralization				
Unilateral	5 (35.7)	6 (60)	0.408	0.37 (0.07–1.97)
Bilateral	9 (64.3)	4 (40)	0.408	2.7 (0.51–14.37)
Location				
Temporal lobe	11 (78.6)	7 (70)		
Mesial temporal lobe	7 (50)	3 (30)		
Lateral temporal lobe	4 (28.6)	5 (50)		
Frontal lobe	6 (42.9)	5 (50)		
Parietal lobe	6 (42.9)	5 (50)		
Occipital lobe	5 (35.7)	5 (50)		
Basal ganglion	0 (0)	4 (40)		
Multiple lobes	11 (78.6)	6 (60)	0.393	2.44 (0.41–14.75)

Categorical variables were presented as n (%).
CI, confidence interval; DWI, diffusion-weighted imaging; FLAIR, fluid-attenuated inversion recovery; OR, odds ratio; SE, status epilepticus.

The limitations of this study are that it was conducted at a single hospital and that the design was retrospective. In addition, the study was started before the availability of recent autoimmune encephalitis screening tests and immunotherapies, which may have affected the outcomes.

In conclusion, we observed that patients with autoimmune SE had a younger age at onset, female predominance, and often presented with psychosis, super-refractory SE and non-convulsive SE. The initial clinical investigations including EEG and MRI only provided limited information about the underlying etiology. CSF tests were helpful in diagnosing bacterial infectious-related SE but had difficulty in differentiating viral encephalitis and autoimmune SE. Since these two etiologies have different treatment strategies and the presenting symptoms are quite similar (12, 29), it is important to differentiate the two conditions as soon as possible. The patient characteristics and presenting features identified in our study may provide clinicians with some clues about the underlying etiology. Empiric treatment can be given based on these clinical clues while waiting for the results of more definitive diagnostic tests such as viral serology tests and neuronal surface auto-antibody screening.

ETHICS STATEMENT

This study is approved by the Chang Gung Medical Foundation Institutional Review Board (IRB No.: 103-3665B and 201800677B0).

AUTHOR CONTRIBUTIONS

All authors have read and approved the final manuscript. C-HL contributed to clinical data analysis and draft of the manuscript. Y-TL, C-JH, and F-YS had contributions to clinical data acquisition and analysis. M-HT had substantial contributions to the conception and design of the study, data analysis, critical revision, and final approval of the manuscript.

FUNDING

This work was supported in part by research grant CMRPG8G0131 to C-HL from Kaohsiung Chang Gung Memorial Hospital, Taiwan.

REFERENCES

1. Bermeo-Ovalle A, Bleck T. Status epilepticus in the intensive care unit. *Semin Neurol.* (2016) 36:550–9. doi: 10.1055/s-0036-1592357
2. Wu YW, Shek DW, Garcia PA, Zhao S, Johnston SC. Incidence and mortality of generalized convulsive status epilepticus in California. *Neurology* (2002) 58:1070–6. doi: 10.1212/WNL.58.7.1070
3. Lv RJ, Wang Q, Cui T, Zhu F, Shao XQ. Status epilepticus-related etiology, incidence and mortality: a meta-analysis. *Epilepsy Res.* (2017) 136:12–7. doi: 10.1016/j.eplepsyres.2017.07.006
4. Glauser T, Shinnar S, Gloss D, Alldredge B, Arya R, Bainbridge J, et al. Evidence-based guideline: treatment of convulsive status epilepticus in children and adults: report of the guideline committee of the American epilepsy society. *Epilepsy Curr.* (2016) 16:48–61. doi: 10.5698/1535-7597-16.1.48
5. Jagoda A, Riggio S. Refractory status epilepticus in adults. *Ann Emerg Med.* (1993) 22:1337–48. doi: 10.1016/S0196-0644(05)80120-9
6. Tsai MH, Chuang YC, Chang HW, Chang WN, Lai SL, Huang CR, et al. Factors predictive of outcome in patients with de novo status epilepticus. *QJM* (2009) 102:57–62. doi: 10.1093/qjmed/hcn149
7. Koubeissi M, Alshekhlee A. In-hospital mortality of generalized convulsive status epilepticus: a large US sample. *Neurology* (2007) 69:886–93. doi: 10.1212/01.wnl.0000269791.96189.70
8. Rossetti AO, Hurwitz S, Logroscino G, Bromfield EB. Prognosis of status epilepticus: role of aetiology, age, and consciousness impairment at presentation. *J Neurol Neurosurg Psychiatry* (2006) 77:611–5. doi: 10.1136/jnnp.2005.080887
9. Seinfeld S, Goodkin HP, Shinnar S. Status epilepticus. *Cold Spring Harb perspect Med.* (2016) 6:a022830. doi: 10.1101/cshperspect.a022830
10. Singh TD, Fugate JE, Rabinstein AA. The spectrum of acute encephalitis: causes, management, and predictors of outcome. *Neurology* (2015) 84:359–66. doi: 10.1212/WNL.0000000000001190
11. Shin JW, Koo YS, Kim YS, Kim DW, Kim KK, Lee SY, et al. Clinical characterization of unknown/cryptogenic status epilepticus suspected as encephalitis: a multicenter cohort study. *J Neuroimmunol.* (2018) 315:1–8. doi: 10.1016/j.jneuroim.2017.12.004
12. Venkatesan A, Tunkel AR, Bloch KC, Lauring AS, Sejvar J, Bitnun A, et al. Case definitions, diagnostic algorithms, and priorities in encephalitis: consensus statement of the international encephalitis consortium. *Clin Infect Dis.* (2013) 57:1114–28. doi: 10.1093/cid/cit458
13. Suthar R, Sankhyan N. Bacterial Infections of the central nervous system. *Indian J Pediatr.* (2018) 86:60–9. doi: 10.1007/s12098-017-2477-z
14. Titulaer MJ, McCracken L, Gabilondo I, Armangue T, Glaser C, Iizuka T, et al. Treatment and prognostic factors for long-term outcome in patients with anti-NMDA receptor encephalitis: an observational cohort study. *Lancet Neurol.* (2013) 12:157–65. doi: 10.1016/S1474-4422(12)70310-1
15. Shin YW, Lee ST, Park KI, Jung KH, Jung KY, Lee SK, et al. Treatment strategies for autoimmune encephalitis. *Ther Adv Neurol Disord.* (2018) 11:1756285617722347. doi: 10.1177/1756285617722347
16. Graus F, Titulaer MJ, Balu R, Benseler S, Bien CG, Cellucci T, et al. A clinical approach to diagnosis of autoimmune encephalitis. *Lancet Neurol.* (2016) 15:391–404. doi: 10.1016/S1474-4422(15)00401-9
17. Armangue T, Leypoldt F, Dalmau J. Autoimmune encephalitis as differential diagnosis of infectious encephalitis. *Curr Opin Neurol.* (2014) 27:361–8. doi: 10.1097/WCO.0000000000000087
18. Sureka J, Jakkani RK. Clinico-radiological spectrum of bilateral temporal lobe hyperintensity: a retrospective review. *Br J Radiol.* (2012) 85:e782–92. doi: 10.1259/bjr/30039090
19. Lancaster E. The diagnosis and treatment of autoimmune encephalitis. *J Clin Neurol.* (2016) 12:1–13. doi: 10.3988/jcn.2016.12.1.1
20. Spatola M, Novy J, Du Pasquier R, Dalmau J, Rossetti AO. Status epilepticus of inflammatory etiology: a cohort study. *Neurology* (2015) 85:464–70. doi: 10.1212/WNL.0000000000001717
21. Brophy GM, Bell R, Claassen J, Alldredge B, Bleck TP, Glauser T, et al. Guidelines for the evaluation and management of status epilepticus. *Neurocrit Care* (2012) 17:3–23. doi: 10.1007/s12028-012-9695-z
22. Ferlisi M, Shorvon S. The outcome of therapies in refractory and super-refractory convulsive status epilepticus and recommendations for therapy. *Brain* (2012) 135(Pt 8):2314–28. doi: 10.1093/brain/aws091
23. Trinka E, Cock H, Hesdorffer D, Rossetti AO, Scheffer IE, Shinnar S, et al. A definition and classification of status epilepticus–Report of the ILAE task force on classification of status epilepticus. *Epilepsia* (2015) 56:1515–23. doi: 10.1111/epi.13121
24. Tuppeny M. Viral meningitis and encephalitis. *Crit Care Nurs Clin North Am.* (2013) 25:363–80. doi: 10.1016/j.ccell.2013.04.003
25. Rossetti AO, Logroscino G, Milligan TA, Michaelides C, Ruffieux C, Bromfield EB. Status Epilepticus Severity Score (STESS): a tool to orient early treatment strategy. *J Neurol.* (2008) 255:1561–6. doi: 10.1007/s00415-008-0989-1
26. Gao Q, Ou-Yang TP, Sun XL, Yang F, Wu C, Kang T, et al. Prediction of functional outcome in patients with convulsive status epilepticus: the END-IT score. *Crit Care* (2016) 20:46. doi: 10.1186/s13054-016-1221-9
27. Hirsch LJ, LaRoche SM, Gaspard N, Gerard E, Svoronos A, Herman ST, et al. American clinical neurophysiology society's standardized critical care EEG terminology: 2012 version. *J Clin Neurophysiol.* (2013) 30:1–27. doi: 10.1097/WNP.0b013e3182784729
28. Heine J, Pruss H, Bartsch T, Ploner CJ, Paul F, Finke C. Imaging of autoimmune encephalitis–Relevance for clinical practice and hippocampal function. *Neuroscience* (2015) 309:68–83. doi: 10.1016/j.neuroscience.2015.05.037
29. Saraya A, Mahavihakanont A, Shuangshoti S, Sittidetboripat N, Deesudchit T, Callahan M, et al. Autoimmune causes of encephalitis syndrome in Thailand: prospective study of 103 patients. *BMC Neurol.* (2013) 13:150. doi: 10.1186/1471-2377-13-150
30. Holzer FJ, Rossetti AO, Heritier-Barras AC, Zumsteg D, Roebling R, Huber R, et al. Antibody-mediated status epilepticus: a retrospective multicenter survey. *Eur Neurol.* (2012) 68:310–7. doi: 10.1159/000341143
31. Gubbels Bupp MR, Potluri T, Fink AL, Klein SL. The confluence of sex hormones and aging on immunity. *Front Immunol.* (2018) 9:1269. doi: 10.3389/fimmu.2018.01269
32. Hao Q, Wang D, Guo L, Zhang B. Clinical characterization of autoimmune encephalitis and psychosis. *Compr Psychiatry* (2017) 74:9–14. doi: 10.1016/j.comppsych.2016.12.006
33. Lim JA, Lee ST, Jung KH, Kim S, Shin JW, Moon J, et al. Anti-N-methyl-d-aspartate receptor encephalitis in Korea: clinical features, treatment, and outcome. *J Clin Neurol.* (2014) 10:157–61. doi: 10.3988/jcn.2014.10.2.157
34. Varley J, Taylor J, Irani SR. Autoantibody-mediated diseases of the CNS: structure, dysfunction and therapy. *Neuropharmacology* (2018) 132:71–82. doi: 10.1016/j.neuropharm.2017.04.046
35. Oyanguren B, Sanchez V, Gonzalez FJ, de Felipe A, Esteban L, Lopez-Sendon JL, et al. Limbic encephalitis: a clinical-radiological comparison between herpetic and autoimmune etiologies. *Eur J Neurol.* (2013) 20:1566–70. doi: 10.1111/ene.12249
36. Lai M, Hughes EG, Peng X, Zhou L, Gleichman AJ, Shu H, et al. AMPA receptor antibodies in limbic encephalitis alter synaptic receptor location. *Ann Neurol.* (2009) 65:424–34. doi: 10.1002/ana.21589
37. Lai M, Huijbers MG, Lancaster E, Graus F, Bataller L, Balice-Gordon R, et al. Investigation of LGI1 as the antigen in limbic encephalitis previously attributed to potassium channels: a case series. *Lancet Neurol.* (2010) 9:776–85. doi: 10.1016/S1474-4422(10)70137-X
38. Hoftberger R, Titulaer MJ, Sabater L, Dome B, Rozsas A, Hegedus B, et al. Encephalitis and GABAB receptor antibodies: novel findings in a new case series of 20 patients. *Neurology* (2013) 81:1500–6. doi: 10.1212/WNL.0b013e3182a9585f
39. Mendes A, Sampaio L. Brain magnetic resonance in status epilepticus: a focused review. *Seizure* (2016) 38:63–7. doi: 10.1016/j.seizure.2016.04.007
40. Limotai C, Denlertchaikul C, Saraya AW, Jirasakuldej S. Predictive values and specificity of electroencephalographic findings in autoimmune encephalitis diagnosis. *Epilepsy Behav.* (2018) 84:29–36. doi: 10.1016/j.yebeh.2018.04.007
41. Dubey D, Blackburn K, Greenberg B, Stuve O, Vernino S. Diagnostic and therapeutic strategies for management of autoimmune encephalopathies. *Expert Rev Neurother.* (2016) 16:937–49. doi: 10.1080/14737175.2016.1189328
42. Kortland LM, Knake S, von Podewils F, Rosenow F, Strzelczyk A. Socioeconomic outcome and quality of life in adults after status epilepticus: a

multicenter, longitudinal, matched case-control analysis from Germany. *Front Neurol.* (2017) 8:507. doi: 10.3389/fneur.2017.00507

43. Holzer FJ, Seeck M, Korff CM. Autoimmunity and inflammation in status epilepticus: from concepts to therapies. *Expert Rev Neurother.* (2014) 14:1181–202. doi: 10.1586/14737175.2014.956457
44. Strzelczyk A, Ansorge S, Hapfelmeier J, Bonthapally V, Erder MH, Rosenow F. Costs, length of stay, and mortality of super-refractory status epilepticus: a population-based study from Germany. *Epilepsia* (2017) 58:1533–41. doi: 10.1111/epi.13837

17

DAT1-Genotype and Menstrual Cycle, but Not Hormonal Contraception, Modulate Reinforcement Learning: Preliminary Evidence

Kristina Jakob[†]*, Hanna Ehrentreich*[†]*, Sarah K. C. Holtfrerich, Luise Reimers and Esther K. Diekhof*[*†]

Department of Biology, Faculty of Mathematics, Informatics and Natural Sciences, Institute of Zoology, Neuroendocrinology Unit, Universität Hamburg, Hamburg, Germany

***Correspondence:**
Esther K. Diekhof
esther.diekhof@uni-hamburg.de

[†]*These authors have contributed equally to this work.*

Hormone by genotype interactions have been widely ignored by cognitive neuroscience. Yet, the dependence of cognitive performance on both baseline dopamine (DA) and current 17ß-estradiol (E2) level argues for their combined effect also in the context of reinforcement learning. Here, we assessed how the interaction between the natural rise of E2 in the late follicular phase (FP) and the 40 base-pair variable number tandem repeat polymorphism of the dopamine transporter (DAT1) affects reinforcement learning capacity. 30 women with a regular menstrual cycle performed a probabilistic feedback learning task twice during the early and late FP. In addition, 39 women, who took hormonal contraceptives (HC) to suppress natural ovulation, were tested during the "pill break" and the intake phase of HC. The present data show that DAT1-genotype may interact with transient hormonal state, but only in women with a natural menstrual cycle. We found that carriers of the 9-repeat allele (9RP) experienced a significant decrease in the ability to avoid punishment from early to late FP. Neither homozygote subjects of the 10RP allele, nor subjects from the HC group showed a change in behavior between phases. These data are consistent with neurobiological studies that found that rising E2 may reverse DA transporter function and could enhance DA efflux, which would in turn reduce punishment sensitivity particularly in subjects with a higher transporter density to begin with. Taken together, the present results, although based on a small sample, add to the growing understanding of the complex interplay between different physiological modulators of dopaminergic transmission. They may not only point out the necessity to control for hormonal state in behavioral genetic research, but may offer new starting points for studies in clinical settings.

Keywords: estrogen, dopamine transporter, reinforcement learning, gender, steroid hormone, hormonal contraception

INTRODUCTION

The sex steroid 17ß-estradiol (E2) increases dopaminergic transmission in the reward system (1) and may enhance behavioral responses to reward and drugs of abuse [e.g., Ref. (2)]. In the animal model, E2 has been found to amplify the dopaminergic response in the striatum by (1) promoting stimulated dopamine (DA) release (3), (2) increasing DA synthesis capacity (4), and (3) decreasing the affinity of inhibitory D2-receptors (DRD2) [(5–7); but also see Ref. (8), who indicate a possible regional specificity of this effect in the striatum that might also lead to an increase]. Recent neuroimaging evidence in humans points in a similar direction. Diekhof and Ratnayake (9) showed that—similar to DA-agonistic drugs (e.g., L-DOPA)—the increase of E2 level during the late follicular phase (FP) of the menstrual cycle had the potential to enhance reward learning capacity at the expense of the ability to learn from negative feedback [see also Ref. (10)]. Previous pharmacological and behavioral genetic evidence already suggested that both intra- and inter-individual variations in dopaminergic capacity may drive differences in reward learning and punishment avoidance capacity [e.g., Ref. (11, 12)]. According to theory, the differential action of DA at two subgroups of DA receptors (DRD1 and DRD2) that are located at the direct and the indirect pathways of the basal ganglia, respectively, may determine the extent to which a person is sensitive to the rewarding as opposed to the punishing outcomes of one's action. Phasic DA release after a rewarded action is thereby assumed to promote learning *via* long-term potentiation at the corticostriatal synapses of the direct "Go-pathway" that mainly expresses DRD1. At the same time, avoidance learning capacity is suppressed through DRD2-dependent long-term depression of the indirect "NoGo-pathway." Conversely, when an action is followed by a dip in tonic DA, such as the one following a negative action outcome or reward omission, the NoGo-pathway is strengthened and avoidance responses are facilitated at the expense of the reward learning capacity (13). Diekhof and Ratnayake (9) found that activation of the dorsal anterior cingulate cortex (dACC) was reduced during processing of negative feedback in the late FP. Assuming that the dACC may particularly optimize action selection during avoidance learning (14), a reduced response of this brain region in a state of heightened E2 may fit well with the proposed properties of E2 in the regulation of DA release (1, 6), which should have strengthened reward learning through weakening DRD2-mediated punishment avoidance capacity.

In addition to that, there is further behavioral evidence for an inverted U-shaped relationship between baseline dopaminergic capacity, cycle-dependent changes in endogenous E2 from the early to the late FP, and reward-related decision making (15, 16) as well as working memory performance in humans (17). Smith et al. (15) assessed the influence of the COMT Met158Val polymorphism (rs4680) as a proxy of prefrontal DA on temporal discounting across the menstrual cycle. Against expectation, they found a reduction of temporal discounting (i.e., the "Now Bias"), when E2 level was increased in the late FP. Diekhof (16) used the Barratt Impulsiveness Scale (BIS) as an indirect proxy of mesolimbic DA. Using a temporal response time adaptation paradigm that is sensitive for differences in striatal DA transmission (18), Diekhof (16) assessed the ability to speed up in order to maximize reward (i.e., a measure of reward sensitivity) and compared it to the capacity to slow down for higher reward (i.e., an indicator of punishment sensitivity). Similar to Smith et al. (15), they found a paradoxical decline in the ability to speed up for higher reward from the early to the late FP, while the capacity to wait for increasing reward value improved from the low to high E2 state. Yet, when looking at inter-individual differences in hormone concentration, they also found a positive correlation between E2 concentration and an enhancement of reward sensitivity as reflected by an improved ability to speed up for higher reward. Interestingly, this correlation only existed at the lower end of the E2 distribution (i.e., in the early FP) and was further specific for subjects with low "trait impulsiveness" in the BIS, who may be characterized by a habitually low baseline DA synthesis capacity (19). In sum, these data are consistent with an inverted U-shaped relationship by showing that only subjects at the lower end of the DA distribution were affected by changes in E2, while subjects with DA levels near the point of optimality, i.e., at the center of the DA distribution, may not show such strong perturbations. Moreover, given the assumption that trait impulsiveness may to some extent mirror one's genetic underpinnings (20–22), this finding points to a possible hormone–genotype interaction in the domain of reinforcement learning.

The present study aimed at elucidating the link between genetic predisposition and the degree to which natural variations in E2 level affect reinforcement learning. It has already been shown that genetic differences can modulate central dopaminergic transmission and cognitive functions (23). Further, individual predisposition may incline the individual to an either more reward- or punishment-sensitive learning style. For example, carriers of genetic polymorphisms, that may be associated with reduced DA autoregulation by DRD2 or an increased DA synthesis capacity, were compromised in their ability to avoid punishment in a probabilistic feedback learning task [e.g., Ref. (12, 24)]. Here, we assessed the interaction between cycle-dependent variations in E2 level and a genetic polymorphism that has been implicated in the reuptake of DA in the striatum. The 40 base-pair (40-bp) variable number tandem repeat polymorphism of the dopamine transporter (DAT1), which has been described in the 3′ untranslated region of the gene SLC6A3, has two common alleles with either 9 or 10 repeats (RP) of the 40-bp sequence The two variants may differentially affect the expression of the DAT in the striatum [(25–28), but see (29) for a null finding], and can also modulate reward-related processing (30–32), although evidence is mixed and it has not been determined, which variant may actually predispose for a higher DAT density. E2 can induce a reversal of DAT function *in vitro*, which is achieved by rapid alterations in several signaling pathways that cause efflux of DA from the DAT instead of DA reuptake (33–35). Given this evidence, the closer examination of a possible E2 by DAT1-genotype interaction and its relation to the model of the inverted U-shape of DA content and reinforcement learning capacity might add to the growing understanding of the baseline dependency of a neurocognitive function that is mediated by DA. When E2 level rises from the early to the late FP, we would predict a reversal of normal DAT function that should result in increased DA transmission in the striatum. By subdividing our sample in carriers of the 9RP allele and homozygotes of the 10RP, we should further be able to identify the genotype of the DAT1-polymorphism (9RP carriers versus subjects that are homozygote for the 10RP variant [10H]) that predisposes a person for a higher DAT density. This is because we would expect that the genetic variant that predisposes one for a higher DAT density and thus a lower DA baseline to begin with, should be more affected by the proposed E2-induced DAT reversal that is expected to happen in the high E2 state of the late FP. For one thing, in the late FP this genotype should become relatively more reward sensitive and should be less able to learn from negative feedback when heightened E2 level might induce a reversal of normal transporter function, which would promote a rise in DA level. Conversely, in the early FP when E2 is still at its nadir, we would expect the same genotype to be relatively more punishment sensitive, because the habitually higher density of DAT and thus more effective DA reuptake, that is unaffected by E2 at this point in time, would promote avoidance learning ability.

In order to test our hypothesis of a possible cycle phase by genotype interaction during reinforcement learning, our subjects performed a probabilistic feedback learning task. This task has been shown to be a sensitive measure for genetic variations in baseline DA (12, 24) and transient variations in DA concentration that were induced by pharmacological intervention [e.g., Ref. (11, 36)]. Two groups of healthy young women were genotyped for the DAT1-polymorphism. The first one had a natural menstrual cycle, while the second group took hormonal contraceptives (HC) on a regular basis. These latter women did not experience natural fluctuations of E2 level over the course of the menstrual cycle, but were influenced by synthetic ethinylestradiol and progestines, which might also affect reinforcement learning capacity. Both groups were tested twice, either in a low versus high E2 phase of the menstrual cycle (i.e., in the early and late FP) or during the "pill break" and the intake phase of HC, respectively.

MATERIALS AND METHODS

Subjects

In total, 85 women were recruited for this study (i.e., 45 participants in the cycle group and 40 subjects in the HC group). Of these, five participants had to be excluded because of either technical problems with the response box or the test protocol, lack of compliance, or drop-out after the first test. Another subject had an exceedingly high E2 level, indicating a possible hormonal disturbance, which also led to exclusion from all further analyses. The remaining 79 healthy women [age (mean ± SEM) = 25.5 ± 0.4 years] had no current or previous psychiatric or neurological diagnosis, reported to have no history of drug abuse or gynecological problems (e.g., endometriosis) and did not have any chronic disorder related to the hormone system (e.g., diabetes, Hashimoto's thyroiditis, PCO). Subjects were of Middle European origin as determined by the place of birth of their parents and grandparents. All subjects gave written informed consent and were paid for participation. The present study was approved by the local ethics committee (*Ethikkommission der Ärztekammer Hamburg*).

The Cycle Group

The cycle group consisted of 39 women, who were free of any medication including hormonal contraception for at least three menstrual cycles in the past and reported to have regular menstrual cycles in the normal range of 24–36 days. Following the procedure applied by former neurobehavioral studies on the effects of E2 across the menstrual cycle (9, 15, 16), subjects from this group were only included in our final analyses if they showed an increase in E2 level from the early to the late FP. This was done because we wanted to assess the effect of rising E2 in the late FP. Ovulation is hidden in humans and the actual extent of follicular development can only be ascertained by vaginal ultrasound. Yet, a rising E2 level during the FP may be an indirect indicator of normal follicular growth. Therefore, an E2 rise from early to late FP in combination with a negative lutropin (LH) ovulation test before testing (see below) was a necessary prerequisite for the late FP test to take place, which left 31 subjects.

Since the goal of the study was to compare DAT1 9-repeat allele carriers and 10-repeat allele homozygotes in their reaction to a natural rise in E2 level and its subsequent impact on reinforcement learning capacity, the participants were also genotyped. In the present sample, 14 subjects were carriers of the 9RP allele (2 of them were homozygote for the 9RP), while the remaining 16 subjects were homozygous for the 10RP variant. There was also one person that carried the rare 11-repeat allele variant in combination with the 9RP (11/9), who was subsequently excluded, leaving the final number of 30 participants in the cycle group [age (mean ± SEM) = 27.5 ± 0.7 years; age range = 21–35 years]. About 38% of the cycle participants were currently in a relationship with a male partner and the majority considered themselves as heterosexual (two bisexual subjects).

The women were tested twice, once during the first 3 days of menstruation (early FP) and once two days before expected ovulation (late FP). The date of expected ovulation was calculated from the expected cycle length individually for each participant. For this we asked the participants to state their expected cycle length and then, upon the onset of menstruation, used the last expected cycle day to determine the optimal test day with a common counting method: for all subjects with a cycle length shorter than 28 days, we subtracted 15 days from the expected cycle end. For subjects with an expected length of 28–31 days, 16 days were subtracted, and for cycle lengths longer than 31 days, 17 days were subtracted to schedule the test in the late FP. Our subjects also determined the daily concentration of LH with a common *in vitro* urine test (One Step® by AIDE Diagnostic Co., Ltd.), starting 2 days before the test date. In case of a positive result before the test day, the test was postponed to the subsequent cycle.

The test design was counterbalanced for cycle phase. Half of the participants started the test protocol in the early FP (i.e., seven carriers of the 9RP variant; eight were 10H). The remaining subjects started in the late FP (same genotype proportion).

The HC Group

The 40 participants of the HC group were recruited when the data collection for the cycle group was almost finished. The HC group allowed us to compare the data from a phase of low hormone availability (pill break) with a phase, during which participants were under the influence of synthetic hormones (intake phase), while the impact of natural hormones was blocked. Participants from the HC group took HC for at least 12 months (mean duration of HC intake = 7.77 ± 0.61 years), but were otherwise free of medication. HC contained ethinylestradiol in the range of 0.015–0.03 mg and different amounts of progestin compounds (e.g., levonorgestrel, dienogest), which are used to suppress follicular growth and ovulation (37). Therefore, we expected no significant change in hormone level between the two test phases, except from a numerical E2 increase or a fall in E2 during the intake phase (38).

The HC group consisted of 20 carriers of the 9RP variant (one of them was homozygote) and 18 subjects were genotyped as 10H. One person in this group also had the rare 11-repeat allele variant combined with the 10RP allele (11/10) and was therefore excluded, leaving a final number of 38 subjects in the HC group [age (mean ± SEM) = 23.5 ± 0.5 years; age range = 19–32 years]. About 87% of the HC participants, i.e., almost three times as many as in the cycle group, were currently in a relationship with a male partner and the majority considered themselves as heterosexual (one bisexual subject).

The HC group had an analogous counterbalanced test design to the cycle group. Twenty participants started the test protocol in the OFF-phase ($n_{9RP} = 10$; $n_{10H} = 10$). The term "OFF-phase" refers to the so-called pill break of 7 days. The test was scheduled for the third or fourth day of the pill break. The second test phase, the "ON-phase," required an intake of HC for at least five consecutive days. In that way, the OFF-phase resembles the early FP in terms of low E2 availability, while the ON-phase might be rather characterized by a slight influence of synthetic hormone content (in this case, the mixture of ethinyestradiol and progestin compounds contained in contraceptive medication). In order to achieve a comparable repeated test schedule to the naturally cycling women, subjects who started in the OFF-phase had the subsequent ON-test approximately 7 days later (mean ± SEM = 7 ± 1.6 days), while the other group had a gap of 18 days (mean ± SEM = 18.5 ± 0.12 days).

Test Procedure

Participants performed a probabilistic feedback task, described in more detail by Diekhof and Ratnayake (9), which is a well-established test of reinforcement learning capacity [see also Ref. (11, 12) for description of the task]. In this task, subjects learned to associate certain stimuli with a higher probability of positive or negative feedback (i.e., a smiley or a grumpy face). During the initial learning phase (session 1), they were confronted with three fixed stimulus pairs of different hiragana and kanji symbols (i.e., pairs AB, EF, CD) from which they had to choose the one symbol that allowed them to maximize reward (positive feedback in form of a smiley) and to avoid frequent punishment (negative feedback of a grumpy face). The task goal was to receive as many smileys as possible. Unbeknownst to the participants, the reward contingencies differed between pairs and stimuli. Among all symbols, A of the pair AB was the best option (80% positive feedback upon selection), while B was the worst option (only 20% positive feedback). The reward contingencies of the remaining symbols lay in between these contingencies (i.e., pair CD: C = 70%, D = 30%; pair EF: E = 60%, F = 50%). After learning, subjects were tested in a transfer phase (session 2) to check whether they had been able to maximize positive outcome through either selection of the better option (i.e., reward learning) or by more effective avoidance of negative feedback (i.e., punishment learning). The individual learning preference cannot be dissociated from the fixed stimulus pairs of session 1, which always combined the same good and bad stimuli (e.g., A and B). This means that in session 1 the preference for the better option (e.g., for the best stimulus A in pair AB) can be equally well driven by approach of the good option A or avoidance of the bad one B. So in the transfer phase, new stimulus pairings (like AC, BD) were presented next to the original ones (AB, CD, EF). These new pairs enabled us to find out whether a subject showed a preference for the best option A (i.e., Choose A performance), which would indicate an enhanced reward learning capacity. Conversely, a participant was classified as having a high punishment learning capacity when she showed more effective avoidance of B in the new stimulus pairs (i.e., Avoid B performance) [see also Ref. (11)]. In the transfer task direct feedback was no longer provided, so that no further learning could take place. The percentage of selections of A from the old pair AB further showed the combined effect of Choose A and Avoid B performance and was thus an indicator of overall learning capacity.

Subjects were tested twice in the two phases, but with different hiragana and kanji symbols for the stimuli A, B, C, D, E, and F on each test day. Tests were scheduled in a counterbalanced sequence that was equally distributed across the two study groups and genotypes (see above).

Genotyping

Genotyping was performed by a commercial laboratory (Bioglobe, Hamburg, Germany). DNA was extracted from buccal swabs and purified with a standard commercial extraction kit. The DAT1-polymorphism was characterized by fragment length determination of PCR products across the variable region. Assignment of genotypes was performed with the software GeneMarker v1.75 (Softgenetics). The PCR amplification procedure used the following primers: AAATAAAACTCCTTGAAACCAGC (forward primer), TGTTGTTATTGATGTGGCACG (backward primer). The distribution of genotypes was in Hardy-Weinberg equilibrium, either when calculated separately for each study group or when looking at the whole group of genotyped subjects.

Collection and Analysis of Salivary E2

Samples of morning saliva were collected on each test day. Subjects started collection at their normal wake-up time and collected five samples in 2 ml Eppendorf tubes at regular intervals over the course of 2 h. No consumption of food or beverages other than water was allowed during this time. This collection method avoided the contamination of samples and controlled for the episodic secretion pattern of steroid hormones, thus providing a representative sample of the free E2 level on the test day. Saliva samples were frozen at −20°C for further analyses. When all samples were collected, aliquots were obtained and processed with a 17beta-Estradiol Luminescence Immunoassay (IBL International, Hamburg, Germany) following the procedure described by Diekhof and Ratnayake (9).

Statistical Analysis

The analysis of the behavioral data was done with the software package IBM SPSS Statistics for Windows (version 22.0; IBM Corp.). Repeated-measures general linear models (GLMs) were performed on the percentage of selections of the better option made in sessions 1 and 2. The specific factors included in the GLMs are further specified in the Section "Results." In order to examine the effect of the cycle phase during which participants entered the study on behavioral outcome in the probabilistic feedback task [see Ref. (39) for a similar procedure], we also re-calculated the GLMs as specified in the Section "Results." For *post hoc* comparisons, either paired or independent *t*-tests were used. Pearson correlations tested for the association between individual differences in hormone level and behavioral preferences. A *p*-value smaller than 0.05 (two-tailed) was considered significant in all tests. If not otherwise indicated, we report the arithmetic mean ± SEM in the text, tables, and figures.

A more fine-grained analysis assessed the more difficult decisions to be made in session 2, which comprised the so-called "WIN-WIN trials" (i.e., pairs "AC," "AE," and "CE") and the "LOSE-LOSE trials" (i.e., "BD," "BF," and "DF"). In the "WIN-WIN trials," the better options A, C, and E were paired with each other and the percentage of selections of the relatively better option was measured. In the "LOSE-LOSE trials," the worse options (B, D, F) were combined with each other and we calculated the percentage of effective avoidance of the relatively worse option. Processing of these options required a finer representation of actual stimulus value and thus indicated the individual sensitivity for more detailed value representations that subjects could have learned from the nature of positive and negative feedback in session 1 (9, 40).

RESULTS

Analysis of E2 Concentration

The cycle group exhibited a significant increase in E2 level from the early to the late FP [$n = 30$; $E2_{early} = 2.42 \pm 0.36$ pg/ml; $E2_{late} = 4.35 \pm 0.48$ pg/ml; $t(29) = -6.16$, $p < 0.001$], while the HC group did not [$n = 38$; $E2_{OFF} = 2.28 \pm 0.24$ pg/ml; $E2_{ON} = 2.63 \pm 0.25$ pg/ml; $t(37) = -1.53$, $p = 0.134$]. This was also reflected by a significant group difference in the phase-related change of E2 level [Delta of $E2_{late-early}$ cycle group = 1.93 ± 0.31 pg/ml; Delta of $E2_{ON-OFF}$ HC group = 0.35 ± 0.23 pg/ml; $t(56) = 4.15$, $p < 0.001$].

Behavioral Data of the Cycle Group

We tested the influence of menstrual cycle phase and thus of the natural rise of follicular E2 on behavior in the probabilistic feedback learning task separately for the learning phase (session 1) and the transfer phase (session2). We found that both overall learning (in session 1) and the capacity for learning from positive as opposed to negative feedback as demonstrated in the transfer phase were affected by the factors "*phase*" and "*DAT1-genotype*" (see **Table 1** for an overview of all main effects and interactions).

For session 1, the GLM with the two within-subject factors "*pair*" (AB, CD, EF) and "*phase*" (early FP versus late FP) and the between-subject factor "*DAT1-genotype*" (9R versus 10H) revealed significant main effects of "*phase*" [$F(1,28) = 6.76$, $p = 0.015$, partial eta squared = 0.19] and "*pair*" [$F(2,56) = 20.53$, $p < 0.001$, partial eta squared = 0.42] as well as a significant two-way interaction between "*phase*" and "*DAT1-genotype*" [$F(1,28) = 6.14$, $p = 0.020$, partial eta squared = 0.18]. All other main effects and interactions in session 1 did not reach the statistical criterion of $p < 0.05$ (see **Table 1**).

Post hoc t-tests showed that subjects exhibited enhanced learning during the early FP [overall selection of the better option across pairs: early FP = 66.69 ± 2.91%; late FP = 59.53 ± 2.45%; $t(29) = 2.25$, $p = 0.032$] and learning success followed the expected pattern of A > C > E, which was in line with the associated reward contingencies (selection of A = 70.1 ± 2.65%; selection of C = 63.46 ± 2.79%; selection of E = 55.77 ± 2.14%; significance of all *post hoc* comparisons: $p < 0.05$).

Finally, carriers of the 9RP variant showed a significant decline in the ability to select the better option during learning in the comparison of the early and late FP [$t(13) = 3.3$, $p = 0.006$], while the 10H were not [$t(15) = 0.09$, $p = 0.927$]. Moreover, during the early FP, the 9RP allele carriers were also significantly better in selecting the better option than 10H [$t(28) = 2.56$, $p = 0.016$], and this difference vanished in the late FP [$t(28) = 0.85$, $p = 0.854$] (see **Table 2** for the descriptive statistics).

For session 2, the GLM with the two within-subject factors "*learning capacity*" (Choose A, Avoid B, old pair AB) and "*phase*" (early versus late FP) and the between-subject factor "*DAT1-genotype*" (9RP versus 10H) revealed a significant main effect of "*learning capacity*" [$F(1.42,39.69) = 5.97$, $p = 0.011$, partial eta squared = 0.18], the two-way interactions of "*phase*" and "*DAT1-genotype*" [$F(1,28) = 4.88$, $p = 0.035$, partial

TABLE 1 | Main effects and interactions in the cycle group ($n = 30$).

Main effect or interaction	*F*-value	Degrees of freedom	*p*-value	Partial eta squared
Learning phase (session 1)				
Phase*	**6.76**	**1, 28**	**0.015**	**0.19**
Phase × DAT1-genotype*	**6.14**	**1, 28**	**0.020**	**0.18**
Pair*	**20.53**	**2, 56**	**<0.001**	**0.42**
Pair × DAT1-genotype	3.10	2, 56	0.053	0.10
Phase × pair	1.49	2, 56	0.235	0.05
Phase × pair × Dat1-genotype	1.25	2, 56	0.295	0.04
DAT1-genotype	2.25	1, 28	0.145	0.07
Transfer phase (session 2)				
Phase	0.49	1, 28	0.488	0.02
Phase × DAT1-genotype*	**4.89**	**1, 28**	**0.035**	**0.15**
Learning capacity*	**5.97**	**1.4, 39.7**	**0.011**	**0.18**
Learning capacity × DAT1-genotype	2.074	1.4, 39.7	0.151	0.07
Phase × learning capacity*	**8.03**	**1.4, 40.1**	**0.003**	**0.22**
Phase × learning capacity × DAT1-genotype*	**3.66**	**1.4, 40.1**	**0.049**	**0.12**
DAT1-genotype	0.13	1, 28	0.723	0.01

**Effects that are significant at p < 0.05 are highlighted in bold and are marked with an asterisk. If required violations of sphericity were corrected with Greenhouse-Geisser.*

TABLE 2 | Descriptive statistics (arithmetic mean ± SEM) of choices during reinforcement learning (session 1) and in the transfer phase (session 2), as well as current E2 level subdivided by study group, DAT1-genotype, and phase.

	Cycle group (n = 30)				HC group (n = 38)			
	9-repeat allele carriers (9/9, 9/10)		10-repeat allele homozygotes (10/10)		9-repeat allele carriers (9/9, 9/10)		10-repeat allele homozygotes (10/10)	
	Early FP	Late FP	Early FP	Late FP	OFF_{HC}	ON_{HC}	OFF_{HC}	ON_{HC}
Learning phase (session 1)								
Choose better option (%)	73.97 ± 4.47	59.04 ± 3.01	60.32 ± 3.11	59.96 ± 3.84	63.51 ± 3.36	63.65 ± 2.72	58.54 ± 2.98	58.93 ± 2.65
Transfer phase (session 2)								
Choose A from new stimulus pairs (%)	50.66 ± 9.10	64.94 ± 6.27	63.12 ± 5.33	75.26 ± 6.37	66.89 ± 5.45	70.39 ± 4.68	63.56 ± 5.29	65.43 ± 4.39
Avoid B in new stimulus pairs (%)	78.32 ± 5.66	52.27 ± 6.70	62.91 ± 4.79	60.96 ± 5.98	68.28 ± 4.72	70.98 ± 5.46	65.56 ± 4.13	59.83 ± 3.26
E2 level (pg/ml)	2.38 ± 0.56	4.24 ± 0.56	2.45 ± 0.48	4.45 ± 0.76	2.27 ± 0.34	2.49 ± 0.31	2.28 ± 0.34	2.78 ± 0.42

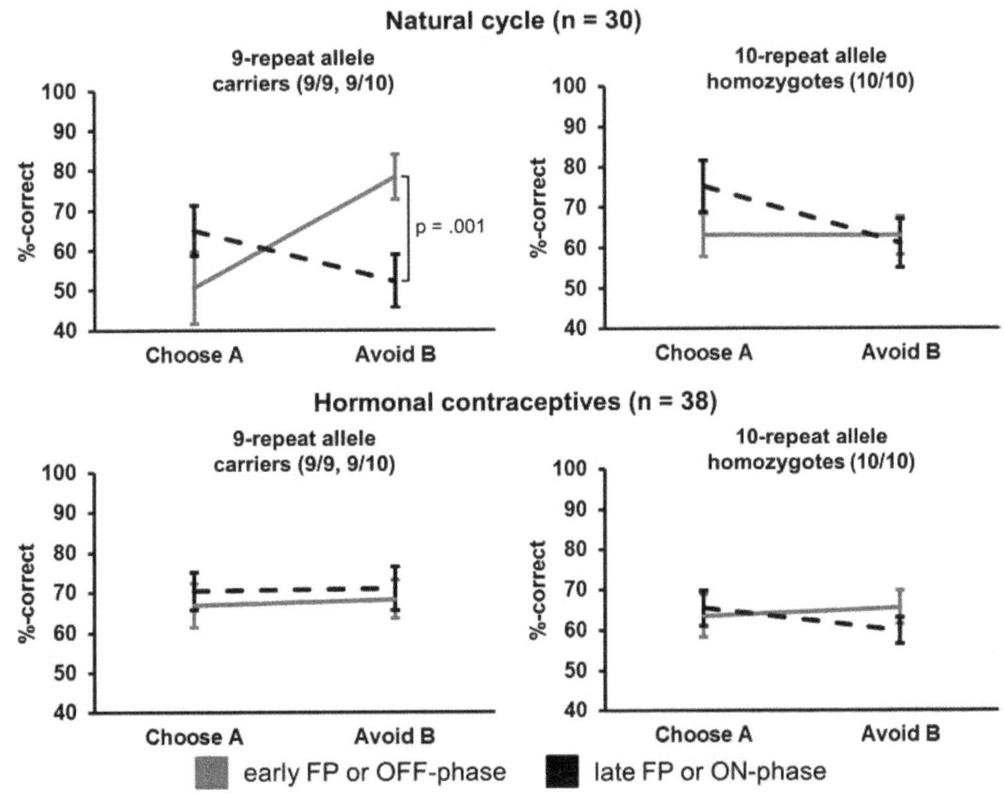

FIGURE 1 | Interaction of "*phase*" × "*preference*" × "*study group*" × "*DAT1-genotype*" in the transfer phase (session 2). Carriers of the 9RP in the cycle group experienced a significant decline in the ability to avoid punishment from the early to the late FP (top left graph). Neither the 10H from the cycle group nor 9RP carriers or 10H from the HC group showed this difference between phases.

eta squared = 0.15], and of "*phase*" and "*learning capacity*" [$F(1.43,40.08) = 8.032$, $p = 0.003$, partial eta squared = 0.22]. The respective *post hoc t*-tests showed that the participants of the cycle group were better at choosing symbol A in the old stimulus pair AB compared to the new pairings ($p < 0.05$ in all *post hoc* comparisons). They were also better at choosing the best option A from all other options in the new stimulus pairs when being in the high E2 state [Choose A performance: early FP = 57.3 ± 5.14%; late FP = 70.44 ± 4.51%; $t(29) = -2.05$; $p = 0.049$], and became significantly worse during avoidance of B in the new stimulus pairs [Avoid B performance: early FP = 70.1 ± 3.88%; late FP = 56.90 ± 4.46%; $t(29) = 2.39$; $p = 0.024$].

Most notably, we also found the hypothesized three-way interaction of "*phase*" by "*learning capacity*" by "*DAT1-genotype*" [$F(1.43,40.08) = 3.66$, $p = 0.049$, partial eta squared = 0.12]. Carriers of the 9RP allele in the cycle group experienced a significant decline in the ability to avoid punishment (i.e., Avoid B performance) from the early to the late FP [$t(13) = 4.53$, $p = 0.001$], while the 10H from the cycle group did not show this difference between phases [$t(15) = 0.24$, $p = 0.816$] (**Table 2**; **Figure 1**). Further, in the direct comparison of genotypes, it became obvious that the difference in learning capacity was not only evident in the Delta between early and late FP, which was significantly bigger in the carriers of the 9RP [Delta Avoid B: $t(28) = -2.34$; $p = 0.024$; Delta Old pair AB: $t(28) = -2.87$; $p = 0.008$], but there was also a significant group difference in the early FP with the 9RP variant carriers outperforming the 10H in avoidance learning [Avoid B performance: $t(28) = 2.10$, $p = 0.045$] and in the Old pair AB [$t(28) = 2.32$, $p = 0.024$] (see also **Figure 2**). These findings suggested that the original two-way interaction of "*phase*" by "*learning capacity*" was most likely driven by the pronounced behavioral change observed in the 9RP allele carriers.

Based on this assumption a more detailed analysis of the value representations in "WIN-WIN-" and "LOSE-LOSE-trials" was performed with the 9RP variant carriers and 10H. In line with the observation of a reduced punishment sensitivity in the late as opposed to the early FP in 9RP allele carriers, we found a reduced ability to avoid the least rewarded symbols in the more difficult "LOSE-LOSE trials" for this genotype [avoidance of worst option from difficult pairs: early FP = 82.48 ± 4.14%; late FP = 64.33 ± 4.30%; $t(13) = 3.95$, $p = 0.002$], but not for the 10H [early FP = 71.76 ± 4.36%; late FP = 72.06 ± 4.14%; $t(15) = -0.43$, $p = 0.966$]. No significant difference emerged in the "WIN-WIN trials" for the 9RP carriers [choice of better option from difficult pairs: early FP = 28.66 ± 6.31%; late FP = 39.74 ± 5.81%; $t(13) = -1.17$, $p = 0.263$], nor the 10H [early FP = 40.52 ± 3.96%; late FP = 49.71 ± 4.33%; $t(13) = -2.09$, $p = 0.055$].

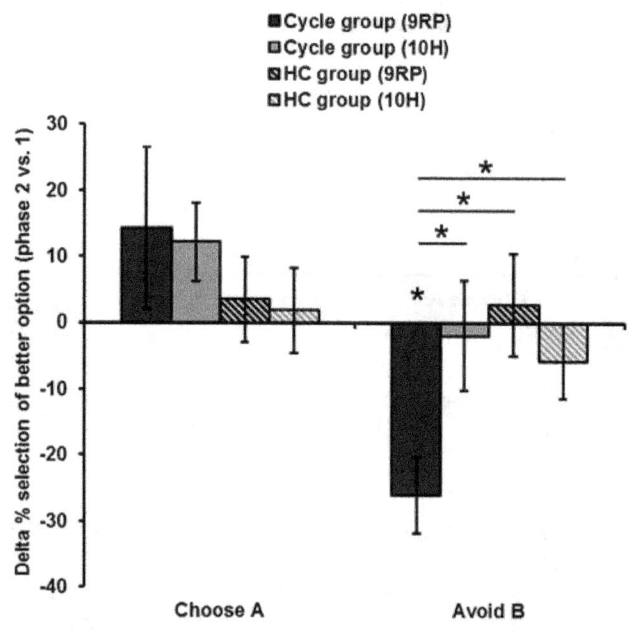

FIGURE 2 | Difference in reinforcement learning capacity between phases (session 2). Displayed is the Delta of the late minus early FP and of the ON- minus OFF-phase, respectively. Only the 9RP genotype showed a significant phase-related change in punishment avoidance capacity. Significant differences ($p < 0.05$, two-tailed) from zero and between genotypes and groups, respectively, are marked with an asterisk. Phase 1, early FP or OFF-phase; phase 2, late FP or ON-phase.

Behavioral Data of the HC Group

In order to find out whether the intake of HC (i.e., synthetic estrogens) may evoke similar changes in reinforcement learning capacity as natural fluctuations in E2 during the FP, we tested this second group of subjects once during the pill break and once during the intake phase of HC. In contrast to the cycle group, we were unable to document a phase-related change in learning performance in session 1 nor was there an effect of HC intake on Choose A and Avoid B performance in session 2. Further, genotype also did not affect performance, whether considered alone or in the interaction with test phase (see **Table 3**).

Group Comparison

For the group comparison (cycle versus HC group), we used the phase-related Deltas of learning performance in the two groups (i.e., Delta of "late–early FP" and Delta of "ON–OFF-phase," respectively). We thereby intended to assess the impact of the between-subject factors "*study group*" (cycle versus HC group) and "*DAT1-genotype*" (9RP allele carriers versus 10H) on the within-subject factor "*Delta learning capacity*," which contained the three Deltas of Choose A, Avoid B, and Old pair AB performance from session 2. The GLM revealed a trend-wise three-way interaction of "*Delta learning capacity*" by "*study group*," and "*DAT1-genotype*," [$F(1.52, 97.23) = 2.93$, $p = 0.072$, partial eta squared = 0.04], a significant two-way interaction of "*Delta learning capacity*" and "*study group*" [$F(1.52, 97.23) = 3.62$, $p = 0.042$, partial eta squared = 0.05] and a significant main effect of "*Delta learning capacity*" [$F(1.52, 97.23) = 6.68$, $p = 0.004$, partial eta squared = 0.10].

Accordingly, 9RP allele carriers of the cycle group showed a stronger phase-related decline in avoidance learning from the low to the high E2 phase [Delta of Avoid B performance in 9RP: cycle group = −26.06 ± 5.74%; HC group = 2.70 ± 7.7%; $t(32) = -2.76$, $p = 0.005$; Delta of Old Pair AB performance in

TABLE 3 | Main effects and interactions in the HC group ($n = 39$).

Main effect or interaction	*F*-value	Degrees of freedom	*p*-value	Partial eta squared
Learning phase (session 1)				
Phase	0.02	1, 36	0.894	<0.01
Phase × DAT1-genotype	0.004	1, 36	0.950	<0.01
Pair*	**24.34**	**2, 72**	**<0.001**	**0.40**
Pair × DAT1-genotype	1.27	2, 72	0.288	0.03
Phase × pair	0.50	2, 72	0.609	0.01
Phase × pair × Dat1-genotype	0.18	2, 72	0.833	<0.01
DAT1-genotype	1,73	1, 36	0.197	0.05
Transfer phase (session 2)				
Phase	0.01	1, 36	0.944	<0.01
Phase × DAT1-genotype	0.59	1, 36	0.447	0.02
Learning capacity*	**9.84**	**1.7, 60.6**	**<0.001**	**0.22**
Learning capacity × DAT1-genotype	0.29	1.7, 60.6	0.713	0.01
Phase × learning capacity	0.29	1.6, 57.1	0.697	0.01
Phase × learning capacity × DAT1-genotype	0.18	1.6, 57.1	0.788	0.01
DAT1-genotype	2.72	1, 36	0.108	0.07

Effects that are significant at $p < 0.05$ are highlighted in bold and are marked with an asterisk. If required violations of sphericity were corrected with Greenhouse-Geisser.

9RP: cycle group = −26.22 ± 6.31%; HC group = 2.15 ± 7.7%; $t(32) = -2.7$, $p = 0.011$] (see also **Figure 2**). Further, in the late FP, 9RP allele carriers of the cycle group were also more compromised in the ability to avoid negative feedback and to choose symbol A from the old stimulus pairs, when being compared to the same genotype in the HC group and the ON-phase [Avoid B performance in 9RP: $t(32) = -2.18$, $p = 0.037$; Old Pair AB performance in 9RP: $t(32) = -2.31$, $p = 0.027$; see also **Table 2** for descriptive statistics].

In contrast, there were no phase-related differences to be found between the 10RP allele homozygotes from the cycle and the HC group. The two *post hoc t*-tests for the main effect and the two-way interaction yielded only weak results. For one thing, in the comparison of the groups there was a nonsignificant, numerical difference between the negative Delta of Avoid B performance [Cycle group = −13.2 ± 5.53%; HC group = −1.29 ± 4.85%, $t(66) = -1.62$, $p = 0.11$] and the positive Delta of Choose A performance [Cycle group = 13.14 ± 6.41%; HC group = 2.73 ± 4.46%, $t(67) = 1.37$, $p = 0.18$], which were both less pronounced in the HC group. Further, when considering all subjects together, there was a significant difference between the mean Delta of Choose A performance (7.32 ± 3.79%) and Avoid B performance (−6.55 ± 3.69%) [$t(67) = 2.46$, $p = 0.016$]. Yet, we presume that any group-related differences had their origin in the strong decline of avoidance learning capacity from the early to the late FP that was rather specific for 9RP variant carriers of the cycle group.

Effect of Initial Test Phase

We also wanted to examine whether the test order may have had a significant influence on reinforcement learning capacity as demonstrated by previous studies. Following the procedure described by Wallen and Rupp (39), we performed two GLMs on the data of the initial test day, when subjects were still naïve with regard to performing the probabilistic feedback task.

For session 1, the GLM included the within-subject factor "*pair*" (AB, CD, EF) and the between-subject factors "*test phase*" (early FP, late FP, OFF-phase, and ON-phase) and "*DAT1-genotype*" (9RP versus 10H). No significant effects emerged. Only the interaction between "*pair*" and "*DAT1-genotype*" reached statistical trend level [$F(2, 120) = 2.54$, $p = 0.083$, partial eta squared = 0.04].

For the transfer phase, the within-subject factor "*learning capacity*" (Choose A, Avoid B, old pair AB) and the two between-subject factors "*test phase*" (early FP, late FP, OFF-phase, and ON-phase) and "*DAT1-genotype*" (9RP versus 10H) we included in the GLM. Here, we found a significant main effect of "*learning capacity*" [$F(1.43, 85.42) = 13.84$, $p < 0.001$, partial eta squared = 0.19] as well as a significant two-way interaction of "*learning capacity*" and "*test phase*" [$F(4.27, 85.42) = 2.66$, $p = 0.018$, partial eta squared = 0.12] and a significant three-way interaction that also included the factor "*DAT1-genotype*" [$F(4.27, 85.42) = 2.93$, $p = 0.023$, partial eta squared = 0.13]. The *post hoc t*-tests confirmed that only the 9RP allele carriers were significantly worse in the avoidance of negative feedback in the LF as opposed to the EF [9RP—Avoid B performance: EF = 87.82% ± 5.59%; LF = 39.56% ± 8.37%; $t(12) = 4.80$, $p < 0.001$], while the 10H were not [10H—Avoid B performance: EF = 64.24% ± 7.47%; LF = 67.28% ± 8.36%; $t(12) = -0.27$, $p = 0.790$]. Moreover, performance was significantly different between genotypes in both the EF [$t(13) = -2.46$, $p = 0.028$] and the LF [$t(13) = 2.33$, $p = 0.036$].

In addition, the women with a natural cycle and the 9RP variant also showed a significant performance decline in the LF (Avoid B = 39.56% ± 8.37%) in comparison to the ON-phase (Avoid B = 79.59 ± 6.51%) [$t(15) = -3.83$, $p = 0.002$]. In contrast, the comparisons of the EF and the OFF-phase in the same genotype and those in the 10H did not yield significant differences in avoidance learning between study groups and phases.

Pearson Correlations between Phase-Dependent E2 Concentration and Performance in the Transfer Phase

To better understand the association between the individual variation in E2 concentration within the different groups and phases and reinforcement learning capacity, we also explored the respective hormone-behavior correlations in the transfer phase [see Ref. (16) for a similar approach]. First, we found a positive correlation between early follicular E2 level and reward sensitivity (i.e., Choose A performance) across genotypes in the cycle group ($n = 30$, $r = 0.39$, $p = 0.034$, two-tailed). No significant correlation emerged in the late FP or in the HC group.

Second, when subdividing the two samples by genotype, only the 9RP carriers of the cycle group exhibited a trend-wise positive correlation in the early FP ($n = 14$, $r = 0.50$, $p = 0.07$, two-tailed), suggesting that this genotype may have primarily driven the positive correlation in the complete cycle group. In contrast, the carriers of the 9RP from the HC group showed the reverse correlation in the OFF-phase ($n = 20$, $r = -0.49$, $p = 0.027$, two-tailed), and the two correlation coefficients were also significantly different (Fisher r-to-z transformation: $z = 2.8$, $p = 0.0051$, two-tailed).

DISCUSSION

Interactions of genotype and hormonal state have been widely ignored by cognitive neuroscience [but see Ref. (15, 17)]. The present study is the first to systematically assess how the natural rise of E2 level in the late FP may interact with DAT1-genotype during reinforcement learning. Our data show that the effect of DAT1-genotype on reinforcement learning may indeed interact with transient hormonal state, but only in women with a natural menstrual cycle. Notably, we found that carriers of the 9RP variant experienced a significant decrease in the ability to avoid punishment from the early to the late FP. No such plasticity emerged in the HC group or in the 10H from either group.

DAT1-Genotype and Avoidance Learning Capacity

Our main finding of a reduced punishment learning capacity in 9RP allele carriers during the high E2 state (i.e., the late FP) conforms to the idea that physiological E2 may act as an endogenous DA-agonist that amplifies central dopaminergic transmission (1, 34, 35). Previous studies have already shown that synthetic drugs that increase striatal DA level may reduce the ability to avoid punishment and may in turn increase reward learning ability (11, 40). A similar effect has also been documented for changes in endogenous hormone level over the course of the menstrual cycle (9, 10, 16). Finally, behavioral genetic studies showed that the sensitivity for negative feedback may be reduced in carriers of polymorphisms associated with a higher DA synthesis capacity and reduced DRD2 density [e.g., the minor A+ allele of the Taq1A polymorphism (12, 24)]. The present study is the first to demonstrate the interactive effect of a state of physiologically increased E2 level (i.e., the late FP) and a genetic polymorphism that might be related to lower striatal DA transmission on intra-individual variations in reinforcement learning capacity. Most previous neuroimaging studies on the DAT1-polymorphism used mixed sex samples and failed to control for menstrual cycle phase in women. It currently remains unclear whether in comparison to the 10RP allele the 9RP variant of the DAT1-polymorphism is associated with a lower (25) or higher density of striatal DAT (26–28), if there is an association with DAT expression at all (29). Behavioral evidence is also mixed, with some studies suggesting that homozygosity of the 10RP allele may enhance reward-related responses [e.g., Ref. (32)], while others found evidence for the opposite with increased activation in 9RP allele carriers [e.g., (30, 31)]. The present data may provide preliminary evidence for the assumption that the 9RP variant may be related to a higher DAT density. If the state of enhanced E2 indeed induced a reversal of normal DAT function that promoted increased DA efflux as suggested by Watson et al. (35), then subjects with the genetic predisposition for a higher density of the DAT should be more strongly affected by this effect of rising E2 in the late FP. This is because the strongest E2-induced DA efflux through the DAT might be expected in individuals carrying the highest density of transporters, which should then also lead to a pronounced behavioral change from the early to the late FP. In addition to that, the same genotype should also have a higher punishment avoidance capacity in comparison to the other variant at cycle onset, when E2 level is at its nadir. Carriers of the 9RP allele of the cycle group fulfilled these two prerequisites, when being compared to homozygotes of the 10RP variant (see **Figure 1**; **Table 2**). Following this logic, the present results may also conform to the model of the inverted U-shape relationship between behavioral performance, baseline DA level, and DA-agonistic substances (41). More specifically, according to this model only subjects with a low baseline DA concentration, who according to our data might be the carriers of the 9RP allele, should be significantly influenced by a physiological rise in E2 level [see also Ref. (16)]. In contrast, the E2 rise in the late FP should have no or only a small effect on punishment learning capacity in subjects with a supposedly higher baseline DA capacity to begin with (as demonstrated here for the 10H).

However, the present observations do not conform to the results of a recent behavioral genetic study that assessed social reward learning capacity in healthy young men. Eisenegger et al. (42) used pharmacological intervention with L-DOPA, which transiently enhances striatal DA levels and assessed the interaction with DAT1-genotype (comparison of carriers of the 9RP allele versus 10H) on learning from economic interactions with either prosocial or antisocial partners. They found an increase of social learning success resulting in enhanced interactions with prosocial partners and higher pay-off under L-DOPA treatment of male 10H. In contrast, male 9RP allele carriers appeared to be impaired in learning from prosocial interactions following treatment with L-DOPA. Yet, there are several differences between the two studies that may explain the divergent findings. First, Eisenegger et al. (42) used a between-subjects design, in which both the pharmacological intervention (L-DOPA versus placebo) and the pairing with a prosocial versus antisocial partner varied between participants. This did not only result in relatively small samples for comparison (e.g., of the group confronted with a prosocial partner, only 16 of the 43 male 9RP allele carriers were treated with L-DOPA), but may have also increased the influence of inter-individual variance. For example, Eisenegger et al. (42) did not control for other genetic polymorphisms in the DA system nor in related neurotransmitter systems (e.g., the serotonin system) that could have significantly affected reinforcement learning capacity or social cognition thus contributing to group differences independent of the pharmacological intervention. When we assessed whether the effects identified in the present study were already evident during the initial, naïve test day, we were also required to use a between-subjects approach. Yet, our finding from the initial test day was in line with the finding that emerged in the within-subject design, which allowed us to rule out these potential confounds related to intersubject variation. Further, the L-DOPA treatment in healthy young men may have induced a supraphysiological DA level. The risk of dopaminergic overstimulation is always immanent when using an effective agent like L-DOPA in healthy young adults. It has already been demonstrated that the effects of supraphysiological stimulation on the DA system are not necessarily comparable to those achieved by stimulation in the physiological range and could even reverse the expected behavioral effects (3), which might explain the discrepant findings of Eisenegger et al. (42). Finally, and most importantly, Eisenegger et al. (42) assessed young men, while the present study was restricted to a female sample. Sex differences in the neural correlates of reward processing have repeatedly been demonstrated [e.g., Ref. (43)]. Further, one may speculate that a high endogenous testosterone concentration in men might have a similar effect on DAT function as rising E2 in women. The DA-agonistic effects of testosterone have repeatedly been documented (44), and testosterone may exert some of its central effect through conversion to E2. It is therefore possible that the DA response of young men, who were at their point of peak fertility, may have also been influenced by their current testosterone level, which may have further contributed to inter-individual differences between subjects. Again, this renders the risk of overstimulation by L-DOPA even more likely and might further explain discrepant findings between the two studies.

It has recently been argued that test order effects may render the interpretation of the results from previous studies on the menstrual cycle difficult (39, 45). For this reason, we analyzed the data from the initial test day separately and found that the results from the analysis of the influence of cycle phase during this naïve test replicated the effects of the repeated-measures design. For this reason, we are confident to assume that the effects identified in this preliminary study could indeed be a consequence of the hypothesized cycle phase by genotype interaction.

Differences between the Cycle and the HC Group

Another important finding of the present study was that the decrease in avoidance learning capacity was restricted to the women from the cycle group who experienced the effect of a natural rise in E2 in the late FP. The HC group showed no behavioral variations between the pill break and the intake phase. Since the intake of HC suppressed the physiological rise in E2 to such an extent that only a slight numerical increase of E2 concentration remained at the group level (**Table 2**), the lack of effect of natural E2 on reinforcement learning ability was not unexpected. Yet, our data also suggest that the women of the HC group remained unaffected by the intake of synthetic hormones. This was in so far surprising as more general differences have been hypothesized to exist between women with a natural menstrual cycle and those that take HC on a regular basis [e.g., Ref. (46)]. The HC sample consisted of women that took HC for at least 1 year, with an average intake duration of more than 7 years. This might have induced profound adaptations to the constant hormonal treatment, such as a compensatory reorganization of neuroanatomy or function that has been demonstrated elsewhere and may also promote behavioral differences (37). When considered as deflections from homeostasis, compensatory long-term adaptations should become particularly evident when the pharmacological agent is with-held (i.e., during the pill break) and may then show up as deflections from homeostasis. Such a mechanism might be comparable to the long-term drug effects on the DA system in substance abuse disorders (47). Yet, the HC subjects from the present study remained quite stable across phases when considering the mean performance in the probabilistic feedback learning task (**Table 2**), which could indicate that long-term HC might have rendered the brain rather unresponsive to the change induced by a short OFF-period. Only the observation of a negative correlation between E2 level and reward sensitivity in the OFF-phase, which contrasted the positive correlation documented in the cycle group, may hint us to the possibility of compensatory long-term adaptations, a speculation, which however needs to be replicated in a bigger sample.

Only a limited number of studies have so far assessed the influence of HC on brain function and anatomy. Bonenberger et al. (48) examined the influence of HC in the context of reward processing in a modified version of the monetary incentive delay task. They demonstrated that the regular intake of HC may slightly alter activation in the anterior insula during reward expectation, but not in the striatum nor in other regions of the mesolimbic DA system. In addition, another two studies suggested HC-related changes in brain regions that are important for various fundamental aspects of cognition (46), which may in part depend on the subtype of HC used [for example in relation to face recognition performance (49)]. In the present sample, 17 women ($n_{9RP} = 9$) used HC containing androgenic progestins, while the remaining 21 subjects ($n_{9RP} = 11$) took HC with anti-androgenic progestins. Exploratory *t*-tests revealed no significant behavioral differences between the HC subtypes at $p < 0.05$ (two-tailed), also not when accounting for the influence of genotype and pill phase. Yet, the present sample was quite small. Since the DA-agonistic properties of androgens have already been demonstrated (44), it might be valuable to readdress the potential impact of HC subtype (androgenic versus anti-androgenic progestins) on reinforcement learning in a bigger sample.

Alternatively, it might also be possible that any changes in reinforcement learning capacity from the OFF- to the ON-phase were masked by a rise in progestin content that accompanied the synthetic estrogen administration. If that was the case, the DA-antagonistic properties of progesterone and its metabolites [e.g., Ref. (50–52); see also Ref. (9)] would have neutralized any E2-related effect on dopaminergic transmission in the ON-phase. Since we did not measure salivary progesterone level, we are unable to rule out this latter possibility.

Finally, other group differences, like the fact that most HC subjects were in a committed relationship, while less then half of the participants from the cycle group indicated to have a partner, could have also contributed to differences in the underlying neurofunctional structure, since partnership has been shown to affect the hormone system, which could indirectly influence brain physiology [e.g., Ref. (53)].

No Evidence of a Cycle Phase by Genotype Interaction in the Context of Reward Learning Capacity—A Possible Relation to Tonic DA?

But why did the 9RP allele carriers become compromised in avoidance learning ability without experiencing an increase in reward sensitivity from the early to the late FP? The functional opponency of reward and punishment learning capacity has been demonstrated repeatedly and can be induced by both variations in central DA transmission [high versus low baseline DA, respectively, e.g., Ref. (11, 13)] and endogenous E2 level (9, 10, 16). The present data indicated a slight rise of the "Choose A" performance from the early to the late FP in both 9RP variant carriers and in 10H in the transfer phase (**Table 2**; **Figure 1**), which, against the background of a decline in "Avoid B" performance, would be in line with the assumption of functionally opponent processes. Yet this increase was not significant. This latter observation may fit with previous evidence suggesting that if tonic DA level is low, the transient upregulation of the phasic DA response can still be observed, which may preserve a normal responsiveness to reward (54). Therefore, even relatively lower levels of DA (e.g., those expected during the early FP) may be sufficient for effective learning from reward through a positive reward prediction error (55). This might have been one explanation for the observation that the rise in E2 level in the late FP had no further enhancing effect on reward learning capacity in the probabilistic feedback task. Diekhof and Ratnayake (9) documented a similar finding, when comparing the late FP and the luteal phase of the menstrual cycle and also found no evidence for a change in striatal processing of positive feedback. In contrast to that, the ability to avoid negative feedback appeared to be more sensitive to variations in tonic DA level. In order to realize effective learning from the negative outcome of an action, a significant depression of tonic DA is required (55, 56). Moreover, the dip in dopaminergic tone has to be strong enough for engaging the respective corticostriatal connections of the indirect NoGo-pathway of the basal ganglia to realize effective punishment learning in the probabilistic feedback task (13). One may assume that in the E2-dominated state of the late FP and the supposedly higher DA content in the striatum, the suppression of dopaminergic tone following a negative feedback would become more difficult. This would decrease the signal-to-noise ratio and thus render the negative prediction error signal less likely, which would ultimately result in a significant decline in punishment learning capacity. Diekhof and Ratnayake (9) demonstrated a significant decline in "Avoid B" performance in the late FP, which was also accompanied by a reduced activation of the dACC by negative feedback. In the present study, the highest sensitivity for more detailed value representations in "LOSE-LOSE trials" was evident in the 9RP allele carriers in the early FP, and this sensitivity declined by 18% when E2 level rose in the late FP. Moreover, carriers of the 9RP variant also showed a cycle phase-related difference in learning performance in session 1. Subjects became particularly worse when learning from pair AB [early FP = 79.3 ± 4.6%; late FP = 62.8 ± 4.8%; $t(13) = 2.77$, $p = 0.016$]. This suggests a reduced ability to identify the least rewarded option already in the fixed stimulus pairs.

Nevertheless, the prediction error theory of dopamine may provide only one possible explanation for the current and previous findings [e.g., Ref. (9)] observed in the probabilistic feedback task. Alternatively, variations in the motivation to act or to engage in goal-directed action might have equally well contributed to the observed differences between cycle phase-related variations in punishment and reward learning capacity [see Ref. (57) for review].

Limitations

First, in this initial study, we tested a relatively small sample of women [in the range of previous behavioral genetic studies; e.g., Ref. (17)] and looked at a single polymorphism that may affect DAT density in the striatum. For these reasons, the present results can only be considered as preliminary and require further replication.

Second, the cycle phase by genotype interaction had a relatively small influence on variations in reinforcement learning capacity, as indicated by the small effect size of the interaction when the factor "*study group*" (HC versus cycle group) was also taken into account (partial eta squared < 0.10). However, the present study used a rather conservative approach by comparing phase-related changes in both a cycle group and a sample including only women that took HC. Most previous studies that assessed the effect of menstrual cycle phase on reward processing did not include such a control sample [e.g., Ref. (15)]. Accordingly, when the cycle group was considered alone in our study, the effect size for the interaction of "*phase*" × "*learning capacity*" × "*DAT1-genotype*" increased from 0.04 to 0.12 (see **Table 1**). Nevertheless, even the smaller effect size of 0.04 is in the range of effect sizes reported by pharmacological intervention studies published in the field. For example, none of the effect sizes reported by Eisenegger et al. (42) for interactions involving the factor "*DA intervention*" and "*DAT1-genotype*" in relation to social reward learning were higher than a partial eta squared of 0.098. When considering the fact that we assessed the impact of the physiological rise in E2 level, our findings indicate that endogenous E2 may be a quite potent modulator of DA transmission with effect sizes comparable to pharmacological agents like L-DOPA. In addition to that, like many of the previous studies on the role of the DAT1-polymorphism in reward processing, our study also did not control for other, potentially relevant genetic polymorphisms that could equally well affect reinforcement learning capacity. Future studies with bigger samples ($n > 200$) should use more advanced behavioral genetic methods like genome-wide association or at least haplotype analysis in order to draw a more comprehensive picture of cycle phase by genotype interactions relevant for inter- and intra-individual variations in reinforcement learning capacity.

Another limitation might be the use of a social feedback (smiley versus grumpy face) in the probabilistic feedback task. This was done to create a design that was comparable to Frank et al. (11), Klein et al. (12), and Diekhof and Ratnayake (9). However, a social feedback may have a lower salience than a monetary reward or loss and may thus lead to a reduced dopaminergic response, i.e., a less effective DA burst or dip, which could have made it easier for variations in E2 to actually tip the balance in favor of reward at the expense of punishment sensitivity. Even though, this thought is currently mere speculation, future studies have to address this potential confound and should test, whether learning from a monetary loss during action selection is equally affected by follicular E2.

Finally, the present study assessed the influence of the rise in endogenous E2 concentration, which precludes any solid inferences on causality. Therefore, placebo-controlled E2 administration studies in young women or a comparison between menopausal women who receive a hormone-replacement therapy or not will be important in that context [e.g., Ref. (58)]. Yet, pharmacological E2 may also have certain disadvantages like the possibility of supraphysiological stimulation in young women, as already outlined above, or the stimulation of a neural structure that might be already compromised by biological aging effects. As an initial step, the understanding of physiological E2 and its role in reinforcement learning may thus be crucial to provide an informed basis for future studies that use pharmacological intervention.

CONCLUSION

Taken together, the present study adds to the growing awareness of the complex interplay between various physiological determinants of dopaminergic transmission. The observed effects on reinforcement learning capacity cannot simply be attributed to cycle phase or genotype alone, but may be a result of their interaction. Furthermore, the present data may provide preliminary evidence for a differential effect of natural and synthetic hormones on reinforcement learning capacity. In that way, they may not only point out the necessity to control for hormonal state and biological sex in behavioral genetics research, but may also offer new ideas for studies in clinical settings.

ETHICS STATEMENT

This study was carried out in accordance with the recommendations of the local ethics committee "Ethikkommission der Ärztekammer Hamburg (Germany)" with written informed consent from all subjects. All subjects gave written informed consent in accordance with the Declaration of Helsinki. The protocol was approved by the "Ethikkommission der Ärztekammer Hamburg (Germany)."

AUTHOR CONTRIBUTIONS

ED designed the research, supervised data collection, analyzed the data, and wrote the paper. KJ collected the data, analyzed the data, and reviewed the manuscript. HE collected the data and reviewed the manuscript. SH supervised data collection and reviewed the manuscript. LR supervised data collection and reviewed the manuscript.

ACKNOWLEDGMENTS

We would like to thank A. Kroll for performing the hormone analysis, M. Langbehn for programming the test protocol and the batches for initial data extraction, F. Starke, J. Schümann, and V. Groenewold for help in data acquisition, as well as all the anonymous participants for their participation. This research did not receive any specific grant from funding agencies in the public, commercial, or non-profit sectors. It was conducted with regular financial resources provided by the Biology Department at the Universität Hamburg.

REFERENCES

1. Becker JB. Gender differences in dopaminergic function in striatum and nucleus accumbens. *Pharmacol Biochem Behav* (1999) 64:803–12. doi:10.1016/S0091-3057(99)00168-9
2. Terner JM, de WH. Menstrual cycle phase and responses to drugs of abuse in humans. *Drug Alcohol Depend* (2006) 84:1–13. doi:10.1016/j.drugalcdep.2005.12.007
3. Xiao L, Becker JB. Effects of estrogen agonists on amphetamine-stimulated striatal dopamine release. *Synapse* (1998) 29:379–91. doi:10.1002/(SICI)1098-2396(199808)29:4<379::AID-SYN10>3.0.CO;2-M
4. Pasqualini C, Olivier V, Guibert B, Frain O, Leviel V. Acute stimulatory effect of estradiol on striatal dopamine synthesis. *J Neurochem* (1995) 65:1651–7. doi:10.1046/j.1471-4159.1995.65041651.x
5. Di Paolo T, Falardeau P, Morissette M. Striatal D2 dopamine agonist bindings sites fluctuate during the rat estrous cycle. *Life Sci* (1988) 43:665–72. doi:10.1016/0024-3205(88)90137-3
6. Lévesque D, DiPaolo T. Rapid conversion of high into low striatal D2-dopamine receptor agonist binding states after an acute physiological dose of 17 beta-estradiol. *Neurosci Lett* (1988) 88:113–18. doi:10.1016/0304-3940(88)90324-2
7. Bazzett TJ, Becker JB. Sex differences in the rapid and acute effects of estrogen on striatal dopamine receptor binding. *Brain Res* (1994) 637:163–72. doi:10.1016/0006-8993(94)91229-7
8. Falardeau P, Di Paolo T. Regional effect of estradiol on rat caudate-putamen dopamine receptors: lateral-medial differences. *Neurosci Lett* (1987) 74(1):43–8. doi:10.1016/0304-3940(87)90048-6
9. Diekhof EK, Ratnayake M. Menstrual cycle phase modulates reward sensitivity and performance monitoring in young women: preliminary fMRI evidence. *Neuropsychologia* (2016) 84:70–80. doi:10.1016/j.neuropsychologia.2015.10.016
10. Reimers L, Büchel C, Diekhof EK. How to be patient. The ability to wait for a reward depends on menstrual cycle phase and feedback-related activity. *Front Neurosci* (2014) 8:401. doi:10.3389/fnins.2014.00401
11. Frank MJ, Seeberger LC, O'Reilly RC. By carrot or by stick: cognitive reinforcement learning in parkinsonism. *Science* (2004) 306:1940. doi:10.1126/science.1102941
12. Klein TA, Neumann J, Reuter M, Hennig J, von Cramon DY, Ullsperger M. Genetically determined differences in learning from errors. *Science* (2007) 318:1642. doi:10.1126/science.1145044
13. Maia TV, Frank MJ. From reinforcement learning models of the basal ganglia to the pathophysiology of psychiatric and neurological disorders. *Nat Neurosci* (2011) 14:154–62. doi:10.1038/nn.2723
14. Ridderinkhof KR, Ullsperger M, Crone EA, Nieuwenhuis S. The role of the medial frontal cortex in cognitive control. *Science* (2004) 306(5695):443–7. doi:10.1126/science.1100301
15. Smith CT, Sierra Y, Oppler SH, Boettiger CA. Ovarian cycle effects on immediate reward selection bias in humans: a role for estradiol. *J Neurosci* (2014) 34:5468–76. doi:10.1523/JNEUROSCI.0014-14.2014
16. Diekhof EK. Be quick about it. Endogenous estradiol level, menstrual cycle phase and trait impulsiveness predict impulsive choice in the context of reward acquisition. *Horm Behav* (2015) 74:186–93. doi:10.1016/j.yhbeh.2015.06.001
17. Jacobs E, D'Esposito M. Estrogen shapes dopamine-dependent cognitive processes: implications for women's health. *J Neurosci* (2011) 31:5286–93. doi:10.1523/JNEUROSCI.6394-10.2011
18. Moustafa AA, Cohen MX, Sherman SJ, Frank MJ. A role for dopamine in temporal decision making and reward maximization in parkinsonism. *J Neurosci* (2008) 28:12294–304. doi:10.1523/JNEUROSCI.3116-08.2008
19. Buckholtz JW, Treadway MT, Cowan RL, Woodward ND, Li R, Ansari MS, et al. Dopaminergic network differences in human impulsivity. *Science* (2010) 329:532–532. doi:10.1126/science.1185778
20. Congdon E, Lesch KP, Canli T. Analysis of DRD4 and DAT polymorphisms and behavioral inhibition in healthy adults: implications for impulsivity. *Am J Med Genet B Neuropsychiatr Genet* (2008) 147B:27–32. doi:10.1002/ajmg.b.30557
21. Forbes EE, Brown SM, Kimak M, Ferrell RE, Manuck SB, Hariri AR. Genetic variation in components of dopamine neurotransmission impacts ventral striatal reactivity associated with impulsivity. *Mol Psychiatry* (2009) 14(1):60–70. doi:10.1038/sj.mp.4002086
22. Colzato LS, van den Wildenberg WP, Van der Does AJ, Hommel B. Genetic markers of striatal dopamine predict individual differences in dysfunctional, but not functional impulsivity. *Neuroscience* (2010) 170:782–8. doi:10.1016/j.neuroscience.2010.07.050
23. Colzato LS, Hommel B. Effects of estrogen on higher-order cognitive functions in unstressed human females may depend on individual variation in dopamine baseline levels. *Front Neurosci* (2014) 8:65. doi:10.3389/fnins.2014.00065
24. Frank MJ, Hutchison K. Genetic contributions to avoidance-based decisions: striatal D2 receptor polymorphisms. *Neuroscience* (2009) 164:131–40. doi:10.1016/j.neuroscience.2009.04.048
25. Heinz A, Goldman D, Jones DW, Palmour R, Hommer D, Gorey JG, et al. Genotype influences in vivo dopamine transporter availability in human striatum. *Neuropsychopharmacology* (2000) 22:133–9. doi:10.1016/S0893-133X(99)00099-8
26. Jacobsen LK, Staley JK, Zoghbi SS, Seibyl JP, Kosten TR, Innis RB, et al. Prediction of dopamine transporter binding availability by genotype: a

preliminary report. *Am J Psychiatry* (2000) 157:1700–3. doi:10.1176/appi.ajp.157.10.1700
27. van Dyck CH, Malison RT, Jacobsen LK, Seibyl JP, Staley JK, Laruelle M, et al. Increased dopamine transporter availability associated with the 9-repeat allele of the SLC6A3 gene. *J Nucl Med* (2005) 46:745–51.
28. van de Giessen E, de Win MM, Tanck MW, van den Brink W, Baas F, Booij J. Striatal dopamine transporter availability associated with polymorphisms in the dopamine transporter gene SLC6A3. *J Nucl Med* (2009) 50:45. doi:10.2967/jnumed.108.053652
29. Martinez D, Gelernter J, Abi-Dargham A, van Dyck CH, Kegeles L, Innis RB, et al. The variable number of tandem repeats polymorphism of the dopamine transporter gene is not associated with significant change in dopamine transporter phenotype in humans. *Neuropsychopharmacology* (2001) 24(5):553–60. doi:10.1016/S0893-133X(00)00216-5
30. Dreher JC, Kohn P, Kolachana B, Weinberger DR, Berman KF. Variation in dopamine genes influences responsivity of the human reward system. *Proc Natl Acad Sci U S A* (2009) 106:617–22. doi:10.1073/pnas.0805517106
31. Aarts E, Roelofs A, Franke B, Rijpkema M, Fernández G, Helmich RC, et al. Striatal dopamine mediates the interface between motivational and cognitive control in humans: evidence from genetic imaging. *Neuropsychopharmacology* (2010) 35:1943–51. doi:10.1038/npp.2010.68
32. Wittmann BC, Tan GC, Lisman JE, Dolan RJ, Düzel E. DAT genotype modulates striatal processing and long-term memory for items associated with reward and punishment. *Neuropsychologia* (2013) 51:2184–93. doi:10.1016/j.neuropsychologia.2013.07.018
33. Alyea RA, Laurence SE, Kim SH, Katzenellenbogen BS, Katzenellenbogen JA, Watson CS. The roles of membrane estrogen receptor subtypes in modulating dopamine transporters in PC-12 cells. *J Neurochem* (2008) 106(4):1525–33. doi:10.1111/j.1471-4159.2008.05491.x
34. Alyea RA, Watson CS. Nongenomic mechanisms of physiological estrogen-mediated dopamine efflux. *BMC Neurosci* (2009) 10:59. doi:10.1186/1471-2202-10-59
35. Watson CS, Alyea RA, Cunningham KA, Jeng YJ. Estrogens of multiple classes and their role in mental health disease mechanisms. *Int J Womens Health* (2010) 2:153–66. doi:10.2147/IJWH.S6907
36. Jocham G, Neumann J, Klein TA, Danielmeier C, Ullsperger M. Adaptive coding of action values in the human rostral cingulate zone. *J Neurosci* (2009) 29:7489–96. doi:10.1523/JNEUROSCI.0349-09.2009
37. Rapkin AJ, Biggio G, Concas A. Oral contraceptives and neuroactive steroids. *Pharmacol Biochem Behav* (2006) 84:628–34. doi:10.1016/j.pbb.2006.06.008
38. van Heusden AM, Fauser BC. Activity of the pituitary-ovarian axis in the pill-free interval during use of low-dose combined oral contraceptives. *Contraception* (1999) 59:237–43. doi:10.1016/S0010-7824(99)00025-6
39. Wallen K, Rupp HA. Women's interest in visual sexual stimuli varies with menstrual cycle phase at first exposure and predicts later interest. *Horm Behav* (2010) 57:263–8. doi:10.1016/j.yhbeh.2009.12.005
40. Jocham G, Klein TA, Ullsperger M. Dopamine-mediated reinforcement learning signals in the striatum and ventromedial prefrontal cortex underlie value-based choices. *J Neurosci* (2011) 31:1606. doi:10.1523/JNEUROSCI.3904-10.2011
41. Cools R, Frank MJ, Gibbs SE, Miyakawa A, Jagust W, D'Esposito M. Striatal dopamine predicts outcome-specific reversal learning and its sensitivity to dopaminergic drug administration. *J Neurosci* (2009) 29:1538–43.
42. Eisenegger C, Pedroni A, Rieskamp J, Zehnder C, Ebstein R, Fehr E, et al. DAT1 polymorphism determines L-DOPA effects on learning about others' prosociality. *PLoS One* (2013) 8:e67820. doi:10.1371/journal.pone.0067820
43. Diekhof EK, Keil M, Obst KU, Henseler I, Dechent P, Falkai P, et al. A functional neuroimaging study assessing gender differences in the neural mechanisms underlying the ability to resist impulsive desires. *Brain Res* (2012) 1473:63–77. doi:10.1016/j.brainres.2012.07.010
44. Wood RI. Reinforcing aspects of androgens. *Physiol Behav* (2004) 83:279–89. doi:10.1016/j.physbeh.2004.08.012
45. Leeners B, Kruger THC, Geraedts K, Tronci E, Mancini T, Ille F, et al. Lack of associations between female hormone levels and visuospatial working memory, divided attention and cognitive bias across two consecutive menstrual cycles. *Front Behav Neurosci* (2017) 4:120. doi:10.3389/fnbeh.2017.00120
46. Pletzer B, Kronbichler M, Aichhorn M, Bergmann J, Ladurner G, Kerschbaum HH. Menstrual cycle and hormonal contraceptive use modulate human brain structure. *Brain Res* (2010) 1348:55–62. doi:10.1016/j.brainres.2010.06.019
47. Koob G, Bloom F. Cellular and molecular mechanisms of drug dependence. *Science* (1988) 242:715. doi:10.1126/science.2903550
48. Bonenberger M, Groschwitz RC, Kumpfmueller D, Groen G, Plener PL, Abler B. It's all about money: oral contraception alters neural reward processing. *Neuroreport* (2013) 24:951–5. doi:10.1097/WNR.0000000000000024
49. Pletzer B, Kronbichler M, Kerschbaum HH. Differential effects of androgenic and anti-androgenic progestins on fusiform and frontal gray matter volume and face recognition performance. *Brain Res* (2015) 1596:108–15. doi:10.1016/j.brainres.2014.11.025
50. Luine VN, Rhodes JC. Gonadal hormone regulation of MAO and other enzymes in hypothalamic areas. *Neuroendocrinology* (1983) 36:235–41. doi:10.1159/000123461
51. Luine VN, Hearns M. Relationship of gonadal hormone administration, sex, reproductive status and age to monoamine oxidase activity within the hypothalamus. *J Neuroendocrinol* (1990) 2:423–8. doi:10.1111/j.1365-2826.1990.tb00427.x
52. Motzo C, Porceddu ML, Maira G, Flore G, Concas A, Dazzi L, et al. Inhibition of basal and stress-induced dopamine release in the cerebral cortex and nucleus accumbens of freely moving rats by the neurosteroid allopregnanolone. *J Psychopharmacol* (1996) 10:266–72. doi:10.1177/026988119601000402
53. Barrett ES, Tran V, Thurston SW, Frydenberg H, Lipson SF, Thune I, et al. Women who are married or living as married have higher salivary estradiol and progesterone than unmarried women. *Am J Hum Biol* (2015) 27(4):501–7. doi:10.1002/ajhb.22676
54. Grace AA. Phasic versus tonic dopamine release and the modulation of dopamine system responsivity: a hypothesis for the etiology of schizophrenia. *Neuroscience* (1991) 41(1):1–24. doi:10.1016/0306-4522(91)90196-U
55. Schultz W. Dopamine neurons and their role in reward mechanisms. *Curr Opin Neurobiol* (1997) 7:191–7. doi:10.1016/S0959-4388(97)80007-4
56. Sutton RS, Barto AB. *Reinforcement Learning*. The MIT Press (1999). Available from: https://mitpress.mit.edu/books/reinforcement-learning
57. Palmiter RD. Dopamine signaling in the dorsal striatum is essential for motivated behaviors: lessons from dopamine-deficient mice. *Ann N Y Acad Sci* (2008) 1129:35–46. doi:10.1196/annals.1417.003
58. Thomas J, Météreau E, Déchaud H, Pugeat M, Dreher JC. Hormonal treatment increases the response of the reward system at the menopause transition: a counterbalanced randomized placebo-controlled fMRI study. *Psychoneuroendocrinology* (2014) 50:167–80. doi:10.1016/j.psyneuen.2014.08.012

Permissions

All chapters in this book were first published by Frontiers; hereby published with permission under the Creative Commons Attribution License or equivalent. Every chapter published in this book has been scrutinized by our experts. Their significance has been extensively debated. The topics covered herein carry significant findings which will fuel the growth of the discipline. They may even be implemented as practical applications or may be referred to as a beginning point for another development.

The contributors of this book come from diverse backgrounds, making this book a truly international effort. This book will bring forth new frontiers with its revolutionizing research information and detailed analysis of the nascent developments around the world.

We would like to thank all the contributing authors for lending their expertise to make the book truly unique. They have played a crucial role in the development of this book. Without their invaluable contributions this book wouldn't have been possible. They have made vital efforts to compile up to date information on the varied aspects of this subject to make this book a valuable addition to the collection of many professionals and students.

This book was conceptualized with the vision of imparting up-to-date information and advanced data in this field. To ensure the same, a matchless editorial board was set up. Every individual on the board went through rigorous rounds of assessment to prove their worth. After which they invested a large part of their time researching and compiling the most relevant data for our readers.

The editorial board has been involved in producing this book since its inception. They have spent rigorous hours researching and exploring the diverse topics which have resulted in the successful publishing of this book. They have passed on their knowledge of decades through this book. To expedite this challenging task, the publisher supported the team at every step. A small team of assistant editors was also appointed to further simplify the editing procedure and attain best results for the readers.

Apart from the editorial board, the designing team has also invested a significant amount of their time in understanding the subject and creating the most relevant covers. They scrutinized every image to scout for the most suitable representation of the subject and create an appropriate cover for the book.

The publishing team has been an ardent support to the editorial, designing and production team. Their endless efforts to recruit the best for this project, has resulted in the accomplishment of this book. They are a veteran in the field of academics and their pool of knowledge is as vast as their experience in printing. Their expertise and guidance has proved useful at every step. Their uncompromising quality standards have made this book an exceptional effort. Their encouragement from time to time has been an inspiration for everyone.

The publisher and the editorial board hope that this book will prove to be a valuable piece of knowledge for researchers, students, practitioners and scholars across the globe.

List of Contributors

Qi Huang, Meigang Ma, Xing Wei, Yuhan Liao, Hengchang Qi, Yuejuan Wu and Yuan Wu
Department of Neurology, First Affiliated Hospital, Guangxi Medical University, Nanning, China

Nicolas Diotel and Christian Lefebvre d'Hellencourt
Université de La Réunion, Institut National de la Santé et de la Recherche Médicale, UMR 1188, Diabète athérothrombose Thérapies Réunion Océan Indien, Saint-Denis de La Réunion, France

Thierry D. Charlier, Joel C. Nicolau, Olivier Kah and Elisabeth Pellegrini
Univ Rennes, Inserm, EHESP, Irset (Institut de recherche en santé, environnement et travail) - UMR_S 1085, Rennes, France

David Couret and Olivier Meilhac
Université de La Réunion, Institut National de la Santé et de la Recherche Médicale, UMR 1188, Diabète athérothrombose Thérapies Réunion Océan Indien, Saint-Denis de La Réunion, France
CHU de La Réunion, Saint-Denis, France

Vance L. Trudeau
Department of Biology, University of Ottawa, Ottawa, ON, Canada

Mika Soma, Jonghyuk Kim and Asami Kato
Department of Cognitive Neuroscience, Faculty of Pharma-Science, Teikyo University, Itabashi, Japan

Suguru Kawato
Department of Cognitive Neuroscience, Faculty of Pharma-Science, Teikyo University, Itabashi, Japan
Department of Urology, Graduate School of Medicine, Juntendo University, Hongo, Japan
Department of Biophysics and Life Sciences, Graduate School of Arts and Sciences, The University of Tokyo, Meguro, Japan

Moeko Kanaya, Masahiro Morishita and Shinji Tsukahara
Division of Life Science, Graduate School of Science and Engineering, Saitama University, Saitama, Japan

Marcia H. Ratner, Vidhya Kumaresan and David H. Farb
Laboratory of Molecular Neurobiology, Department of Pharmacology and Experimental Therapeutics, Boston University School of Medicine, Boston, MA, United States

Graziano Pinna
The Psychiatric Institute, Department of Psychiatry, College of Medicine, University of Illinois at Chicago, Chicago, IL, United States

Emese Domonkos
Faculty of Medicine, Institute of Molecular Biomedicine, Comenius University, Bratislava, Slovakia

Daniela Ostatníková
Faculty of Medicine, Institute of Physiology, Comenius University, Bratislava, Slovakia

Július Hodosy
Faculty of Medicine, Institute of Molecular Biomedicine, Comenius University, Bratislava, Slovakia
Faculty of Medicine, Institute of Physiology, Comenius University, Bratislava, Slovakia

Peter Celec
Faculty of Medicine, Institute of Molecular Biomedicine, Comenius University, Bratislava, Slovakia
Faculty of Medicine, Institute of Pathophysiology, Comenius University, Bratislava, Slovakia
Department of Molecular Biology, Faculty of Natural Sciences, Comenius University, Bratislava, Slovakia

Yang Zheng, Yinxi Zhang, Mengting Cai and Meiping Ding
Department of Neurology, Second Affiliated Hospital, School of Medicine, Zhejiang University, Hangzhou, China

Nanxi Lai
Department of Pharmacology, Key Laboratory of Medical Neurobiology of the Ministry of Health of China, College of Pharmaceutical Sciences, School of Medicine, Zhejiang University, Hangzhou, China

Zhong Chen
Department of Neurology, Second Affiliated Hospital, School of Medicine, Zhejiang University, Hangzhou, China
Department of Pharmacology, Key Laboratory of Medical Neurobiology of the Ministry of Health of China, College of Pharmaceutical Sciences, School of Medicine, Zhejiang University, Hangzhou, China

Matthew C. S. Denley, Nicholas J. F. Gatford and Katherine J. Sellers
Department of Basic and Clinical Neuroscience, Maurice Wohl Clinical Neuroscience Institute, London, United Kingdom

Deepak P. Srivastava
Department of Basic and Clinical Neuroscience, Maurice Wohl Clinical Neuroscience Institute, London, United Kingdom
MRC Centre for Neurodevelopmental Disorders, King's College London, London, United Kingdom

Yi Guo, Xin Tian and Zheng Xiao
Department of Neurology, The First Affiliated Hospital of Chongqing Medical University, Chongqing Key Laboratory of Neurology, Chongqing, China

Xuefeng Wang
Department of Neurology, The First Affiliated Hospital of Chongqing Medical University, Chongqing Key Laboratory of Neurology, Chongqing, China
Center of Epilepsy, Beijing Institute for Brain Disorders, Beijing, China

Toshiya Funabashi
Department of Physiology, Yokohama City University School of Medicine, Yokohama, Japan
Department of Physiology, St. Marianna University School of Medicine, Kawasaki, Japan

Fumiki Hirahara
Department of Obstetrics and Gynecology, Yokohama City University School of Medicine, Yokohama, Japan

Hideya Sakakibara
Department of Obstetrics and Gynecology, Yokohama City University School of Medicine, Yokohama, Japan
Department of Gynecology, Yokohama City University Medical Center, Yokohama, Japan

Fukuko Kimura
Department of Physiology, Yokohama City University School of Medicine, Yokohama, Japan
Tanaka Clinic Yokohama-Koen, Yokohama, Japan

Sabina Bhatta and Jeffrey A. Blair
School of Biomedical Sciences, Kent State University, Kent, OH, United States

Gemma Casadesus
School of Biomedical Sciences, Kent State University, Kent, OH, United States
Department of Biological Sciences, Kent State University, Kent, OH, United States

Dumitru A. Iacobas
Center for Computational Systems Biology, Prairie View A&M University, Prairie View, TX, United States
DP Purpura Department of Neuroscience, Albert Einstein College of Medicine, New York, NY, United States

Sanda Iacobas
Center for Computational Systems Biology, Prairie View A&M University, Prairie View, TX, United States
Department of Pathology, New York Medical College, Valhalla, NY, United States

Nino Nebieridze
Department of Cell Biology & Anatomy, New York Medical College, Valhalla, NY, United States

Libor Velíšek
Department of Cell Biology & Anatomy, New York Medical College, Valhalla, NY, United States
Department of Pediatrics, New York Medical College, Valhalla, NY, United States
Department of Neurology, New York Medical College, Valhalla, NY, United States

Jana Velíšková
Department of Cell Biology & Anatomy, New York Medical College, Valhalla, NY, United States
Department of Neurology, New York Medical College, Valhalla, NY, United States
Department of Obstetrics & Gynecology, New York Medical College, Valhalla, NY, United States

Kazuhiro Sano, Chihiro Morimoto, Mariko Nataka, Mumeko C. Tsuda and Sonoko Ogawa
Laboratory of Behavioral Neuroendocrinology, University of Tsukuba, Tsukuba, Japan

Sergei Musatov
Laboratory of Molecular Neurosurgery, Department of Neurological Surgery, Weill Cornell Medical College, New York, NY, United States

Naoko Yamaguchi
Department of Medicine, Aichi Medical University, Nagakute, Japan

Toshiro Sakamoto
Department of Health Sciences, Kyoto Tachibana University, Kyoto, Japan

Zulvikar Syambani Ulhaq and Mitsuyo Kishida
Graduate School of Science and Technology, Kumamoto University, Kumamoto, Japan

Chih-Hsiang Lin, Yan-Ting Lu, Chen-Jui Ho and Meng-Han Tsai
Department of Neurology, Kaohsiung Chang Gung Memorial Hospital, College of Medicine, Chang Gung University, Kaohsiung, Taiwan

Fu-Yuan Shih
Department of Neurosurgery, Kaohsiung Chang Gung Memorial Hospital, College of Medicine, Chang Gung University, Kaohsiung, Taiwan

Kristina Jakob, Hanna Ehrentreich, Sarah K. C. Holtfrerich, Luise Reimers and Esther K. Diekhof
Department of Biology, Faculty of Mathematics, Informatics and Natural Sciences, Institute of Zoology, Neuroendocrinology Unit, Universität Hamburg, Hamburg, Germany

Index

www.ingramcontent.com/pod-product-compliance
Lightning Source LLC
LaVergne TN
LVHW082151200926
848484LV00008B/2143